FOUNDATIONS OF AURAL REHABILITATION

Children, Adults, and Their Family Members

2nd Edition

Nancy Tye-Murray, Ph.D.

Washington University School of Medicine
St. Louis, Missouri

THOMSON

DELMAR LEARNING™

Australia Canada Mexico Singapore Spain United Kingdom United States

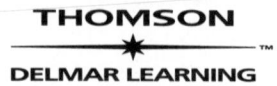

THOMSON

DELMAR LEARNING

Foundations of Aural Rehabilitation: Children, Adults, and Their Family Members, 2nd Edition
by Nancy Tye-Murray

Vice President, Health Care Business Unit:
William Brottmiller

Editorial Director:
Cathy L. Esperti

Acquisitions Editor:
Kalen Conerly

Developmental Editor:
Juliet Byington

Marketing Director:
Jennifer McAvey

Channel Manager:
Lisa Osgood

Marketing Coordinator:
Chris Manion

Editorial Assistant:
James Duncan

Production Manager:
Barbara A. Bullock

Art and Design Specialist:
Robert Plante

Project Editor:
David Buddle

Production Coordinator:
Kenneth McGrath

Library of Congress Cataloging-in-Publication Data
Tye-Murray, Nancy
Foundations of aural rehabilitation : children, adults, and their family members / Nancy Tye-Murray.--2nd ed.
    p. cm.
Includes bibliographical references and index.
ISBN 0-7668-6329-8
1. Hearing impaired--Rehabilitation.
2. Deaf--Rehabilitation. 3. Hearing impaired children--Rehabilitation. 4. Audiology. I. Title
RF297.T94 2004
617.8'9--dc22   2003070074

NOTICE TO THE READER

Publisher does not warrant or guarantee any of the products described herein or perform any independent analysis in connection with any of the product information contained herein. Publisher does not assume, and expressly disclaims, any obligation to obtain and include information other than that provided to it by the manufacturer.

The reader is expressly warned to consider and adopt all safety precautions that might be indicated by the activities described herein and to avoid all potential hazards. By following the instructions contained herein, the reader willingly assumes all risks in connection with such instructions.

The publisher makes no representation or warranties of any kind, including but not limited to, the warranties of fitness for particular purpose or merchantability, nor are any such representations implied with respect to the material set forth herein, and the publisher takes no responsibility with respect to such material. The publisher shall not be liable for any special, consequential, or exemplary damages resulting, in whole or part, from the readers' use of, or reliance upon, this material.

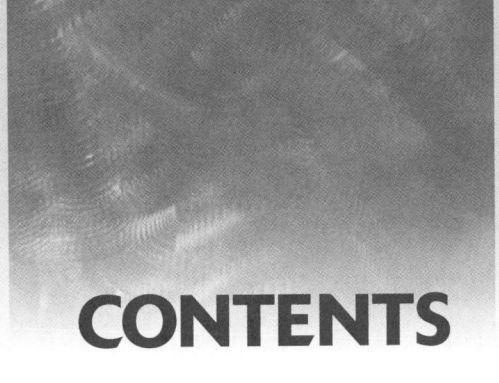

CONTENTS

Preface

What exactly is aural rehabilitation? The answer to this question can conceivably include almost every aspect of audiology and deaf education. Under the rubric of aural rehabilitation may fall any of the following topics: identification and diagnosis of hearing loss and other hearing-related communication difficulties, patient and family counseling, selection and fitting of listening devices, follow-up services for the prescribed listening devices, communication training, noise protection, tinnitus, speech and language therapy, literacy promotion, classroom management, parent instruction, and speech perception training.

If a survey of textbooks for aural rehabilitation is any indication, increasingly, a primary component (if not the essence) of what we define as aural rehabilitation has come to mean the provision and maintenance of appropriate listening devices. This indeed is an important activity in any aural rehabilitation service delivery model. However, this textbook represents a bit of a departure from many current texts and, to some extent, a return to the roots of aural rehabilitation. Although it includes chapters and sections on identification and quantification of hearing loss, and on hearing aids and other listening devices, these topics are not the book's primary focus. Instead, the emphasis is placed on three other topics: (1) understanding the patients who are served by speech and hearing professionals, (2) providing them with appropriate professional support and counseling, and (3) maximizing their communication success in their everyday environments, once they have received appropriate amplification.

When I wrote the first edition of *Foundations of Aural Rehabilitation: Children, Adults, and Their Family Members,* I had two overriding

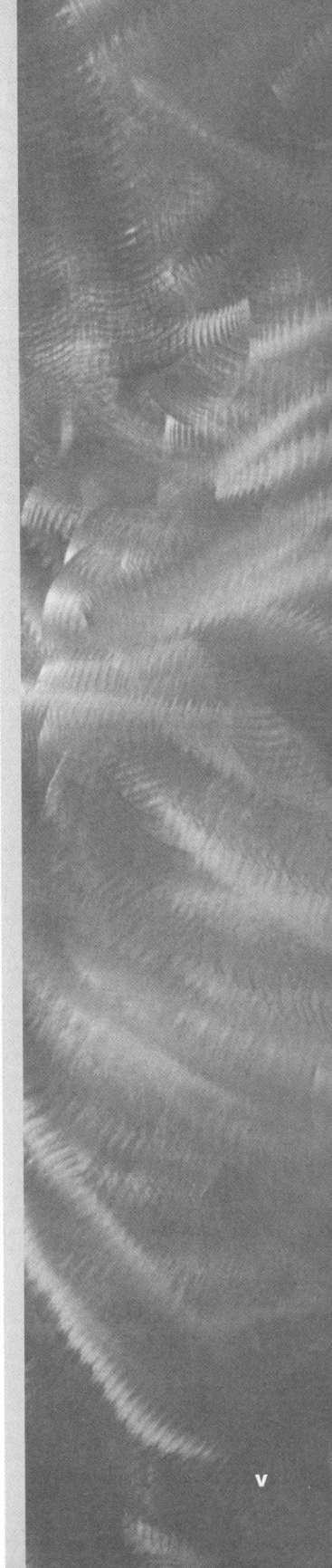

v

goals. First, I wanted to write a book that would interest students in and excite them about the profession of aural rehabilitation. Many textbooks that are written for health-care professions lay out the science and the procedures in such a way that students never intuit the rewards involved in delivering services to real-life people. They focus on the data and the chronology of research that has preceded a particular practice, but the books fail to connect readers to the target patient population—the people behind the data. In a profession like aural rehabilitation, where the personal and professional rewards of interacting with persons who have hearing loss can be enormous, it seems imperative that students leave their reading with a sense of, *This seems like something I want to do in my professional career.* To achieve this first goal, I adopted what I believe to be an interactive and engaging writing style, and I interwove anecdotes and popular culture items with descriptions of the research and the procedures.

My second goal in writing the first edition was to prepare students to provide aural rehabilitation to their patients. To this end, the chapters describe how speech and hearing professionals might go about developing an aural rehabilitation strategy for a particular individual, why they might make particular choices, and how to go about the nuts-and-bolts of service delivery. This book is a reference that readers can return to again and again once they launch their careers as speech and hearing professionals.

The popularity of the textbook has been gratifying and has far exceeded my expectations. Adherence to the two original goals is no doubt the reason why *Foundations of Aural Rehabilitation* has found such a wide audience. In writing the second edition, I again let these two goals serve as my guide, along with a third goal. To respond to comments from professors and students in North America, Europe, and Australia, I expanded the coverage of the original topics and included additional topics. In sum, my guiding goals for writing this second edition have been as follows: *Make it interesting; make it useful; make it comprehensive.*

ORGANIZATION

The first half of the book concerns the components of aural rehabilitation, and the second half concerns the persons we serve. Each half is divided into two, so the book has four parts.

Part I of this book deals with conversation, communication-strategies training, and counseling and related issues. Communication strategies and conversational styles are considered, and data from both speech and hearing and sociolinguistics literature are reviewed. This information provides a firm foundation for a consideration of assessment procedures for conversational fluency and communication handicap and for developing specific intervention protocols for both adults and children.

Part II concerns speech recognition: How to assess speech recognition, how to maximize speech listening through the use of technology, and how to develop speech perception skills. The chapters on speech perception training do not take us back to the days when speechreading training was the sole component of aural rehabilitation. However, it is recognized that speech perception training still has an important place in the arsenal of speech and hearing professionals, particularly when they provide intervention for young children. Although adults may not receive as much benefit from speech perception training per se, it is important that they and their families understand the difficulty of the speech recognition task in the presence of reduced auditory capabilities.

The third part of the book concerns the adult population with hearing loss. Part III begins with individuals who are under the age of 60 years and then discusses adults who are older. Comprehensive descriptions of the patient groups are provided, as are specific tactics for developing aural rehabilitation plans. The guiding theme in this section is that aural rehabilitation services must be tailored to meet the needs of the individual.

Part IV deals with children. Topics include hearing loss and assessment, the design of an intervention plan, and speech, language, and literacy achievement. A chapter is devoted to each of two especially timely topics. Chapter 17 pertains to parent-centered conversation and language instruction, whereas Chapter 18 deals with patient management and cochlear implants in children.

The structure of the text has three notable features. First, supplemental or tangential information to the main text is provided in shaded inserts. These inserts are meant to provide an added dimension to the text and add interest for the student. In addition, final remarks appear at the end of every chapter, and important concepts are summarized. Finally, key terms in the text are defined in the margins.

NEW FEATURES

In comparison with the first edition, the coverage of topics in this second edition is more comprehensive, but not unwieldy. More topics are covered within each chapter; for example, Chapter 15 (Aural (Re)Habilitation Plans for Children) now includes a section on education law. The second edition also includes a new chapter devoted to counseling and related issues, Chapter 5 (Counseling, Psychosocial Therapy, and Assertiveness Training). This book may be the first aural rehabilitation text to devote so many pages to psychosocial therapy and assertiveness training, but it probably will not be the last to do so.

Readers will find multiple choice questions at the end of each chapter. Several years ago, I participated in writing the examination that certifies audiologists to practice in the United States (the examination for the Certificate of Clinical Competence–Audiology, or the CCC-A). Although none of the multiple choice questions that comprise that examination appear in this text, the questions mimic their nature and spirit. In the same way that students prepare for such college entrance examinations as the SAT or the GRE, I believe it is important that students practice for the certification examination by completing review questions such as those in this book. Completing these questions is a great way for students to test their own knowledge and to decide whether they need to re-read sections of a chapter.

Most of the chapters now include one or more case studies. Case studies demonstrate how procedures may be implemented, and they enhance the readability of the material. They also provide a stimulating springboard for class discussion.

The key resources sections of many of the chapters contain additional materials in this second edition. In particular, readers will find examples of questionnaires, tests, and self-assessment instruments; example syllabuses for group intervention programs; additional references; and training activities.

TARGET AUDIENCE

This book was designed to be used by both undergraduate and beginning graduate students in audiology and speech-language pathology. In addition, it may serve as a text for training programs in deaf education, special education, medicine, nursing, occupational therapy, and vocational rehabilitation counseling.

■ THE CURRENT ERA

This is an exciting time to be involved with aural rehabilitation. We know more about hearing loss and how to manage its consequences than ever before. Advances in hearing measurement and hearing-related technology and increased understanding in the areas of sociolinguistics, psychology, speech acquisition, and speech perception have created a climate in which providing aural rehabilitation is both rewarding and challenging to the speech and hearing professional.

About the Author

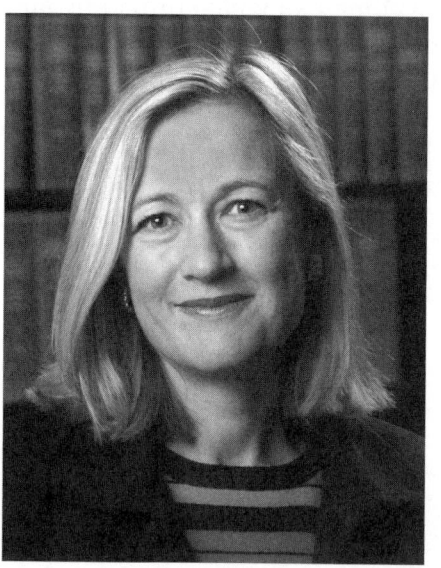

Nancy Tye-Murray is a professor at the Washington University School of Medicine in St. Louis, Missouri, and the principal investigator of an RO1 grant from the National Institutes of Health and co-principal investigator of a second. Her research interests include the effects of aging on speech perception, conversational fluency, the efficacy of aural rehabilitation, and the speech production and perception of children who have hearing loss. Tye-Murray founded and ran both the aural rehabilitation program for adult cochlear-implant users and the children's speech and language project at the University of Iowa Hospitals. At Central Institute for the Deaf, she taught the graduate level aural rehabilitation class at Washington University, helped assess the psychosocial therapy program for adult cochlear implant users, and for six years served as department head of the research program, which was composed of the Center for the Biology of Hearing and Deafness and the Center of Childhood Deafness and Adult Aural Rehabilitation. She has written six nonfiction books, including, *Let's Converse! A How-To Guide to Expand the Conversational Skills of Children and Teenagers Who Have Hearing Loss* and *Cochlear Implants and Children: A Hand-*

book for Parents, Teachers, and Speech and Hearing Professionals (Alexander Graham Bell Association Publishing). Tye-Murray has published extensively in such peer-reviewed journals as *Ear and Hearing, Journal of Speech-Language-Hearing, Journal of the Acoustical Society of America,* and *Journal of the Academy of American Audiology.* She developed the CD-ROM aural rehabilitation series *Conversation Made Easy: Speechreading and Communication Training* (published by Central Institute for the Deaf). She is the former president of the Academy of Rehabilitative Audiology and the former chief editor of *Volta Review.*

Dedication

For Ellen Thornber Murray and Aubrey Fox Murray

CHAPTER 1

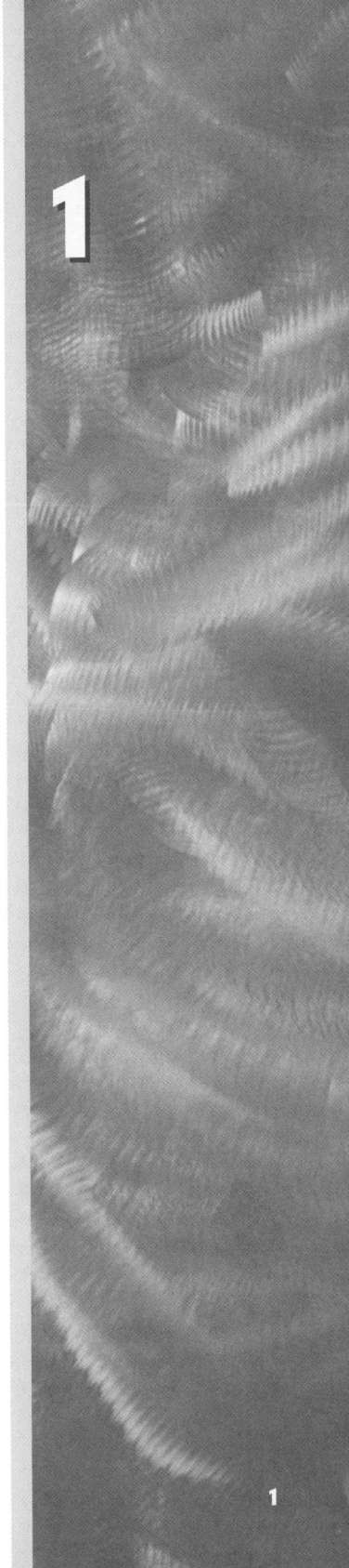

Introduction

TOPICS

- Definitions of aural rehabilitation and communication handicap
- Hearing loss
- Relevance of aural rehabilitation
- Final remarks
- Key chapter points
- Multiple choice questions
- Key resources
- Appendix 1-1
- Appendix 1-2

Hearing loss often has been called the "invisible condition," yet its impact may be anything but invisible. The consequences of hearing loss may be manifested in a broad spectrum of an individual's life. For example, everyday communication may be difficult and, for some persons, impossible without a great deal of effort. The adult may feel the ramifications of hearing loss at home, in the workplace, and in the community. The young child may share similar difficulties in everyday communication, and may also experience delays in speech, language, educational achievement, and social development.

In this introductory chapter, we will consider prevalence of hearing loss in today's world and define what we mean by the term *aural rehabilitation*. We will do so in the context of considering relevance. That is, why is aural rehabilitation so necessary in the service delivery models provided by speech and hearing professionals?

The answer to the question of the relevance of aural rehabilitation is two-pronged. First, the ranks of persons who have hearing loss continue to swell, and they include individuals who are both old and young. The demand for aural rehabilitation is likely to demonstrate a concomitant growth. Second, aural rehabilitation can improve the quality of life for individuals who have hearing loss, and can minimize the negative consequences of this invisible disability, in a manner that is cost-effective.

Aural rehabilitation is intervention aimed at minimizing and alleviating the communication difficulties associated with hearing loss.

DEFINITIONS OF AURAL REHABILITATION AND COMMUNICATION HANDICAP

Rehabilitation services are designed to help individuals overcome the challenges posed by a disability. The logic behind rehabilitation is to provide an individual with the most appropriate technological support and then to help the person build skill levels in functioning. Skill levels are developed in small increments and in a way that is not overwhelming. For instance, a patient who has a knee injury may first receive a knee brace. A physical therapist may then help the patient perform simple leg extensions early on in a rehabilitation program. Much later, the patient may progress to one-legged hopping.

"Better Hearing Institute in USA estimates that untreated hearing loss costs the American society a total of 56 billion dollars annually. This is an equivalent of 216 dollars per American each year."
— *Hear-it Organization 2003*

Similarly, much of what we do in aural rehabilitation is designed to provide appropriate technical support and then develop the individual's skill levels step-by-step. For example, a child with a profound hearing loss may receive a cochlear implant. Initially, a speech and hearing professional may help the child learn to detect the presence or absence of sound. Only later will the child learn to identify words. Mastering this, the child may then progress to an even more advanced skill level, and learn to comprehend ongoing discourse.

What Is Aural Rehabilitation and What Are the Goals?

The goals of aural rehabilitation are to:

- Alleviate the difficulties related to hearing loss and
- Minimize its consequences

The concrete outcome of achieving these goals is enhanced conversational fluency, a concept that will be developed more fully in Chapter 2, and reduced hearing disability and communication handicap.

ENHANCED CONVERSATIONAL FLUENCY

One of the most deleterious effects of hearing loss is impaired ability to communicate with other people during everyday life activities. For example, the person with hearing loss may miss out on casual conversations, on conversations that establish intimacy and friendship, and on conversations that convey important information or promote life goals. Everyday activities that persons with normal hearing take for granted, such as using the telephone or listening to a store clerk, may be effortful and frustrating. If the hard-of-hearing person is a child, the difficulties may relate not only to hearing spoken messages, but also to formulating and expressing messages in light of limited speech and language skills. In the wake of a successful aural rehabilitation plan, persons with hearing loss should be able to converse with the people in their home, work, school, and social environments and achieve success in their communication efforts. Much of the content of this textbook revolves around ways to promote conversational fluency.

REDUCED HEARING DISABILITY AND COMMUNICATION HANDICAP

A **communication handicap** consists of the psychosocial disadvantages that result from hearing loss.

An **impairment** is a structural or functional impairment of the auditory system.

A **disability** is a loss of function imposed by hearing loss.

Difficulty in participating in conversations contributes heavily to an individual's hearing disability and ***communication handicap***. The World Health Organization (WHO, 1980) makes a clear distinction between the terms impairment, disability, and handicap. In their nomenclature, an ***impairment*** is defined as an abnormality in the structure or the function of the ear. Someone who has a dead region in the cochlea has a hearing impairment. The term implies a lack of normal function, as manifested by elevated audiometric thresholds, impaired frequency resolution or poor speech discrimination. ***Disability*** results from impairment, for example, a person may not be able to talk on the telephone because of the hearing impairment. Disability is not an attribute of the individual per se, but rather, arises from a complex collection of conditions, some of which stem from the individual's real-world environment. A disability might mean that the individual experiences problems when trying to listen in a noisy conference room. Whereas disability is the functional consequence of impairment, a *handicap* is its social consequence. A person may have a hearing handicap because he or she has had to make a job change because of the hearing loss, or may experience extreme feelings of isolation. The handicap effect on a person's life might be marital stress, reduced chance of promotion in the workplace, or social withdrawal. In this classification system, it is possible for a person to have an impairment while experiencing neither a disability or a handicap. This classification system has been updated (WHO, 1999). The dimensions of functioning have been expanded to include those of activity (the nature and extent of functioning and how they may be limited in nature, duration, or quality), participation (the extent to which participation in life situations may be restricted in nature, duration, or quality), and context (the physical, social, and attitudinal environments in which a person lives).

In this text, we will consider the difficulties stemming from hearing loss and the accompanying consequences to have an impact on both an individual's ability to converse in everyday life and with everyday communication partners and to have an impact on his or her internal state, meaning the person's psychosocial adjustment and self-image, emotional well-being, and communication behaviors. Thus, the goal of aural rehabilitation is to enhance everyday conversational fluency and to promote personal adjustment in the presence of hearing loss. This is an ecological interpretation of aural rehabilitation (e.g., Borg, 2000), meaning that we will take into account the individual, the person's self-image and perceived reality, his or her interpersonal interactions, and the components of the communication process within the context of the person's environment.

Figure 1-1 presents a model of communication handicap that is based on both the World Health Organization's definition of handicap and an ecological interpretation of aural rehabilitation. In this figure, the solid lines indicate an exacerbation and dotted lines indicate an alleviation. Four factors (i.e., disability, lifestyle, frequent communication partner, and psychosocial) contribute directly to communication handicap.

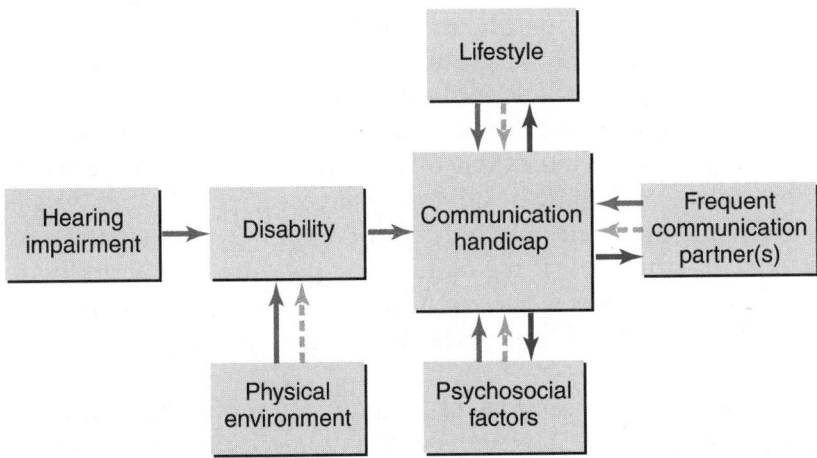

FIGURE 1-1. A model of communication handicap.

The impairment of hearing has a direct effect on the disability experienced, which in turn affects handicap. One goal of the aural rehabilitation plan is to minimize the impact of hearing loss through the provision of appropriate listening devices such as hearing aids or cochlear implants and through the provision of other listening aids such as assistive listening devices.

The magnitude of disability has a direct impact on communication handicap. In turn, disability can be either positively or negatively affected by the physical environment, as when the environment is either noisy or sound-treated. Another goal of the aural rehabilitation plan is to help patients and the persons who have input to their listening environments tailor the listening situation to optimize conversation success and to use other strategies to lessen disability.

Lifestyle may have a major effect on the experience of handicap. For instance, a male computer programmer and a salesman may have the same degree of hearing loss as measured audiometrically, yet the consequences for either one may differ. The programmer, who works alone at a computer monitor, may rarely experience conversational difficulties as a result of hearing loss. His typical day revolves around reading, problem solving at his desk, and working at the keyboard. On the other hand, the salesman must contact customers throughout the workday and may be devastated by a similar degree of hearing loss. He may frequently misunderstand an order, he may not be able to use the telephone effectively, and he may feel helpless to handle his communication difficulties at group meetings. The goal of the aural rehabilitation plan is to identify the effects of a patient's communication handicap on lifestyle and to implement effective means to overcome it. To the extent that the handicap cannot be overcome, the lifestyle may be adversely affected, as indicated by the reciprocal solid line leading from *communication handicap* to *lifestyle* in Figure 1-1. If the handicap experienced by an individual is great, the person may withdraw from lifestyle activities that formerly were found to be rewarding or pleasurable.

The behaviors and attitudes of frequent communication partners (the people the patient interacts with at home, in the workplace, or during social activities) also affect communication handicap. For instance, a frequent communication partner who mumbles, who resents the patient's hearing loss, and who feels burdened and cheated out of a high quality of life because of the patient's hearing loss serves to exacerbate communication handicap experienced by the patient, whereas a partner who is empathetic and who actively promotes effective communication will lessen the handicap. Other attitudes of the frequent communication partner that may exacerbate communication handicap include four different approaches to the hearing loss (Hallberg & Barrenas, 1993): (1) pretending that the hearing loss does not exist, (2) playing down the effects of hearing loss, (3) controlling or dominating the hard-of-hearing person and the person's communication problems, and (4) separating or isolating her- or himself from the patient. This relationship is a reciprocal one. Many times, the patient's communication handicap has an adverse effect on the quality of life experienced by the frequent communication partner. For instance, a man who refuses to attend parties or other social events because of his hearing loss may limit the social interactions of his wife by insisting they stay home. Another common aim of an aural rehabilitation plan is to enhance the interaction between a patient and the communication partner.

Psychosocial factors refer to two distinct components. *Psychological* factors pertain to the patient's attitudes toward the disability (e.g., to some persons a hearing loss might be a source of shame, whereas to others it may seem inconsequential in comparison to other life events), the patient's self-image, the patient's motivation to participate in aural rehabilitation, and the patient's assertiveness (see Stephens, 1996). For example, as will be noted in Chapter 2, an assertive person may effectively use communication strategies but a passive person may not, leading each to experience different degrees of communication handicap. *Social* factors (also referred to as cultural factors) are the prevailing viewpoints of the society in which the patient lives and operates. If the prevailing view is that hearing loss is a negative state, as when it is an indicant of aging in a youth-oriented society or it is a sign of inadequacy to maintain performance in the workforce, then the concomitant communication handicap increases. The relationship between psychosocial factors and communication handicap is reciprocal. For instance, just as a person's self-image may affect communication handicap (e.g., "I'm a strong personality, I can handle this."), communication handicap can affect self-image (e.g., "I'm not as valuable to my children because I can no longer interact with their friends and teachers like I once did."). An effective aural rehabilitation plan might focus on the patient's psychosocial issues and sometimes on those of the frequent communication partner.

SERVICES INCLUDED IN THE AURAL REHABILITATION PLAN

Table 1-1 presents components of several services often included in an aural rehabilitation plan and brief descriptions of each. These services help to alleviate hearing impairment, disability, and communication handicap and are described more fully in the remaining chapters of this textbook.

Table 1-1. Components of a typical aural rehabilitation program.

COMPONENT	DESCRIPTION
Diagnostics and quantification of hearing loss	Assessment of the hearing loss and speech-recognition skills
Provision of appropriate listening device	Provision of hearing aid(s) or tactile aid or participation on a team that results in cochlear implantation and follow-up services
Assistive listening devices (ALDs)	Explanation and dispensing of devices that supplement or replace a hearing aid or that serve to lessen communication handicap
Auditory training	Structured and unstructured listening practice
Communication strategies training	Teaching of strategies that enhance communication and minimize communication difficulties (facilitative strategies, repair strategies, environmental management)
Informational/educational counseling	Instruction about normal hearing, hearing loss, listening device technology, speech perception, available services
Rational acceptance counseling	Intervention to enhance the management of hearing loss and communication difficulties
Psychosocial adjustment counseling	Addressing the psychological and social impact of hearing loss on the person with hearing loss, family, and friends (may include stress management and relaxation techniques)
Frequent communication partner training	Communication training for the spouse, partner, family, friends, or co-workers
Speechreading	Training speech recognition via both auditory and visual channels
Speech-language therapy	For children primarily, training that emphasizes developing strategies to monitor one's own speech production and developing vocabulary, syntax, and pragmatics
Inservice training	Specialized training for other professionals, such as teachers in the public school system or caretakers in senior citizen centers

Source: Adapted from Prendergast, S. G., and Kelley, L. A. (2002). Aural rehab services: Survey reports who offers which ones and how often. *The Hearing Journal, 55,* 30–35.

A typical aural rehabilitation plan may include diagnosis and quantification of the hearing loss and the provision of appropriate listening devices. In addition, aural rehabilitation for an adult may include communication strategies training; counseling related to hearing loss; assertiveness training; psychosocial therapy; and counseling and instruction for family members, colleagues, or caretakers. Less commonly, an aural rehabilitation program for an adult may also include speech perception training, such as speechreading training. For a child, aural rehabilitation may include diagnostics, provision of appropriate amplification and communication aids, and speech perception and communication strategies training, as well as intervention related to speech, language, and academic achievement. Children's family members and teachers may also receive services under the umbrella of the aural rehabilitation plan.

A recent survey of the membership of the American Academy of Audiology (AAA) suggested that respondents most typically provided the following three services to adult patients: (1) information on assistive listening devices (84% of the 110 respondents), (2) communication strategies training (83%), and (3) information/education counseling (82%) (Prendergast & Kelley, 2002). About half of the 110 respondents reported they provided coping strategies training and psychosocial adjustment counseling, and 38% reported providing frequent communication partner training. Auditory training and speechreading training were the two services reported as least frequently provided.

Similar kinds of data are not readily available for children who have hearing loss, as aural rehabilitation interventions often are folded into their everyday school experiences. For example, speechreading practice might be provided in the context of learning vocabulary for a history lesson. The teacher might focus the children's attention on the way the words *Civil War*, or *Gettysburg*, or *Lincoln*, appear on the mouth when she speaks them during a unit about the Civil War. One piece of data that relates to this issue comes from Geers and Brenner (2003). They considered only the provision of auditory training and speech-language therapy for children who use cochlear implants, and found that, on average, children who use cochlear implants receive an hour and a half of individual therapy a week, for at least 4 years following implantation.

Aural habilitation is intervention for persons who have not developed listening, speech, and language skills.

Other Terms Related to Aural Rehabilitation

Sometimes the terms aural habilitation or audiologic rehabilitation are used when discussing the provision of services related to alleviating the problems associated with hearing loss. The term *aural habilitation* instead of aural rehabilitation is used when the person receiving the services is a child rather than an adult. This is because in the strict sense, *rehabilitation* means to restore something that was lost. When we provide speech perception training or speech and language therapy to children who have hearing loss, we are not aiming to restore lost function, but rather, to develop (that is, to habilitate or furnish) skills that were not present beforehand. Although this is a cogent distinction between the terms rehabilitation and habilitation, in this text, we shall use the two synonymously for simplicity's sake.

The term audiologic rehabilitation closely parallels the term *aural rehabilitation,* but it usually encompasses a narrower breadth of services. The term *audiologic rehabilitation* implies an emphasis on the diagnosis of hearing loss and the provision of listening devices and a lesser emphasis on follow-up support services, such as communication strategies training.

Audiologic rehabilitation is a term often used synonymously with aural rehabilitation or aural habilitation; may entail greater emphasis on the provision and follow-up of listening devices and less emphasis on communication strategy and speech perception training.

Where Does Aural Rehabilitation Occur?

Now that we have defined what aural rehabilitation may encompass, let us consider where it might be provided. Aural rehabilitation may occur in a variety of locales. For example, it may be provided in any of the following settings:

- A university speech and hearing clinic
- An audiology private practice
- A hearing-aid dealer's private practice
- A hospital speech and hearing clinic
- A community center or nursing home
- A school (Figure 1-2)
- An otolaryngologist's office
- A speech-language pathologist's office
- Consumer organization meetings
- The home, with the aid of a computer

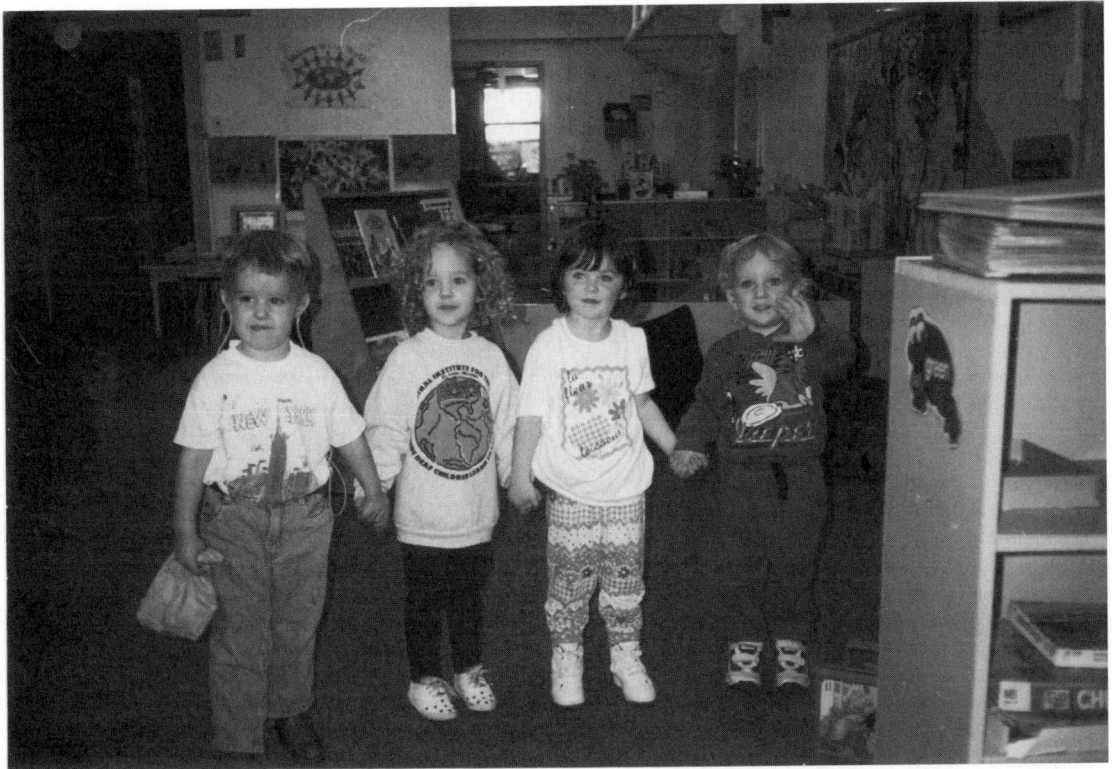

FIGURE 1-2. Aural rehabilitation for young children often occurs in educational settings. *(Photograph by Julia Rottjakob, courtesy of Central Institute for the Deaf.)*

Who Provides Aural Rehabilitation?

Aural rehabilitation might be provided by an audiologist, a speech-language pathologist, or a teacher for the hard-of-hearing and deaf. Typically, an audiologist takes a lead role in developing an individual's aural rehabilitation plan and coordinates the services provided by other professionals. Particularly with adults, the audiologist is the primary health-care professional in the management of the hearing loss.

In some cases, however, the speech-language pathologist may play the lead role for a child, especially in a school environment. For instance, the speech-language pathologist is most likely to provide speech and language therapy and often is the professional who provides auditory and speechreading training.

Whereas the audiologist may fit and maintain a child's hearing aids and equip the classroom with appropriate assistive listening devices, the speech-language pathologist may be the person who has extended one-on-one contact with a child, and the one who knows the child well. The American Speech-Language-Hearing Association (ASHA) convened a working group on audiologic rehabilitation (ASHA, 2002). Its charge was to summarize the knowledge and skill sets that audiologists and speech-language pathologists should have if they are to provide aural rehabilitation. These outlines are presented in Appendix 1-1 (audiologists) and Appendix 1-2 (speech-language pathologists).

In addition to a general knowledge about basic communication processes, audiologists who provide aural rehabilitation are expected to understand the auditory system function and disorders; developmental status, cognition, and sensory perception; audiologic assessment procedures; speech and language assessment procedures; evaluation and management of listening devices; effects of hearing impairment on functional communication; case management; interdisciplinary collaboration and public advocacy; and hearing conservation and acoustic environments.

In addition to general knowledge about the basic communication processes, speech-language pathologists are expected to have a broad knowledge of auditory system function and disorders; developmental status, cognition, and sensory perception; audiologic assessment procedures; assessment of communication performance; listening devices; effects of hearing loss on psychosocial, educational, and vocational functioning; management; interdisciplinary collaboration and public advocacy; and acoustic environments.

◼ HEARING LOSS

Individuals who have hearing loss represent a heterogeneous group. They vary in the nature of their hearing loss and in their aural rehabilitation needs. In this section, we will briefly consider how hearing loss may be parameterized (Figure 1-3).

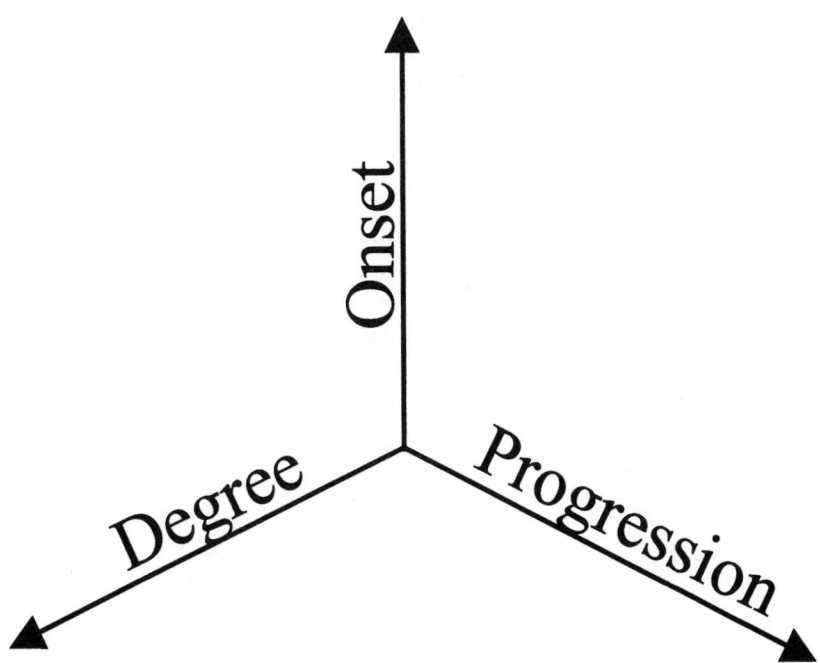

FIGURE 1-3. Hearing loss can be parameterized on three dimensions: onset, degree, and time course.

Hearing loss may be categorized along three dimensions: degree, onset, and time course. In terms of degree, hearing loss may be characterized as mild, moderate, moderate-to-severe, severe, or profound (Chapter 6).

Degree of hearing impairment is often defined by the *pure tone average* (PTA) (Chapter 6), the average of the individual's pure-tone frequencies at 500, 1000, and 2000 Hz obtained with supra-aural earphones. In describing the degree of hearing loss, you may take into consideration the *configuration* of the loss. Config-uration of hearing loss reflects the extent of hearing loss at each of the audiometric frequencies (audiograms measure hearing sensitivity at the frequencies of 250, 500, 1000, 2000, 4000, and 8000 Hz) and provides an overall picture of hearing sensitivity. For example, a person who has normal hearing for the frequen-cies 250–2000 Hz and then reduced sensitivity for the frequencies 4000–8000 Hz may be described as having a "high-frequency hearing loss." A person who has equal sensitivity across the audiometric frequencies has a "flat hearing loss" (see Figure 1-4). Other descriptors associated with degree of hearing loss include the following:

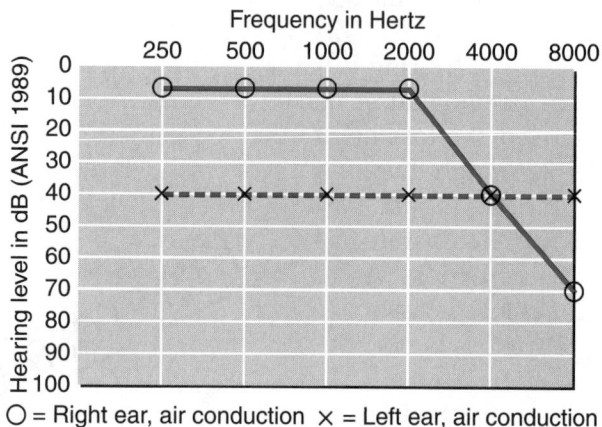

FIGURE 1-4. Example of an audiogram. This person has an *assymetrical* hearing loss, meaning that the degree and configuration of loss in one ear is different than the degree and configuration in the other ear. The left ear has a "flat" hearing loss; the right ear has a "high-frequency" hearing loss.

■ *Bilateral versus unilateral.* Bilateral hearing loss means both ears have reduced sensitivity, whereas unilateral means only one ear is affected.
■ *Symmetrical versus asymmetrical.* Symmetrical hearing loss means the degree and configuration of hearing loss are the same in each ear, whereas asymmetrical means the two ears differ.
■ *Fluctuating versus stable.* Sometimes a person's hearing sensitivity may fluctuate (for example, if a child has fluid in the ear), whereas at other times sensitivity remains stable.

Hard-of-hearing means having a hearing loss; usually not used to refer to a profound hearing loss.

A person who has a mild, moderate, or moderate-to-severe hearing loss (i.e., a hearing loss between 26 and 70 dB) is often called **hard-of-hearing**. Sometimes the term *hearing-impaired* is used in lieu of the term hard-of-hearing. Many persons dislike it as it connotes that they may be exactly that, impaired, even though they may function effectively in their everyday lives. A person who has a severe or profound hearing loss (i.e., hearing loss greater than 70 dB) may sometimes be called *deaf*. People who belong to the deaf community, often people who were born deaf or who grew up with deaf family members, may refer to themselves as *Deaf*. The capital "D" denotes their membership in the Deaf Culture.

Deaf: having minimal or no hearing.

In terms of onset, a hearing loss may be described as prelingual, perilingual, or postlingual. A person who has a *prelingual* hearing loss incurred the loss before the acquisition of spoken language skills. Although there is no universally agreed cut-off time as to when the prelingual phase ends, generally, when a child incurs a hearing loss before the age of 2 years, he or she is said to have a prelingual loss. A *congenital* hearing loss is thought to be present at birth or associated with the birthing process. An *acquired* hearing loss is not present at birth but is incurred later, either as a child or as an adult. A child who lost the hearing after acquiring some spoken language but before acquisition was complete is said to have a *perilingual* hearing loss. Finally, a *postlingual* loss is one that occurred after the acquisition of speech and language. Again, there is no agreed-on age at which the perilingual stage ends and the postlingual stage begins, but it may be around the age of 5 years. The postlingual distinction may be further divided into four additional cohorts. These are:

Prelingual refers to a hearing loss acquired before the acquisition of spoken language.

A label of *congenital* implies the hearing loss was present at birth.

A label of *acquired* implies the hearing loss was incurred after birth.

- Prevocational (around the ages 5–17 years)
- Early working age (18–44 years)
- Later working age (45–64 years)
- Retirement age (65 years and older)

Perilingual refers to a hearing loss acquired during the stage of acquiring spoken language.

Postlingual refers to a hearing loss incurred after the acquisition of spoken language.

Depending on a patient's membership in a cohort, his or her aural rehabilitation needs may vary. For instance, someone who is prevocational may benefit from having a special amplification system available in the classroom, and the child's family may benefit from communication strategies training. Another person of later working age, someone who before hearing loss may have been able and competent in every respect, may require personal adjustment counseling and even psychosocial therapy to accept his or her change in abilities.

Finally, a hearing loss may be categorized as progressive or sudden. An individual who has a hearing loss that occurs over the

A **progressive hearing loss** is a hearing loss that increases over time.

A **sudden hearing loss** is a hearing loss that has an acute and rapid onset.

course of several months or years has a ***progressive hearing loss***. An individual who lost hearing suddenly, say as a result of head trauma, has a ***sudden hearing loss***.

We will consider in more detail levels of hearing loss and onset in Chapters 6 and 14, respectively. As we shall see, an aural rehabilitation plan for an individual patient may vary as a function of the degree, age of onset, and progression of the hearing loss.

▦ RELEVANCE OF AURAL REHABILITATION

Now let us tackle the issue of relevance. Aural rehabilitation is an important component of the speech and hearing professionals' service delivery program for at least two reasons. These reasons relate to demographics and cost-effectiveness.

Demographics and Service Needs

Many different segments of our society require aural rehabilitation:

"Working adults and the elderly have been largely without services. Working adults often face not only the growing challenges to their hearing, communication, and linguistic abilities brought by the information society, but also the negative psycho-social effects of impaired hearing. . . . Preventive work with senior citizens can promote extended independent living and better quality of life."

Huttunen, 2001, p. 89

OLDER PERSONS

With the aging of the "baby boom" population, age-related hearing loss (which is called presbycusis, Chapter 13) is affecting an increasing percentage of our citizens (Figure 1-5). These individuals often are unwilling to, nor should they be expected to, sit on the sidelines of life because they are unable to communicate with those around them. They have a demand for services that will enhance their ability to communicate with their families and friends, to participate in community activities and volunteer work, and to stay in touch with their world via multimedia technology. Some desire to continue in their professional careers and postpone retirement. With increased awareness of preventative medicine routines and a growing sophistication in medical practice, an ever-growing number of older persons are living longer, and many have few health problems other than hearing loss that restrict their day-to-day functioning.

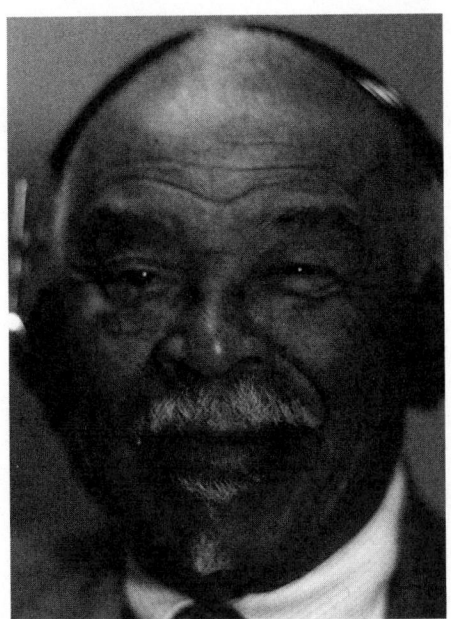

FIGURE 1-5. Older persons have a demand for aural rehabilitation services to enhance their abilities to communicate with their families and friends and to stay in touch with their world via multimedia technology. *(Photograph by Marcus Kosa, courtesy of Central Institute for the Deaf.)*

INFANTS AND CHILDREN

On the other end of the life cycle, advances in neonatology and critical-care medicine have led to better survival rates of high-risk babies. Infants who might have died in earlier times now survive, often with a myriad of medical conditions that might include hearing loss. Families of babies who have hearing loss desire and expect assistance and support that will enable their children to grow up and achieve their full potential. Public policy reflects these trends. There is now a greater emphasis on earlier identification and service provision for young children who have hearing loss, under the auspices of Public Law 94-142 (Chapter 14).

ADULTS

In addition to the youngest and oldest members of our society, individuals in the center of the life cycle also may desire aural rehabilitation services. They have learned that, with appropriate support, they can make meaningful contributions in both the workplace and in their communities. Indeed, this realization helped lead to the passage of the Americans with Disabilities Act, which is landmark legislation that calls for equal access for all persons with disabilities (Chapter 10).

FAMILY AND FREQUENT COMMUNICATION PARTNERS

A primary goal of any aural rehabilitation plan is to develop and enhance communication between the person with hearing loss and his or her family and communication partners. Implicitly, this goal suggests that the plan must target not only the individual, but also the people with whom the individual interacts during everyday activities. For an adult patient, the aural rehabilitation might include those persons in the home, social/avocational settings, and the work place. Figure 1-6 shows these communication realms as intersecting, as some communication partners may interact with the individual in both work and social environments. For a child, the plan might target the communication partners in the school system, social and extracurricular activities, and the home.

Communication partners of persons with hearing loss can acquire techniques for optimizing communication. For example, a wife may learn how to speak slowly and clearly so that her husband might better speechread her vocalizations. A father might develop techniques for stimulating conversation between himself and his son. In addition, communication partners sometimes need additional support from the aural rehabilitation specialist. A mother may need personal adjustment counseling as she reconciles herself to her baby's hearing loss. A husband may need to adjust to the changed hearing status of his wife who may have just received a cochlear implant.

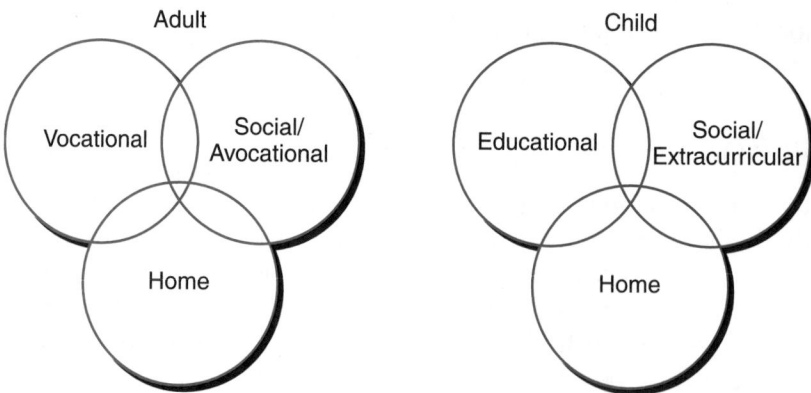

FIGURE 1-6. The aural rehabilitation plan addresses the individual's communication realms.

UNSERVED AND UNDERSERVED

There is evidence from the Institute on Rehabilitation Issues that individuals who have hearing loss are currently unserved or underserved (Robards-Armstrong & Stone, 1994). *Unserved* means this population is a group that is not served as a result of policy, practice, or environmental barriers. *Underserved* denotes a population that is inadequately served, in part because of:

An **unserved** population refers to a group of patients in need of but not receiving services.

An **underserved** population is a group of patients receiving less than ideal services.

- A dearth of outreach and immediate or extended support services
- The attitudes of service delivery personnel
- The lack of reimbursement policies for aural rehabilitation
- Communication or environmental barriers

Increasingly, persons with hearing loss and their families are exerting pressure on lawmakers and policy makers to ensure that more services are provided to individuals who have hearing loss and deafness. There will be a need for aural rehabilitation specialists to provide these services.

The Importance of Aural Rehabilitation Training for Speech-Language Pathologists

Because aural rehabilitation is provided to persons who have a hearing loss, we sometimes think that only audiologists provide it. As the following except from a letter to *ASHA Leader* indicates, this supposition is not true. Speech-language pathologists often play a major role:

The changes taking place in the profession and populations served will require speech-language pathologists who are prepared to deal with issues in aural rehabilitation. Universal neonatal hearing screening is rapidly becoming a reality in many states and will result in a dramatic increase of hearing impaired babies and their families entering early intervention programs. Because the hearing loss will be identified so early, the children will be staying in the system for nearly three years— longer than if they had been identified at a later

(continues)

age. Babies with milder degrees of hearing loss will be identified, as well as those who are deaf. Cochlear implants are also becoming a reality for many young hearing impaired children with implantation occurring at an earlier age. These children are the "hard of hearing deaf" who, once destined for schools for the deaf, will most likely be mainstreamed into regular classrooms. In both these settings, early intervention programs and the public schools, the only professional on hand who is expected to have any training in hearing impairment is the speech-language pathologist.

At the end of the age spectrum, the fastest growing segment in our society is the over 80 year olds, a population with a high percentage of hearing loss. Again, the speech-language pathologist in the nursing home or rehabilitation facility will be the only one with any credible training in hearing disorders and appropriate intervention.

The demand for skilled clinicians who are competent to plan and implement appropriate and effective aural (re)habilitation programs across the life span will become greater in the near future. (Letter to the editor, David Luterman and Ellen Kurtzer-White, *ASHA Leader*, February 17, 1998)

Incidence

Statistics underscore the fact that a significant number of persons have hearing loss. About 28 million people in the United States have some degree of reduced hearing sensitivity. Of this number, about 80% have an irreversible hearing loss. In the Scandinavian countries of Denmark, Finland, Norway, and Sweden, and in the United Kingdom, hearing loss also has high incidence. For instance, in a review article of surveys performed on adult populations, Maki-Torkko et al. (2001) suggest that the incidence of hearing loss increases with age, and the proportion of people over the age of 65 who have hearing loss may fall somewhere between 15 and 60%, depending on how one defines the age group and how one defines degree of hearing loss.

CHILDREN AND INFANTS

Data suggest that one of every 22 infants born in this country has some kind of hearing problem. One in every 1,000 infants has a severe or profound hearing loss, which means hearing thresholds that are poorer than 70 dB HL. With respect to school-age children, for every 1,000 children in the United States, 83 have what can be described as an "educationally significant hearing loss" (National Dissemination Center for Children with Disabilities, 2003).

ADULTS AGES 18–64 YEARS

Hearing loss is a significant issue not only for children and older persons, but for adults between the ages of 18 and 64 as well. For example, 4.6% of persons between the ages of 18 and 44 have some degree of hearing loss. This percentage rises to 14% for adults between the ages of 45 and 64 (Benson & Marano, 1998).

ADULTS AGE 64 AND OLDER

The incidence of hearing loss increases with age. Fifty-four percent of adults over the age of 64 have hearing loss, while one in three persons over the age of 65 has decreased hearing. In fact, hearing is the third most prevalent chronic condition in the older population (National Institute of Deafness and Communication Disorders, 2002).

Cost-Effectiveness and Costs

Cost-effectiveness also relates to the relevance of aural rehabilitation, whereas the costs of providing services relate to the reality of providing services in an environment where health-care expenses are spiraling, and services are being cut for economic purposes.

COST-EFFECTIVENESS

In recent years, there has been a growing awareness of the importance of rehabilitation services for individuals who have acute or chronic disabilities. We have learned that rehabilitation can promote an individual's quality of life and increase his or her productivity in the home, workplace, and community. In the case of children, appropriate rehabilitation can promote success in school as well.

In areas other than aural rehabilitation, such as occupational therapy and physical therapy, we have documented that rehabilitation is cost-effective. By providing appropriate support services, we can reduce dramatically medical and education costs, as well as other costs related to supporting individuals who are not as productive and independent as they might be.

We are realizing gradually that this also is true with aural rehabilitation. For instance, children who receive cochlear implants and abundant aural rehabilitation, particularly auditory speech stimulation are more likely to demonstrate benefit than those who do not receive such follow-up support (Osberger, Robbins, Todd, & Riley, 1994). Spitzer (1997) reviewed evidence that demonstrates the cost-effectiveness of providing a cochlear implant and related support services to adult patients.

Compelling support for aural rehabilitation has come from research performed with new hearing aid users. About 16% of people who receive hearing aids choose not to use them, and a similar percentage of people describe their experiences with hearing aids as "unsatisfactory" (Kochkin, 2000), suggesting the need for follow-up programs. An even more discouraging statistic is that only 20% of persons who could benefit from receiving a hearing aid actually get one (Holmes, 1995; Kochkin, 1999). This lack of use in hearing aids suggests that it is not enough to simply fit and dispense the devices. A well rounded management plan must include proper counseling and follow-up programs. Research has shown that when counseling and follow-up programs are provided, patients are less likely to return their hearing aids to the audiologist than when they are not provided (Northern and Beyer, 1999).

COSTS AND REIMBURSEMENTS

Perhaps the primary obstacle to providing aural rehabilitation pertains to the short-term costs of service provision. Aural rehabilitation can be expensive for two reasons: Listening device technology is often costly, and providing services such as communication strategies training is labor-intensive. Often these kinds of costs are not covered by insurance companies and must be borne by the individual.

Insurance policies can be classified as private (e.g., Health Maintenance Organizations [HMOs]), state (e.g., Blue Cross and Blue Shield), or federal plans (e.g., Medicare). Sometimes when insurance plans provide coverage for services following receipt of a listening device, they do so only when the services are provided by a speech-language pathologist rather than an audiologist. If coverage is provided for a hearing aid or cochlear implant, follow-up services may not be included. In these instances, it is not unusual for an audiologist to bundle aural rehabilitation costs into the price of the listening device.

FINAL REMARKS

In the following chapters, we will review both traditional and cutting-edge practices in aural rehabilitation. In the first half of the text (Parts I and II), we will consider some of the components of an aural rehabilitation service delivery model, including communication strategies training, diagnostics and assessment, provision of listening devices, and speech perception training. In the second half (Parts III and IV), we will consider specific populations and how an aural rehabilitation plan can be customized to meet the needs of individual patients.

A number of professional journals deal with aural rehabilitation. These journals are listed in Key Resources at the end of each chapter. They can provide interested readers with additional and timely information about the topics covered in this text.

KEY CHAPTER POINTS

✔ Individuals may experience hearing impairment, disability, or communication handicap.
✔ Hearing loss can affect several aspects of an individual's daily life at home, at work, in school, and in social situations.
✔ Aural rehabilitation for the adult may include diagnosis and quantification of hearing loss, provision of appropriate

listening devices, training in communication strategies, counseling related to hearing loss, vocational counseling, noise protection, and counseling and instruction for family members. It may or may not include speech perception training.

✔ Aural rehabilitation for the child may include diagnostics; provision of appropriate amplification; speech perception training; communication strategies training; family training; and intervention related to speech, language, and educational development.

✔ Aural rehabilitation may occur in a variety of locales, including university speech and hearing clinics and audiology private practices.

✔ Aural rehabilitation may be provided by an audiologist, speech-language pathologist, or educator.

✔ Hearing loss may be categorized by degree, onset, and time course.

✔ The aural rehabilitation plan includes the communication realms of the person who has hearing loss.

✔ Aural rehabilitation is relevant for two general reasons: demographics and cost-effectiveness.

▉▉▉ MULTIPLE CHOICE QUESTIONS

1. In the World Health Organization nomenclature, a disability is:
   a. An abnormality of a body function or structure
   b. A psychosocial consequence of hearing loss
   c. A functional consequence of an impairment
   d. A handicap

2. A person has lost hearing in the right ear, presumably as a result of exposure to gun blasts during duck hunting season. This person may best be described as:
   a. Deaf
   b. Hard-of-hearing with a flat hearing loss
   c. Hearing-impaired
   d. Unilaterally hard-of-hearing

3. A teacher and school speech-language pathologist wish to develop an aural rehabilitation plan for a 6-year-old child. They might search the audiological records for information concerning:

   a. Hearing loss degree, onset, and progression
   b. Hearing configuration, handicap, and function
   c. Activity, participation, and context
   d. Disability, impairment, and handicap

4. If someone says to you, "The aural rehabilitation plan will address the patient's communication realms," you might interpret this statement as:

   a. The plan must optimize communication in the workplace through provision of hearing aids, assistive listening devices, and other technology.
   b. The family and the patient's frequent communication partners will be included in the aural rehabilitation plan.
   c. The patient will participate in communication strategies training, auditory and speechreading training, and psychosocial therapy.
   d. Counseling will be provided to family members.

KEY RESOURCES

Professional Journals

Advance for Audiologists
Advance for Speech-Language Pathologists and Audiologists
American Annals of the Deaf
American Journal of Audiology: A Journal of Clinical Practice
American Journal of Speech-Language Pathology: A Journal of Clinical Practice
ASHA (American Speech-Language Hearing Association)
Audiology
Australian and New Zealand Journal of Audiology
British Journal of Audiology

Contact

Deafness and Education

Ear and Hearing

Educational Audiology

Hearing Journal

Hearing Review

International Journal of Audiology (formerly *Audiology, British Journal of Audiology, & Scandinavian Audiology*)

Journal of the Academy of Rehabilitative Audiology

Journal of the American Academy of Audiology

Journal of Child Language

Journal of Communication Disorders

Journal of Deaf Studies and Deaf Education

Journal of Speech, Language and Hearing Research

Language and Speech

Language, Speech, and Hearing Services in the School

Noise and Health

Noise Regulation Report

Scandinavian Audiology

Seminars in Hearing

Seminars in Speech and Language

Speech Communication

Tinnitus Today

Topics in Language Disorders

Trends in Amplification

Volta Review

Volta Voices

APPENDIX 1-1

Knowledge and skills for audiologists providing aural rehabilitation (AR) services (reprinted from ASHA, Supplement No. 22, April 16, 2002, pp. 90–92. Copyright by the American Speech-Language Hearing Association. Reprinted with permission.)

▰ BASIC AREAS OF KNOWLEDGE AND SKILLS

Audiologists who provide AR services demonstrate knowledge in the basic areas that are the underpinnings of communication sciences and disorders. These include the following:

I. General Knowledge

  A. General psychology; human growth and development; psychosocial behavior; cultural and linguistic diversity; biological, physical, and social sciences; mathematics; and qualitative and quantitative research methodologies.

II. Basic Communication Processes

  A. Anatomic and physiologic bases for the normal development and use of speech, language, and hearing (including anatomy, neurology, and physiology of speech, language, and hearing mechanisms);

  B. Physical bases and process of the production and perception of speech and hearing (including acoustics or physics of sound, phonology, physiologic and acoustic phonetics, sensory perceptual processes, and psychoacoustics);

  C. Linguistic and psycholinguistic variables related to the normal development and use of speech, language, and hearing (including linguistics, [historical, descriptive, sociolinguistics, sign language, second language usage], psychology of language, psycholinguistics, language and speech acquisition, verbal learning and verbal behavior, and gestural communication);

  D. Dynamics of interpersonal skills, communication effectiveness, and group theory.

■ SPECIAL AREAS OF KNOWLEDGE AND SKILLS

Audiologists who provide AR have knowledge in the following special areas and demonstrate the itemized requisite skills in those areas:

III. Auditory System Function and Disorders

    A. Identify, describe, and differentiate among disorders of auditory function (including disorders of the outer, middle, and inner ear; the vestibular system; the auditory nerve and the associated neural and central auditory system pathways and processes).

IV. Developmental Status, Cognition, and Sensory Perception

    A. Provide for the administration of assessment measures in the client's preferred mode of communication;

    B. Verify adequate visual acuity for communication purposes;

    C. Identify the need and provide for assessment of cognitive skills, sensory perceptual and motor skills, developmental delays, academic achievement, and literacy;

    D. Determine the need for referral to other medical and nonmedical specialists for appropriate professional services;

    E. Provide for ongoing assessments of developmental progress.

V. Audiologic Assessment Procedures

    A. Conduct interview and obtain case history;

    B. Perform otoscopic examinations and ensure that the external auditory canal is free of obstruction, including cerumen;

    C. Conduct and interpret behavioral, physiologic, or electrophysiologic evaluations of the peripheral and central auditory systems;

    D. Conduct and interpret assessments for auditory processing disorders;

    E. Administer and interpret standardized self-report measures of communication difficulties and of psychosocial and behavioral adjustment to auditory dysfunction;

F. Identify the need for referral to medical and nonmedical specialists for appropriate professional services.

VI. Speech and Language Assessment Procedures

A. Identify the need for and perform screenings for effects of hearing impairment on speech and language;

B. Describe the effects of hearing impairment on the development of semantic, syntactic, pragmatic, and phonologic aspects of communication, both in terms of comprehension and production;

C. Provide for appropriate measures of speech and voice production;

D. Provide for appropriate measures of language comprehension and production skills and/or alternate communication skills (e.g., signing);

E. Administer and interpret appropriate measures of communication skills in auditory, visual, auditory-visual, and tactile modalities.

VII. Evaluation and Management of Devices and Technologies for Individuals with Hearing Impairment (e.g., hearing aids, cochlear implants, middle ear implants, implantable hearing aids, tinnitus maskers, hearing assistive technologies, and other sensory prosthetic devices)

A. Perform and interpret measures of electroacoustic characteristics of devices and technologies;

B. Describe, perform, and interpret behavioral/psychophysical measures of performance with these devices and technologies;

C. Conduct appropriate fittings with and adjustments of these devices and technologies;

D. Monitor fitting of and adjustment to these devices and technologies to ensure comfort, safety, and device performance;

E. Perform routine visual, listening, and electroacoustic checks of clients' hearing devices and sensory aids to troubleshoot common causes of malfunction;

F. Evaluate and describe the effects of use of devices and technologies on communication and psychosocial functioning;

G. Plan and implement a program of orientation to these devices and technologies to ensure realistic expectations; to improve acceptance of, adjustment to, and benefit from these systems; and to enhance communication performance;

H. Conduct routine assessments of adjustment to and effective use of amplification devices to ensure optimal communication function;

I. Monitor outcomes to ensure professional accountability.

VIII. Effects of Hearing Impairment on Functional Communication

A. Identify the individual's situational expressive and receptive communication needs;

B. Evaluate the individual's expressive and receptive communication performance;

C. Identify environmental factors that affect the individual's situational communication needs and performance;

D. Identify the effects of interpersonal relations on communication function.

IX. Effects of Hearing Impairment on Psychosocial, Educational, and Occupational Functioning

A. Describe and evaluate the impact of hearing impairment on psychosocial development and psychosocial functioning;

B. Describe systems and methods of educational programming (e.g., mainstream, residential) and facilitate selection of appropriate educational options;

C. Describe and evaluate the effects of hearing impairment on occupational status and performance (e.g., communication, localization, safety);

D. Identify the effects of hearing problems on marital dyads, family dynamics, and other interpersonal communication functioning;

E. Identify the need and provide the psychosocial, educational, family, and occupational/vocational counseling in relation to hearing impairment and subsequent communication difficulties;

    F. Provide assessment of family members' perception of and reactions to communication difficulties.

X. AR Case Management

    A. Use effective interpersonal communication in interviewing and interacting with individuals with hearing impairment and their families;

    B. Describe client-centered, behavioral, cognitive, and integrative theories and methods of counseling and their relevance in AR;

    C. Provide appropriate individual and group adjustment counseling related to hearing loss for individuals with hearing impairment and their families;

    D. Provide auditory, visual, and auditory-visual communication training (e.g., speechreading, auditory training, listening skills) to enhance receptive communication;

    E. Provide training in effective communication strategies to individuals with hearing impairment, family members, and other relevant individuals;

    F. Provide for appropriate expressive communication training;

    G. Provide appropriate technological and counseling intervention to facilitate adjustment to tinnitus;

    H. Provide appropriate intervention for management of vestibular disorders;

    I. Develop and implement an intervention plan based on the individual's situational/environmental communication needs and performance and related adjustment difficulties;

    J. Develop and implement a system for measuring and monitoring outcomes and the appropriateness and efficacy of intervention.

XI. Interdisciplinary Collaboration and Public Advocacy

    A. Collaborate effectively as part of multidisciplinary teams and communicate relevant information to allied professionals and other appropriate individuals;

B. Plan and implement in-service and public-information programs for allied professionals and other interested individuals;

C. Plan and implement parent-education programs concerning the management of hearing impairment and subsequent communication difficulties;

D. Advocate implementation of public law in educational, occupational, and public settings;

E. Make appropriate referrals to consumer-based organizations.

XII. Hearing Conservation/Acoustic Environments

A. Plan and implement programs for prevention of hearing impairment to promote identification and evaluation of individuals exposed to hazardous noise and periodic monitoring of communication performance and auditory abilities (e.g., speech recognition in noise, localization);

B. Identify need for and provide appropriate hearing protection devices and noise abatement procedures;

C. Monitor the effects of environmental influences, amplification, and sources of trauma on residual auditory function;

D. Measure and evaluate the environmental acoustic conditions and relate them to effects on communication performance and hearing protection.

APPENDIX 1-2

Knowledge and skills for speech-language pathologists providing aural rehabilitation (AR) services (reprinted from ASHA, Supplement No. 22, April 16, 2002, pp. 92–95. Copyright by the American Speech-Language Hearing Association. Reprinted with permission.)

■ BASIC AREAS OF KNOWLEDGE AND SKILLS

Speech-language pathologists who provide AR services demonstrate knowledge in the basic areas that are the underpinnings of communication sciences and disorders. These include the following:

I. General Knowledge

   A. General psychology; human growth and development; psychosocial behavior; cultural and linguistic diversity; biological, physical, and social sciences; mathematics; and qualitative and quantitative research methodologies.

II. Basic Communication Processes

   A. Anatomic and physiologic bases for the normal development and use of speech, language, and hearing (including anatomy, neurology, and physiology of speech, language, and hearing mechanisms);

   B. Physical bases and process of the production and perception of speech and hearing (including acoustics or physics of sound, phonology, physiologic and acoustic phonetics, sensory perceptual processes, and psychoacoustics);

   C. Linguistic and psycholinguistic variables related to the normal development and use of speech, language, and hearing (including linguistics, [historical, descriptive, sociolinguistics, sign language, second language usage], psychology of language, psycholinguistics, language and speech acquisition, verbal learning and verbal behavior, and gestural communication);

   D. Dynamics of interpersonal skills, communication effectiveness, and group theory.

American Speech-Language Hearing Association. Knowledge and Skills for Providing Aural Rehabilitation, Supplement No. 22 (Rockville, MD: American Speech-Language Hearing Association, April 15, 2002). Copyright by American Speech-Language Hearing Association. Reprinted with permission.

■ SPECIAL AREAS OF KNOWLEDGE AND SKILLS

Speech-Language pathologists who provide AR have knowledge in the following special areas and demonstrate the itemized requisite skills in those areas:

III. Auditory System Function and Disorders

　A. Identify, describe, and differentiate among disorders of auditory function (including disorders of the outer, middle, and inner ear; the vestibular system; the auditory nerve and the associated neural and central auditory system pathways and processes).

IV. Developmental Status, Cognition, and Sensory Perception

　A. Provide for the administration of assessment measures in the client's preferred mode of communication;

　B. Verify adequate visual acuity for communication purposes;

　C. Identify the need and provide for assessment of cognitive skills, sensory perceptual and motor skills, developmental delays, academic achievement, and literacy;

　D. Determine the need for referral to other medical and nonmedical specialists for appropriate professional services;

　E. Provide for ongoing assessments of developmental progress.

V. Audiologic Assessment Procedures

　A. Conduct audiologic screening as appropriate for initial identification and/or referral purposes;

　B. Describe type and degree of hearing loss from audiometric test results (including pure tone thresholds, immittance testing, and speech audiometry);

　C. Refer to and consult with an audiologist for administration and interpretation of differential diagnostic procedures (including behavioral, physiological and electrophysiological measures).

VI. Assessment of Communication Performance

    A. Provide for assessment measures in the client's preferred mode of communication;

    B. Identify and perform screening examinations for speech, language, hearing, auditory processing disorders, and reading and academic achievement problems;

    C. Identify and perform diagnostic evaluations for the comprehension and production of speech and language in oral, signed, written or augmented form;

    D. Provide diagnostic evaluations of speech perception in auditory, visual, auditory-visual, or tactile modalities;

    E. Identify the effects of hearing loss on speech perception, communication performance, listening skills, speechreading, communication strategies, and personal adjustment;

    F. Provide for clients' self-assessment of communication difficulties and adjustment of hearing loss;

    G. Monitor developmental progress in relation to communication competence.

VII. Devices and Technologies for Individuals with Hearing Loss (e.g., hearing aids, cochlear implants, middle ear implants, implantable hearing aids, hearing assistive technologies, and other sensory prosthetic devices)

    A. Describe candidacy criteria for amplification or sensory-prosthetic devices (e.g., hearing aids, cochlear implants);

    B. Monitor clients' prescribed use of personal and group amplification systems;

    C. Describe options and applications of sensory aids (e.g., assistive listening devices) and telephone/telecommunication devices;

    D. Identify the need and refer to an audiologist for evaluation and fitting of personal and group amplification systems and sensory aids;

    E. Implement a protocol, in consultation with an audiologist, to promote adjustment to amplification;

F. Perform routine visual inspection and listening checks of clients' hearing devices and sensory aids to troubleshoot common causes of malfunctioning (e.g., dead or corroded batteries, obstruction or damage to visible parts of the system);

G. Refer on a regularly scheduled basis clients' personal and group amplification systems, other sensory aids, and assistive listening devices for comprehensive evaluations to ensure that instruments conform to audiologists' prescribed settings and manufacturers' specifications;

H. Describe the effects of amplification on communication function;

I. Describe and monitor the effects of environmental factors on communication function.

VIII. Effects of Hearing Loss on Psychosocial, Educational, and Vocational Functioning

A. Describe the effects of hearing loss on psychosocial development;

B. Describe the effects of hearing loss on learning and literacy;

C. Describe systems and methods of educational programming (e.g., mainstream, residential) and facilitate selection of appropriate educational options;

D. Identify the need for and availability of psychological, social, educational, and vocational counseling;

E. Identify and appropriately plan for addressing affective issues confronting the person with hearing loss;

F. Identify appropriate consumer organizations and parent support groups.

IX. Intervention and Case Management

A. Develop and implement a rehabilitative intervention plan based on communication skills and needs of the individual and family or caregivers of the individual;

B. Provide for communication and counseling intervention in the client's preferred mode of communication;

    C. Develop expressive and receptive competencies in the client's preferred mode of communication;

    D. Provide speech, language, and auditory intervention (including but not limited to voice quality and control, resonance, phonologic and phonetic processes, oral motor skills, articulation, pronunciation, prosody, syntax/morphology, semantics, pragmatics);

    E. Facilitate appropriate multimodal forms of communication (e.g., auditory, visual, tactile, speechreading, spoken language, Cued Speech, simultaneous communication, total communication, communication technologies) for the client and family;

    F. Conduct interviews and interact effectively with individuals and their families;

    G. Develop and implement a system to measure and monitor outcomes and the efficacy of intervention.

X. Interdisciplinary Collaboration and Public Advocacy

    A. Collaborate effectively as part of multidisciplinary teams and communicate relevant information to allied professionals and other appropriate individuals;

    B. Plan and implement in-service and public-information programs for allied professionals and other interested individuals;

    C. Plan and implement parent-education programs concerning the management of hearing impairment and subsequent communication difficulties;

    D. Plan and implement interdisciplinary service programs with allied professionals;

    E. Advocate implementation of public law in educational, occupational, and public settings;

    F. Refer to consumer-based organizations.

XI. Acoustic Environments

    A. Provide for appropriate environmental acoustic conditions for effective communication;

B. Describe the effects of environmental influences, amplification systems, and sources of trauma on residual auditory function;

C. Provide for periodic hearing screening for individuals exposed to hazardous noise.

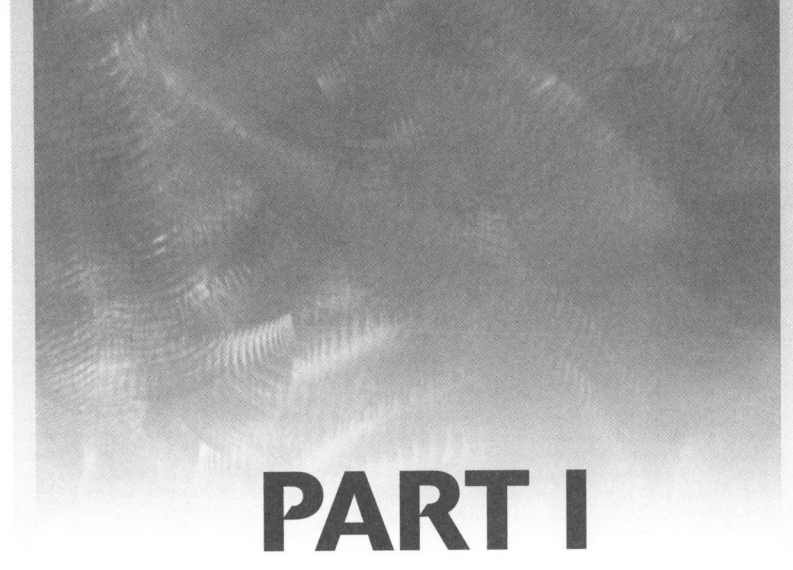

PART I
Conversation and Communication Behaviors

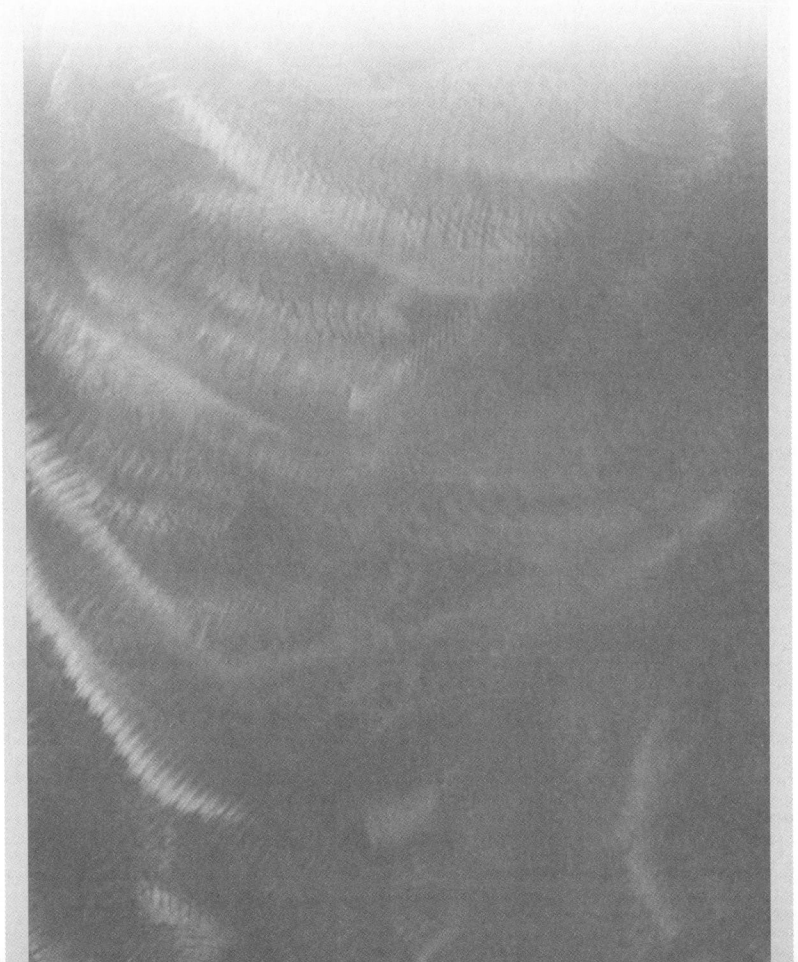

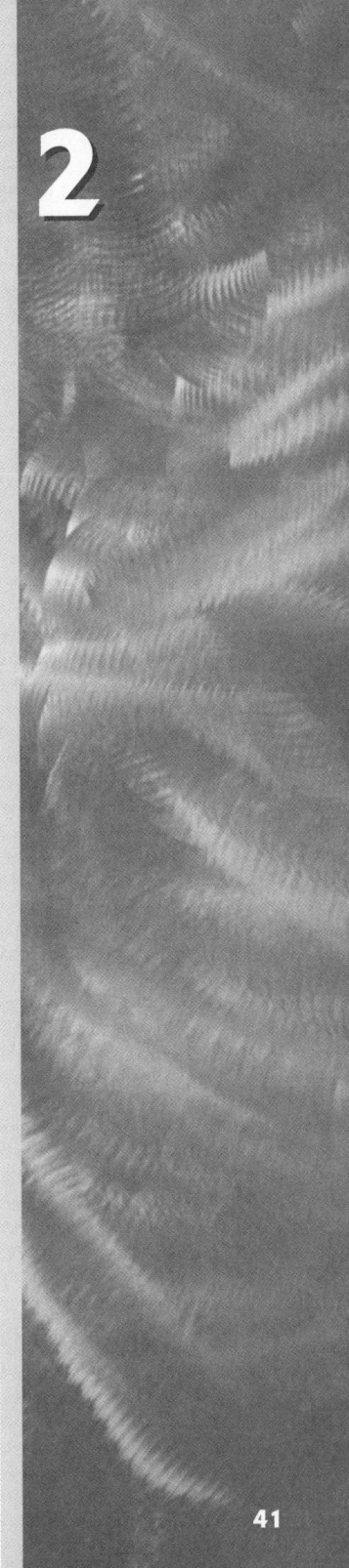

CHAPTER 2

Communication Strategies and Conversational Styles[1]

TOPICS

- Conversation
- Classes of communication strategies
- Factors that influence reception of spoken messages
- Facilitative communication strategies
- Repair strategies
- Stages in repairing a communication breakdown
- Research related to communication strategy use
- Conversational styles and behaviors
- Final remarks
- Key chapter points
- Multiple choice questions

[1] The transcripts of conversation in this chapter are based on actual interchanges. Some have been edited for the sake of brevity or clarity.

Communication strategies training is instruction provided to a person with a hearing loss to maximize his or her communication potential.

With this chapter, we begin our consideration of communication training in the aural rehabilitation setting. *Communication strategies training* is a catchall term used to denote communication strategies, auditory, and speechreading training collectively. Ideally, all speech and hearing-related professionals offer communication training to their patients. In reality, however, communication training is not proffered universally, and when it is, it is often provided in a cursory fashion.

Successful everyday communication for individuals with hearing loss is influenced by many variables, including the effectiveness of their listening device, their lipreading skills, and the amount of residual hearing. In addition, success in communication is affected greatly by how well people use communication strategies. A *communication strategy* is a course of action taken to facilitate a conversational interaction or to rectify a problem that arises during conversation. During communication strategies training, patients receive instruction about how to manage their conversational interactions effectively. In recent years, many hearing professionals have recognized that communication strategies training is a powerful way to enhance individuals' abilities to manage everyday listening problems.

A **communication strategy** is a course of action taken to enhance communication.

In this chapter, the foundation will be laid for subsequent chapters about communication assessment and communication training. We will consider briefly general issues related to conversation, and then we will focus on communication strategies and conversational styles.

▬ CONVERSATION

Much of the fabric of human relationships is woven by our conversations—by what we say, how we say it, and how we listen. We engage in conversation for several reasons (Figure 2-1):

- To share ideas
- To relate experiences
- To tell stories
- To express needs
- To effect a result
- To instruct
- To influence
- To establish intimacy

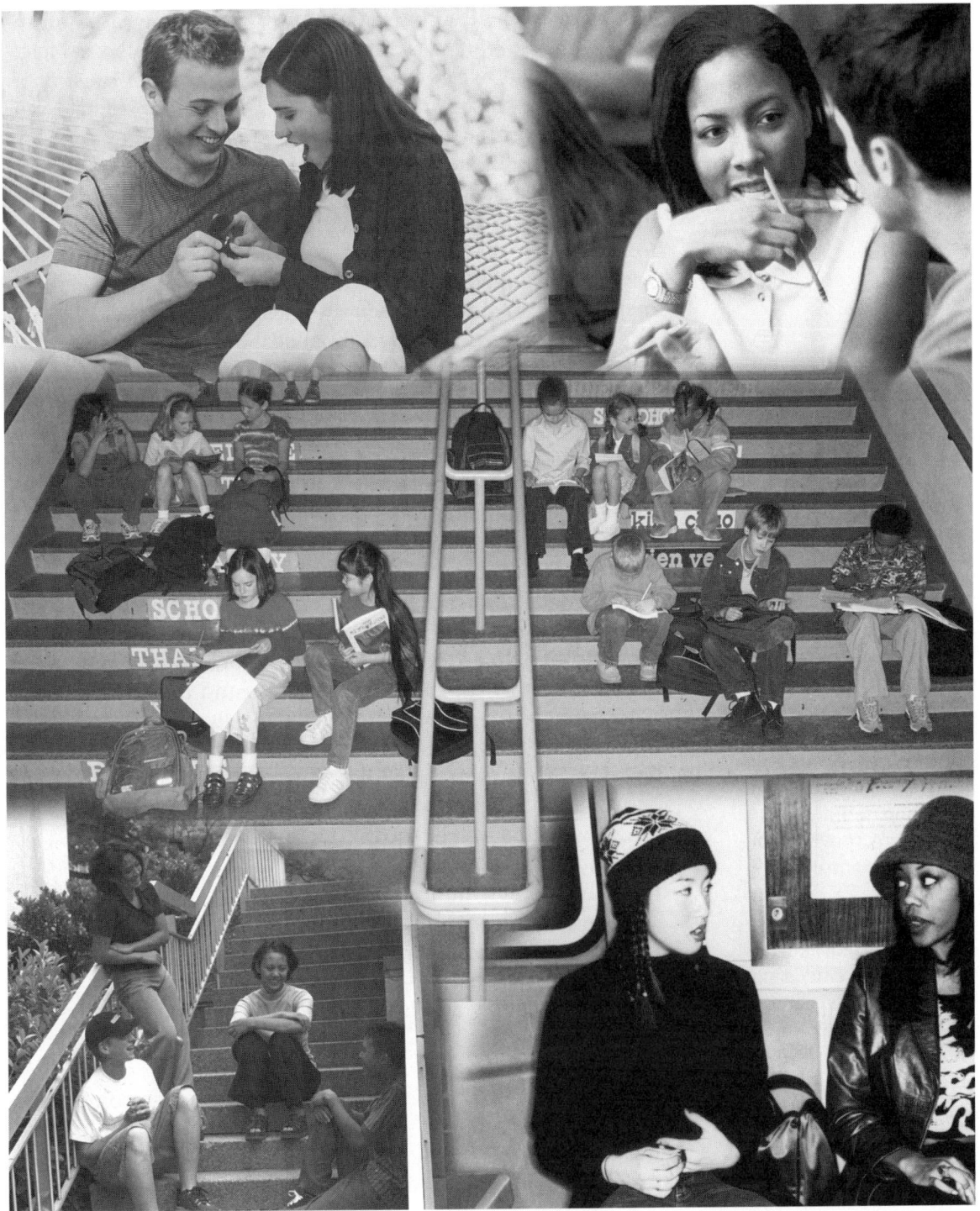

FIGURE 2-1. We engage in conversation for a variety of reasons, for example, to share, to inform, or to instruct.

Conversational rules are implicit rules that guide the conduct of participants in a conversation.

The way we talk with others is guided by our knowledge of implicit *rules of conversation*. If you reflect in a metaphysical fashion about the way we converse, you may realize that most of us typically adhere to culturally established conventions. For example, when two or more people begin a conversation, they each:

- **Tacitly agree to share one another's interests.** We commit our mental resources to attending to our communication partner's message, and respond to the messages in a way that furthers the discussion.
- **Ensure that no single person does all of the talking.** We do not dominate the conversation with our own talking, and we do not expect our communication partners to bear the onus of continuing the conversation alone. We share speaking turns.
- **Participate in choosing what to talk about, and participate in developing the topic.** Typically, there is not a "chief" who leads the conversation, and who alone decides what is talked about and how that subject is developed. Rather, all participants play a role, at some point or other, in deciding what is talked about and in shaping the direction in which the discussion progresses.
- **Take turns in an orderly fashion.** Everyone should have a chance to contribute to the conversation and to end a contribution before someone else begins their speaking turn. This means that interruptions do not occur too often.
- **Try to be relevant to the topic of conversation.** If a conversation is centered on automobiles and someone abruptly begins to talk about a recipe for cornbread, that individual has violated an implicit rule of conversation by not being relevant to the discussion.
- **Provide enough information to convey a message without being verbose.** In a conversation, we expect our communication partners to deliver their messages in a fairly succinct way and in a manner that maintains our interest in listening.

"For successful conversation between any two people, there must be mutual interest, cooperation, and sensitivity. For successful conversation between a normal-hearing person and a hearing-impaired partner, the same basic requirements exist. Greater time, effort, and awareness may be required, however, to reach the same level of understanding."

– N.P. Erber, 1993, p. 109

If one participant in a conversation has a hearing loss, some of the rules of conversation may have to be modified or adapted. For instance, interruptions may occur more frequently because the individual must frequently ask for clarification of a misperceived message. Other participants may have to exert a greater effort to ensure that the person has an opportunity to contribute to a topic's development. If he or she did not understand or misunderstood something that has been said, the hard-of-hearing person may sometimes contribute remarks that are not relevant to the ongoing discussion. The person with hearing loss may also have to use communication strategies, ideally in a way that does not violate the more universally established rules of conversation.

Erber (1996, p. 20) suggests that conversations involving someone who has a hearing loss may have any of the following characteristics:

- **Disrupted taking of turns.** When we come to an end of speaking turn, we often begin to speak slower and our intonation contour begins to fall. The person with hearing loss may not hear these signals and, thus, inappropriate silences may occur because he or she does not initiate a conversational turn on cue.
- **Modified speaking style.** A communication partner may speak slowly with precise articulation in order to facilitate speech recognition for the hard-of-hearing person.
- **Inappropriate topic shifts.** The hard-of-hearing person may not recognize previous remarks and may inadvertently (and inappropriately) change the subject.
- **Superficial content.** Because speech recognition is difficult for the hard-of-hearing individual, the participants in a conversation may avoid certain topics for discussion and avoid topics that might evoke unusual vocabulary or complex syntax.
- **Frequent clarification.** Misunderstandings are commonplace in conversations, even when all participants have normal hearing. When someone has a hearing loss, misunderstandings may become even more frequent. Both the hard-of-hearing person and communication partner may need to engage in clarification more often, and diversions from the topic may occur regularly.
- **Violation of implicit social rules** (Hétu, 1996). The hard-of-hearing person may talk too loudly and may appear as "not paying attention" or as "not caring about what is said."

CLASSES OF COMMUNICATION STRATEGIES

Now that we have considered how conversations may unfold when one of the participants has a hearing loss, let us review strategies that can be used to modify conversational interactions. Persons with hearing loss may use two kinds of communication strategies during the course of a conversation to minimize or prevent communication difficulties, facilitative and repair. Individuals use *facilitative strategies* to influence the talker, the structure of the message, the environment, or themselves. *Receptive repair strategies* provide explicit instruction to the communication partner about what to do immediately following a communication breakdown. A *communication breakdown* is an instance in which one person says something and another person does not recognize the message.

Facilitative strategies include instructing the talker and structuring the listening environment, to enhance the listener's performance.

A **receptive repair strategy** is a tactic used by an individual when he or she has not understood a message.

A **communication breakdown** occurs when one communication partner does not recognize another's message.

FACTORS THAT INFLUENCE RECEPTION OF SPOKEN MESSAGES

Before we consider communication strategies in depth, it is important to analyze the factors that influence how successfully a hard-of-hearing person participates in conversation. Four such factors are the talker, the message, the environment, and the listener. As we will learn in the next section, facilitative strategies are used to influence these four factors.

The Talker

How a communication partner delivers the message, and whether the partner uses appropriate speaking behaviors affect message reception. For instance, the sentence, "Geeze, yashoul-daseendagameFridee, it'dovblownyaway!" would be difficult for a hard-of-hearing individual to understand for at least three reasons: The talker spoke quickly, blurred together word boundaries, and omitted some of the words' component sounds. If the talker had been chewing gum, or had covered his face with his hand (Figure 2-2), recognition would have been even more difficult.

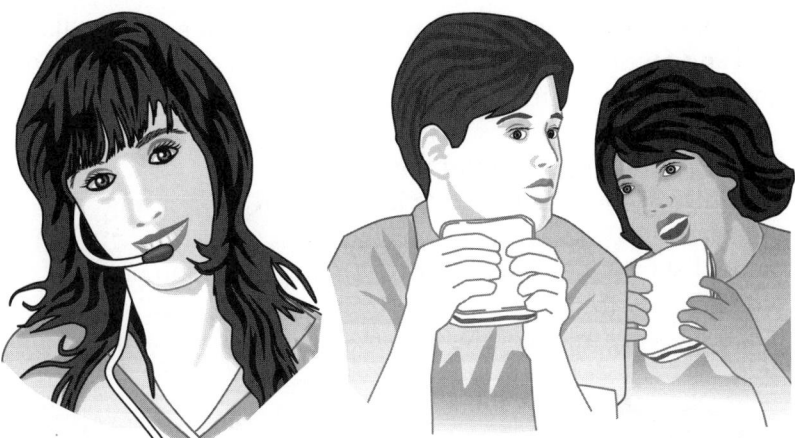

FIGURE 2-2. Chewing or obstructions in front of a talker's mouth can decrease a hard-of-hearing person's ability to recognize a spoken message.

The Message

The second factor that influences someone's ability to recognize a message is the message itself. For example, the sentence on the previous page spoken slowly is, "Geeze, you should have seen the game Friday, it would have blown you away." This sentence could be revised to make it even easier to recognize. The talker might say instead, "I saw the baseball game Friday. The game was great." This alternative version is easier for a hard-of-hearing person to recognize because this version has the following characteristics:

- Simple syntax
- Repetition of an important keyword, *game*
- Two sentences rather than a single, long one
- No ambiguous references, such as *it*
- No colloquialisms, such as *blown you away*

Environment

The third factor that influences an individual's speech recognition performance is the environment. It is not hard to imagine that a person with hearing loss will experience difficulty when attempting to communicate in a dimly lit room with loud music playing in the background. Most hard-of-hearing persons have an especially difficult time recognizing speech in the presence of background noise, particularly when they cannot see the talker's mouth and face clearly to speechread. Environments that have the following characteristics are much more suitable:

- Quiet, without background noise
- Well-lit, without light shining into the hard-of-hearing person's eyes
- Good distance (i.e., 4–6 ft) from the communication partner
- No visual distractions
- Good viewing angle of the talker

The Patient

The final factor that influences message reception is the patients themselves. An individual who is inherently a good speechreader will recognize more of a spoken message than someone who is not. Someone with a mild hearing loss will recognize more than someone who has a severe loss, unless that person uses amplification and receives excellent benefit. Of course, someone who has appropriate amplification and corrected vision will recognize speech better than someone who has similar hearing and visual capabilities, but which are untreated.

How well an individual concentrates on the message also influences message reception. For example, a hard-of-hearing person may feel anxious, stressed, or fatigued while engaging in conversation. "Oh no," he or she may think, "I'm not getting any of this; they are going to think I'm stupid or not interested." These kinds of emotional states are self-defeating. One's ability to recognize speech decreases when a person allocates mental resources to considerations other than comprehending the message being spoken at the moment.

▬ FACILITATIVE COMMUNICATION STRATEGIES

Table 2-1 summarizes four types of facilitative communications strategies. Each type is designed to influence each of the four factors we have just considered, factors that impinge on message recognition success.

Table 2-1. Facilitative and repair strategies.

Facilitative strategies may be used to influence:

■ **Patient's speech recognition skills**
 Adaptive strategies: the individual with hearing loss implements relaxation techniques.
 Attending strategies: the individual pays attention to situational, linguistic, and facial cues for the purpose of inferring partially recognized messages.
 Anticipatory strategies: the individual prepares for conversational interactions in advance by anticipating conversational content and potential listening difficulties.

■ **Communication Environment**
 Constructive strategies: a person structures the environment to optimize communication by minimizing background noise and ensuring a favorable view of the talker.

■ **Communication partner**
 Instructional strategies: a person influences the communication partner's speaking behaviors by asking the partner to speak clearly, facing forward.

■ **Message**
 Message-tailoring strategies: individuals encourage communication partners to use short sentences or they control the topic of conversation.

Source: Adapted from Tye-Murray, N., Knutson, J. F., and Lemke, J. (1993). Assessment of communication strategies use: Questionnaires and daily diaries, *Seminars in Hearing, 14,* 338–353.

Strategies That Influence the Talker

Hard-of-hearing persons use *instructional strategies* to influence communication partners' speaking behaviors. A person asks the talker to change the delivery of the message, as in these examples:

In an **instructional strategy**, the listener asks the talker to change the delivery of the message.

■ "Slow down."
■ "When you cover your mouth with your hand, I have a hard time speechreading you."
■ "Could you face me please?"
■ "Please slow down your talking. I understand more that way."

To use instructional strategies, hard-of-hearing persons must identify behaviors that impede their speech recognition efforts. Then they may instruct the communication partner about how to change the behavior.

Strategies That Influence the Message

Message-tailoring strategy: phrasing one's remarks to constrain the response of a communication partner.

Message-tailoring strategies, the second kind of facilitative strategy, influence the way someone constructs a message. A person might ask, "Did you go swimming or biking last night?" This question sets the stage for one of two responses, *swimming* or *biking.* Alternatively the individual may not use a message-tailoring strategy, and instead ask, "What did you do last night?" which opens the floodgate for a multitude of answers and a greater likelihood of communication breakdown.

Using a message-tailoring strategy requires some meta-communication skills. That is, persons must be able to think about not only what they want to say, but also, how best to say it in order to effect the desired result.

Strategies That Influence the Environment

Constructive strategy: a tactic designed to optimize the listening environment for communication.

John Dooling, a father who has a significant hearing loss, is talking to his daughter in the kitchen. His son is running water in the sink, the refrigerator is humming, the dishwasher is gurgling, and their dog is barking. John motions toward the living room and says to his daughter, "Let's go into the living room and finish talking about your plans for the weekend." In this instance, John employed a **constructive strategy** to enhance the communication environment. Constructive strategies are a third kind of facilitative strategy and are used to effect a modification in environmental listening conditions.

The success of constructive strategies hinges on the ability of the person to analyze the communication environment and identify those elements that can be modified or exploited to optimize communication. Table 2-2 presents a list of other constructive strategies that patients may use to optimize communication.

Table 2-2. Examples of constructive strategies that can be used to optimize the listening and speechreading task. This list might be provided to the person who has hearing loss.

- If possible, ensure that the talker is well-lit so that you watch the talker's face.
- If the talker is far away, move closer.
- If background noise is present, try to either reduce the noise or move to a quieter setting.
- Try to avoid rooms or auditoriums that have sound reverberation. You might request that a meeting be held in a room with good acoustics; typically, a room that has carpet, draperies, and minimal noise from air conditioners and radiators.
- Arrive early so that you can get favorable seating, near the talker.
- Eliminate visual distracters, such as a curtain flapping in an open window.

Maladaptive Strategies

Sometimes people who are hard of hearing adopt *maladaptive strategies* to cope with their communication difficulties. These strategies include bluffing and pretending to understand, social withdrawal to avoid communication difficulties, dominating conversations so as to be aware of what is being talked about, and succumbing to feelings of anger, hostility, or self-pity. Some individuals become unduly anxious and tense, either as they anticipate an upcoming communication interaction (such as a meeting with their boss), or during the interaction itself, as problems in understanding begin to arise. It is well within the purview of a communication strategies training program to encourage alternative behaviors in lieu of maladaptive strategies.

Maladaptive strategy: an inappropriate behavioral mechanism for coping with the difficulties caused by hearing loss in a conversation.

Strategies That Influence the Patient's Reception of the Message

Adaptive, attending, and anticipatory strategies are ways in which persons can adapt to their hearing losses and minimize communication difficulties. These strategies influence a person's reception of a message.

Adaptive and attending strategies: methods of counteracting maladaptive behaviors that stem from hearing loss.

Adaptive and *attending strategies* serve to counteract maladaptive behaviors and include relaxation techniques and other means of dealing with emotions and negative behaviors that stem from hearing loss. For example, some hard-of-hearing persons feel anxious during a conversation with someone who is unfamiliar to them, and they worry about what they might miss or what their communication partners think of them. In these instances, they might have to take a deep breath, consciously relax, purposefully redirect their thoughts toward the present conversation, and attend to the talker's lip movements. This adaptive behavior not only can decrease anxiety, but also enhance message recognition.

Ready? Set? Go!

People with hearing loss can implement anticipatory strategies prior to a communication interaction and enhance their probability of recognizing spoken messages. Examples of anticipatory strategies are listed below:

- Obtain a synopsis of a play before going to see it. Knowing the plot may help you follow the dialogue that occurs between the play's characters.
- Learn the names of key players and products before you go on a job interview. These words will then likely be more recognizable on the talker's face. Also know how job interviews are structured, from beginning, to middle, to end. This information will help you anticipate what may be said during each segment.
- Keep abreast of current events and movies. If these topics arise during group conversations, you will be better able to fill in the blanks when you miss words here and there.
- Read the textbook before a subject is covered in class (good advice for any student). Knowing the subject matter in advance will help you to follow it in class.

Aside from enhancing actual speech recognition, there may be psychological advantages to using anticipatory strategies. If you have hearing a hearing loss, you might feel more comfortable during an interaction if you have practiced speechreading the vocabulary that might occur and if you have obtained some background information. Moreover, simply having a definitive course of action may make you feel more in charge of your communication interactions.

An individual uses an *anticipatory strategy* to prepare for a communication interaction. These strategies include anticipating potential vocabulary and conversational content. For example, before a job interview, a person with hearing loss might study related information about the company, such as employee handbooks or news clippings. The individual might buy books about recruitment procedures and learn what kinds of questions are standard during interviews. Should the interviewer mention names of key employees, the person may thus recognize the names because they are already familiar. When the interviewer asks routine questions, they also may be easier to recognize because the person has the appropriate framework in which to listen. More global preparatory work may include considering what vocabulary is likely to occur (e.g., "popcorn" at a movie theater concession stand) and then practice speechreading that vocabulary with a partner (e.g., Kaplan, Bally, & Garretson, 1985, Tye-Murray, 1992e). Erber (1996) suggested that patients can anticipate spoken remarks by attending to situational cues (e.g., talking with a ticket seller at a movie theater). They can make predictions on the basis of "knowledge of a partner's typical conversational style (e.g., use of colloquialisms or gestures); common conversational sequences (e.g., as in greeting rituals); and expected responses to utterances of particular types (e.g., to choice questions)" (p. 42).

Anticipatory strategies are methods of preparing for a communication interaction.

Resolving Difficulties in Speech Recognition by Using Facilitative Strategies

Figure 2-3 summarizes the process that hard-of-hearing persons might engage in when they experience difficulty in recognizing speech during conversation. The individual identifies the source of difficulty, implements a facilitative strategy, and determines whether the difficulty is resolved. If it is, then the conversation can continue. If it is not, the person might implement another strategy.

REPAIR STRATEGIES

Now that we have reviewed the various facilitative communication strategies, we will now consider repair strategies. As we have noted, a *communication breakdown* occurs when one communication partner speaks a message and another does not recognize it. After signaling the occurrence of a communication breakdown,

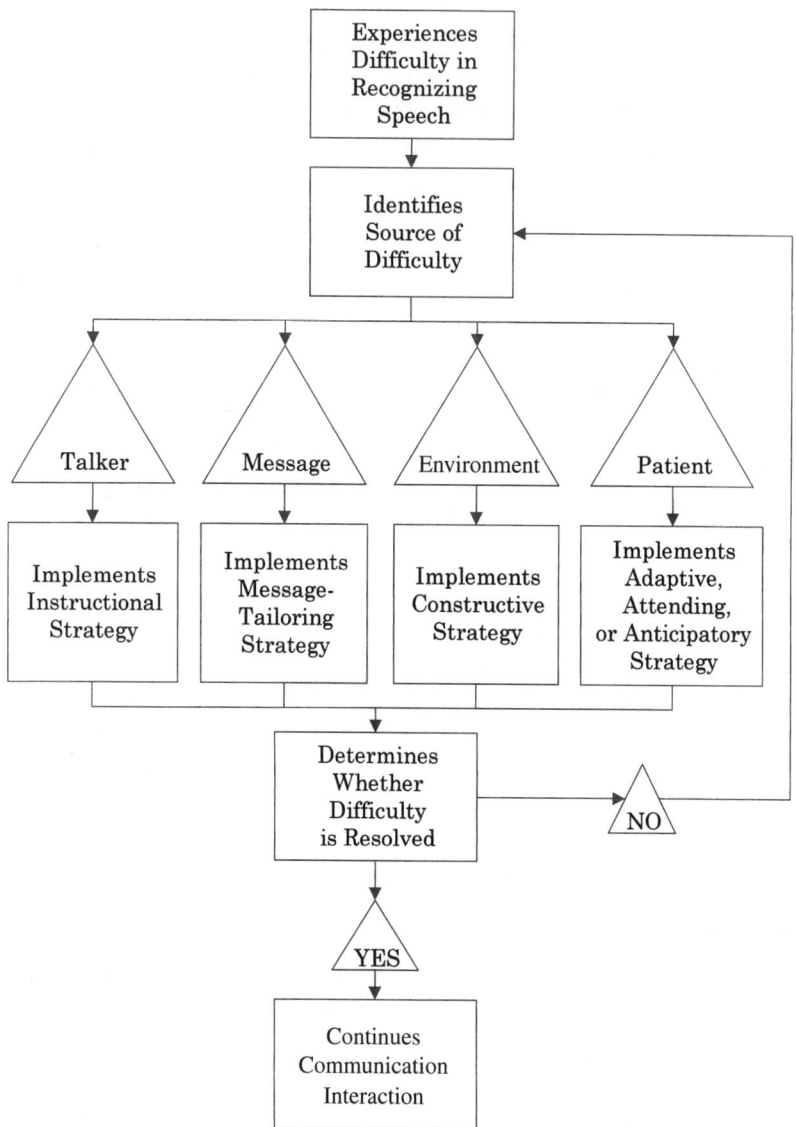

FIGURE 2-3. Process someone may follow when encountering a communication difficulty.

Receptive repair strategy: a tactic used by a listener when the message presented by a communication partner is not understood.

people can request information by using one of many possible *receptive repair strategies* (Table 2-3). The word *receptive* indicates that the repair strategy is used to rectify a communication breakdown when the recipient of a message (in this case, a hard-of-hearing person) does not recognize the sender's (talker's) message. Examples include: "Could you say that again?" (the *repeat*

Table 2-3. Repair strategies that can be used by individuals who are hard-of-hearing to repair breakdowns in communication.

Specific repair strategies request the communication partner to:
- Repeat all or part of message
- Rephrase the message
- Elaborate the message
- Simplify the message
- Indicate the topic of conversation
- Confirm the message
- Write
- Fingerspell

Nonspecific repair strategies ask:
- What?
- Huh?
- Pardon?

---

repair strategy), "Who is going to give you a ride?" (the *request for information repair strategy*) and, "I missed that completely, what are you talking about?" (the *key word repair strategy*). An individual also might ask for more information (the *elaborate repair strategy*): "Tell me more; I didn't catch that."

Depending on how well individuals know their communication partners, they might feel comfortable in asking them to write, use gestures and hand signals, or to spell important topic words. Selection of a particular repair strategy may hinge on a variety of factors, including how useful a particular strategy has been in the past, how much of the message was understood, and an assessment of how well a communication partner might follow the instructions.

■ STAGES IN REPAIRING A COMMUNICATION BREAKDOWN

Figure 2-4 indicates there are at least three stages involved in repairing a communication breakdown. First, the breakdown must be detected by either the hard-of-hearing person or the

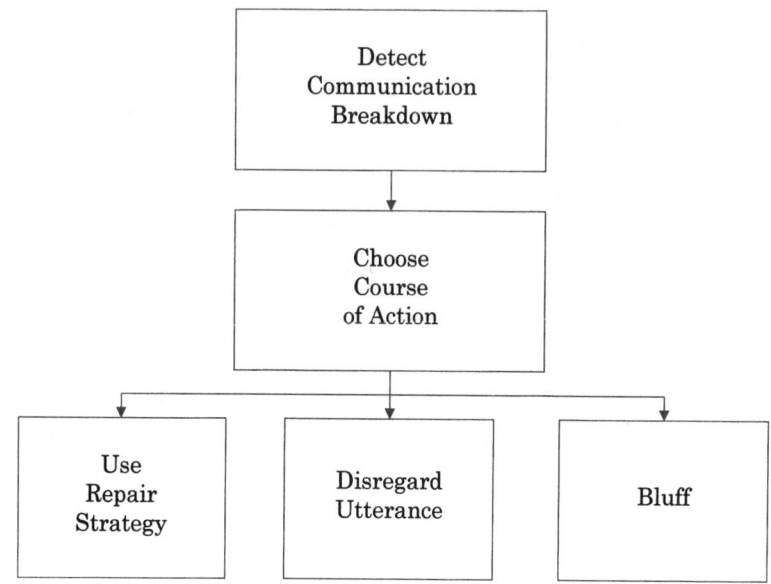

FIGURE 2-4. Stages associated with communication repair.

communication partner. The person may have missed all of the message, missed only a part of the message, or perceived it incorrectly.

Once the communication breakdown has been detected, one of the communication partners must initiate a repair of the breakdown (Stage 2). If the hard-of-hearing person initiates repair, he or she first chooses a course of action and then implements it. The individual might choose to attempt repair, decide that the message was not important enough to pursue understanding, or bluff and pretend to understand. The action is then implemented (Stage 3). If the individual chooses to implement a repair strategy, and the strategy leads to successful repair, the conversation carries on. If the hard-of-hearing person still does not understand, the repair process must continue.

Detection of a Communication Breakdown (Stage 1)

Stage 1 of the model depicted in Figure 2-4 is detection of a communication breakdown. When communication breakdowns occur, hard-of-hearing persons might detect immediately that they did not recognize the message. In such cases, an individual might alert the partner and seek repair. "Hold on," the person might say, "I missed that."

Sometimes, a person might recognize that his or her response to a remark was inappropriate, perhaps by his or her communication partner's facial expression or by attempts at clarification. For example, a communication partner may ask, "What are you reading?" If the hard-of-hearing person responds, "Chicken salad," the communication partner might then say, "Not 'eating;' I said 'reading.' "

It sometimes happens that an individual does not realize a breakdown has occurred until much later in the conversation, as in the following example:

Professor (who has hearing loss):	"What was your last assignment?"
Film student:	"I did a 10-minute educational film on Arctic moss."
Professor:	(thinking the film student said Arctic *moths*) "Oh, you must have had to do that over the summer then."
Film student:	"Believe it or not, some species live embedded in ice crystals, so we did some shots in early November."
Professor:	"What do they do, live in caverns?"
Film student:	"Huh?"
Professor:	(beginning to wonder whether he has missed something) "Live in caverns?"
Film student:	"Well, I guess there's some moss in caverns up there, but I've never seen any caves."
Professor:	"*Moss?*" (blushing) "Oh, I thought we were talking about *moths!*"

As the professor sensed an incongruence between the film student's and his own remarks, he gradually realized that he misunderstood an utterance earlier on in the conversation. This is a prime example of not realizing that a breakdown has occurred at its onset.

Dealing With a Breakdown in Communication (Stages 2 and 3)

The second and third stages of the model depicted in Figure 2-4, which shows the stages associated with communication breakdown and repair, are choosing a course of action and then implementing it. We will consider what may happen when someone uses a repair strategy and what may happen when someone bluffs.

USING A REPAIR STRATEGY

Once a misunderstanding becomes apparent, an individual might alert the communication partner and provide instruction about how to repair it. For instance, he or she may ask about the topic of conversation (e.g., "What are you talking about?").

Usually, breakdowns are repaired with the use of one or two repair strategies. There are occasions, however, especially when one of the participants has a severe or profound hearing loss, when several exchanges are required to repair a communication breakdown. In the worst of circumstances, these interchanges can be awkward for all parties involved in the conversation, as in the following example in which a husband and wife (who recently received a cochlear implant) talked while seated in a speech and hearing test room:

Husband:	"Laura is going to catch the train on Tuesday."
Wife:	"What? I didn't catch any of that."
Husband:	"I said, Laura is going to catch the train on Tuesday."
Wife:	"No, none of it."
Husband:	"Laura . . ."
Wife:	"Something about more?"
Husband:	"No, watch me. Laura is going to get the train."
Wife:	"Oh, yeah. I got 'train'."
Husband:	"Yes, a train. Laura is . . ."
Wife:	(shaking her head) "Nope, nope, none of it. Spell it."
Husband:	"L-A-U-R-A"
Wife:	"Oh Laura! What about Laura and the train?"

At this point, several repair strategies have been implemented and the message is still not conveyed. This is an example of an ***extended repair***, because many repair strategies are needed before the breakdown is resolved. It would be easy for both participants in the conversation to abandon repair, and say, "Never mind, it's not that important." Indeed, in situations such as this, that is often exactly what happens.

Extended repair: when many repair strategies are needed to mend a communication breakdown.

It is important that use of a repair strategy does not create a concomitant disruption of conversation. Sometimes when someone uses a repair strategy to repair a breakdown in communication, the topic of conversation can shift, as indicated in Figure 2-5. Ideally, people use repair strategies in such a way that they do not cause the conversation to stagnate or veer off into a different direction. For example, a student with a hearing loss, Janet, did not use a repair strategy effectively in the following exchange:

Cynthia: "I got my grades in the mail last Saturday."

Janet: "Grapes? Why are you getting grapes in the mail?"

Cynthia: "No, I said *grades*, not *grapes*."

Janet: "Oh, I know you make wine, so I thought you had joined some kind of mail-order program. By the way, when am I going to get my bottle?"

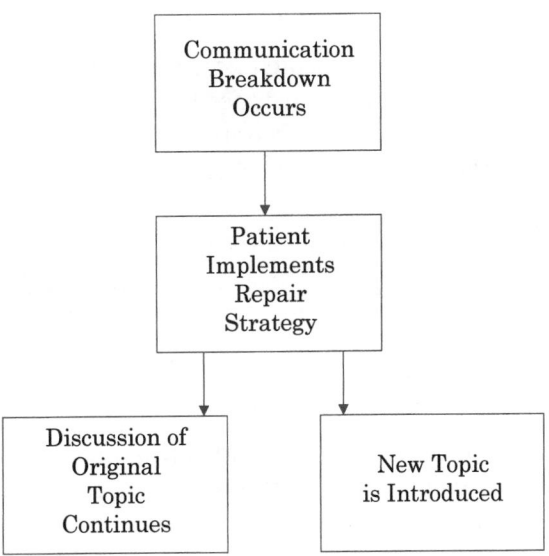

FIGURE 2-5. Possible effects of using a repair strategy.

The problem with this interchange is that the topic of conversation changed inappropriately (from grades to a promised bottle of wine) as a result of the repair strategy used. A seemingly more cooperative and congenial way to repair this communication breakdown is as follows:

Cynthia: "I got my grades in the mail last Saturday."

Janet: "Grapes?"

Cynthia: "No, I said *grades*."

Janet: "Oh, you got your grades in the mail. How did you do?"

In this latter version, Janet asked for confirmation and then steered the conversation back on track.

BLUFFING

Sometimes patients bluff and pretend to understand following a communication breakdown, nodding and smiling in agreement with what they do not know. The consequences of bluffing can be unpleasant. The person may appear insensitive, uninterested, dull, or inattentive. He or she may begin to feel powerless to manage communication difficulties. When bluffing is used excessively, conversation may leave the person feeling like a failure or angry at him- or herself.

The following conversation, which occurred between two women who had just met, presents an instance in which bluffing led to the appearance of insensitivity. Woman 2 has just said that she is about to take a trip. Woman 1 has a hearing loss:

Woman 1:   "Where are you going?"

Woman 2:   "To Portland to see my daughter. She is having a baby."

Woman 1:   (nodding; she understood the word *baby*, but not much else) "I see."

Woman 2:   "She has been bedridden for several weeks because she has diabetes and high blood pressure, and now the doctor says they are going to have to induce or the baby you know might be in trouble if it goes much longer than it's been going, even

	though it will be 4 weeks premature which we are pretty worried about especially since it's her first."
Woman 1:	(lost by the length and convoluted syntax of her partner's utterance, and still not understanding much) "Oh, how nice."
Woman 2:	"No, not really, this is pretty serious."

Inadvertently, Woman 1 has created an unfavorable impression because she bluffed and pretended to understand instead of repairing the communication breakdown. There are at least two reasons why people bluff extensively as in the example conversation: (1) reluctance to acknowledge a hearing loss, and (2) spirit of cooperation.

Many people are reluctant to admit a hearing loss (e.g., Hines, 2000). The first reason someone may bluff is because use of a repair strategy may require a person to acknowledge a hearing loss. For instance, an individual might say, "Can you say that again please?" and the communication partner might respond, "What's the matter?" For some people, it is difficult to acknowledge, "I have hearing loss, and I can't always catch all that is said to me."

I'll Never Tell

The following summary was included in a report about the communication problems experienced by hard-of-hearing persons who were inpatients at a hospital. This section dealt with reluctance to admit a hearing loss:

> Patients who conceal their hearing loss do so for a variety of reasons, but the most common one is self-consciousness. Some go to great lengths to conceal their disability. Some are very skillful at this concealment, not appreciating how dysfunctional it is. Female patients often adopt hairstyles that cover their hearing aids. One patient admitted that she disliked wearing a hearing aid, because her hair was no longer thick enough to cover it. Many hearing-impaired people pretend to understand what is being said, rather than admit to their difficulties. This can be very misleading and create many problems. One patient said: "My reticence to make my hearing loss known made me the victim of my own vanity." A patient who finally decided to admit to his problem was agreeably surprised that both the doctors and nurses were helpful and understanding. In some cases patients' deceptions were unexpectedly exposed. (Hines, 2000, p. 35)

We could devote an entire chapter to issues regarding the difficulty of acknowledging hearing loss. Many persons are reluctant to admit a hearing loss, in part because of personal vanity and perceived social stigmata (Blood, Blood, & Danhauer, 1978; Danhauer, Johnson, Kasten, & Brimacombe, 1985; Hétu, Riverin, Getty, Lalande, & St-Cyr, 1990). Unfortunately, many people have stereotypical views of hard-of-hearing persons. Some see them as difficult to communicate with or as deserving pity. For many people, revealing a hearing loss to someone who does not know they have one can be a daunting challenge and, hence, they may be reluctant to use repair strategies. Hallberg (1996) suggests that the driving force for all coping strategies, including bluffing and pretending to understand, lies in an individual's efforts to maintain a positive and "I am normal" self-image and to avoid being considered as deviant or deficient by others. Acknowledging a hearing loss, and putting a spotlight on the loss by signaling communication breakdowns and using repair strategies, may result in a spoiled self-identity. These behaviors may also lead others to view the hard-of-hearing person as an undesirable social deviation from a normal state, a situation that most people would like to avoid. In addition, Hallberg suggests that the reluctance to admit a hearing loss might stem from self-deception (or, a distortion of reality). There may be a discrepancy between a person's desired self-image and actual circumstances, and the self-deception protects the self-image and helps the individual maintain a positive or normal self-image in the face of hearing loss. "(T)he consequence is a less realistic view of the situation." (p. 28).

A second reason why people may bluff relates to a desire to be cooperative and agreeable. Some people are unwilling to use repair strategies and bluff because they feel guilty and embarrassed about introducing difficulties into a conversation. Typically, when we converse, we try to ensure that a conversation is as pleasant and rewarding an experience for our communication partner(s) as it is for ourselves. If someone frequently halts the conversation for clarification, it may become less pleasant and less rewarding (Figure 2-6).

If you were a participant in the following conversation, you probably would conclude that Richard, who, unknown to you, has a hearing loss, is both uncooperative and troublesome, and not a lot of fun to talk with:

> "For the hearing impaired, to achieve understanding and acceptance of others may be more important in creating involvement and solidarity than employing successful hearing tactics."
>
> —Stephens, Jaworski, Lewis, & Aslan, 1999, p. 25

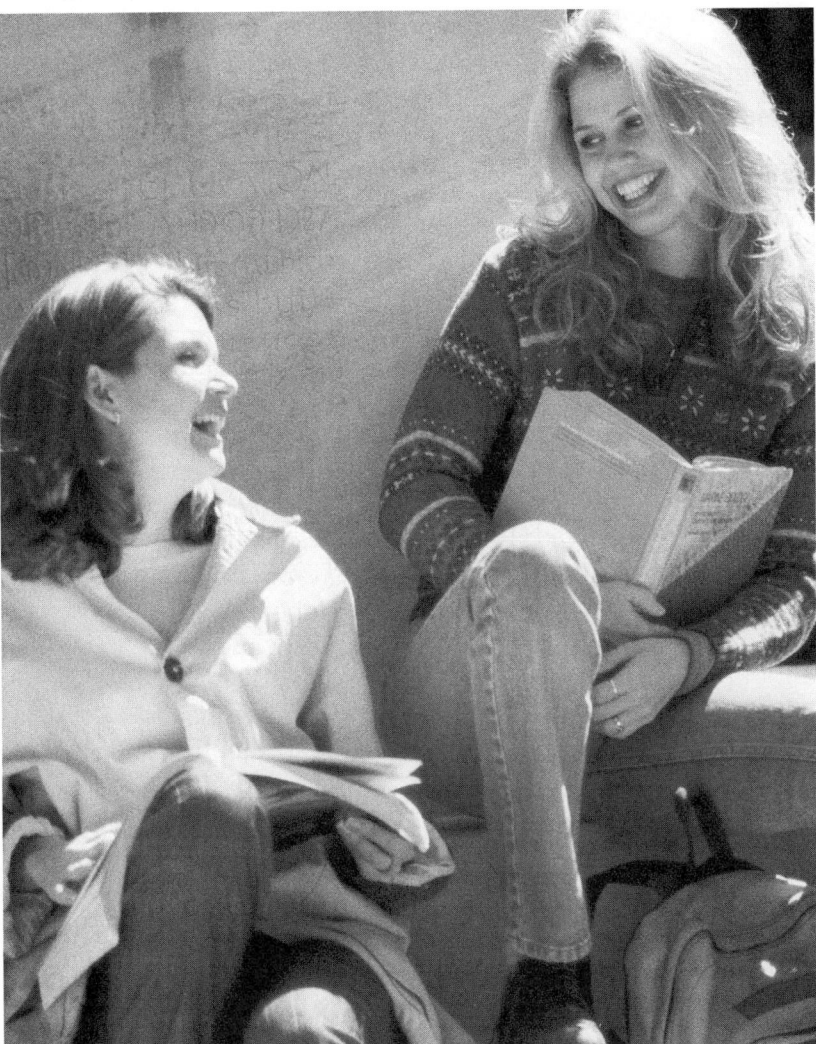

FIGURE 2-6. When we engage in a conversation, we usually try to be cooperative and help make the conversation a pleasurable or meaningful experience for all participants.

Patrick:	"I am going on spring break next week."
Richard:	"Huh?"
Patrick:	"I said *spring break*."
Richard:	"Oh."

Patrick:	"We are driving to Florida in Jason's parents' car."
Richard:	"Huh?"
Patrick:	"We are driving to Florida in Jason's parents' car."
Richard:	"Oh."
Mary:	"I wish I were going somewhere."
Richard:	"Huh?"
Mary:	"I wish I were going somewhere."
Richard:	"Yeah, me too."

As the interchange unfolds, the spontaneity of the conversation becomes stifled by Richard's continual requests for clarification. Maintaining continued conversation will prove laborious and effortful for all involved. It is for such reasons that many hard-of-hearing people opt to bluff, particularly when talking to people they do not know well.

Interruptions

Research has shown that frequent requests for clarifications may lead a communication partner to view a hard-of-hearing person unfavorably. Robinson and Reis (1989) found that people who interrupted their communication partners were perceived as less sociable than those who did not. Gagné, Stelmacovich, and Yovetich (1991) and Tye-Murray, Witt, Schum, and Sobaski (1995) found that a hard-of-hearing person was perceived more favorably when few communication breakdowns occurred during the course of a conversation. More research is needed about communication breakdowns and repair strategies. We need to explore how the hard-of-hearing person might gracefully indicate that a communication breakdown has occurred, when it is important for the individual to alert the communication partner (which might not be necessary in every instance of communication breakdown), and how long a hard-of-hearing person should attempt to repair the breakdown before giving up or moving on.

Expressive Repair Strategies

Heretofore, discussion has centered around receptive repair strategies, that is, a course of action someone may take when he or she does not recognize (receive) a spoken message. In addition to using receptive repair strategies, many children who have hearing loss need to use expressive repair strategies. *Expressive repair strategies* are used to rectify a communication breakdown that occurs because the hard-of-hearing person (the sender) produces an unintelligible utterance, and the conversational partner (the receiver) is unable to recognize it.

Expressive repair strategies are used when the sender produces an unintelligible utterance and the conversational partner cannot understand it.

Many children who have hearing impairments have limited language skills or poor articulation. As a result, their conversational partners often may not recognize their spoken messages. Thus, it is important for them to learn how to cope with these kinds of communication breakdowns by using expressive repair strategies. Expressive repair strategies include repeating their original message using their best speech (e.g., they might slow down their speaking rate and emphasize important key words), breaking their longer sentences into shorter sentences, using another communication modality such as writing or mime, and using hand gestures, such as pointing. For instance, a child may say, "Hu mah meh mah," and her communication partner might respond, "Huh?" The child then may repeat the message using her best speech, "He make me *mad*." In this example, the child has implemented an expressive repair strategy. She has articulated her words more precisely and emphasized the keyword *mad*.

■ RESEARCH RELATED TO COMMUNICATION STRATEGY USE

Several investigators have studied how hard-of-hearing individuals use repair strategies and have converged on interesting conclusions. This research provides an important theoretical substratum for the content of a communication strategies training program.

When Do Communication Breakdowns Occur?

Although communication breakdowns may occur in any conversation for any variety of reasons, certain conditions increase the likelihood of their occurrence. As we considered earlier, environmental conditions, message content, and speaking behaviors all influence how well a person with hearing loss recognizes a spoken message. A study by Cassie (2002) suggests that the dynamic nature of the conversation also affects when communication breakdowns are most likely to occur. For instance, if two people are engaged in a conversation, and they limit themselves to talking about a single topic, they are less likely to experience communication breakdowns than if they jump from one topic to the next. This adherence to a single topic is called *topic maintenance.* As the two individuals exchange remarks on their chosen topic, there is more contextual information available to resolve potential misunderstandings.

Abruptly shifting from one topic to another is more likely to cause communication difficulties than discussing only one topic. Interestingly, even more disruptive than topic changing is topic shading. *Topic shading* happens when a new topic is introduced, but is a direct offshoot of something that was just being discussed, as in the following example:

Janice (who has hearing loss):	"I'm going to Chicago tomorrow."
Robert:	"Are you driving or flying?"
Janice:	"Flying."
Robert:	"I've got to get my tickets for my New York trip."
Janice:	"Huh?"

In this example, the two participants are still talking about traveling when the topic shifts, but instead of talking about Janice's trip they are now talking about Robert's need to purchase airline tickets. It may be that when an entirely new topic is introduced, the hard-of-hearing person can contribute a relevant comment, even if she or he has not understood every word. For example, if instead of mentioning his airline tickets, Robert had said, "What are you doing tonight?" Janice might have caught the general gist of his message and might have responded with an appropriate response (e.g., "Not much."). When topics shift subtlety, individuals may request clarification to ensure they are following the direction the conversation is veering toward (Cassie, 2002).

The Repeat Repair Strategy and Nonspecific Repair Strategies

One issue investigators have addressed pertains to which repair strategies are used most commonly. The findings reveal that most individuals are more likely to ask their communication partners to repeat a message following a communication breakdown than to simplify it, restructure it, or elaborate (Cassie & Gibson, 1997; Tye-Murray et al., 1993; Tye-Murray, Purdy, Woodworth, & Tyler, 1990; Tye-Murray & Witt, 1996). Moreover, their most common repair tactic is to say, "What?" "Huh?" or "Pardon?" This kind of repair strategy (i.e., what-huh-pardon) is called a *nonspecific*, as opposed to a *specific repair strategy*. When using a *specific repair strategy*, the hard-of-hearing person provides explicit instruction to the communication partner about how to repair the breakdown.

Specific and nonspecific repairs: Providing explicit instructions to the communication partner about how to repair the breakdown, as opposed to simply indicating lack of understanding.

Another issue that researchers have examined is what happens after particular repair strategies are used. For instance, when a person says, "Pardon?" how is a communication partner likely to respond? One of the most noteworthy findings pertains to the use of the repeat repair strategy and nonspecific repair strategies. When these are used following a communication breakdown, the communication partners typically repeat the original message verbatim (Cassie & Gibson, 1997; Tye-Murray, Witt, Schum, & Sobaski, 1995). Thus, if someone says "Huh?" to you, there is a high probability that you will repeat exactly what you have just said.

Interestingly, additional research suggests that someone is more likely to understand a message following a communication breakdown if the communication partner restructures it rather than simply repeating it (Gagné & Wyllie, 1989), especially if the talker already has repeated the message one time and the hard-of-hearing person still has not recognized it. Suppose someone says, "I bought a new car," and your patient responds "Huh?" Then the person repeats, "I bought a new car." A third verbatim repetition may be less helpful to the patient than if the person had rephrased the message as, "I bought a Buick." New words, especially the more visible word *Buick* as opposed to *car*, may be easier for the patient to recognize audiovisually. Cassie and Gibson (1997) found that the most effective repair of communication breakdowns occurred when conversational partners either paraphrased or confirmed the message. They showed that repeating the message one time was almost equally effective. The least effective strategies used by partners appeared to be elaboration.

These findings suggest that many persons with hearing impairment typically use repair strategies that are apt to elicit the least effective response from their communication partners. That is, they often say "Huh?" and, in turn, receive a verbatim repetition of the very message they did not understand the first time.

The results of another set of investigations suggest there may be another drawback to using nonspecific repair strategies. When persons often say "What?" or "Huh?" during a conversation to rectify communication breakdowns, their communication partners are more likely to perceive them unfavorably and to enjoy the interaction less (Gagné, Stelmacovich, & Yovetich, 1991; Tye-Murray, Witt, Schum, & Sobaski, 1995). Some laboratory studies have found that individuals who asked "What?" or "Huh?" following a breakdown in communication are more likely to be perceived unfavorably. In the experimental paradigm that was used in these experiments, audiovisual recordings were made of spontaneous conversations between two people, one of whom had a real or simulated hearing loss. The recordings were then shown to a team of judges who were asked to view the recordings and rate the person with hearing loss on a personality 6-point rating scale (e.g., *this person is competent-incompetent*). The judges also rated the hard-of-hearing persons on a scale of emotional responses, using a second 6-point rating scale (e.g., *this person makes me feel composed-irritated*). The results revealed that, when individuals used nonspecific instead of specific repair strategies, they were rated unfavorably, and they elicited unfavorable reactions from the judges. Thus it appears that some hard-of-hearing persons often tend to use the very repair strategies (nonspecific) most likely to elicit an unfavorable response from their communication partners.

Before we conclude our review of this area of research, two caveats must be appended. First, communication breakdowns that occur during spontaneous conversation between adults in which one partner has a hearing loss often are resolved after the use of a single repair strategy, even if it is a nonspecific strategy (Tye-Murray, Witt, Schum, & Sobaski, 1995). These data suggest that nonspecific repair strategies can be effective. Second, a nonspecific repair strategy is minimally disruptive to the flow of ongoing conversation. For instance, when an individual asks,

"Huh?" he or she assumes the speaking floor briefly, and the communication partner can easily continue a speaking turn. However, when someone uses other repair strategies, such as, "I missed that, can you tell me what you are talking about?" and uses them frequently, a conversation can become stilted and less fluent. By using a nonspecific repair strategy, the individual takes a phantom speaking turn and may appear more cooperative in the conversational interchange.

Who Uses Repair Strategies, When, and What Are the Benefits?

Some research has focused on how the use of communication strategies relates to attitudinal variables and social-interaction indices, how repair strategy use varies as a function of whether the communication partner is familiar or unfamiliar, and the characteristics of hard-of-hearing adults who are most likely to use repair strategies. Hard-of-hearing persons have been surveyed about their use of communication strategies, and their responses have then been related to attitudinal variables, social-interaction indices, audiograms, or demographic variables.

These kinds of studies have yielded the following results. People are generally more likely to use communication strategies if their communication partner is familiar rather than unfamiliar. For instance, if they know the person, they might ask, "Can you tell me what you are talking about?" If they do not know the person, they may pretend to understand.

Some individuals are more likely than others to use a repair strategy than to say nothing following a communication breakdown. Individuals who use repair strategies also are less likely to feel frustrated with their speechreading skills and less likely to avoid social interactions than individuals who say nothing.

Persons who are least likely to use communication strategies tend to share certain characteristics (Tye-Murray, Purdy, & Woodworth, 1992; Tye-Murray et al., 1993):

- They have attained lower levels of education.
- They have experienced a sudden hearing loss.
- They receive minimal benefit from their listening devices.

In summary, research data suggest that an important component of an aural rehabilitation program might be provision of practice in using types of repair strategies other than nonspecific strategies. Nonspecific repair strategies comprise one of the most commonly used class of repair strategies but are the least effective. Moreover, patients should practice communication strategies with both familiar and unfamiliar communication partners, because some persons use strategies differently depending on who they are talking with. Finally, some persons may have a greater need for communication strategies training than others, for example, people who have experienced sudden hearing loss.

Informing a Communication Partner About a Hearing Loss

As noted earlier, some people are reluctant to use repair strategies because they do not want their communication partners to know they have hearing losses. One investigation examined what happened when adults who use cochlear implants talked with someone they did not know, and who did not know about the hearing loss (Tye-Murray & Witt, 1996). In this investigation, one patient was seated at a table with someone who had normal hearing. The normally hearing person was told that he or she was participating in a study about conversation, but did not know that his or her communication partner had a hearing loss. Each dyad tested in the experiment talked for 10 minutes. The conversations were videotaped and later analyzed.

Analyses showed that only 44% of the patients revealed their hearing losses, even though most experienced many communication breakdowns during the course of the 10-minute conversation. What is perhaps most interesting is what happened when a patient did reveal a loss. Once the patient did so, the conversation began to center around the topic of hearing loss and difficulties associated with hearing loss, rather than other shared topics of interest. This change may be yet another reason why people are reluctant to reveal a hearing loss—they do not want the loss to become the focus of discussion.

Effectiveness of Anticipatory Strategies

There are mixed findings about the effectiveness of anticipatory strategies. Recall that an anticipatory strategy entails preparing for an upcoming conversational interaction. Persons with hearing loss may consider vocabulary and statements that may occur and might practice recognizing them either by speaking into a mirror or interacting with a partner. One study showed that anticipatory strategies are not effective in enhancing speech recognition when a person is about to enter into a familiar communication situation, as when preparing for an appointment with a physician or a visit to a bank or a gas station (Tye-Murray, 1992e). However, when the situation is unfamiliar, use of anticipatory strategies appear to be effective in preparing individuals to recognize speech (Rubinstein, Cherry, Hecht, & Idler, 2000). For instance, if people learn the plot of a heretofore unfamiliar story, they will later recognize sentences about the story better than if they had not reviewed it.

> "The value of anticipatory strategy training lies in teaching clients to increase their knowledge about upcoming unfamiliar communication contexts."
> —*Rubinstein et al., 2000, p. 54*

You Say, I Say

When hard-of-hearing persons implement a repair strategy, they invite a response from their communication partners, thereby establishing a linked speaking turn. Schegloff and Sacks (1973) call linked speaking turns *adjacency pairs.* Examples of adjacency pairs include question-answer (e.g., "Who asked?"—"Bob asked.") and greeting-greeting combinations (e.g., "Hey there."—"Hi."). Particular repair strategy-response adjacency pairs often emerge when a hard-of-hearing person interacts with a normally hearing person. These include:

Adjacency pairs: linked speaking turns

1. *Nonspecific repair strategy-message repetition response.* When a hard-of-hearing individual implements a nonspecific repair strategy following a communication breakdown, the communication partner typically repeats the original message.
2. *Request for information repair strategy-provide information response.* When a hard-of-hearing person requests specific information, the communication partner typically provides it.
3. *Confirmation repair strategy-feedback response.* When a hard-of-hearing person restates the message content, the communication partner usually either confirms or corrects the statement (see Tye-Murray and Witt, 1996, p. 467).

Research with Children

Some research has concerned children's use of specific kinds of repair strategies and communication breakdown management (e.g., Ciocci & Baran, 1998; Givens & Greenfeld, 1982; Most, 2002). Findings suggest that children who are hard-of-hearing and deaf tend to revise utterances that their communication partners do not understand. In addition, they often rely on non-linguistic responses when seeking clarification of their partner's messages; for instance, they might signal a misunderstanding by a confused look or a shoulder shrug. In contrast, children with normal hearing are more likely to repeat than revise their utterances and more likely to use linguistic responses when seeking clarification.

We examined the conversations of 181 children who use cochlear implants and compared their performance to 24 children who have normal hearing, using both objective and subjective measuring procedures (Tye-Murray, 2003). The children engaged in conversations with a clinician, using an oral mode of communication. Audio-videotapes of the conversations were analyzed to yield the following measures: percent of time the child and clinician spent trying to repair a breakdown in communication, percent of time the two spent sitting in silence, and the ratio between the amount of time the child spoke and the amount of time the clinician spoke (as we shall see in the next chapter, these measures are related to a construct called *conversational fluency*). We found that cochlear implant users spent significantly more time in communication breakdown and in silence than did the children with normal hearing, and children who are in an educational placement that emphasizes oral communication spent less time in breakdown than children who are in educational placements that use both speech and sign. Speech intelligibility and receptive language were the best predictors of communication breakdown, with children who had better speech and language skills experiencing fewer and shorter breakdowns in communication. These results underscore the importance of providing explicit instruction to manage communication difficulties (Chapter 4), as even children who have state-of-the-art listening technology still experience more difficulties than children who have normal hearing.

CONVERSATIONAL STYLES AND BEHAVIORS

Many communication training curricula include materials that are aimed at developing desirable conversational styles and conversational behaviors. Although there are no right and wrong ways per se of engaging in conversation, and what is appropriate will vary with the situation, some conversational styles and behaviors are nonetheless more effective when communication is hampered by the presence of hearing loss than are other styles and behaviors.

Conversational Styles

Kaplan et al. (1985, pp. 19–20) described three kinds of conversational styles that adults with significant hearing impairment may exhibit: (1) passive, (2) aggressive, and (3) assertive. A person with a *passive conversational style* is someone who often does the following:

> A person with **passive conversational style** tends to withdraw from conversations and social interactions rather than attempt to repair conversations.

- Withdraws from conversation
- Frequently bluffs and pretends to recognize utterances
- Avoids social interactions and group gatherings in order to avoid communication difficulties

Someone who sits at the bridge table, smiling and quietly nodding, is probably someone who can be characterized as having a passive conversational style. The person gains little by being in the game, and may begin to feel frustration and helplessness.

A person with an *aggressive conversational style* is the opposite extreme of the person with a passive conversational style. He or she may exhibit some of the following characteristics during conversation:

> A person with an **aggressive conversational style** may blame others for misunderstanding.

- Hostility
- Belligerence
- Bad attitude

The person may inadvertently embarrass, hurt, or anger his or her communication partners and often blame others for their communication difficulties. "Quit mumbling, and try to help me out!" someone may demand, or "I may as well not be here; you're talking to everyone but me." The first utterance is a tacit insult (i.e., it implies, "You could help me out but you have chosen not to"), whereas the second is demanding ("I have hearing loss and no one else does, so you should accommodate me"). These kinds of utterances have the potential to alienate communication partners and may result in the hard-of-hearing person being ineffective and even avoided.

During communication training, patients often are encouraged to minimize their use of a passive or aggressive conversational style and instead implement an assertive style. Persons who adopt an *assertive conversational style* usually follow these guidelines during conversation. They:

A person who adopts an **assertive conversational style** takes responsibility for managing communication difficulties in a way that is considerate of communication partners.

- Respect the rights of their communication partners, while honestly and openly expressing their own needs and emotions
- Take responsibility for managing communication difficulties, but do so in a way that is considerate of their communication partners

"Let's get a seat away from the stereo speaker," an assertive person may suggest, "and then you won't have to repeat everything you say." This remark is courteous and provides direct explanation of how to remedy a communication problem.

These three types of conversational styles (passive, aggressive, and assertive) are often reviewed in a communication training program. Hard-of-hearing persons can learn to develop assertive ways of dealing with communication problems and minimize their passive or aggressive responses.

Sometimes, the aural rehabilitation plan includes psychosocial therapy (e.g., Hogan, 2001). One of the primary goals of this type of intervention is to encourage assertive behaviors. Participants explore the psychological and social ramifications of hearing loss and some of the underlying reasons why they may not engage in assertive behaviors. For instance, some people who behave passively may do so because they feel they burden other people when they ask for assistance. These underlying assumptions are challenged during psychosocial therapy.

Communication Behaviors

Figure 2-7 presents three constellations of behaviors that complement the model of conversational styles described by Kaplan et al. (1985) (Tye-Murray & Witt, 1996). The model consists of three circles that are labeled interactive, noninteractive, and dominating.

Persons who fall within the *interactive behavior* circle use cooperative conversational tactics, which are consistent with an assertive conversational style. These individuals share responsibility with their conversational partners for advancing a topic of conversation and selecting topics of conversation. They do not dominate discussion, and they show interest in what their communication partners say and attempt to respond appropriately to their remarks.

Psychosocial therapy challenges erroneous assumptions and develops self-image.

Interactive behavior is the use of cooperative conversational tactics, consistent with an assertive conversational style.

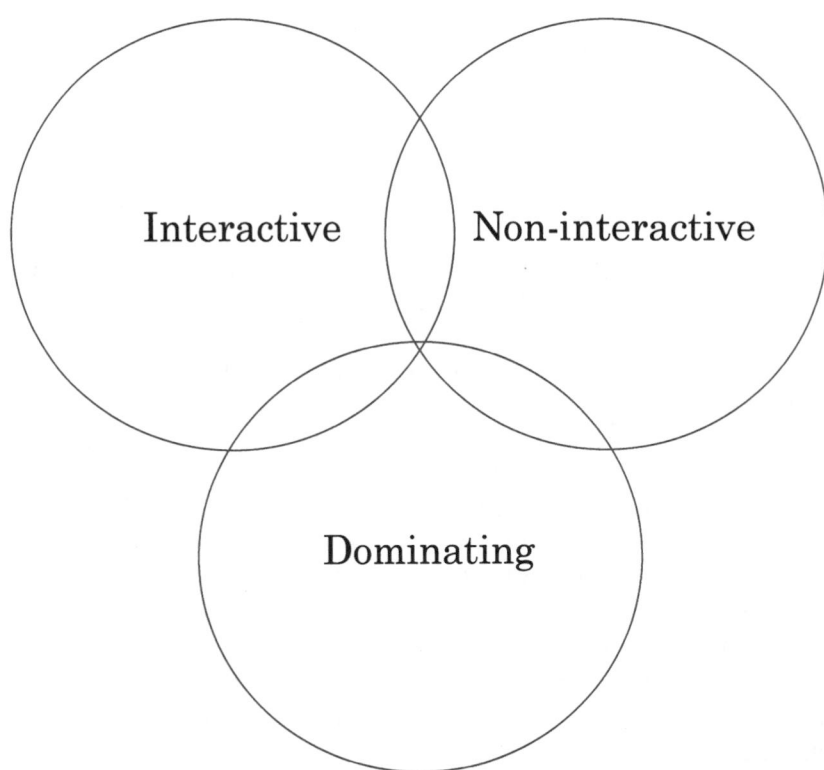

FIGURE 2-7. Constellations of behaviors that characterize some hard-of-hearing persons.

Noninteractive behavior is characteristic of a passive behavioral style.

Persons who fit the ***noninteractive behavior*** constellation often can be characterized as having a passive conversational style. They may bluff following a communication breakdown. They may not contribute much to the development of a conversation topic, and they may not participate in selecting a topic to talk about. They also may not respond to turn-taking signals. For instance, a communication partner may say, "So . . . you know . . . hmmm," hoping that the person with hearing impairment will contribute a remark. The following interchange illustrates a noninteractive conversational style (exhibited by Rose, who has a hearing loss):

Marie:	"I saw a great movie last night."
Rose:	"Oh."
Marie:	"It was on the old movies channel on cable."
Rose:	"Hmmm."
Marie:	"It had Fred Astaire and Ginger Rogers, lots of dancing and, you know, that kind of old movie stuff . . ."
Rose:	(nods)
Marie:	"I just love that . . ."
Rose:	(nods)
Marie:	"I guess it takes me back to when I was going to the movies as a kid."

In this interchange, Rose does not express interest in Marie's remarks and does not share in advancing the topic. Marie begins to talk more in order to fill in the silences.

A noninteractive conversational style often yields unfavorable consequences. In a series of interviews with hard-of-hearing adults, Cowie and Douglas-Cowie (1992) were told by one participant, "There are many occasions when I would like to ask questions, but in case I don't hear the answer I just don't do it. I think that probably gives the impression that I'm not interested which isn't the case, it's just to save embarrassment" (p. 269). An individual's withdrawal can elicit negative reactions from communication partners and create an internal source of stress for oneself.

There is some evidence that two characteristically passive behaviors, avoidance and pretending to understand, are commonly used by persons who have hearing loss. Stephens et al. (1999) provided a questionnaire to 100 consecutive patients attending their audiological rehabilitation clinic in Cardiff, Wales. The patients were asked how often they exhibited certain behaviors in eleven different communication interactions. The most commonly cited behavior (in addition to asking people to repeat a misunderstood message) was *avoidance,* defined as "deliberately avoiding conversations with other people in certain circumstances to avoid the embarrassment of having to ask them to repeat what they say." Another commonly cited behavior was *pretend,* defined as pretending "they are hearing even when they don't, to avoid asking people to repeat themselves."

The final constellation in Figure 2-7 denotes a constellation of ***dominating conversational behaviors***, which are characteristic of an aggressive conversational style. Persons who fall into this circle may take extended speaking turns, interrupt, and use abrupt topic changes. They may try to dominate the conversation, in order to always be aware of what is being talked about. Sometimes they will avoid asking questions so that they do not have to give up the speaking floor to hear the answers. Here is an excerpt from one conversation in which Deidre, an older woman with hearing loss, was conversing with her friend's daughter, Carrie:

Dominating conversational behaviors are characteristic of an aggressive conversational style.

Deidre: "Sharon says you are going on vacation."

Carrie: "Yes, I am flying with my brother to . . ."

Deidre: (interrupting) "Oh, I went on a plane once, to see my brother in South Carolina. He has a house down there, one he built himself on a lake."

With one remark, the two are suddenly talking about Deidre's plane trip and her brother rather than Carrie's upcoming travels.

As is the case with a passive conversational style, a dominating conversational style also may have undesired effects. One participant in the interviews conducted by Cowie and Douglas-Cowie (1992) reported, "I have to dominate the meeting, I make myself the artificial center of attention so that people will just speak to me

. . . instead of speaking to the chairman they would be speaking to me" (p. 269). One can surmise that colleagues (or at least the chairman) might react unfavorably to such a dominating conversational style.

In the model illustrated in Figure 2-7, the three circles overlap because an individual usually demonstrates behaviors that are characteristic of more than one constellation. An individual's use of conversational behaviors may vary during a conversation, as the person becomes more comfortable or the dynamics of the interchange are established. Behavior may vary as a function of the familiarity of the communication partner too, as well as the circumstances in which the conversation is occurring.

FINAL REMARKS

In this chapter, we have considered communication strategies and conversational styles and behaviors. Patients have a myriad of means for managing their communication difficulties. Although many of the strategies we considered in this chapter seem like common sense, it is surprising that many people either have not explicitly thought about them or do not use them effectively. Moreover, many people are not aware they may be using a conversational style or conversational behaviors that alienate their communication partners. Although these behaviors may have been adopted as a means of coping with hearing-related difficulties, they may create problems in and of themselves.

KEY CHAPTER POINTS

✔ The accepted rules of conversation often must bend when one of the conversational partners has a hearing loss. The overall quality of conversation also may be diminished. For instance, there may only be superficial content.
✔ There are two classes of communication strategies, facilitative and repair. Within each of these classes are several kinds of strategies that hard-of-hearing individuals can use to facilitate conversational interchanges.

✔ There are at least three stages involved in repairing a communication breakdown: detection, selection of a course of action, and implementation.

✔ Hard-of-hearing persons often bluff and pretend to understand. They may do this because they are reluctant to admit a hearing loss or because they do not want to appear uncooperative.

✔ Much research has centered on the use of repair strategies. One conclusion that emerges is that the most commonly used repair strategy is the repeat strategy.

✔ Anticipatory strategies are more effective when used before unfamiliar communication interactions than when used before familiar ones.

✔ Hard-of-hearing persons may be passive, assertive, or aggressive during conversation.

✔ Psychosocial therapy encourages the development of assertive conversational behaviors.

▰▰ MULTIPLE CHOICE QUESTIONS

1. Marcus Jones has a significant hearing loss. The tacit rules of conversation may be violated when he talks to an unfamiliar communication partner because:

   a. Marcus will slow his speaking rate.

   b. Marcus will probably shift topics inappropriately.

   c. The communication partner will repeatedly confirm that Marcus has recognized her message.

   d. The communication partner will provide too much information and border on verbosity.

2. Two classes of communication strategies are:

   a. Anticipatory and facilitative

   b. Environmental and corrective

   c. Specific and nonverbal

   d. Facilitative and repair

3. Which of the following messages might be easiest for a person with hearing loss to recognize?
   a. John gave the baseball to Tom and asked him to take it home last night.
   b. He took it home.
   c. He tossed the baseball to Tom. "Take it home," he said.
   d. John had the baseball. John gave the baseball to Tom.

4. Which question might reflect a message-tailoring strategy?
   a. Who did you see at the game?
   b. Where were you this morning?
   c. Did you find my list?
   d. How do you get to Toledo?

5. Moving close to the podium during a lecture is an example of:
   a. An anticipatory strategy
   b. A constructive strategy
   c. An instructional strategy
   d. An attending strategy

6. Which of the following is a disadvantage of using a nonspecific repair strategy following a communication breakdown?
   a. Your communication partner may react unfavorably to the conversation.
   b. You might elicit a simplified version of what was originally said.
   c. You take a "phantom" speaking turn.
   d. You are viewed as taking away your communication partner's speaking turn.

7. A person who frequently interrupts may be said to have what kind of conversational style?
   a. Passive
   b. Assertive
   c. Uncooperative
   d. Aggressive

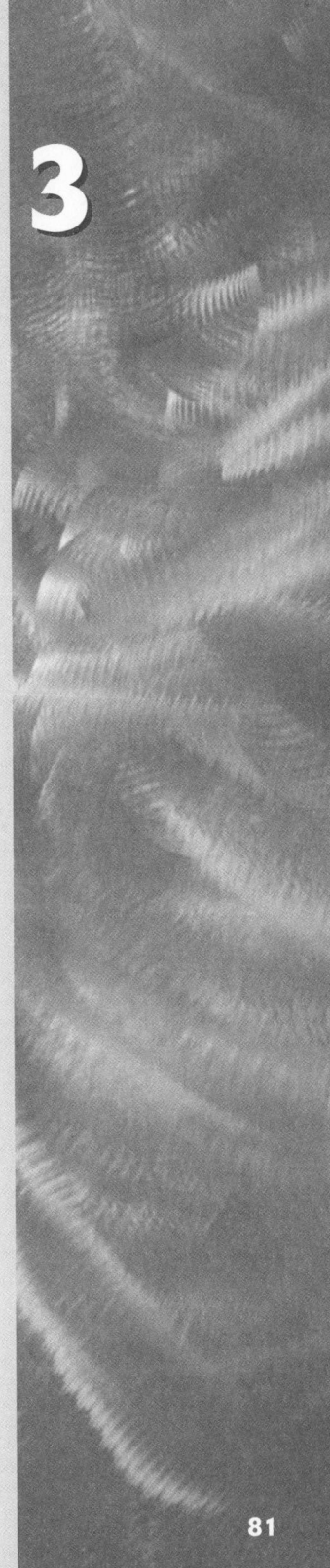

CHAPTER 3

Assessment of Conversational Fluency and Communication Handicap

TOPICS

Typically, a communication strategies training program begins and ends with an assessment of individuals' conversational fluency and communication handicap. The goals of the initial assessment are to:

- Determine the communication demands placed on individuals in their everyday life.
- Evaluate the impact of hearing loss on daily activities.
- Identify the settings in which communication problems arise.
- Document the kinds of social activities in which a person is likely to engage.
- Assess how effectively they use communication strategies in a variety of settings.
- Chronicle their employment responsibilities.

The goals of assessment will guide your selection of which measures you administer. For example, if the goal of assessment is to identify communication problems that are especially troublesome, you might interview the patient or administer a questionnaire. On the other hand, if the goal is to document conversational fluency, you might determine how well information can be exchanged between two communication partners, while maintaining a give-and-take dialogue. Assessment techniques for this purpose may include structured communication interactions or informal conversations.

The final assessment indicates whether a person's actual or perceived conversational fluency and communication handicap have improved as a result of training. Some of the original measures might be repeated to determine whether performance has changed. One-time-only measures also might be administered, such as a questionnaire, in which participants can critique the success of an aural rehabilitation plan.

You will want to know what the patient's audiogram looks like, both aided and unaided. In addition, you will assess his or her ability to recognize words in an audition-only condition and in an audition-plus-vision condition. In Chapter 6, we consider the audiogram and assessment of word recognition. In this chapter, we consider those assessment instruments that pertain to communication difficulties in everyday situations and conversational fluency.

■ CONVERSATIONAL FLUENCY

Now we consider conversational fluency. *Conversational fluency* relates to how smoothly conversation unfolds. The following factors help to define conversational fluency (Erber, 1996, pp. 204–205; Erber, 1998):

■ Time spent in repairing communication breakdowns. If during the course of a conversation, numerous communication breakdowns occur and they require many interchanges between the hard-of-hearing person and communication partner before they are resolved, then conversational fluency is low. On the other hand, if need for clarification is minimal, conversational fluency is high. When analyzing communication breakdowns, consider (Erbert & Yelland, 1998, p. 78) (a) the proportion of time spent in communication breakdowns, (b) the total number of breakdowns, and (c) the average duration of a breakdown.

■ Exchange of information and ideas. If the participants in a conversation successfully and easily share information and ideas, and the conversation seems to them to be spontaneous and not stilted, then conversational fluency is high.

■ Sharing of speaking time. When conversation is smooth-flowing, participants have ample opportunity to speak, and no one person dominates with protracted speaking times. Prolonged silences or frequent interruptions are not characteristic of fluent conversations.

■ Time spent in silence. If the participants sit in awkward silence for an inordinate amount of time, then conversational fluency is poor.

Sociolinguists (scientists who study conversational interactions and how they are influenced by social and cultural factors) often index the sharing of speaking time with a measure called *mean length turn ratio (MLT ratio)*. To determine this ratio, *mean length of speaking turn (MLT)* is first computed for each participant in a conversation by determining the average number of words each person speaks for some set number of conversational turns (often 50 turns). A *conversational turn* begins when one communication partner starts to speak. The turn ends when the person stops talking, and someone else responds to the remark. The MLT ratio is computed by taking a ratio between the MLTs of the two communication partners. Table 3-1 illustrates how MLT and MLT ratio are determined.

Conversational fluency relates to how smoothly conversation unfolds.

Sociolinguistics is a branch of linguistics that studies the effects of social and cultural differences within a community on its use of language and conversational patterns.

Mean length turn ratio (MLT ratio) is the ratio of the MLTs of two speakers in a conversation.

Mean length (speaking) turn is computed by determining the average number of words spoken during a set number of conversational turns.

Conversational turn is the period during which a participant delivers a contribution to the conversation.

Table 3-1. Dialogues that illustrate two levels of conversational fluency. Example 1 presents a sample with high conversational fluency, whereas Example 2 presents a sample with poor conversational fluency.

Example 1

Joan: "Has your new furniture arrived yet?"
Ann: "Yes, and I'm thrilled with it."
Joan: "You said that it was going to be French regency."
Ann: "No, I didn't go with that. My husband wanted a deco look."
Analysis: Joan's MLT = 8.0 words (16 words divided by 2 utterances)
   Ann's MLT = 9.0 words (18 words divided by 2 utterances)
   MLT ratio: 0.9, where 1.0 = equal length speaking turns

Example 2

Martha: Has your new furniture arrived yet?"
Tom: "Huh?"
Martha: "Your furniture?"
Tom: (looks around, shakes head)
Martha: "How are you doing? How is your wife? . . . Mary?"
Tom: "Fine."
Analysis: Martha's MLT = 5.6 words (17 words divided by 3 utterances)
   Tom's MLT = 0.7 (2 words divided by 3 utterances)
   MLT ratio: 6.2, where 1.0 = equal length speaking turns

MLT = mean length turn

The dialogues in Table 3-1 also illustrate two different levels of conversational fluency. In the first example, conversational fluency is high. The two communication partners exchange information with ease, and they share responsibility in advancing the topic of discussion. They talk about a content-dense subject, period furniture. The MLT ratio for this conversation is approximately equal, which is often characteristic of fluent interchanges.

The second conversational excerpt in Table 3-1 presents a sample of low conversational fluency. The topic of discussion quickly becomes superficial, as communication breakdowns occur. In this conversation, Martha bears the onus of responsibility for advancing the conversation. She must fill in the awkward silences and develop the topic. Conversational fluency of this type is not uncommon when one of the conversational partners has a significant hearing loss.

Traditional Audiologic Tests Versus Measures of Conversational Fluency

There are at least three reasons why traditional tests of word recognition sometimes do not index how well patients perform in real-world conversational interactions. "First, most audiologic test lists present unrelated speech stimuli. In typical conversations, utterances are related by linguistic, and often situational, context. Second, clients usually must repeat what they hear verbatim. In everyday conversation, they listen more often for the gist of the message and not for the purpose of repeating every word. Finally, clients usually interact with their conversational partners during the give and take of an ongoing conversation. If a client does not recognize an utterance, the individual can ask the partner to repeat or modify the message. Clients who repair communication breakdowns effectively might experience fewer difficulties in conversations than standard audiologic test results would predict; clients who do not repair breakdowns very well might experience more difficulties" (Tye-Murray, Witt, & Castelloe, 1996, p. 396).

■ COMMUNICATION HANDICAP AND DISABILITY

An issue closely related to conversational fluency is that of communication handicap. *Communication handicap* refers to the psychosocial disadvantages that result from hearing loss. These disadvantages include limitations that occur in performing activities of daily life. When we discuss how well a patient can talk to a business associate on the telephone, we are considering that person's communication handicap.

A **communication handicap** consists of the psychosocial disadvantages that result from hearing loss.

As noted in Chapter 1, the term *communication handicap* contrasts with the term *communication disability,* which is any restriction resulting from hearing impairment to perform an activity in the range that is considered normal (WHO, 1980). When we say that a person cannot detect the /s/ sound in the word *soup,* we are talking about that person's disability.

A **communication disability** is a loss of function.

■ GENERAL CONSIDERATIONS FOR EVALUATING CONVERSATIONAL FLUENCY AND COMMUNICATION HANDICAP

Conversational fluency and communication handicap can be challenging for a speech and hearing professional to assess for a number of reasons. First, conversational fluency and success in managing communication difficulties vary as a function of the conversational setting and situation and as a function of the communication partner. For instance, conversational fluency may be high when an individual talks with a seasoned speech and hearing professional but poor when the person converses with an unfamiliar store clerk. The speech and hearing professional is likely to be accustomed to talking to persons with hearing loss and probably speaks slowly and clearly and checks for comprehension. The store clerk may not know how to facilitate speech recognition for the person with hearing loss, may turn away when talking (and hence limit the hard-of-hearing person's ability to speechread), and may speak quickly. A measure of conversational fluency taken from the same hard-of-hearing individual probably would be high for the first communication partner but low for the second.

A second reason that assessment of conversational fluency may be problematic is because measures vary with the topic of discussion. For instance, conversational fluency may be high for a superficial topic such as the weather but low for a topic centering on local politics. Thus, depending on what you talked about, you might rate conversational fluency with a particular patient as either high or low.

A third reason conversational fluency and communication handicap are difficult to assess is because communication difficulties do not always arise during a conversation. A person may experience numerous difficulties in conversing in the workplace, but none while talking to a family member in a speech and hearing clinic test room. If communication breakdowns do not occur during the course of an assessment, a speech and hearing professional may not gain an appreciation of how an individual manages communication difficulties.

Finally, conversational fluency and communication handicap are difficult to index because no one measure can capture adequately the "construct" of conversational fluency or communication handicap, because both are defined by several dimensions. That is, both are abstractions that reflect a multitude of factors, such as those we considered previously for conversational fluency (i.e., the occurrence of breakdowns and pauses,

Table 3-2. Some general procedures for measuring conversational fluency and communication needs, and one advantage and disadvantage of each.

PROCEDURE	ADVANTAGE	DISADVANTAGE
Interview	Yields patient-specific information	Difficult to quantify information
Questionnaire	Quick and easy to administer	May miss patient-specific information
Daily log	Provides quantitative information about an extended time period	Can be a reactive procedure
Group discussion	Stimulates patients to introspect and reflect	Some patients may be reluctant to participate
Structured communication interaction	Has good face validity because assessment is based on actual conversational interactions	Can be time-consuming to score
Unstructured communication interactions	Good ecological validity because it best mimics real-world interaction	Results may vary as a function of the communication partner

the fluidity of conversation, MLT ratio, amount of time spent in silence, and the superficiality of discussion). A number of measures must be performed, and the results must be aggregated and then interpreted.

For all these reasons, assessment can be challenging. In the next sections, we consider specific assessment procedures that may be used. These procedures are listed in Table 3-2, along with some of their advantages and disadvantages.

■ INTERVIEWS

The most straightforward assessment procedure is the *interview.* Individuals talk about their conversational problems, and they consider possible reasons as to why communication breakdowns happen (Figure 3-1). They comment on their subjective impressions of conversational fluency in a variety of settings (e.g., the workplace, the home). "Are you able to use the telephone?" a clinician might ask, or the clinician might ask a more open-ended question, such as, "Tell me about your listening difficulties." People's answers will indicate their particular concerns and their

Interviews are a basic assessment procedure used to elicit information about specific information about each individual's hearing problem.

"Functional tests cannot tell the story of disabilities and handicaps, since these are to do with the person's actual experiences in the world. Thus that experience must be tapped, and the only way to do it is by asking people to make accounts of it."

—W. Noble, 1996, p. 9

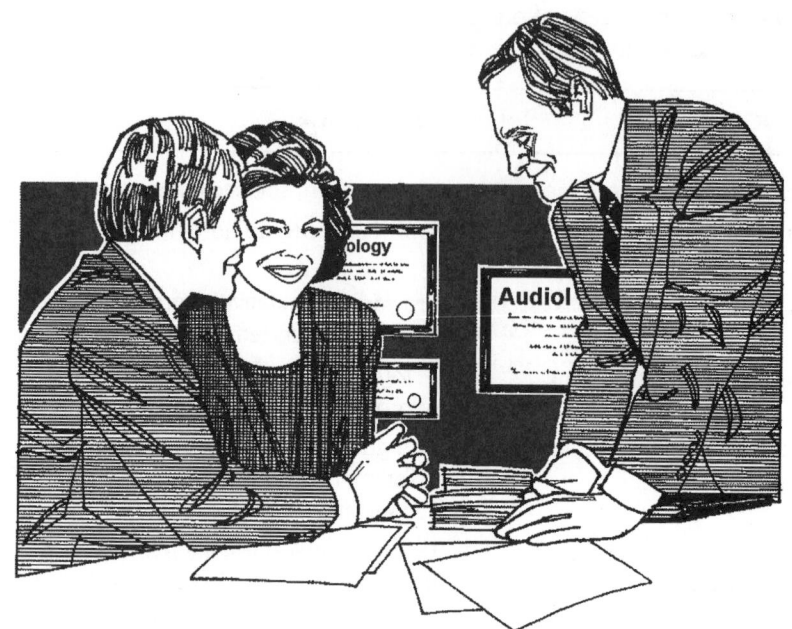

FIGURE 3-1. A clinician may interview the patient or the patient and a family member to learn about communication difficulties that are being experienced.

perceptions of their situation and problems. As you interact with the patient, you will acquire a sense of how well the patient can converse informally.

Interviews are effective because they elicit information that is specific to an individual. For instance, you may learn that one individual has difficulty communicating during office conferences, whereas another experiences problems while watching television. An open-ended discussion about the workplace may trigger a patient to reflect about particular instances in which communication was difficult in his or her recent past and may provide direction for the aural rehabilitation plan.

The disadvantage of interviews is that remarks cannot be quantified. This is problematic when changes in communication behaviors that result from intervention must be documented (Stephens & Hétu, 1991). Documentation is essential when you seek reimbursement for providing training to patients from third party health care providers.

■ CONDUCTING THE INTERVIEW

When interviewing a patient, engage in "generous listening." Listen in a way that lets people know they are being heard, without being judged. Provide positive attention, regard, and acknowledgment. Here are specific tips to keep in mind as you interview a patient for the first time (Gitles, 1999):

- "Do not get involved writing information and do not turn away from the patient. Continue to look at the person, and, most important, listen as if your life depended on it. Listen as if you have never heard any of this before, because you haven't, not from this person.
- If the patient pauses, stifle the impulse to ask the next question, interpret what the person is saying, or change the subject. Instead say something like, 'Is there anything else?' or 'What else can you tell me about that?' or 'Tell me more about that.'
- Use how, what, and when questions and avoid why questions. People will reveal more to you if they do not feel the need to justify their actions or defend their behavior.
- Encourage patients to talk until they have nothing left to tell you.
- When people answer questions, the more you listen, the greater the depth of the information they will reveal. That is where connectedness and relatedness occur. The more that patients reveal, the more they feel it is safe to talk to you, the more they get to weave and listen to their own story about their hearing (which they may have never told a soul), and the greater realization they have of the extent of their problem. As a result, the less reluctant they are about receiving help and the more they begin to let you help them.
- Listen to patients without judgment, evaluation, or opinions. Listen for the emotion and feelings in their expression and be aware of what is *not* being said. Acknowledge patients for having the courage to come in for help and let them know you will support them in whatever way you can.
- The more that you, as a professional, reveal your passion and commitment to helping people—perhaps through a personal story about someone you have helped—the greater the intimacy and relatedness with your patient" (pp. 54–56).

Excerpts from two sample interviews demonstrate the potency of the tips just listed. In the first interview, presented next, the clinician asks a preponderance of yes-no questions. You get the sense that she knows the answer before the patient even responds. In particular, note how a following question is not influenced by the patient's response to a previous question. By the end of the interview, the clinician has gained little information about the patient's communication handicap or conversational fluency, and the patient feels like he has been cycled through a pat list of questions that the clinician fires away at everyone who comes in for a hearing test.

Clinician:	(Leads Mr. Brown to the testing suite. When he is seated in the testing chair, the clinician begins the interview). "So, you think you have a hearing loss?"
Mr. Brown:	"My wife seems to think I do."
Clinician:	(The clinician makes a tick mark with her pen on the yellow note pad she is holding). "You have trouble hearing at home?"
Mr. Brown:	"I do okay."
Clinician:	(The clinician makes a tick mark). "What about work?"
Mr. Brown:	"Yeah, that's okay too."
Clinician:	(The clinician makes a tick mark). "You can use the telephone?"
Mr. Brown:	"Yeah."
Clinician:	(The clinician makes a tick mark, tucks the pad of paper under her arm). "Fine. Let's test your hearing and see what we find."

In contrast, in the excerpt from the second interview, which appears next, the clinician adheres to the tips described by Gitles (1999). She engages in "generous listening." She asks open-ended questions and encourages the patient to elaborate on his responses. Because there is a genuine dialog occurring, the clinician has a first person opportunity to observe the patient experience a communication breakdown, giving her some insight as to how the individual handles breakdowns and the ease with which they can be repaired.

Clinician:	(Greets the patient in the waiting room and asks him to follow her to her office for a conversation). "Good morning, Mr. Andrews. What brings you here today?"
Mr. Andrews:	"My wife says I have a hearing loss."
Clinician:	(Nods, continues to look Mr. Andrews in the eye).
Mr. Andrews:	"I think she mumbles a lot. But then again, I guess I'm cranking up the volume of the TV too high. That probably means something."
Clinician:	"What happens when she tries to talk to you from another room?"
Mr. Andrews:	"Huh?"
Clinician:	"Say you are in the living room. Your wife is talking to you from the hallway. What happens?"
Mr. Andrews:	"I can't hear her. Same as when she's talking in the kitchen with the water running. I can't hear her."
Clinician:	"Tell me more about listening at home."
Mr. Andrews:	(Describes his difficulties with hearing the doorbell and listening on the telephone. They then discuss the challenges he encounters when listening in the workplace).

Simply by listening, and treating the person as a unique individual and not as Mr. or Mrs. Joe/Jane client, you will learn much about your patient's communication difficulties. Moreover, you will establish a bond of human contact that lets the individual know you genuinely care about his or her hearing health and communication needs.

▬ QUESTIONNAIRES

Another assessment instrument that is used to assess conversational fluency and communication handicap is the questionnaire. *Questionnaires* might query respondents about how often communication breakdowns occur and whether they typically attempt to repair communication breakdowns and how. Questionnaires are a means of gathering general information easily and quickly (Figure 3-2).

Questionnaires are procedures used to gain subjective conversational fluency and communication handicap from respondents.

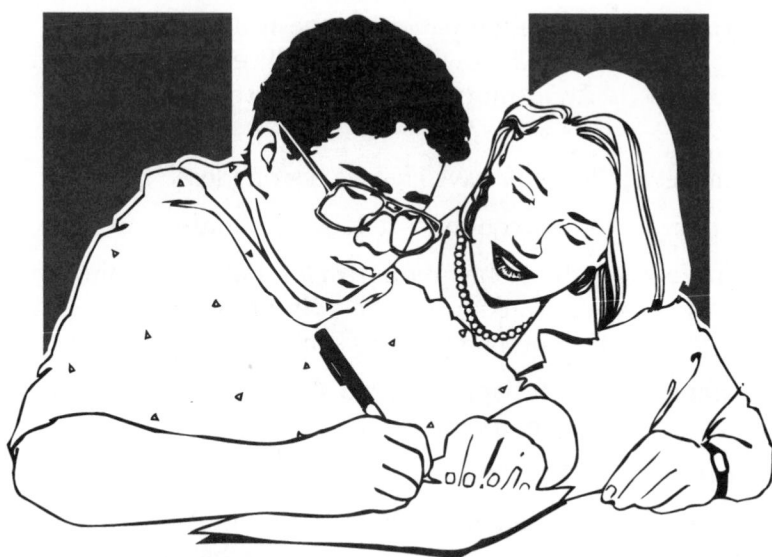

FIGURE 3-2. Questionnaires are an effective means of obtaining information about communication and conversation in an easy and fast way.

One drawback in using questionnaires is that it is possible to miss important information about communication difficulties that are specific to an individual simply because they are not covered by items in the questionnaire (Stephens & Hétu, 1991). For instance, a true/false statement such as, *I always verify what I understood during a meeting with a co-worker afterwards*, is irrelevant to the respondent who does not work or does not attend meetings. Moreover, responses to questionnaires may not reflect the importance of each communication difficulty or communication situation to the individual. For example, an inability to talk on the telephone may be devastating to the lifestyle of one person but only a minor annoyance to another.

A number of self-assessment questionnaires have been developed. Members of the Academy of Rehabilitative Audiology consider four instruments to be most valid and useful, the Hearing Handicap Inventory for the Elderly, the Self-Assessment of Communication, the Hearing Handicap Inventory for Adults, and the Communication Profile for the Hearing Impaired (Dancer & Gener, 1999). The first three appear in the appendixes at the end of this chapter, and the fourth is available for purchase (CPHI Services, P.O. Box 444, Simpsonville, MD, 21150-0444). Bentler and Kramer (2000) provide a table of available self-report questionnaires and discuss guidelines for choosing a measure. An adapted version of their work appears in Table 3-3.

Table 3-3. A list of self-report questionnaires.

TEST	PURPOSE	REFERENCES
Abbreviated Profile of Hearing Aid Benefit (APHAB) 24 items, 4 subscales (ease of communication, reverberation, background noise, aversiveness of sounds)	To measure the disability associated with hearing loss and the amount by which use of hearing aid reduces disability. Example: *(answered with and without hearing) I can communicate with others when we are in a crowd. (Always, almost always, generally, half the time, occasionally, seldom, never.)*	Cox & Alexander (1995) Paul & Cox (1995)
Amsterdam Inventory for Auditory Disability and Handicap 30 items, 6 factors (detection of sounds, distinction of sounds, auditory localization, intelligibility in noise and in quiet, intolerance of noise)	To identify factors that affect the patient in daily life and to assess hearing handicap. Example: *Can you carry on a conversation with someone in a busy street? (Almost never, occasionally, frequently, almost always.)*	Kramer, Kapteyn, Festen, & Tobi (1995) Kramer, Kapteyn, Festen, & Tobi (1996) Kramer, Kapteyn, & Festen (1998)
Client Oriented Scale of Improvement (COSI) 16 standardized listening situations	To identify up to five areas of listening difficulty and the degree of benefit obtained compared to that expected for similar persons in similar situations.	Dillon, James, & Ginis (1997) Dillon, Birtles, & Lovegrove (1999)
Communication Profile for the Hearing Impaired (CPHI) 145-item questionnaire dealing with 4 areas: communication performance, communication environment, communication strategies, and personal adjustment	To assess a broad range of communication problems. Example: *One way I get people to repeat what they said is by ignoring them (5-point scale ranging from "rarely" to "almost always").*	Demorest & Erdman (1987)
Communication Scale for Older Adults 72 items divided into 2 scales: communication strategies and communication attitudes	To provide in-depth information about the effects of aural rehabilitation on daily life and to evaluate use of communication strategies and an individual's feelings about hearing loss. Example: *I become angry when people do not speak clearly enough for me to understand (scale ranging from "always" to "never").*	Kaplan, Bally, Brandt, Busacco, & Pray (1997)
(Revised) Communication Self Assessment Scale Inventory for Deaf Adults (CSDA) 125 items, 4 scales (difficult communication situation, importance of each situation, communication strategies, communication attitudes)	To measure the communication abilities of adults who have prelingual deafness. Example: *You have difficulty hearing music when it is loud enough for other people (Almost always, sometimes, almost never).*	Kaplan, Bally, & Brandt (1995)

(continues)

Table 3-3. (continued)

TEST	PURPOSE	REFERENCES
Denver Scale of Communication Function-Modified (DSCF-M) 34 items concerning 4 areas (attitudes towards peers, socialization, communication, difficult listening situations)	To assess communication skills of older patients. Example: *The people I live with are annoyed with my hearing loss (5-point scale ranging from "definitely agree" to "definitely disagree").*	Kaplan, Feeley, & Brown (1978)
Glasglow Hearing Aid Benefit Profile (GHABP) 4 prespecified/4 subject specified items across 6 dimensions (disability, handicap, hearing aid use, benefit, satisfaction, residual disability)	To measure disability/handicap and benefit from use of hearing aid(s). Example: *The people I live with are annoyed with my hearing loss (5-point scale ranging from "not satisfied at all" to "delighted with it").*	Gatehouse (1999)
Gothenburg Profile (GP) 20 items, 2 scales: Experienced disability (being able to hear speech, being able to localize sounds) and experienced handicap (impact of hearing impairment, how you perform and react)	To measure experienced hearing disability and handicap. Example: *Do you find hearing problems an obstacle to your social life? (11-point scale, ranging from "never" to "always")*	Arlinger, Bellermark, Oberg, Lunner, & Hellgren (1998) Ringdahl, Eriksson-Mangold, & Andersson (1998)
Hearing Aid Needs Assessment (HANA) 11 items, 3 ratings per item: (1) How often (hardly ever, occasionally, frequently); (2) How much trouble (very little, some, very much); (3) How much help expected (very little, some, very much)	To compare perceived communication needs with actual benefit eventually achieved with hearing aids. Example: *You are at home listening to your stereo system (Ratings for how often, how much trouble, and how much help expected).*	Schum (1999)
Hearing Attitudes in Rehabilitation Questionnaire (HARQ) 40 items, 7 scales measure attitudes toward: hearing impairment (e.g., personal distress, hearing loss stigma, minimization of hearing loss); hearing aid (e.g., hearing aid stigma, hearing aid not wanted, pressure to be assessed, positive expectation of aid)	To measure older people's attitudes toward hearing loss and use of a hearing aid. Example: *If I wear a hearing aid, people will probably think I'm a bit stupid: (1) not true, (2) partly true, (3) true.*	Hallam and Brooks (1996)

Table 3–3. (continued)

TEST	PURPOSE	REFERENCES
Hearing Coping Assessment (HCA) 21 multiple choice items covering problem-focused coping and emotion-focused coping	To evaluate how well the patient thinks he or she can cope with hearing impairment. Example: *(1) I never had any problem talking to one person . . . (4) I have much trouble talking to one person.*	Andersson, Melin, Lindberg, & Scott (1995)
Hearing Disabilities and Handicaps Scale (HDHS) 20 items, 3 factors (speech perception, nonspeech sounds, handicap)	To assess the severity of the most common disabilities and handicaps associated with hearing impairment. Example: *Is it difficult for you to ask people to repeat themselves? (Never, seldom, often, always)*	Hétu, Getty, Philibert, Desilets, Noble, & Stephens (1994) Hallberg (1998)
Hearing Handicap and Disability Inventory (HHDI) 40 items, 4 scales (performance, emotional response, social withdrawal, perceived reaction of others)	To assess the consequence of hearing impairment in the elderly and to identify aural rehabilitative needs and effect of intervention. Example: *My hearing loss discourages me from using the telephone (Almost never, sometimes, often, almost always).*	VanderBrink (1995)
Hearing Handicap Inventory for Adults (HHIA) 25 items with two subscales (emotional consequences, social and situational effects)	To quantify perceived handicap and to assess benefit of hearing aids. Example: *Does a hearing problem cause you to feel embarrassed when meeting new people? (Yes, sometimes, no)*	Newman, Weinstein, Jacobson, & Hug (1990) Newman, Weinstein, Jacobson, & Hug (1991)
Hearing Handicap for the Elderly (HHIE) 25 items with 2 subscales (emotional consequences, social and situational effects)	To assess older person's perceptions of hearing loss, used with noninstitutionalized individuals. Example: *Does a hearing problem cause you to use the phone less often than you would like? (Yes, sometimes, no)*	Ventry and Weinstein (1982) Weinstein, Spitzer, & Ventry (1986)
Hearing Handicap Scale (HHS) 20 items	To measure disadvantage caused by the presence of hearing loss during everyday listening. Example: *When you ask someone for directions, do you understand what he or she says (5-point scale, ranging from "practically always" to "almost never").*	High, Fairbanks, & Glorig (1964) Tannahil (1979)

(continues)

Table 3-3. (continued)

TEST	PURPOSE	REFERENCES
Hearing Performance Inventory (HPI) 158 items that assess understanding of speech, speech intensity, response to auditory failure, and social, personal, and occupational issues	To evaluate problem areas experienced during everyday living. Example: *You are with a male friend or family member and several people are talking nearby. Can you understand him when his voice is loud enough and you can see his face?* (4-point scale ranging from "practically always" to "practically never")	Giolas, Owens, Lamb, & Schubert (1979)
Open-ended Problems Questionnaire 1 item is used to assess various groups (e.g., cochlear implant users, frequent communication partners)	To measure what people consider are the main problems as a result of hearing impairment. Example: *Please make a list of difficulties you may have as a result of your hearing loss. List them in order of importance starting with the biggest difficulties. Write down as many as you can think of.*	Barcham & Stephens (1980) Stephens, Jaworski, Kerr, & Zhao (1998)

Source: Adapted from Bentler, R. A., and Kramer, S. E. (2000). Guidelines for choosing a self-report outcome measure. *Ear and Hearing, 21,* 375–495.

The recent popularity of these instruments relates in part to the fact that subjective impressions of communication difficulties often do not correspond to patients' audiograms (Brainerd & Frankel, 1985; Demorest & Walden, 1984; Speaks, Jerger, & Trammell, 1970; Weinstein & Ventry, 1983). For example, an audiogram may indicate that a person has a significant hearing loss. However, the individual, when completing a questionnaire, may describe the loss as a minor nuisance, but not overly problematic. In considering the discrepancy that sometimes exists between audiological and questionnaire information, Erdman (1994) notes:

> Self-reports simply constitute different measures; the method of measurement differs as does the content of the measurement. Audiometric tests assess maximum potential or best performance of the central or peripheral hearing mechanism. Self-report instruments, on the other hand, assess typical performance in behavioral utilization of hearing ability. (p. 69)

Questionnaires may yield either quantitative or qualitative information, depending on the design of the questionnaire items.

Open-ended questions typically elicit qualitative data. Examples of open-set items include the following:

- *Describe the situations wherein you typically have problems communicating.*
- *What do you usually do when you do not understand someone?*

Open-ended questions elicit qualitative information.

Closed-ended questions may be used to gather quantitative information. An example of a quantitative questionnaire item appears next. On this item, the respondent's task is to write a number between 1 and 10 on each response blank, where *1* means *never* and *10* means *always:*

Closed-ended questions are used to gather quantitative information.

> *I am at a department store. The clerk asks me a question, but I do not understand her. I am most likely to:*
> _____ *ask the clerk to repeat the question*
> _____ *ask the clerk to say the question in a different way*
> _____ *shake my head to indicate that I missed what the clerk said*
> _____ *say and do nothing*

Both kinds of questionnaire items offer advantages and disadvantages. Open-ended items are less restrictive and might yield information from a patient that could not have been anticipated. However, sometimes answers to open-ended items are rambling or off-topic, and they may be difficult to quantify, which may be important if a clinician desires to compare pre- and postintervention performance. Closed-ended items allow for a quantitative analysis of responses. However, important information may be missed if the questionnaire does not include items that tap information relevant to a patient's communication difficulties.

■ DAILY LOGS

In completing a *daily log,* respondents perform a self-monitoring procedure regarding behaviors of interest, and provide self-reports. For example, they may log how many times a day they experience communication difficulties, and in which communication settings (e.g., the home, the workplace). In completing logs, patients may answer a series of questions about their communication difficulties or behaviors every day for a set number of days. Example items from a daily log appear in Table 3-4.

Daily logs are self-reports of behavior used by respondents for self-monitoring.

Table 3-4. Example items from a daily log designed to monitor someone's communication behaviors.

1. **Think about your communication interactions today. For the following situations, circle the term *(never, a few times, many times)* that best describes how much time you spent a talking today (beyond a greeting). Circle one response for each condition:**

In a quiet place	Never	a few times	many times
In a noisy place	Never	a few times	many times
On the telephone	Never	a few times	many times
From another room	Never	a few times	many times
In a group of people	Never	a few times	many times

2. **For the following two situations, write down a number between 0 to 100 (0 = nothing and 100 = everything) that indicates how much of what was said to you today you believe you understood.**

   _____ while watching the talker and listening

   _____ while listening only

3. **Did you ever indicate that you did not understand a spoken message today (Yes or No)?**

   _____

4. **What did you do when you did not understand a message? (Check all that apply.)**

   _____ I asked the talker to repeat the message.

   _____ I said "Huh" or "Pardon."

   _____ I asked the talker to rephrase the message.

   _____ I asked the talker to indicate what he or she was talking about.

   _____ I decided the message was not important enough to keep trying.

   _____ I asked the talker to spell or write the message.

   _____ Other (describe) _____

5. **Consider the conversations that you had with relatives today. Check all of the statements below that apply.**

   _____ I felt anxious when I tried to talk with my relative today.

   _____ I was able to understand my relative's spoken messages.

   _____ I felt satisfied with the success of our communication interactions.

   _____ I avoided talking about unimportant topics.

When patients complete a log for several consecutive days, their responses provide a general index of their daily use of communication strategies, their conversational fluency, and their communication handicap. Responses also may provide information about their aural rehabilitation needs. For example, if an individual reports that he never spoke on the telephone during 6 consecutive days, it might be inferred that this person may be unable to use the telephone successfully, and therefore avoids telephone conversations. The aural rehabilitation plan may thus be designed to provide telephone training and a telephone receiver amplifier.

Individuals can perform a daily log activity before and after participating in a communication strategies training program, and trends in responses can be compared before and after training. For example, if after completing a communication strategies training program and after receiving a telephone receiver amplifier, the man just discussed reported he used the telephone an average of two times every day (as compared to never), then it might be concluded that intervention provided some benefit to this individual.

Guidelines for Constructing a Daily Log

Few examples of daily logs for aural rehabilitation applications are available in the literature. Therefore, you may have to design your own and tailor them to track the pertinent activities and behaviors of each patient. Next are five guidelines you might consider when developing a daily log:

1. Include detailed instructions at the beginning of the daily log and at the start of each section that initiates a new format. Make the instructions clear and concise.
2. Use active sentences rather than passive sentences when writing daily log items.
3. Log items should have a minimum of prepositional phrases.
4. Avoid professional jargon or terms often used within the speech and hearing communication field but not by the general public.
5. Limit the number of items in a daily log to a maximum of seven. Otherwise, it may be too taxing for your client to complete or too much of an imposition in the daily routine.

Self-monitoring can provide a **reactive** procedure as it may influence how a person uses communication behaviors and strategies.

Self-monitoring can be a ***reactive*** procedure because it may influence a person's communication behaviors and how he or she uses communication strategies. For example, researchers have shown that when individuals complete self-monitoring diaries, they often improve their academic performance, reduce their consumption of alcohol, or decrease the number of cigarettes smoked (e.g., Johnson & Wilhite, 1971; McFall, 1970). Similarly, by monitoring use of communication strategies, patients may actually improve their use of them. As such, the use of daily logs can be used as a training procedure as well as an assessment procedure. However, for this very reason, it can be problematic when one is trying to assess the effects of an intervention program.

■ GROUP DISCUSSION

Group discussion provides a forum for class members to discuss communication issues.

In a ***group discussion*** (Figure 3-3), usually convened on the first meeting of a communication strategies training program, members of the class construct a list of their communication problems

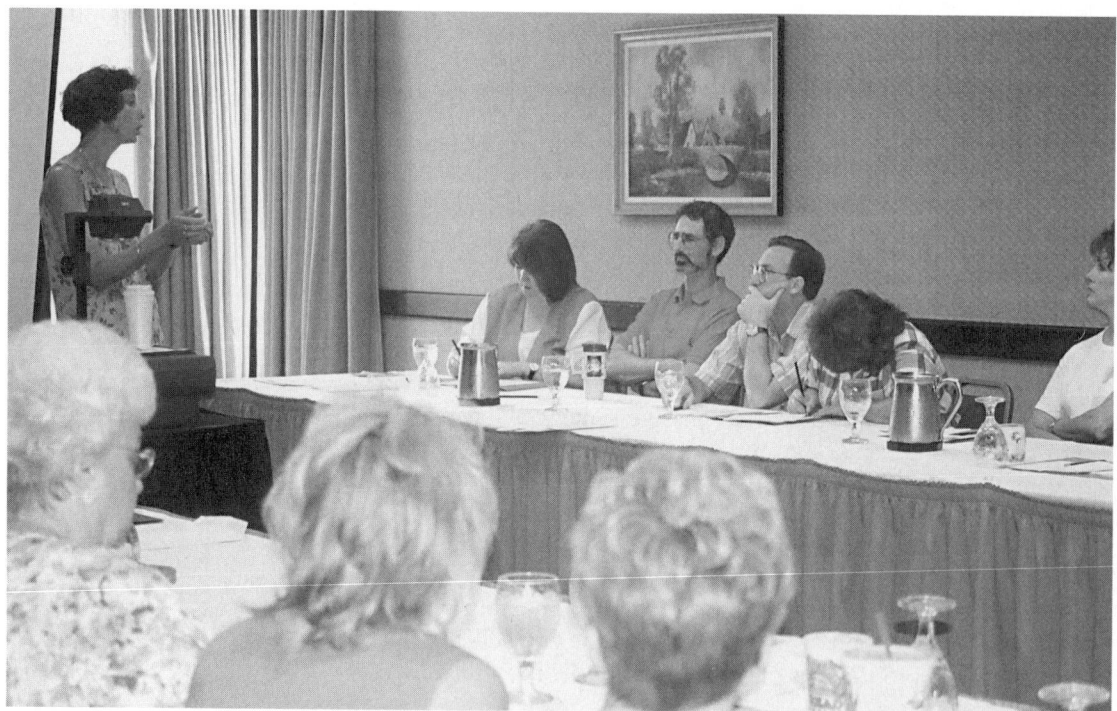

FIGURE 3-3. The success of a group discussion may well hinge on the skill of the group leader. In this session, the clinician is using an overhead projector to record the group participants' comments. (Photo by Kim Readmond, courtesy Central Institute for the Deaf.)

Table 3-5. Common concerns that might by identified during a group discussion.

Difficulty talking on the telephone

Impatience on the part of a spouse

Inability to manage communication breakdowns effectively

Avoidance by old friends

People talk to my spouse instead of me

Feelings of isolation and loneliness

Feelings of incompetence and anger

Difficulty conversing in noisy settings

Difficulty in communicating with my co-workers

Anxiety about not being able to hear warning signals

Frustration that family does not understand my hearing loss

Frustration that most people do not know what it is like to have a hearing loss

Feelings of being "left out"

Source: Adapted from Trychin, S. (1994). Helping people cope with hearing loss. In J. G. Clark and F. N. Martin (Eds.), *Effective counseling in audiology: Perspectives and practice* (pp. 247–277). Englewood Cliffs, NJ: Simon and Schuster Co.

and the topics they would like included in the syllabus. The remainder of the program then focuses on these issues. This procedure is excellent, and can be used any time that instruction occurs in a group setting as opposed to one-on-one. Table 3-5 lists some concerns that have emerged during this kind of group session.

Tips on Conducting a Group Discussion

The success (or failure) of a group discussion often hinges on the skill of the speech and hearing professional who conducts the session. Next are a list of suggestions that might be followed when conducting a group discussion:

- Encourage everyone to participate in the discussion, perhaps by asking group members to take turns one at a time around the table.
- Record remarks on a chalkboard, on an overhead projector slide, or on an oversized hanging notebook, even if they seem off-topic or minor.
- Make sure that no one is made to feel embarrassed or foolish for making a contribution.
- Ask some questions that guide the discussion and engage the students in the discussion. For example, you might say, "Mrs. Smith, you work in a pharmacy. What kinds of listening difficulties do you experience when you are behind the counter?"
- Come to the class prepared to draw specific material from the participants.

STRUCTURED COMMUNICATION INTERACTIONS

Structured communication interactions are simulated conversations used to reflect a patient's communication difficulties.

TOPICON is an example of a structured communication interaction activity.

Structured communication interactions also can be used during both assessment and training. ***Structured communication interactions*** are simulated conversations that reflect some of the difficulties that actually occur in a patient's typical day. ***TOPICON*** (Erber, 1988) is an example of a structured communication interaction activity that may be used for both assessment and training purposes. In this procedure, the patient carries on a conversation with the clinician. The clinician monitors and evaluates conversational difficulties that occur. Afterwards, the clinician and student discuss the fluency of the interaction. They talk about the problems that arose and alternative ways of handling them. They consider who spoke more during the interaction and why. They discuss the direction of information flow, and they identify which communication strategies were applied and whether or not they were effective. Conversation fluency can be evaluated with a consideration of the following: (1) number of prolonged pauses, (2) number of restarts, (3) number of topic shifts, (4) interruptions of turn-taking, (5) level of abstraction and superficiality, (6) presence of self-consciousness, and (7) the degree of understanding (Erber, 1988, p. 79).

Quest?AR is a structured communication procedure that can be used to assess communication difficulties.

Question-Answer Sessions (Quest?AR)

Quest?AR is a structured communication procedure that can be used to assess communication difficulties. In the procedure, the clinician asks a series of scripted questions, and the patient responds. Occasionally, listening difficulties are added to induce communication breakdowns. Performance is then evaluated in terms of the frequency of communication breakdowns, and the patient's facility in repairing them. An example of the procedure is presented next (quoted from Erber & Lind, 1994, p. 280).

	Difficulty Added	Difficulty Identified
1. Why did you go there?		
2. When did you go?	fast	no

(continues)

	Difficulty Added	Difficulty Identified
3. How many people went with you?	_____	_____
4. Who were they (relations/names)?	soft	yes
5. What did you take with you?	long	yes
6. Where is (the place where you went)?		
7. How did you get there?	_____	_____
8. What did you see on the way?	fast	yes
9. What time did you get there?	_____	_____

■ UNSTRUCTURED COMMUNICATION INTERACTIONS

As the name implies, an unstructured communication interaction is a fairly spontaneous interaction that has few external constraints. Typically, it is a free-flowing conversation between a patient and a communication partner that is most often scored after the fact, although sometimes it is evaluated as it unfolds. At least three ways have been developed to evaluate unstructured communication interactions: transcription analysis, ratings, and *Dyalog*. All three ways typically entail obtaining an audio-videotape recording of the patient engaged in conversation with a communication partner (although sometimes for the rating procedure or *Dyalog*, the analysis is scored on the spot). The partner might be a frequent communication partner, such as a spouse, a child, or a parent; an unfamiliar communication partner, such as a clinician; or a naïve communication partner. This latter kind of partner is someone who is unfamiliar to the hard-of-hearing person and someone who is also naïve about hearing loss. The naïve communication partner has interacted little if at all with hard-of-hearing persons and may not know that the patient being evaluated has a hearing loss. The use of different types of conversational partners may indicate how conversational dynamics vary as a function of the familiarity of the partner.

The conversation sample is typically recorded in a quiet room or a room with background noise (e.g., music playing on a radio to induce communication breakdowns). The camera is mounted on a tripod, turned on, and then the camera operator leaves the room so the patient and communication partner can begin to converse. The conversation might be stimulated with the use of "conversation cards" that list topics to talk about. For example, topics might consist of the following:

- What did you do last weekend?
- Where are you going this summer?
- What's your favorite restaurant?
- Do you have any hobbies?
- Tell me about your family.

In the transcription analysis method of evaluation, the conversation is transcribed word-for-word, and then analyzed. The analysis might reveal information such as the number of communication breakdowns, the number of turn exchanges required to resolve the breakdowns, the number of interruptions, the number of fillers, mean length turn ratio, and number of different topics discussed (see Tye-Murray, Witt, & Schum, 1995, and Tye-Murray, Witt, Schum, & Sobaski, 1995, for examples).

A second way to analyze an unstructured communication interaction is to obtain ratings from trained students or clinicians. The observer watches the sample and then assigns a number from 1 *(poor)* to 4 *(good)* to indicate how smoothly the conversation flows without the need for clarification (Erber, 1996). This kind of rating gives a gross assessment of overall fluency and has proven to be a reliable measure both within and between raters.

Finally, a computer-based technique called *Dyalog* (Erber, 1998) permits relatively fast analyses of unstructured communication interactions. It is a software package that loads onto most computers. The clinician watches the conversation from one (Erber, 1998) to three times (Tye-Murray, 2003), depending on how much information is desired. In the three-times version, the clinician first watches it for the purpose of recording talk time for the patient. Every time the patient begins talking, the clinician presses the space bar of the computer keyboard. When the patient stops talking, the clinician releases the computer keyboard. In the second viewing, the clinician records the intervals in which the communication partner talked. Finally, for the third viewing (and the first viewing if only watching one time), the clinician, who by now is well familiarized with the interaction, presses the space bar at the onset of a communication breakdown and releases it at the offset of the breakdown. The program then can be used to compute the following information: mean length turn for the patient, mean length turn for the communication partner, mean length turn ratio, time spent in silence, time spent in communication breakdown, and average length of communication breakdown.

FINAL REMARKS

In this chapter, we have considered a variety of ways to assess conversational fluency and communication handicap. Each procedure has advantages and disadvantages, and a major challenge for a speech and hearing professional may lie in the optimum selection and use of the measurement procedures. It is not uncommon for clinicians to use a test-battery approach and employ more than one type of assessment procedure. This approach can provide a more well-rounded portrait of communication difficulties than the use of a single measure. However, you need to be careful not to overwhelm patients with assessment procedures. For example, if they spend their entire first class of communication training with assessment, and do not perceive they have benefitted by attending, they are not likely to show up for a second class.

KEY CHAPTER POINTS

✔ Most communication strategies training programs begin and end with an assessment of conversational fluency and communication handicap. Conversational fluency relates to how smoothly conversation unfolds. Communication handicap pertains to the psychosocial disadvantages related to the hearing loss.
✔ Conversational fluency and communication handicap are difficult to assess for many reasons. For example, conversational fluency may vary as a function of the communication partner (Is the person familiar? Is the person experienced with talking to hard-of-hearing people?) and with the topic of conversation.
✔ A variety of assessment procedures are available. These procedures include interviews and questionnaires. Each offers both advantages and disadvantages. Often, clinicians opt to use a test-battery approach.

■ MULTIPLE CHOICE QUESTIONS

1. Which of the following is not one of the reasons why you might want to assess conversational fluency and communication handicap at the onset of an aural rehabilitation program?

   a. To verify the audiogram

   b. To determine the communication demands placed on an individual during everyday life

   c. To chronicle a person's employment responsibilities

   d. To document the kinds of social activities in which a person is likely to engage

2. What is mean length turn ratio?

   a. The number of years a person has had a hearing loss divided by the person's age in years

   b. The ratio of MLTs of two speakers in a conversation

   c. The average length of time a person talks during a conversational turn

   d. The ratio between amount of time spent in silence and the amount of time spent in talking during a conversation

3. All but one of the following are reasons that conversational fluency is difficult to measure clinically:

   a. Fluency varies with topic of conversation.

   b. Fluency varies as a function of the conversational partner.

   c. Communication difficulties may not arise.

   d. There are no valid assessment procedures and/or instruments.

4. If you wanted to informally assess someone's conversational fluency, the most direct way might be to:

   a. Administer a questionnaire

   b. Ask the patient to complete a daily log

   c. Stage a structured communication interaction

   d. Conduct an interview using open-ended questions

5. The term *generous listening* is used to describe:
    a. Instances in which you listen more than you talk
    b. Instances in which you listen while providing positive regard, attention, and acknowledgment
    c. Instances in which you employ an assistive listening device to ensure that the patient can understand what you have to say
    d. A term used to describe a component of conversational fluency

6. One disadvantage of using a questionnaire to assess communication handicap is that:
    a. The information is redundant with results from speech audiometry.
    b. It is possible to miss important information about communication difficulties because the wrong questions are asked.
    c. So few are available.
    d. Most have not been normalized.

7. Which procedure requires the patient to repeat the process on several consecutive days?
    a. Interview
    b. Questionnaire
    c. Daily log
    d. Structured interaction

8. The following item is included on a daily log: "Think about your communication interactions today. Indicate how many times you implemented a facilitative strategy." This item is:
    a. Inappropriate because it contains professional jargon (*facilitative strategy*)
    b. Appropriate because it asks about a specific behavior
    c. Appropriate because it provides information that tells you whether communication strategies training is needed
    d. Inappropriate because the item has active verb tense

9. Three means of assessing conversational fluency or communication handicap include:

a. Unstructured communication interactions, the NU-6 Test, and Dyalog

b. Unstructured communication interactions, daily logs, and essays

c. Unstructured communication interactions, structured communication interactions, and bi-structured communication interactions

d. Daily logs, questionnaires, and interviews

KEY RESOURCES

The Hearing Handicap Inventory for the Elderly (HHIE)

(Reproduced with permission by Ventry, I. J., and Weinstein, B. (1982). The hearing handicap inventory for the elderly: A new tool. *Ear and Hearing, 3,* 128–134).

The purpose of this scale is to identify the problems your hearing loss may be causing. Answer YES, SOMETIMES, or NO for each question. Do not skip a question if you avoid a situation because of your hearing problem. If you use a hearing aid, please answer the way you hear without the aid.

Hearing Handicap Inventory for the Elderly

		YES (4)	SOMETIMES (2)	NO (0)
S-1	Does a hearing problem cause you to use the phone less often than you would like?			
E-2	Does a hearing problem cause you to feel embarrassed when meeting new people?			
S-3	Does a hearing problem cause you to avoid groups of people?			
E-4	Does a hearing problem cause make you irritable?			
E-5	Does a hearing problem cause you to feel frustrated when talking to members of your family?			
S-6	Does a hearing problem cause you difficulty when attending a party?			

(continues)

Hearing Handicap Inventory for the Elderly (continued)

		YES (4)	SOMETIMES (2)	NO (0)
E-7	Does a hearing problem cause you to feel "stupid" or "dumb"?			
S-8	Do you have difficulty hearing when someone speaks in a whisper?			
E-9	Do you feel handicapped by a hearing problem?			
S-10	Does a hearing problem cause you difficulty when visiting friends, relatives, or neighbors?			
S-11	Does a hearing problem cause you to attend religious services less often than you would like?			
E-12	Does a hearing problem cause you to be nervous?			
S-13	Does a hearing problem cause you to visit friends, relatives, or neighbors less often than you would like?			
E-14	Does a hearing problem cause you to have arguments with your family members?			
S-15	Does a hearing problem cause you difficulty when listening to TV or radio?			
S-16	Does a hearing problem cause you to go shopping less often than you would like?			
S-17	Does any problem or difficulty with your hearing upset you at all?			
S-18	Does a hearing problem cause you to want to be by yourself?			
S-19	Does a hearing problem cause you to talk to family members less often than you would like?			
E-20	Do you feel that any difficulty with your hearing limits or hampers your personal or social life?			
S-21	Does a hearing problem cause you difficulty when in a restaurant with relatives or friends?			
S-22	Does a hearing problem cause you to feel depressed?			
S-23	Does a hearing problem cause you to listen to TV or radio less often than you would like?			
E-24	Does a hearing problem cause you to feel uncomfortable when talking to friends?			
E-25	Does a hearing problem cause you to feel left out when you are with a group of people?			

For clinicians use only: Total score: _____

Subtotal E: _____

Subtotal S: _____

Self-Assessment of Communication (SAC)

(Reprinted by permission from Schow, R. I., and Nerbonne, M. A. (1982). Communication screening profile: Use with elderly clients. *Ear and Hearing, 3*, 135–147.)

Name _____

Date _____

Raw Score _____ × 2 = _____ − 20 = _____ × 1.25 _____%

Please select the appropriate number ranging from 1 to 5 for the following questions. Circle only one number for each question. If you have a hearing aid, please fill out the form according to how you communicate when the hearing aid is not in use.

Disability

Various Communication Situations

1. Do you experience communication difficulties in situations when speaking with one other person? (for example, at home, at work, in a social situation, with a waitress, a store clerk, with a spouse, boss, etc.)
   - (a) almost never (or never)
   - (b) occasionally (about ¼ of the time)
   - (c) about half of the time
   - (d) frequently (about ¾ of the time)

2. Do you experience communication difficulties in situations when conversing with a small group of several persons? (for example, with friends or family, co-workers, in meetings or casual conversations, over dinner or while playing cards, etc.)
   - (a) almost never (or never)
   - (b) occasionally (about ¼ of the time)
   - (c) about half of the time
   - (d) frequently (about ¾ of the time)
   - (e) practically always (or always)

3. Do you experience communication difficulties while listening to someone speak to a large group? (for example, at a church

or in a civic meeting, in a fraternal or women's club, at an educational lecture, etc.)

    (a) almost never (or never)

    (b) occasionally (about ¼ of the time)

    (c) about half of the time

    (d) frequently (about ¾ of the time)

    (e) practically always (or always)

4. Do you experience communication difficulties while participating in various types of entertainment? (for example, movies, TV, radio, plays, night clubs, musical entertainment, etc.)

    (a) almost never (or never)

    (b) occasionally (about ¼ of the time)

    (c) about half of the time

    (d) frequently (about ¾ of the time)

    (e) practically always (or always)

5. Do you experience communication difficulties when you are in an unfavorable listening environment? (for example, at a noisy party, where there is background music, when riding in an auto or bus, when someone whispers or talks from across the room, etc.)

    (a) almost never (or never)

    (b) occasionally (about ¼ of the time)

    (c) about half of the time

    (d) frequently (about ¾ of the time)

    (e) practically always (or always)

6. Do you experience communication difficulties when using or listening to various communication devices? (for example, telephone, telephone ring, doorbell, public address system, warning signals, alarms, etc.)

    (a) almost never (or never)

    (b) occasionally (about ¼ of the time)

    (c) about half of the time

    (d) frequently (about ¾ of the time)

    (e) practically always (or always)

Handicap

Feelings About Communication

7. Do you feel that any difficulty with your hearing limits or hampers your personal or social life?
    (a) almost never (or never)
    (b) occasionally (about ¼ of the time)
    (c) about half of the time
    (d) frequently (about ¾ of the time)
    (e) practically always (or always)

8. Does any problem or difficulty with your hearing upset you?
    (a) almost never (or never)
    (b) occasionally (about ¼ of the time)
    (c) about half of the time
    (d) frequently (about ¾ of the time)
    (e) practically always (or always)

Other People

9. Do others suggest that you have a hearing problem?
    (a) almost never (or never)
    (b) occasionally (about ¼ of the time)
    (c) about half of the time
    (d) frequently (about ¾ of the time)
    (e) practically always (or always)

10. Do others leave you out of conversations or become annoyed because of your hearing?
    (a) almost never (or never)
    (b) occasionally (about ¼ of the time)
    (c) about half of the time
    (d) frequently (about ¾ of the time)
    (e) practically always (or always)

Hearing Handicap Inventory for Adults (HHIA)*

Instructions: The purpose of the scale is to identify the problems your hearing may be causing you. Check YES, SOMETIMES, or NO for each question. Do not skip a question if you avoid a situation because of a hearing problem.

		YES (4)	SOMETIMES (2)	NO (0)
S-1	Does a hearing problem cause you to use the phone less often than you would like?			
E-2	Does a hearing problem cause you to feel embarrassed when meeting new people?			
S-3	Does a hearing problem cause you to avoid groups of people?			
E-4	Does a hearing problem make you irritable?			
E-5	Does a hearing problem cause you to feel frustrated when talking to members of your family?			
S-6	Does a hearing problem cause you difficulty when attending a party?			
S-7	Does a hearing problem cause you difficulty hearing/understanding co-workers, clients, or customers?			
E-8	Do you feel handicapped by a hearing problem?			
S-9	Does a hearing problem cause you difficulty when visiting friends, relatives, or neighbors?			
E-10	Does a hearing problem cause you to feel frustrated when talking to co-workers, clients, or customers?			
S-11	Does a hearing problem cause you difficulty in the movies or theater?			
E-12	Does a hearing problem cause you to be nervous?			
S-13	Does a hearing problem cause you to visit friends, relatives, or neighbors less often than you would like?			
E-14	Does a hearing problem cause you to have arguments with family members?			
S-15	Does a hearing problem cause you difficulty when listening to TV or radio?			

(continues)

*Reprinted with permission from Newman, C. W., Weinstein, B. E., Jacobson, G. P., et al. (1991). Test-retest reliability of the Hearing Handicap Inventory for Adults. *Ear and Hearing, 12*, 355–357.

		YES (4)	SOMETIMES (2)	NO (0)
S-16	Does a hearing problem cause you to go shopping less often than you would like?			
E-17	Does any problem or difficulty with your hearing upset you at all?			
E-18	Does a hearing problem cause you to want to be by yourself?			
S-19	Does a hearing problem cause you to talk to family members less often than you would like?			
E-20	Do you feel that any difficulty with your hearing limits or hampers your personal or social life?			
S-21	Does a hearing problem cause you difficulty when in a restaurant with relatives or friends?			
E-22	Does a hearing problem cause you to feel depressed?			
S-23	Does a hearing problem cause you to listen to TV or radio less often than you would like?			
E-24	Does a hearing problem cause you to feel uncomfortable when talking to friends?			
E-25	Does a hearing problem cause you to feel left out when you are with a group of people?			

For clinicians use only: Total score: _____
                              Subtotal E: _____
                              Subtotal S: _____

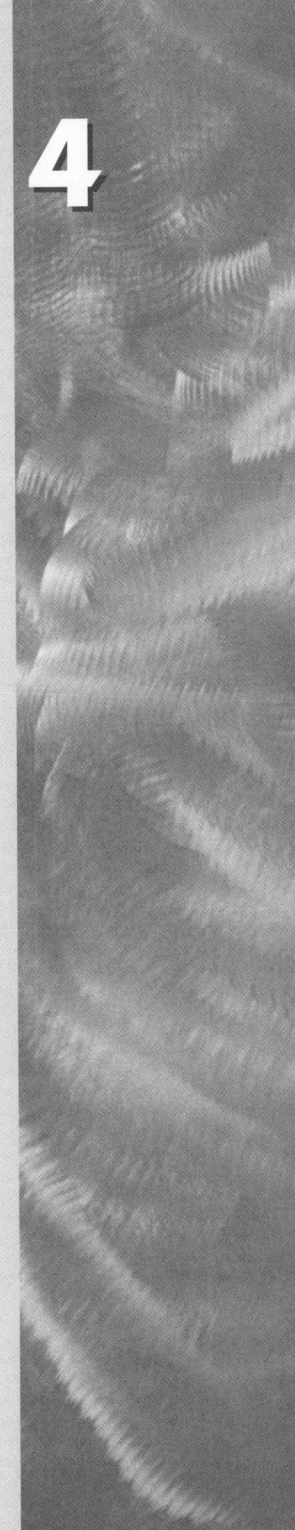

CHAPTER 4

Communication Strategies Training

TOPICS

- General program content
- Issues to consider when developing a training program
- Model for training
- Getting started
- Short-term training
- Communication strategies training for frequent communication partners
- Communication strategies training for children
- Efficacy of training
- Final remarks
- Key chapter points
- Multiple choice questions
- Appendix 4-1
- Appendix 4-2
- Appendix 4-3

There are many ways to provide training in the use of communication strategies. Current practices range from simply making printed materials available in the clinic waiting room to presenting a weekly program that may extend several weeks or even months. Training activities may include paper and pencil tasks, role-playing, group discussions, and workbook exercises. When possible, the training program should be designed to meet the participants' expectations, age, socioeconomic background, lifestyle, and particular communication problems.

In the following sections, we consider the stages of a communication strategies training program and training activities for each stage. Because it is not always feasible to implement this model, we also consider alternative models.

Sensitivity to People's Self-Perceptions

"[Speech and hearing professionals] may find it particularly helpful when working with hard-of-hearing adults and their families to remember that how people perceive communication problems (i.e., their meaning or significance to the people involved) is a very important factor to consider. For example, some hard-of-hearing people believe that, due to their hearing loss, they are a burden on other people, and this belief leads them to withdraw from social contact and also probably leads to depression. As another example, many people believe that hearing aids correct hearing problems to the same degree that glasses correct visual problems. It is difficult for people holding this belief to understand why a person wearing hearing aids does not understand what is being said, and it does not occur to them to think about doing anything else to remedy the situation. So, included in the [communication strategies training] programs I conduct are some ways to help people separate fact from fiction pertaining to hearing loss, and methods for helping hearing-impaired people develop a more realistic appraisal of themselves and their hearing problem" (Trychin, 1994, p. 248).

GENERAL PROGRAM CONTENT

The content of a communication strategies training program typically concerns problems specifically related to hearing loss and how these problems can be minimized. Excessive sympathy for individuals is not expressed, and personal problems unrelated to hearing loss are not considered. Content may include training for the two types of communication strategies, facilitative and repair (see Chapter 2). During this training, individuals learn to modify the four factors that affect communication success (the talker, the message, the environment, themselves), and learn to rectify breakdowns in communication. They typically learn about assertive versus nonassertive behaviors too, and work on developing their skills to deal assertively with communication difficulties. We revisit assertiveness training in the next chapter.

ISSUES TO CONSIDER WHEN DEVELOPING A TRAINING PROGRAM

In developing a training program, several nuts-and-bolts issues must be considered. One issue is the optimum program length. Some persons will have minimal time to devote to a communication strategies training program, and 1 hour may be all that is available. Standard programs usually require 12 to 40 hours, and are presented in one of two formats. The course may provide intensive instruction during a weekend-long period, meeting 4 to 7 hours per day or may be spread over an 8 to 15 week period, with each session lasting several hours each week.

Another issue to consider is the class format. Communication strategies training may be provided during a one-on-one class, a couple's session, or in a group. Common wisdom suggests that the most effective means is the group setting, where people interact with other persons who have hearing loss, and also interact with their family members. Defenses and recriminations between a hard-of-hearing person and a family member may subside when they recognize that other families share common experiences and when they share solutions with individuals who are in similar situations.

When you work with a group, it is important to develop a group spirit and esprit de corps. Table 4-1 presents attributes of a class group where participants receive optimal benefit from participation.

Other issues to consider include the participants' gender, age, life stage, culture, motivation to participate in training, and specific

Table 4-1. Attributes of an optimal class spirit.

---

1. Every class member accepts every other class member with an appreciation of the individual's strengths and a tolerance of the individual's quirks and weaknesses.

2. There is a familiarity of approach among the members of the class, with an awareness of each person's hearing difficulties and backgrounds.

3. Contributions from each class member are encouraged and recognized.

4. Class members can communicate easily with one another, possibly with the use of assistive listening devices.

5. There is acceptance of and conformity to a code of behavior (e.g., "only one person may speak at a time"), usually involving courtesy, mutual respect, and empathy.

6. There is an ability to recognize and use wisely the experiences of individual class members to educate other participants in the class.

7. There is a clear definition of the class agenda and format so each individual knows what to expect.

8. Discussion remains focused, and comments are not made to distract the class.

9. Class members are encouraged to be specific and to use examples.

Source: Adapted from Houle, C. O., (1997). *Governing boards.* San Francisco, CA: Jossey-Bass Publishers.

communication difficulties. The program material and the teaching activities may need to be modified to meet these variables.

▰ GETTING STARTED

Before the first session, the clinician usually develops a curriculum and collects materials that will be used during the program. Sample curriculums include those presented in *Learning to Hear Again with a Cochlear Implant* (Wayner & Abrahamson, 1998) and *Learning to Hear Again* (Wayner & Abrahamson, 1996). Although a curriculum provides a loose blue print of what will happen in the class, it should be flexible enough to meet the needs of the class participants. A cardinal rule for a communication strategies training program, or any aural rehabilitation plan, is that it should cater to the specific concerns of the patient(s), experienced at the point of time that he or she engages in the program. Thus, a business woman who has received a cochlear implant, after having been deaf for many years, may have different needs than a young mother who has recently been diagnosed as having a hearing loss. Whereas the business woman might be interested in using the telephone and learning effective telephone conversational strategies, the young mother may benefit from an introduction to facilitative strategies, particularly within the context of using them in her home and with her husband and baby. Find out at the beginning of the program the needs and expectations of the patients, and tailor the curriculum accordingly.

Materials that might be needed to conduct the program may include name tags, handouts, diagrams, whiteboard and whiteboard markers, videotapes, planned communication scenarios for role-playing, FM or infrared system, overhead projector, snacks, and pencil and paper. The program may include workbooks and homework materials.

A program may begin with setting ground rules for group interactions (e.g., *Only one person speaks at a time. Let us know when you are finished speaking by nodding your head. You have a right to pass on a question. Everything said in this room is confidential.*) It's extremely important to establish a secure and safe environment at the onset of a communication strategies program so that participants feel comfortable in sharing their feelings and their solutions with one another.

After introductions, for adult patients (and their frequent communication partners, if they are in attendance), a common way to begin a communication strategies program is to ask participants to identify those situations or predicaments in which they most commonly experience communication difficulties. In a group setting, this may be done by going around the table person by person, asking each one talk about why he or she is attending the class, and when and where and with whom each experiences communication difficulties. For instance, one person may feel that group meetings at work pose the greatest challenge. Another person may remark that listening to her granddaughter on the telephone is frustrating. These specific examples can be the focus of problem-solving exercises. Participants can brainstorm how to facilitate communication within specific environments that are problematic for them and how to facilitate communication with specific people they may interact with on a regular basis. By incorporating a consideration of their unique environmental, social, and cultural factors that contribute to communication handicap, patients will leave the program with a better understanding of how to minimize their particular communication difficulties. For children, a common procedure is to ask them to think about how they communicate, and what is the nature of communication breakdowns.

Model for Training

The model presented in Figure 4-1 provides a useful framework for conceptualizing the stages of communication strategies training (Tye-Murray, 1992a; modified by Witt, 1997). The first stage entails formal instruction. The second stage centers around guided learning, and the third stage involves realworld practice. In the ideal program, students move through the three stages sequentially, with one stage providing the foundation for the next. Sometimes a student may revisit a previous stage before advancing to the next one, perhaps to review or refresh important concepts.

Formal Instruction

Formal instruction provides individuals with information about various types of communication strategies and appropriate listening and speaking behaviors; the first stage in a communication strategies training program.

During *formal instruction,* the first stage in the model presented in Figure 4-1, individuals are introduced to the various types of communication strategies and other appropriate listening and speaking behaviors, and they receive examples of each. In a group setting, you might ask people to talk about ways they manage their communication difficulties. You might do so in the context of the communication difficulties that the group has just identified. For example, someone in a group might say, "I have difficulty understanding speech in a noisy restaurant. Since I

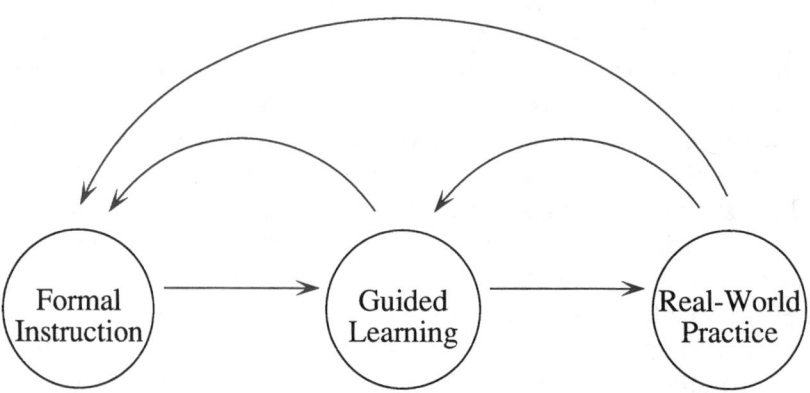

FIGURE 4-1. A framework for conceptualizing the stages of communication strategies training. (From: Witt, S. [1997]. *Effectiveness of an intensive aural rehabilitation program for adult cochlear implant users: A demonstration project.* Unpublished master's thesis, University of Iowa, Iowa City. Reprinted with permission.)

have to eat out a lot as part of my job, this is a big problem." This remark serves as a springboard for a discussion about facilitative strategies. Participants can suggest strategies they have found to be helpful in this specific situation. Their suggestions can lead to a consideration of constructive strategies (strategies to modify environmental listening conditions) and instructional strategies (strategies to influence the communication partner's speaking behaviors). For each solution generated, the group should analyze and evaluate its potential benefits, drawbacks, feasibility, and acceptability.

In the curriculum described by Wayner and Abrahamson (1998), the clinician conducts this kind of formal exercise by asking each person to write down a communication situation that he or she wants to improve. The discussion is then guided until a minimum of 15 possible solutions is generated for each situation. Beforehand, the group reviews a printed handout listing communication guidelines that can enhance communication. The participants in the program take turns reading each guideline aloud. The group discusses why each guideline would help to improve communication. The guidelines include suggestions like, *"Pick the best spot to communicate by avoiding areas that are poorly lit and very noisy," "Look for visual clues to what is being said,"* and, *"Anticipate difficult situations and plan how to minimize problems."*

You may find it valuable to write participants' ideas and responses on a chalkboard or an oversized hanging notebook to stimulate contributions to an ongoing discussion. Formal instruction usually is most effective when the clinician engages everyone in a dialogue as opposed to making a formal presentation, as might occur in a typical university classroom. You will quickly discover that a long-winded lecture and advice-giving alienate (and anesthetize) students (Trychin, 1994).

Guided Learning

The purpose of *guided learning,* the next stage in the model depicted in Figure 4-1, is to encourage people to use conversational strategies in a structured setting. Activities for guided learning include modeling, role-playing, analysis of videotaped scenarios, continuous discourse tracking, attention, and drill activities. Any number or combination of these activities can be included.

In **guided learning,** the second stage in a communications strategies training program, students use conversational strategies in a structured setting.

Example of a Formal Instruction Training Activity

When sections on passive, aggressive, and assertive behaviors are included in the content of a communication strategies training program, participants must reflect on their own styles of handling communication difficulties and consider alternative, perhaps more effective, styles. Below is a paper-and-pencil exercise from Kaplan, Bally, and Garretson (1985) that asks respondents to identify communication styles exhibited in each situation. Answers and discussion are provided afterwards.

A. "Penny entered the office of her boss, the dean. She noticed it was dark and probably it would be hard to speechread. She pushed past the dean's desk (he was sitting at it!) and opened the blinds. Then she sat down and said, 'Let's get this meeting over with.'"

B. "Wilma replaced the battery in her hearing aid and entered the classroom for the course she signed up for, Feminism in the Deaf Community. She immediately noticed that the room was arranged with desk-chairs in a circle. She was relieved to think that this would facilitate speechreading. However, when the rapid-fire discussions began, she had difficulty identifying which of the 22 participants was speaking. Although she was really interested in the topic, she dropped the course the next week."

C. "Harry stopped at his instructor's office after the first day of his geometry class. He was feeling really frustrated because he was unable to understand the questions being asked of the instructor by class members in front of him; he couldn't see their lips. The instructor suggested he move to the front row and look back at the questioners. The next day he was back again. 'I still have a problem,' he admitted. 'I can't identify the speaker quickly enough to speechread. Could we ask the questioners to identify themselves by holding up their hands a little bit longer?' Harry was able to follow class discussions after that."

Answers

A. "Aggressive. Penny's behavior was both rude and demanding.
B. Passive. Wilma didn't try to solve her problem; she gave up on it.
C. Assertive. Harry recognized his problem and worked it out with his instructor" (pp. 37–38).

Modeling

Modeling is a technique often used with children. After a formal consideration of good listening behaviors or communication strategies, the clinician or teacher might demonstrate them through modeling. When modeling, the clinician explicitly points out what is appropriate and inappropriate about the modeled behaviors and does not assume students will automatically recognize this independently. During modeling, the clinician might ask someone in the group or class to help demonstrate the use of a repair strategy. She might pretend to misunderstand a remark spoken by the person. She might then turn to the group and say, "I didn't understand what she said, did you? I'm going to ask her to tell me what she is talking about." *(The asking for a keyword repair strategy.)*

ROLE-PLAYING

A hypothetical conversational interaction is staged during *role-playing.* Participants practice using communication strategies and other assertive listening behaviors. If possible, the situation parallels one that is relevant to the participants' everyday experiences. The use of props helps to make the role-playing more realistic, as if the interaction was really occurring.

In **role-playing,** individuals participate in hypothetical real-world situations and interactions.

For older children and adults, a clinician might set up a restaurant, using a menu as a prop. The clinician can play the part of the waiter, and a member of the group can play the part of the customer. The student is charged with ordering dinner for the family. As the student sits at a chair, examining the menu prop, the clinician asks several questions, such as whether the family wants to order drinks, do they want to hear about the nightly specials, and how would they like their meat prepared. The clinician might occasionally speak with inappropriate speaking behaviors, such as mumbling or speaking in profile. The student must respond to the questions, and when necessary, use facilitative and repair strategies to promote communication. At the end of a role-playing interaction, the clinician and group members review it. They talk about what happened, what worked and what did not work, and what communication strategies were implemented. Sometimes, an effective role-playing scenario is a home living room, where a patient and his or her spouse play themselves and talk about a hypothetical problem. Other situations for role-playing in a group setting include the following:

- Movie theater, where the clinician plays the part of a concession stand worker, and a patient plays the role of a customer
- Bank, where the clinician plays the part of a concession stand worker, and a patient plays the role of a customer
- Party, where a frequent communication partner of one patient pretends to be the spouse of another patient
- Kitchen, where a frequent communication partner and a patient talk about grocery shopping

ATTENTION

The clinician can reinforce formal instruction by focusing group members' attention on both identifying and rectifying environmental problems and appropriate talker behaviors. For instance, a hard-of-hearing man and his normal-hearing wife might be participants in the class. Before speaking, the wife might flicker her fingers and ensure that her husband has turned toward her and is watching her mouth. The clinician might observe to the group, "That was an effective strategy in helping him to speechread. She got his attention first, before speaking, so he could watch her lips."

ANALYSIS OF VIDEOTAPES AND COMPUTER-BASED INTERACTIONS

Videotaped scenarios
provide examples of communication interactions that can be used to discuss communication strategies and stimulation techniques.

Videotaped scenarios help patients identify and talk about their communication problems by providing concrete examples. Individuals view videotaped scenarios that contrast inappropriate with appropriate use of communication strategies (Trychin, 1987a, 1987b). For instance, one scenario might show a couple in the living room. One person has a hearing loss, the other one does not. The person with normal hearing talks behind a newspaper to the other one. The hard-of-hearing person accuses the talker of mumbling and leaves the room in anger. The videotape is stopped at this point so that the class can discuss how the hard-of-hearing person might have effectively implemented an instructional strategy in this context. After the discussion, the class views a second videotape scenario, where the hard-of-hearing person demonstrates how to use an instructional facilitative strategy appropriately.

A CD-ROM-based program, *Conversation Made Easy* (Tye-Murray 2002), demonstrates the use of repair strategies and facilitative strategies. In a typical exercise scenario, a talker appears on the computer monitor and speaks a sentence. Afterward, one of four pictures appear, one of which illustrates the sentence. If the student picks the right picture, the text of the sentence is provided on the screen, the talker then repeats the sentence, and the next sentence in the exercise is presented. If the student picks the wrong picture (by entering a choice onto the computer keyboard), five repair strategies are offered: repeat, speak a keyword, rephrase, simplify, and elaborate (i.e., speak two sentences). Whatever strategy is selected, it happens right away. The talker reappears on the computer monitor and performs the strategy. Occasionally, a listening difficulty occurs. For example, the talker might speak while chewing gum or music might be playing in the background. In these instances, the student can ask that the talker "not chew gum" or "turn off the music." If one of these facilitative strategies is selected, it happens right away, for example, the talker reappears and speaks the sentence without chewing gum. These exercises can be used either in group situations with the clinician and patient, or by the patient practicing communication strategies alone at home or in a classroom or clinical setting. Three versions of the program are available: one for adults and teenagers, one for children who have high level language, and one for children who have low level language.

CONTINUOUS DISCOURSE TRACKING

Continuous discourse tracking is another means to provide guided learning. In *continuous discourse tracking* (DeFillipo & Scott, 1978), the clinician plays the role of *sender* and the patient plays the role of *receiver*. The sender reads a selection from a book, phrase by phrase. After each phrase, the receiver attempts to repeat it verbatim. If the receiver cannot recognize it, then he or she must bear the onus of repair and be responsible for using a repair strategy. For instance, the receiver may say, "Can you tell me in a different way?" The instructor provides coaching and suggestions in how to select and implement particular repair strategies effectively.

Continuous discourse training is an aural rehabilitation technique in which the listener attempts to repeat verbatim text presented by a sender.

Sender: an individual who presents a message.

Receiver: an individual who receives a message from a sender.

Example of a Guided Learning Training Activity

After the patient views the picture in Figure 4-2, a clinician will ask him or her to perform a continuous discourse tracking procedure, with the clinician assuming the role of sender and the patient assuming the role of receiver. The following passage corresponds to the picture (Tye-Murray, 1997). The sender reads it sentence by sentence, and the receiver attempts to repeat it verbatim. When unable to do so, the sender encourages the receiver to use a repair strategy, and request an alteration of the passage so that it can be tracked correctly.

PASSAGE: At Camp Eagle, children learn how to ride horses. Every morning, they arrive at the barn and saddle their mounts. They fall in line behind their camp counselor. The morning ride lasts about four hours. They ride through the forest. Sometimes they pass a lake. Other times, they ride into the mountains. Halfway through the ride, they stop and eat a hearty breakfast. The camp counselor prepares the breakfast over a campfire.

This is what might happen during a continuous discourse tracking exercise:

Sender:	"At Camp Eagle, children learn how to ride horses."
Receiver:	"Something about children and horses."
Sender:	"Yes. Children learn how to ride horses."
Receiver:	"Children learn how to ride horses."
Sender:	(nods) "At Camp Eagle, children learn how to ride horses."
Receiver:	"Didn't get that first part."
Sender:	"Camp."
Receiver:	"Camp?"
Sender:	(nods) "At Camp Eagle . . ."
Receiver:	"At Camp Eagle?"
Sender:	"At Camp Eagle, children learn how to ride horses."
Receiver:	"At Camp Eagle, children learn how to ride horses."
Sender:	"Every morning . . ."
Receiver:	"Every morning . . ."
Sender:	(Presents the rest of the sentence.)

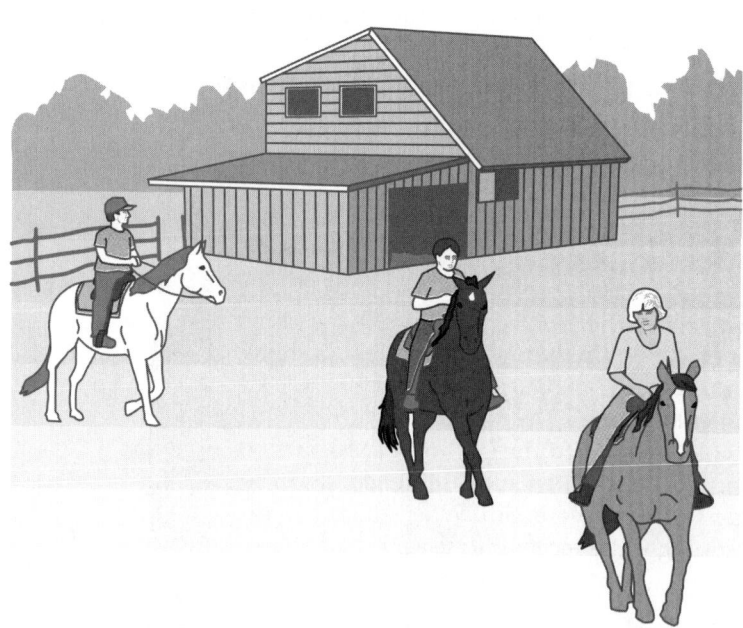

FIGURE 4-2. A picture that provides a context for a continuous discourse tracking task.

Exercise drills also can provide guided learning. An example of a *drill activity* is a sentence identification task (Tye-Murray, 1997), which proceeds as follows. The clinician reads a sentence from a printed text (Table 4-2). A four- or nine-split picture page (Figure 4-3) is laid before the client. The patient's task is to choose the picture that illustrates the sentence. The pictures in a picture-split share similar actors or actions, therefore, the individual must identify more than one or two words in order to respond correctly. Patients must use repair strategies if they are unable to identify the correct picture (e.g., "What about the girl?").

Drill activity: repeated exercises and rote activities.

Table 4-2. For a drill activity, the clinician presents the sentences below. The sentences correspond to the picture set shown in Figure 4-3.

Upper Left Corner

- The man by the maple tree is raking leaves
  The man is raking leaves. (simplify)
  The man rakes the lawn. (rephrase)

- The maple tree is very colorful in the autumn.
  The tree is colorful. (simplify)
  The leaves on the tree have changed color. (rephrase)

Upper Right Corner

- The woman by the fence is raking leaves.
  The woman is raking leaves. (simplify)
  The woman is raking the lawn. (rephrase)

- The picket fence encloses the lawn.
  The fence is around the lawn. (simplify)
  The lawn is bounded by a fence. (rephrase)

Lower Left Corner

- The man is on a ladder picking apples.
  The man picks apples. (simplify)
  The man climbed the ladder to pick apples. (rephrase)

- The ladder is propped against the apple tree.
  The ladder is against the tree. (simplify)
  The man propped the ladder against the tree. (rephrase)

Lower Right Corner

- The woman is mowing the grass with a lawn mower.
  The woman mows the grass. (simplify)
  The woman pushes the lawn mower over the grass. (rephrase)

- Pushing a lawn mower can be hard work.
  Mowing is hard work. (simplify)
  It is difficult to push a lawn mower. (rephrase)

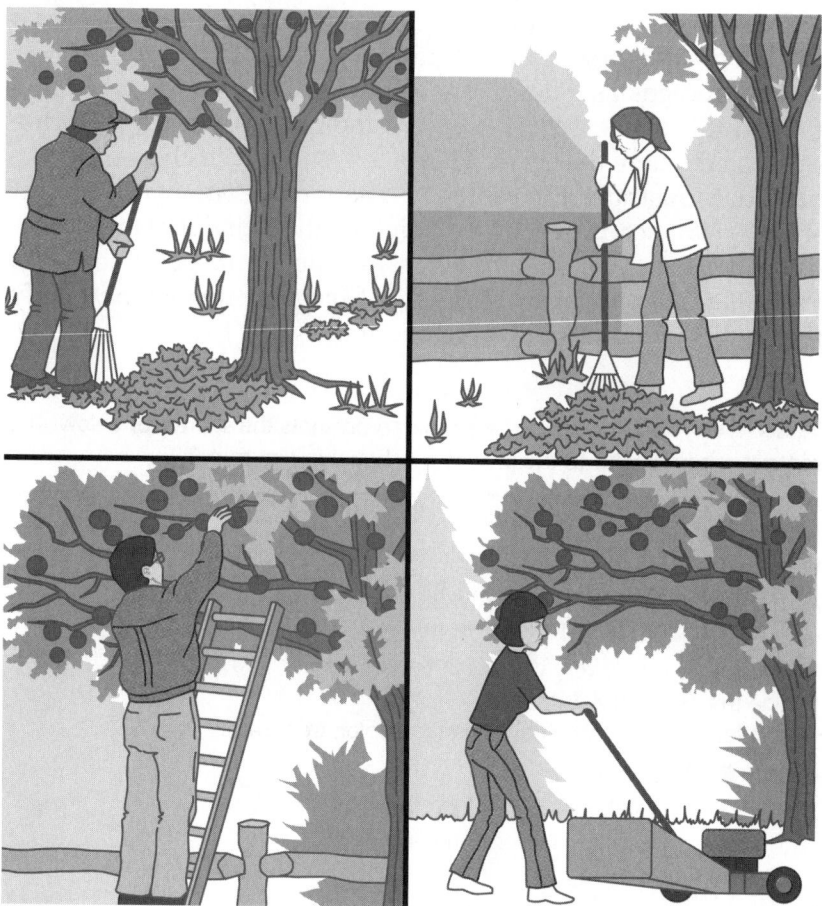

FIGURE 4-3. A four-split picture set that can be used during a guided learning exercise.

In performing this activity, the clinician occasionally may speak with an inappropriate behavior (e.g., while turned away from the student) or in an unfavorable listening environment (e.g., while music from a radio plays loudly in the background). In these instances, the patient can ask the clinician to avoid the speaking behavior or request that the listening difficulty be corrected. This training thus provides practice in using facilitative communication strategies, as well as repair strategies. Frequent communication partners can also engage in guided learning activities. Appendix 4 presents sample workbook pages that promote the effective use of repair strategies.

Real-World Practice

The final stage of the training model shown in Figure 4-1 is real-world practice. ***Real-world practice*** includes activities that students have performed successfully in the classroom and also some activities that require them to communicate in a setting that is highly motivating, such as the office or a social gathering. Individuals can report back to the class about their successes and problems, and they can share ideas of how to handle problems in the future. Instructions for the activity should be provided to the students in written form, in language that is simple and easily understood. The students should have a means to record their experiences and to share them later with their instructor and other members of their communication strategies training group.

In **real-world practice,** the third stage in a communications strategies training program, students practice a new skill or behavior in an everyday environment.

For adults, a real-world training activity might entail completing a worksheet at home. The worksheet might ask the student to select an upcoming communication interaction and to consider possible problems that might arise (e.g., poor lighting or background noise). They list these problems on the worksheet. Then they list possible solutions or preventive measures. After engaging in the interaction, they summarize in writing which solutions they implemented and how well they worked. This worksheet is brought to the next class and shared with the clinician and other class participants.

A patient might maintain a calendar like that shown in Table 4-3. The days of the week are listed in the left-most column, and the

Table 4-3. A calendar for recording a real-world practice activity.

When Did You Repair a Communication Breakdown?			
	WIFE	**SON**	**SISTER**	**CO-WORKER**
Monday	At dinner			Eating lunch in cafeteria
Tuesday		Watching TV		Weekly meeting
Wednesday		Watching TV		On telephone
Thursday	On the drive home from shopping			
Friday			In the car	
Saturday				
Sunday				

patient's frequent communication partners are listed in the row across the top. The patient's task is to indicate when he or she repaired a breakdown in communication by asking the communication partner for a repair. After 1 week, the group leader or the group as a whole can review the calendar with the patient.

Example of a Real-World Training Activity

Topic = Listening for Directions

Instructions: Ask a partner to hide an object somewhere in your house. Then ask your partner for directions for finding it. Only listen as the directions are told to you, and ask for clarification if necessary. After finding the object, answer the following questions:

1. Did you understand the directions?
2. Did you ask for clarification about any part of the directions? If yes, what did you say? How did your partner respond?
3. Did you have any problems in finding the object? If yes, did you ask for more information from your partner? What did you say?

SHORT-TERM TRAINING

So far we have considered procedures for conducting an intensive, relatively lengthy communication strategies training program. The clinician leads an individual or group through three distinct phases, formal instruction, guided learning, and real-world practice, using a variety of procedures and activities.

For many reasons, an extended program such as the one we have considered may not be feasible. A person may not have time to commit to a longer program, or the clinic may not have the personnel available to conduct training. In these situations, short-term approaches are available for providing brief communication strategies training. One approach is to provide materials and self-directed instruction. Another approach is to provide a short tutorial.

Materials Approach

The *materials approach* for providing communication strategies training during a brief time interval includes providing printed and recorded materials to the hard-of-hearing person about communication strategies. This might be accomplished by means of a clinic library, an audio-videotape station, and printed pamphlets.

The library can be established in a small room adjacent to the clinic waiting room or in the waiting area itself. It might include periodicals and books about hearing loss, communication strategies, speech and auditory training activities, and assistive devices. The materials can be read in the waiting room before or after an appointment, or even checked out and returned by mail. A video cassette player also might be placed in the library or waiting room. Individuals can view videotapes about hearing loss and communication strategies.

Short Tutorial

Another way to provide a brief communication strategies training program is by means of a short tutorial. **WATCH** is an acronym that Montgomery (1994) coined to describe his short-tutorial communication strategies training program. This program requires about 1 hour to administer. The acronym represents the following concepts:

WATCH: a brief communication strategies training program.

W = **Watch the talker's mouth, not his eyes.**

A = **Ask specific questions.**

T = **Talk about your hearing loss.**

C = **Change the situation.**

H = **Acquire health care knowledge.**

The clinician discusses with the patient each of these concepts in this order.

During the "W" component, the clinician encourages the patient to focus on the talker's mouth for speechreading, as opposed to hand gestures or other items in the communication setting.

During the "A" component, the patient is taught to use specific rather than nonspecific repair strategies. A clinician might dramatize this point by speaking with a low voice or slurred speech, and then ask the person to use specific repair strategies.

During the "T" component of the program, the clinician discusses the importance of revealing a hearing loss to one's communication partners. A patient can then manage the communication interaction more effectively and implement instructional strategies.

The clinician asks the patient to identify situations in which communication is problematic during the "C component." Together, they consider possible ways to overcome these problems.

Finally, the clinician provides information about health care and hearing loss resources during the "H" component of the program.

A short program such as WATCH may not always result in a momentous change in how a patient uses communication strategies. However, much of the program's value lies in the fact that simple ideas have been reviewed. The individual might reflect on these ideas and develop them or even become motivated to enroll in a more extended communication strategies training program.

■ COMMUNICATION STRATEGIES TRAINING FOR FREQUENT COMMUNICATION PARTNERS

Two parents, Mrs. Ansley and Mrs. Kemp, were asked to instruct their children (cochlear implant users) to perform simple tasks, including unwrapping a mint candy (Tye-Murray & Kelsey, 1993; Tye-Murray, 1994b, pp. 89–90). Each parent and her child sat before a table that held a variety of objects. The goal of the investigation was to determine what would happen in those instances that children misunderstood instructions. Would the parents repeat the message? If so, would these repetitions help their child to recognize the instruction?

In both instances, neither child understood the instruction, *Unwrap the mint,* after their mothers presented it for the first time. Here is what happened next.

Speech

The acronym SPEECH presents a short tutorial about communication strategies for significant others (Schow, 2001, p. 20):

■ **S**potlight your face and keep it visible. Keep your hands away from your mouth so that the hearing-impaired person can get all the visual cues possible. Be sure to face the speaker when you are talking and be a good distance (5 to 10 feet). Avoid chewing gum, cigarettes, and other facial distractions when possible. And be sure not to talk from another room and expect to be heard.

■ **P**ause slightly between the content portions of sentences. Slow exaggerated speech is as difficult to understand as fast speech. However, speech at a moderate pace with slight pauses between phrases and sentences can allow the hearing-impaired person to process the information in chunks.

■ **E**mpathize and be patient with the hearing-impaired person. Try plugging both ears and listen for a short while to something soft that you want to hear in an environment that is distracting and noisy. This may help you appreciate the challenge of being hard of hearing and it should help you be patient if the responses seem slow. Rephrase if necessary to clarify a point and remember, empathy, patience, empathy!

■ **E**ase their listening. Get the listener's attention before you speak and make sure you are being helpful in the way you speak. Ask how you can facilitate communication. The listener may want you to speak more loudly or more softly, more slowly or faster, or announce the subject of discussion, or signal when the topic of conversation shifts. Be compliant and helpful and encourage the listener to give you feedback so you can make it as easy as possible for him or her.

■ **C**ontrol the circumstances and the listening conditions in the environment. Maximize communication by getting closer to the person. If you can be 5 to 10 feet away, that is ideal. Also, move away from background noise and maintain good lighting. Avoid dark restaurants or windows behind you that blind someone watching you.

■ **H**ave a plan. When anticipating difficult listening situations, set strategies for communication in advance and implement them as necessary. This might mean that at a restaurant you communicate with a waitress/waiter instead of having your hard-of-hearing family member or friend do so."

After saying it the first time, Mrs. Ansley repeated the original instruction, "Unwrap the mint." Her daughter, Libby, picked up a red block and threw it gently. "Unwrap the mint," Mrs. Ansley repeated again. Libby gave her a puzzled expression. "Unwrap the mint," her mother said again. Libby picked up a cup and set it on a cardboard box. "No, unwrap the mint." Libby shook a sheet of plastic. "Unwrap the mint," her mother said in response. This interchange continued for 1 minute, until Mrs. Ansley gave up trying to convey the instruction.

In this interaction, the repeat repair strategy was ineffective. No matter how many times Mrs. Ansley repeated the instruction, Libby never understood that she was to unwrap the candy.

The second mother, Mrs. Kemp, adopted a different tact. When her son, Tim, did not understand the instruction, she used different words and said, "Take the paper off the candy." When he still did not comprehend the instruction, Mrs. Kemp said, "Tim, where's the candy?" Tim picked up the mint. "Open it, " Mrs. Kemp instructed. Tim looked at his mother and started to open the candy. "Mmmm," she said encouragingly, "Open it." Tim then unwrapped the mint.

Unlike Mrs. Ansley, Mrs. Kemp used repair strategies other then repetition. She rephrased the instruction (i.e., "Take the paper off the candy."), she emphasized an important keyword ("Where's the *candy*?"), and provided feedback when her son began to understand the message ("Mmmm."). By using a variety of repair strategies, she was able to convey the message successfully.

This investigation, which also included other parents of cochlear implant users, illustrates two important points. First, the repeat repair strategy is not always the optimal strategy to use in repairing communication breakdowns, a topic that we covered in Chapter 2. Second, and of relevance to the current chapter, is that frequent communication partners often do not have an intrinsic knowledge of communication strategies, even if they have lived with a hard-of-hearing person for many years.

Persons with whom the hard-of-hearing person converses with frequently also may benefit from receiving communication strategies training. A frequent communication partner may be a spouse, a son or daughter, a close friend, or a health-care provider. If the hard-of-hearing person is a child, this person may be a parent or guardian. An entire chapter in this text (Chapter 18) is devoted to instruction for parents. The goals of communication strategies training for frequent communication partners are to foster empathy for the difficulty of the speechreading task, encourage the use of appropriate speaking behaviors, learn how to tailor messages so they are easy to recognize, and learn how to repair communication breakdowns effectively.

In many ways, the topics included in a communication strategies training program for frequent communication partners mirrors the content for hard-of-hearing individuals. Table 4-4 summarizes topics that may be reviewed. Frequent communication partners can learn to present their messages with appropriate speaking behaviors. For example, they can learn to speak clearly and slowly and to make sure their faces are clearly visible so the hard-of-hearing person can speechread. Frequent communication partners also can learn to organize their messages. They can learn simple principles for message organization, such as those summarized in Table 4-4. For example, they can avoid verbosity and use semantically simple sentences. Finally, they can learn to use repair strategies (see also Chapter 18).

Communication strategies training for frequent communication partners often is provided at the same time that the hard-of-hearing individual receives training, frequently within the same class. In addition to receiving communication strategies training, they also may receive support and counseling from the speech and hearing professional about adjusting to the changes in life quality that occur because of their relatives' or friends' hearing losses. For instance, frequent communication partners often detect changes in their life quality after the patient incurs a hearing loss (Stephens & Hétu, 1991). Sometimes they report feeling stressed by excessive noise in the home, such as a loud television volume or loud speaking. They may experience annoyance, irritation, or tension as a result of this noise and also as a result of recurring misunderstandings between themselves and the person with hearing loss. Social interactions outside the home may decrease, and feelings of social isolation and loneliness may set in. The frequent communication partner also may have to assume extra tasks as a result of the patient's hearing loss, such as interpreting for the person during group conversations or acting as intermediary for the person's telephone calls. In many cases,

Table 4-4. Content that may be included in a communication strategies training program for frequent communication partners.

Appropriate Speaking Behaviors
Frequent communication partners may be encouraged to:

- Speak clearly and slowly.
- Speak with their faces toward the hard-of-hearing individual.
- Avoid putting objects in or near their mouths while speaking.
- Stand away from windows or bright light sources when talking to someone who has a hearing loss.

Empathy
Frequent communication partners may be asked to consider:

- The difficulty of the speech recognition task when one must rely on a degraded audio signal, perhaps with the use of filtered speech samples.
- The difficulty of the lipreading task.
- How stress and anxiety levels may rise when someone has a hearing loss, and how persons with hearing loss often may experience fatigue and desire social withdrawal.

Organized Messages
Frequent communication partners may be asked to:

- Avoid verbosity, and to use concise and syntactically simple sentences. For example, they might say, *Let's go to a movie,* rather than *I haven't really thought much about it, but I know we aren't doing much on Saturday, so maybe let's go to a movie.*
- Avoid ambiguity by using precise terminology. For example, they may say, *The sweater is Sarah's,* rather than, *It's hers.*

Comprehension
Frequent communication partners may be encouraged to:

- Ask their partner often if he or she comprehended a message.
- Ask for verification and listen to the hard-of-hearing person repeat or paraphrase what they have just said.
- Provide feedback about whether the individual correctly recognized the message.

Repair of Communication Breakdowns
The frequent communication partner may receive coaching about how to use repair strategies optimally. Following a communication breakdown, they might:

- Repeat their messages.
- Rephrase their messages, and say it in a different way. For example, the sentence, *I left* may be rephrased as *I went home.*

Table 4-4. (continued)

■ Repeat a keyword, to indicate the topic of conversation. For example, if the sentence, *Tom fell down* was not recognized, the communication partner might repair the communication breakdown by saying, *Tom. Tom fell down.*

■ Simplify the message by using fewer words or by using more commonplace words. For example, the sentence, *Jane bought a brown bowler hat* might be simplified to *Jane bought a hat.*

■ Elaborate, by providing more information and repeating important key words. For instance if the sentence, *I cut the paper* was misunderstood, the frequent communication partner might say, *I have some scissors. I cut the paper with the scissors.*

■ Build from the known, by presenting information that can easily be recognized to establish a context. For instance, the original sentence might have been, *Please put the wallet in my purse.* In repairing a communication breakdown, the communication partner may say, *Please put the wallet* (and then point to the wallet) *in my purse* (with a gesture toward a purse).

---

communication strategies training, along with counseling, can enhance and accelerate the adjustment process that frequent communication partners may have to undergo.

■ COMMUNICATION STRATEGIES TRAINING FOR CHILDREN

Children who have hearing impairments also may benefit from communication strategies training. The program content may focus on facilitative and repair communication strategies, as we have been discussing for adults in the foregoing sections.

Facilitative and Receptive Repair Strategies

CD-ROM-based training programs and one-on-one printed programs are currently available for providing training for facilitative strategies and receptive repair strategies (Tye-Murray, 2002b). Often, programs for children are simplified when compared to those designed for adults. For example, children might receive instruction for only three repair strategies (e.g., *Say it again, Tell me in a different way, What are you talking about?*), because other strategies, such as asking for an elaboration, may involve abstract concepts that are too difficult for them to grasp.

FORMAL INSTRUCTION

Formal instruction for children might include a review of effective listening behaviors (e.g., *Pay attention, Watch the talker's face, Try to identify key points*) and how to ask talkers to clarify a message (e.g., *When you don't understand a message, ask the talker to say just one word. This will tell you what he or she is talking about.*). Most children will experience great difficulty in applying concepts learned during formal instruction to the give-and-take of everyday conversation. Indicating that a communication breakdown has occurred in a gracious and socially acceptable manner can be challenging for even the most accomplished conversationalists. Moreover, finding the words to instruct the talker is not easy. Children will need abundant opportunity to practice repairing communication breakdowns, and the clinician probably should reiterate formally taught concepts many times in an informal way, in many different contexts.

As an example of formal instruction, a group leader might ask her young students to consider the basic nature of the communication process (Elfenbein, 1994, pp. 129–132). The group leader explains that communication entails a transmission of a message. The group might then generate examples of communication, with the group leader listing each item on the whiteboard: for example, a dog growling at another dog, two children speaking together, a gym teacher signaling that recess is over. Through this process, children realized that they play two roles in the communication process, *sender* (expressing themselves) and *receiver* (understanding messages generated by others). This discussion lays the foundation for an exploration of communication breakdowns and reasons why messages are not understood and what children can do to prevent or rectify breakdowns. The group leader might show videotaped scenes of different kinds of communication breakdowns and why they might occur to stimulate discussion (Table 4-5). Whereas some sources of communication breakdown may be obvious to students (e.g., "I can't hear when the TV is turned up too loud.") other sources may not be obvious (e.g., the sender used an ambiguous pronoun to specify the subject of a sentence).

Table 4-5. Causes of communication breakdown that might be generated by children during a group discussion.

- "The TV is too loud."
- "I can't see the talker's lips."
- "I'm sitting too far back in class. Can't hear and can't see very well."
- "She talks funny."
- "I don't know those words."

GUIDED LEARNING

Guided learning for children focuses the child's attention on good listening behaviors and communication strategies. The child practices the behaviors and strategies in a structured setting, via modeling and role-playing. As with adults, in *modeling,* a child might watch the clinician as he or she demonstrates the desired behavior and then try to imitate it. In role-playing, as with adults, a hypothetical listening situation is created, wherein the child must listen and use communication strategies. When setting up a scene for role-playing, the speech and hearing professional should select situations that are important to the child, for example, a department store or movie theater. The props should be as realistic as possible so that the child feels as if the interaction was really occurring (Tullos, 1990).

In **modeling,** an instructor demonstrates a behavior and the student attempts to imitate it.

Example of a Guided Learning Activity for Children

To foster an understanding of the communication process, "have the children create scrapbooks that contain examples of the ways people communicate. Use a combination of the children's own drawings, photographs, and representative items such as a birthday card. Include situations from home, school, and community. Discuss each entry. Decide what the message is, what modality or modalities were used, and who the senders and receivers were." (Elfenbein, 1994, p. 140)

Table 4-6. Guidelines for developing real-world practice activities for children.

A. Assign a real-world practice activity that the child has performed successfully during guided learning practice.

If the child is to ask someone to repeat a message following a communication breakdown, the youth first should practice asking for clarification in the classroom or clinical setting. Then the child can be asked to attempt the strategy in for example, art class. Although not necessary, the art teacher can be briefed beforehand that the child will practice repair strategies with her or him.

B. Select a communication situation in which the child will feel motivated to communicate.

For instance, a young child might be asked to use repair strategies when ordering food at a fast food restaurant.

C. Select an interaction that allows the child to experience some success.

For example, you might ask the child to interact with a familiar teacher before asking the youth to try using repair strategies with an unfamiliar store clerk.

D. Provide instructions for the activity. Present the instructions with simple language and vocabulary.

The purpose of a homework activity might be to listen for the main points of a one-paragraph narrative. The clinician might provide the following written instructions:

This envelope contains a story. Ask your mother to read it to you. Watch and listen carefully. If you do not understand the story, ask questions. Draw a picture about the story.

E. Provide a means for the child to record the experience.

In the activity described in letter D above, the record is the child's drawing.

Source: Adapted from Glennon, S. L. (1990). Homework activities for social skills training. In P. J. Schloss and M. A. Smith (Eds.), *Teaching social skills to hearing-impaired students* (pp. 85–90). Washington, DC: Alexander Graham Bell Association for the Deaf.

REAL-WORLD PRACTICE

Once a child has practiced communication strategies in structured settings, he or she may apply them to everyday experiences. Real-world practice activities help children transfer their use of communication strategies to natural settings. Activities should require them to interact with different talkers, in a variety of contexts. Guidelines for developing real-world activities for children are presented in Table 4-6.

Expressive Repair Strategies

In addition to learning how to use facilitative and receptive repair strategies, children also can learn to use expressive repair strategies. Expressive repair strategies may be appropriate to use when the child presents a message, usually with speech, and the communication partner does not recognize it. The child then

Table 4-7. Five-step plan of action from teaching children to use communication strategies.

Step 1. Understanding Basic Communication Processes
A. Sender-message-receiver relationship
B. Ways to communicate (e.g., speech, sign, writing, mime, gesture)

Step 2. Understanding Communication Breakdowns
A. Definitions and examples
B. Causes of communication breakdown
C. Ways people signal confusion

Step 3. Message Formulation
A. Information to be transmitted
B. Evaluation of the receiver's position (e.g., background knowledge)
C. Evaluation of sender's abilities (e.g., speech proficiency)
D. Environmental constraints (e.g., background noise)
E. Social constraints (e.g., conventions of politeness and etiquette)

Step 4. Introduction of Communication Repair Strategies
A. Receiver's responsibilities
   1. Acknowledge confusion
   2. Identify causes of breakdown
   3. Implement receptive repair strategies
B. Sender's responsibilities
   1. Be alert to signals of confusion
   2. Identify causes of a communication breakdown
   3. Implement expressive repair strategies

Step 5. Practice Using Communication Repair Strategies
A. Move from sheltered environments to the real world
B. Move from transmission of simple to complex more complex messages
C. Discuss feelings associated with communication breakdown

Source: Adapted from Elfenbein, J. (1994). Communication breakdowns in conversations: Child-initiated repair strategies, In N. Tye-Murray (Ed.), *Let's converse: A how-to guide to develop and expand the conversational skills of children and teenagers who are hearing impaired* (pp. 123–146). Washington DC: Alexander Graham Bell Association for the Deaf.

repairs the communication breakdown, perhaps by trying again using his or her best speech or by adding hand gestures.

Table 4-7 summarizes a five-step training plan of action for teaching children to use expressive repair strategies (Elfenbein, 1994). Formal instruction and guided learning can be provided during the first four steps. Real-world practice is provided in the fifth step.

In this plan, children begin by reviewing principles of basic communication processes and consider the sender–message receiver relationship and the various ways of communicating. Children may create a book about the ways people communicate, tearing pictures from old magazines for illustrations.

The next step, Step 2, entails talking about communication breakdown: What happens when a breakdown occurs? how can you tell that it has happened? Why did it happen? Here, children might generate a list of the ways that people signal a breakdown.

Step 3 focuses on message formulation. In this step, the group leader asks the children to consider how best to formulate and transmit their messages. This entails considering the needs of the communication partner, such as how much information does the receiver already have. For instance, if the child uses the pronoun, *he*, will the receiver know who is the referent? If the child talks about last summer's vacation, will the receiver know anything about the locale visited? In addition to considering the needs of the receiver, children also are asked to consider their own abilities. What kind of language will they need to express themselves? Do they have the speech skills necessary to convey their message or should they use another modality to express themselves? Finally, during this step, children are asked to be aware of environmental factors. Is there background noise? Will the receiver rely on speechreading to understand what they say? Is the lighting adequate? In an exercise to develop these skills associated with Step 3, children might consider why an abbreviated form of a message, such as *chocolate milkshake*, might work in one context, such as when ordering at a fast-food restaurant, but not in another, such as when riding in a car and the child wants to ask his or her mother to make a chocolate milkshake when they arrive at home.

Step 4 focuses on introduction of expressive repair strategies. This is a step in which children learn that both sender and receiver share responsibilities in the communication process. The receiver's responsibility is to signal when a breakdown occurs and how it might be repaired. The sender's responsibility is to enact the repair. A variety of repair strategies are considered, and children practice revising their own messages using different words and practice modifying their listening environments (e.g., turning off a radio). One of the most important messages conveyed during this step is that children share responsibility in managing their conversational interactions, and they have a variety of options available to them for rectifying their communication breakdowns.

Children might play a game in which they are assigned a particular expressive repair strategy, such as mime. Communication breakdowns can be simulated, and children can implement their assigned repair strategy.

The final step in the model presented in Table 4-7 provides practice in using communication repair strategies. At this time, children might talk about their feelings and responses to communication breakdown. Often, it is reassuring to learn that their classmates have experienced similar frustration and embarrassment following a communication breakdown. They can be videotaped using a repair strategy during a conversation with a school secretary or another teacher. Later, the class can view the videotape and critique the interaction. In practicing repair strategies, children progress through increasingly difficult settings: role-playing, then sheltered environments, then real-world situations. Children do not advance to the next context until they have mastered the preceding one. Having a conversation with a schoolteacher is an example of a sheltered environment; using repair strategies at the corner drug store is an example of a real-world situation. In these practice sessions, children first work in pairs or in teams—having a buddy along enhances confidence and resourcefulness—and then later, alone. The group leader provides coaching as needed. After each interaction, the class discusses the tactics and strategies used during an interaction (e.g., Did this work? Were you comfortable doing this?) and some of the feelings that the children experienced during the event.

■ EFFICACY OF TRAINING

Few experimental investigations have focused on the efficacy of communication strategies training. So the question remains, is training beneficial to those who receive it? Preliminary data suggest the answer to this question is *yes*. Abrahamson (1991) reported that 89% of the patients who began a 6-week communication strategies training program completed it. Attendance rates at the classes averaged 85%. Their willingness to stay with the program suggests that participants were benefitting from it. Another investigation showed that patients changed how they used repair strategies after participating in a communication strategies training program that concentrated on repair-strategy use (Tye-Murray, 1991). Following training, subjects began to use the repair strategies they found were especially helpful during their training sessions. For example, if during the course of training an individual found that asking for the topic of conversation helped him or her to understand an unrecognized message, then the individual was more likely to begin using that strategy. Finally, Kricos and Holmes (1996) provided active listening training to a group of older adults with hearing loss. The program included both speech perception training and emphasis on use of communication strategies. Following training, subjects showed improved speech recognition and enhanced psychosocial functioning.

Little if any work has focused on the efficacy of communication strategies training for children.

▬ FINAL REMARKS

Communication strategies training can empower many students to manage their communication environments more effectively. However, students will vary in the extent to which they benefit. Some individuals are incapable of changing their communication behaviors. Some do not have the meta-communication skills to examine their conversational styles and may not be able to monitor how they interact with their communication partners, regardless of the quality or amount of instruction. For example, an elderly woman might not use communication strategies and might deal with communication problems with excessive aggression, but these behaviors are a part of her personality and likely will not change with aural rehabilitation intervention. In these instances, it is critical that individuals who interact frequently with the hard-of-hearing person receive instruction as well.

▬ KEY CHAPTER POINTS

✔ A communication strategies training program should be tailored to accommodate a patient's expectations, age, socioeconomic background, life style, and particular communication problems.

✔ The content of a communication strategies training program centers around problems specifically related to hearing loss and how these problems can be minimized. Training may be provided for facilitative and repair communication strategies. Patients may also consider assertive versus nonassertive listening behaviors.

✔ One model for a training program includes three stages: formal instruction, guided learning, and real-world practice. A variety of exercises and activities can be used for each stage.

✔ A communication strategies training program for children can include instruction for the use of expressive repair strategies in addition to the use of receptive repair strategies and facilitative communication strategies.

▇ MULTIPLE CHOICE QUESTIONS

1. When designing a communication strategies training program (select the statement that best applies):
    a. A clinician can implement any one of many available published curricula, which are applicable to almost all patients.
    b. A clinician typically designs a curriculum for patients and another one for frequent communication partners.
    c. A clinician tailors the intervention according to the specific concerns of the patient, experienced at the point of time at program entry.
    d. A clinician decides whether to focus on repair or facilitative strategies.

2. At the beginning of a communication strategies training program, the clinician often reviews rules for group interactions. The reason for this is:
    a. To establish a safe and secure environment where patients feel comfortable in sharing their feelings and their solutions
    b. Because there are always time constraints, to ensure that people do not digress once the class gets going, and that the extensive curriculum content is covered in the limited time available

    c. To ensure that frequent communication partners understand their role in the program

    d. To serve as an ice-breaker and an exercise in assertive behavior

3. A clinician stands up at a whiteboard and lectures the group about how to manage the communication environment. During the presentation, slides and overheads are used to supplement the talk. Which statement best describes this technique for formal instruction?

    a. A prelude to real-world practice

    b. A good way to conduct formal instruction because visual aids support the spoken message, and persons with hearing loss can easily follow the lecture

    c. A means to ensure that both the patient and the frequent communication partner share the same information, and hence, start from the same playing field

    d. An ineffective way to convey information to a communication strategies training group

4. Which of the following activities is something that might happen during guided learning?

    a. Patients describe their most difficult listening situations.

    b. Patients practice ordering in a restaurant in a simulated interaction.

    c. Patients take a multiple choice test.

    d. Frequent communication partners quiz patients on the night before each class about what they learned at the last communication strategies training class.

5. What is continuous discourse tracking?

    a. A way to track one's use of repair strategies during real-world conversations

    b. An example of a guided learning activity

    c. A way to assess conversational content

    d. A communication strategy in which patients inform their frequent communication partners about what they understood

6. A classroom teacher says to a student, "Mary, you told me what you heard. Now I know what information you missed. I find that helpful in helping to understand what I just said." This is an example of:

   a. Modeling

   b. Role-playing

   c. Formal instruction

   d. Attention technique

7. For real-world activities, students should:

   a. Have a means of recording their experiences so they can later share the results with the group

   b. Select a situation that will be challenging enough to test the limits of their abilities

   c. Never be asked to do something that might lead to an unsuccessful communication interaction

   d. Develop the activity at home, as a homework assignment

8. Mr. K. lives in a rural town in Illinois. His clinician lives several hours away. The most feasible intervention for Mr. K. might be, at least initially:

   a. Guided learning drill activities that he can do at home

   b. A workbook and set of how-to pamphlets

   c. A short tutorial

   d. A correspondence course

9. One of the key principles that children learn during an expressive communication strategies training program is that:

   a. The general public does not understand the nature of hearing loss.

   b. They can take charge in managing their communication difficulties.

   c. The most effective way to receive a message is to ask people to speak slowly.

   d. Nonverbal communication entails fewer communication breakdowns than verbal communication.

APPENDIX 4-1

A guided learning activity for frequent communication partners.

■ USING THE REPHRASE REPAIR STRATEGY

Suppose you said the following sentences to your hard-of-hearing family member. Indicate how you would repair the communication breakdown if the person did not recognize your message.

You say: "The cereal is on the counter."
Your family member says: "Huh?"
You say (using words better specified by context): _____

You say: "I'm going to the mall on Saturday."
Your family member says: "I didn't get that."
You say (using a different sentence structure): _____

You say: "We'll drive to the grocery store."
Your family member says: (nothing. Shrugs shoulders)
You say (using a different sentence structure): _____

You say: "Get the soda cans from downstairs."
Your family member says: "What?"
You say (using words that are more visible on the lips): _____

When this worksheet is completed, the participants might discuss the responses. The clinician might point out that instead of saying cereal in the first communication breakdown, the frequent communication partner might have used the name of the cereal (e.g., Frosted Cornflakes). The use of a more specific word, in context (i.e., when the box of Frosted Cornflakes is visible to the hard-of-hearing person) is often more recognizable than the use of a more generic word. In the second and third breakdowns, the frequent communication partner might have said, "This weekend, I'll go to the mall," and "I'll drive you to the grocery store." In the last example, the partner might say, "The pop cans are in the basement." The word *pop* is more visible on the mouth than the word *soda*. The word *basement* is more visible on the mouth than the word *downstairs*. Hence, both alternative words would be easier for a hard-of-hearing person to speechread.

APPENDIX 4-2

An example of a guided learning activity for frequent communication partners.

USING THE SIMPLIFY REPAIR STRATEGY

In the following paragraph, circle the words that you might omit if your family member did not understand you the first time that you spoke it.

Janice put the hamburger condiments on the table just before lunch. So all you have to do is bring out the paper plates and napkins. Meanwhile, I'll be working at the barbecue cooking the meat patties.

Here is an example of how a frequent communication partner might simplify the paragraph above:

Janice put the condiments on the table. You bring out the paper plates and napkins. I'll barbecue the meat.

APPENDIX 4-3

An example of a guided learning activity for frequent communication partners, in this instance, parents or guardians (taken from Tye-Murray, 1994b, p. 111).

USING THE KEYWORD REPAIR STRATEGY

The situation in which the conversation is occurring may influence what keywords you select to repeat. Below, the same sentence has been spoken in two different contexts. How would you use the keyword repair strategy to repair the communication breakdown in each setting?

You are standing by a closet. In the closet is a small school box, a paper sack, and a backpack. You say, "The calculator is in your backpack." Your child does not understand the sentence. You say (using the keyword repair strategy):

_____

_____

Your child is trying to figure out how much he has earned from his garage sale. He has a small pile of receipts. You say, "The calculator is in your backpack." Your child does not understand the sentence. You say (using the keyboard repair strategy):

_____

_____

_____

In the first situation, you might have selected the word *backpack* to repeat (e.g., "Backpack. The calculator is in your backpack.") to distinguish between the three options of a school box, a paper sack, and the backpack. In the second situation, you might have selected the word *calculator* to repeat because you want to focus your child's attention on what to look for in the backpack.

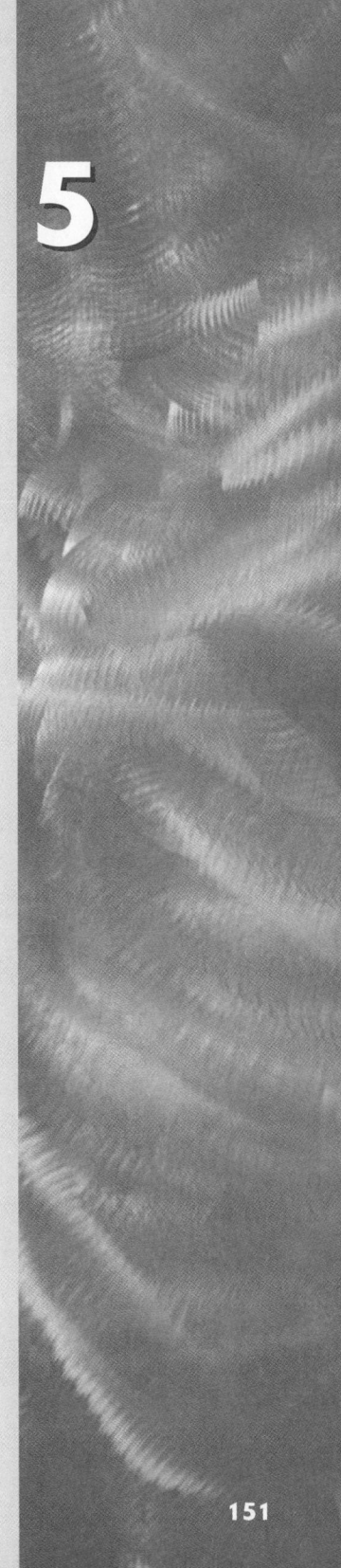

CHAPTER 5

Counseling, Psychosocial Therapy, and Assertiveness Training

TOPICS

- Who provides counseling, psychosocial therapy, and assertiveness training?

- Counseling

- Psychosocial therapy

- Assertiveness training

- Related research

- Case study

- Final remarks

- Key chapter points

- Multiple choice questions

- Key resources

In Chapter 4, "Communication Strategies Training," we considered the nuts and bolts of providing communication strategies training, or how to put tools in the toolbox of conversation management. In some respects, this is a simplistic view of the problems that hard-of-hearing people encounter and the solutions they can enact. Individuals can have the tools, but if they do not have the confidence, motivation, self-esteem, or wherewithal to use them, then the tools are not much use. In this chapter, we review counseling, psychosocial therapy, and assertiveness training as they pertain to hearing loss.

One goal of an aural rehabilitation plan often is to help patients and frequent communication partners realize the effect of hearing loss on their lives and to develop the skill sets and self-acceptance to carry on conversations with each other, using communication strategies effectively. Counseling techniques, psychosocial therapy, and assertiveness training are means to achieve this goal.

There is a fine line between counseling, psychosocial therapy, and assertiveness training, and often the boundary between where one begins and the next ends is gray. Whereas counseling may center only on issues directly related to hearing loss, psychosocial therapy may dig deeper and delve into the realms of a person's self-image and personal relationships. Assertiveness training may focus on conversational behaviors and effective means for interacting with other people. In the following discussion, we consider general counseling principles, psychosocial therapy, and assertiveness training.

■ WHO PROVIDES COUNSELING, PSYCHOSOCIAL THERAPY, AND ASSERTIVENESS TRAINING?

The aural rehabilitation specialist often provides counseling to patients and their frequent communication partners. This person might be an audiologist, speech-language pathologist, or a teacher of the hard-of-hearing. Sometimes the patient may receive counseling from another health-care professional, such as a physician, nurse, or occupational therapist. Counseling might be provided in the context of an audiological examination or during the development of an individualized family service plan, or it may be provided during times specifically designated for this purpose, such as when a group of adults enroll in a communication strategies training class.

Aural rehabilitation specialists may also participate in providing psychosocial therapy. When this happens, the aural rehabilitation specialist often teams up with a certified psychosocial therapist or a clinical psychologist. The goals of psychosocial therapy are often interwoven with the goals of communication strategies training. Similarly, the aural rehabilitation specialist may provide assertiveness training in the context of communication strategies training or may team up with a mental health care professional. Advantages of a team approach are that patients benefit from receiving the expertise of two types of professionals, and the two professionals can model and role-play desirable behaviors. In cases when the participants have profound losses, and assistive listening devices cannot be used, one professional can write notes on a whiteboard or hanging easel, while the other professional leads the discussion. Disadvantages relate to the cost of labor and the logistics of arranging for the professionals to be at the same place at the same time.

■■ COUNSELING

There are many reasons to include counseling in an aural rehabilitation plan. Counseling often provides patients with the following benefits (Erdman, 2000):

Counseling may target the head, the heart, or the behaviors of an individual.

- Enhanced understanding of hearing loss and its effects on communication
- Better self-disclosure and self-acceptance
- Greater knowledge about how to manage communication difficulties
- Reduced stress and discouragement
- Increased satisfaction with aural rehabilitation services
- Increased motivation to minimize listening problems
- Stronger adherence/compliance with the aural rehabilitation plan, including use of amplification

Types of Counseling

Clinicians often provide three kinds of counseling: informational, rational acceptance and adjustment, and emotional acceptance and adjustment (Alpiner & Garstecki, 1996; Wylde, 1982). These are summarized in Figure 5-1.

After a hearing test, an audiologist often explains the nature and degree of hearing loss to the patient, usually in conjunction with a review of the person's audiogram. There also may be a discussion of the benefits and limitations provided by a hearing aid and

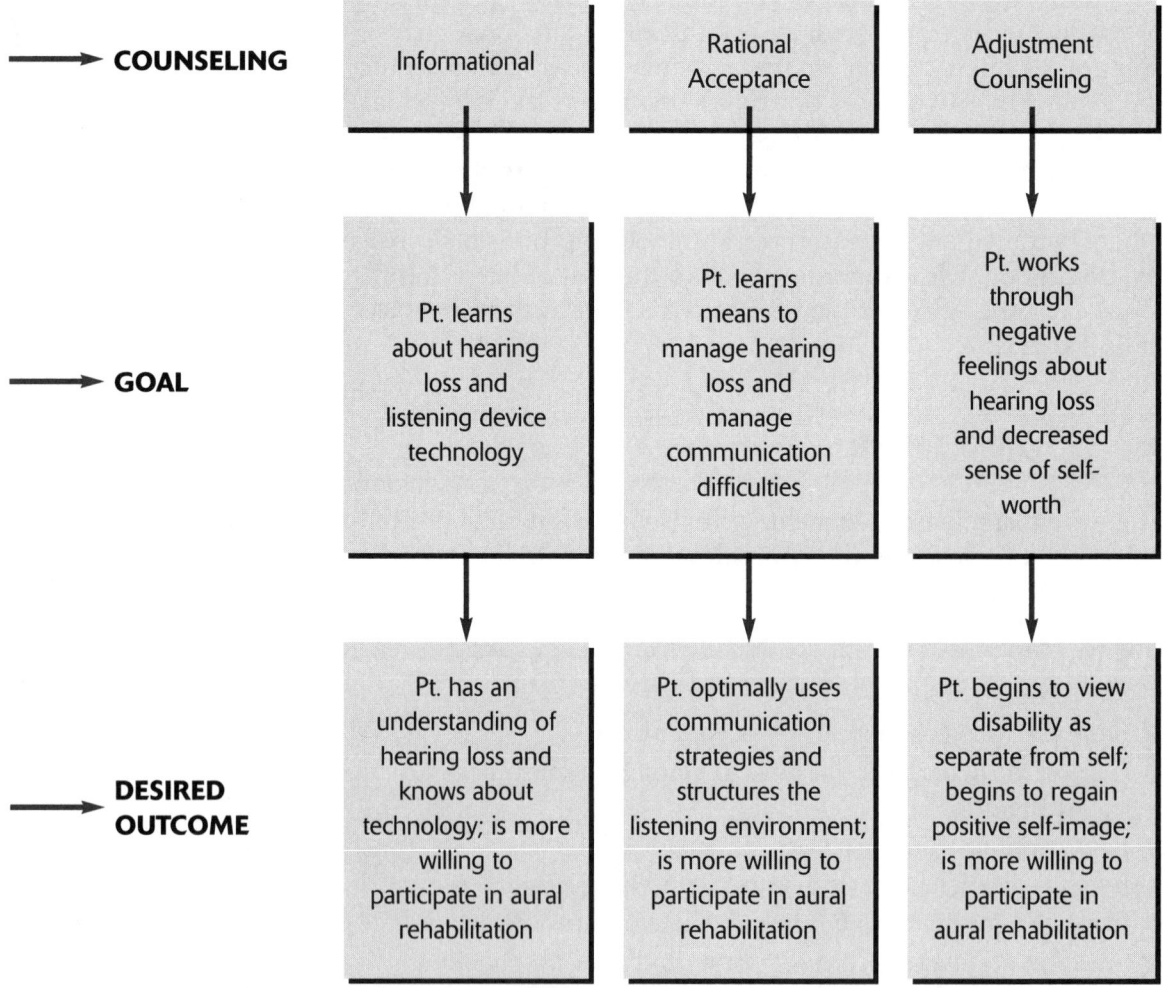

COUNSELING	Informational	Rational Acceptance	Adjustment Counseling
GOAL	Pt. learns about hearing loss and listening device technology	Pt. learns means to manage hearing loss and manage communication difficulties	Pt. works through negative feelings about hearing loss and decreased sense of self-worth
DESIRED OUTCOME	Pt. has an understanding of hearing loss and knows about technology; is more willing to participate in aural rehabilitation	Pt. optimally uses communication strategies and structures the listening environment; is more willing to participate in aural rehabilitation	Pt. begins to view disability as separate from self; begins to regain positive self-image; is more willing to participate in aural rehabilitation

FIGURE 5-1. Three kinds of counseling provided in the aural rehabilitating setting. (Pt. = Patient)

possibly a hands-on demonstration. In this interaction, the audiologist provides ***informational counseling.*** The professional instructs, guides, and gives expert information.

Patients and their clinicians may discuss communication strategies and ways to improve communication at home and at school. During ***rational acceptance and adjustment counseling,*** clinicians focus on the permanence of the hearing loss and may introduce concrete means for managing communication difficulties. For instance, an audiologist might recommend specific assistive devices to use, such as a telephone amplifier.

Central Tenets

Although there are many different counseling techniques, at least three central tenets of Roger's person-centered counseling theory are often appropriate for use with adults in the aural rehabilitation setting (Rogers, 1980). These tenets as they apply to audiologic counseling are considered by J. G. Clark (1994) and summarized here.

A first tenet of person-centered counseling is ***congruence with self.*** This tenet means that clinicians act as themselves and do not assume an imposing facade of professionalism. Instead of saying to a first-time patient: "Your audiogram indicates a mild-to-moderate sensorineural hearing loss bilaterally with a conductive component," a pronouncement replete with professional jargon, an audiologist might instead say, "I know you are worried about your hearing. My tests seem to agree with your impression that you are not hearing as well as you used to hear. I'd like to answer your questions." With the former statement, the audiologist might inadvertently increase the patient's anxiety. With the latter approach, the audiologist has validated the patient's own opinions and allowed the patient to share the lead in discussing the test results.

A second tenet to follow when providing counseling is ***unconditional positive regard.*** The clinician assumes that patients know best and that they have the inner resources to overcome their communication difficulties. The professional accepts patients as human beings of stature; respects them regardless of their employment or social status; and brings appropriately placed empathy, sincerity, and caring to the interaction.

Informational counseling includes imparting information about the hearing loss and the benefits and limitations of amplification.

Rational acceptance and adjustment counseling focuses on the permanency of the hearing loss and concrete means of managing communication problems.

Congruence with self is the first tenet of person-centered counseling in which clinicians act as themselves in interactions with patients and do not assume a facade of professionalism.

In **unconditional positive regard,** the second tenet of person-centered counseling, clinicians assume that patients know best and assume that they have the inner resources to overcome their conversation difficulties.

Empathetic understanding is the third tenet of person-centered counseling. The counselor listens to the patient's concerns and feelings about the hearing problem, reflects them back to the patient, and helps the patient identify solutions.

Roger's third tenet is *empathetic understanding.* The clinician listens carefully as patients perhaps rationalize or deny their hearing difficulties, as they talk about their concerns and feelings, and as they express their ideas and solutions. The professional establishes the patient's viewpoints, reflects them back, and then helps the patient identify solutions. For example, a person might cite the soft presentation level as a reason for poor performance on a word discrimination test. In this instance, the audiologist would probably not say, "I presented the words at a normal conversational level, Mr. Smith. There is no doubt you have a word discrimination problem."

Instead, in order to show empathy and respect for the patient's feelings, the audiologist might respond, "I know the words were not very loud for you. Are there occasions during your typical day when speech seems too soft to hear?" With this remark, the patient's impressions are acknowledged, and the test results are related to situations that are relevant.

Counseling Techniques

Although there probably as many different approaches to counseling as there are professional counselors, the various approaches can be broadly sorted into three general categories: approaches aimed at modifying thought process *(cognitive)*, approaches aimed at modifying behavior *(behavioral)*, and approaches aimed at modifying emotions *(affective)* (Erdman, 2000). In practice, most counseling entails a combination of these approaches.

A cognitive approach to counseling (e.g., Ellis & Grieger, 1977; Beck & Emery, 1985) relies on intellectual means for addressing problems related to hearing loss. In this approach, faulty thought processes are assumed to underlay inappropriate emotional responses to hearing loss and to underlay erroneous assumptions and self-image difficulties. The aural rehabilitation specialist implements logic to direct and redirect individuals' thoughts, belief systems, perceptions, values, ideas, and opinions. This educational experience is designed to increase self-worth and decrease inferiority feelings and discouragement. For instance, a woman with hearing loss may believe she can no longer serve on a charitable board because her hearing loss prevents her from understanding everything that is said during meetings. The clinician might

Gathering Information

Effective counselors learn how to listen to and observe their patients. This approach means attending to both the patient's verbal and nonverbal messages, and doing so in a way that is nonjudgmental and accepting. Effective counselors also listen to the message behind the message, instances when patients may say one thing but mean something else (Luterman, 1996, calls this "listening with the third ear"). When listening to verbal messages (Citron, 2000):

■ Make eye contact.
■ Fully face the patient.
■ Lean forward about 20° so your forearms can rest on your thighs.
■ Be consistent in your attending postures so as to communicate interest in the patient and what the patient has to say.

When observing nonverbal messages, consider (Citron, 2000; Madell, 2000):

■ The patient's appearance. For example, a slovenly appearance, slow body movements, and a sad expression may suggest low energy level and minimal readiness for help.
■ The patient's behavior. A seemingly uncooperative or sour person may be feeling ill-equipped to cope with the communication situation and the hearing loss.
■ The patient's punctuality. Patients who are chronically late for appointments or miss them may lack motivation for services.
■ Where is the hearing aid? Parents who carry their child's hearing aid in a purse when they arrive for an appointment may be expressing their distress or frustration.

Some messages your "third" ear may detect include (Citron, 2000, p. 468):

■ *"I'm not vain but. . . ."* The patient may be telling you that he or she would never wear a hearing aid that is visible to others.
■ *"I would never spend that. . . ."* The patient might be using financial considerations as an excuse not to confront the hearing problem or to try a hearing aid.
■ *"If everyone talked like you. . . ."* The patient may believe that his or her communication difficulties are not due to hearing loss, but rather, due to other people not speaking clearly.

counter this by asking her to consider her experience and expertise, which brought her to serve on the board in the first place, and then by asking her to consider some of the ways she might enhance the communication setting during meetings. Sometimes the clinician is passive in a process like this, and at other times, the clinician might direct a counseling session using didactic questioning that may be both accepting and confrontational at the same time. The goal is to eliminate cognitive distortions and arbitrary assumptions and to replace them with positive thoughts and positive perspectives. Techniques that are used in cognitive approaches include questioning, interpreting, goal setting, creation of contracts, and homework assignments. An example of a homework assignment appears in Figure 5-2, and an example of a contract appears in Figure 5-3.

---

1. Choose a person at work, a friend or neighbor, or someone in your extended family and tell the person that you have just received a new hearing aid.

2. Explain to this person the benefits and limitations you perceive your hearing aid will afford you.

3. You might use the results of the speech tests that we collected during your appointment today to explain how well you now understand speech.

FIGURE 5-2. A counseling homework assignment.

Personal Contact

Name:_____

Clinician:_____

Before I return to my next appointment, I will:

■ Explain to people that I have a hearing loss

■ Use repair strategies when I do not understand a spoken message

■ Not scold myself when I do not recognize a message

■ Remind my wife to use optimal speaking behaviors so that I may understand her, using language that is assertive but not aggressive

Signed: _____

Date: _____

FIGURE 5-3. Example of a contract that might be issued during a counseling session.

Skinnerian learning theory (Skinner, 1953, 1971) forms the basis for most behavioral approaches to counseling. This approach often focuses on observable and measurable behavior foremost, with the idea that changes in cognitive and emotional adjustment will follow behavioral changes. For example, a businessman might hyperventilate before major meetings because he fears he may not understand the other participants' remarks. The clinician may first ask him to identify those physical symptoms he experiences in response to stress (Figure 5-4), and then introduce him to relaxation techniques, such as that described in Figure 5-5. Behavioral techniques such as this work directly on the physical response to stress.

Right before a major meeting, I worry that I will not understand what is said at the conference table. I experience the following physical symptoms of stress:

My head pounds.

My palms sweat.

My heart beat races.

My stomach churns.

I feel short of breath.

My neck aches.

I feel dizzy as I walk toward the conference room.

My mouth goes dry.

After the meeting, I think about my performance. Once I get home, I feel the following emotions:

Depression

Anxiety

A sense of being on edge

Anger

FIGURE 5-4. A behavioral approach to counseling may include asking a business man who has hearing loss to identify his stress-reactions to business meetings.

- Focus on point one inch below navel, in the middle of your body

- Breath deeply

- Expand lower abdomen as you breathe in

- Flatten abdomen as you breathe out

- Perform exercise for 10–20 minutes

FIGURE 5-5. Relaxation techniques can reduce stress responses. These techniques may be reviewed in a behavioral counseling approach (Hogan, 2001).

Finally, in addition to cognitive and behavioral approaches, counseling might take an affective approach. An affective approach (e.g., Rogers, 1980) centers on feelings and on fostering emotional adjustment to hearing loss. The clinician creates an empathetic, accepting environment in which patients can evaluate self-concepts and their reactions to hearing loss. The goal is phenomenologic: Patients change how they view themselves and their place in the world, even though their circumstance may remain the same. By receiving unconditional positive regard from the clinician, the patient develops a sense of being loved and cared for because the patient is who he or she is. As noted in the previous section, central tenets of Rogers' affective approach are congruence, positive regard, and empathetic understanding.

Targeting Counseling

As you develop your aural rehabilitation strategy and implement a plan, you will want to consider how best to target counseling for particular concerns. For example, one hard-of-hearing patient, Candice Brown, commented to her audiologist, "I worry that I can't be there for my 13-year-old daughter the way I want to be. It's too much of an effort for her to talk to me, she says. Lately, she just tunes me out." In this case, the aural rehabilitation plan might include the following counseling tactics:

- Provide informational counseling by enrolling Candice and her daughter in a group communication strategies training program. Thus, both Candice and her daughter will learn about difficult listening situations, appropriate speaking behaviors, and communication strategies.

- Provide rational acceptance and adjustment counseling, and help Candice understand that communication between a teenage daughter and her parent is universally problematic and not just an issue for a hearing-impaired mother. Encourage Candice in the optimal use of amplification and appropriate assistive devices such as telephone amplifiers.
- Provide emotional acceptance and adjustment counseling by involving the daughter and Candice in aural rehabilitation group sessions, where both will have an opportunity to share their frustrations, feelings, and ideas for solutions.

■ PSYCHOSOCIAL THERAPY

Counseling may be expanded to include psychosocial therapy in some instances. Psychosocial therapy is particularly valuable when patients' emotional responses to hearing loss are negative and when they have experienced communication failure and other people's disapproving attitudes. The goal of therapy is to facilitate emotional adjustment in the context of the aural rehabilitation plan. The outcome is increased self-acceptance, increased self-confidence, and more effective use of communication strategies.

Losing one's hearing can be devastating, particularly if the loss is severe enough to result in isolation from society. The loss, and concomitant changes in how the hard-of-hearing person relates to family, friends, and co-workers, can decrease one's self-confidence and foster a negative self-image, which may be reinforced by others' reactions, including their stigmatization. Because acquired hearing loss may cause a restriction in one's activities and create unsatisfactory interactions, depression may follow (Kerr & Cowie, 1997). For example, Knutson and Lansing (1990) showed that profoundly deaf adults were likely to be depressed, introverted, lonely, and experience social anxiety, particularly if they had inadequate communication strategies. Hétu and Getty (1991) found a prevalence of a negative self-image among individuals with hearing loss.

Individuals who suffer a hearing loss, whether it is sudden or gradual, often develop a sense that they have gone from being "able-bodied" to being "abnormal." They no longer are able to communicate as easily as they once did, and they may no longer be able to perform their professions and daily responsibilities as effectively because of hearing loss. Their social and emotional interactions may be less rewarding than before, and they may have lost or diminished their sense of independence and self-sufficiency. One woman, when asked how she was different now that she had a hearing loss, responded, "I feel like the world dumped on me." A man, asked the same question, responded, "I feel like I'm a piece of driftwood drifting away."

Individuals who are born with hearing loss, or who acquire hearing loss early, may also experience isolation and a negative self-image, especially as they begin to realize they are in some ways different from others in their social and school environments. Preadolescents and teenagers who are mainstreamed into hearing classrooms, in particular, may experience self-adjustment issues. If the hearing loss has been present since birth, the individual may have developed a self-image of being different, and perhaps, less capable than others.

Because hearing loss has a deleterious impact on interactions with others, the hard-of-hearing individual may have a psychological experience that is closely related with the social consequences of the disability. These consequences may include being ostracized by peers; loss of job opportunities; changes or limitations in everyday roles (e.g., as a spouse, a parent, a friend); and attendant levels of stress, anxiety, isolation, and fatigue (Getty & Hétu, 1991; Hétu & Getty, 1991; Hogan, 2001). A psychosocial feedback loop may develop, where the impaired social, vocational, or academic function related to the hearing loss stimulates a negative self-image (e.g., "I'm inadequate."). A person's coping responses may in turn deteriorate or not develop, and the person may experience limited confidence and feelings of help-lessness and unworthiness (Heydebrand, Binzer, Mauzé, Tye-Murray, & Skinner, submitted; Hogan, 2001).

For many deaf and hard-of-hearing persons, the stress that re-sults from their communication difficulties and their perceived inabilities is debilitating. One reason they may seek psychosocial therapy is to understand who they are, what has happened to them, and to get their lives moving forward. Raymond Hétu and Louis Getty at the University of Montreal performed some of the seminal work on developing a psychosocial therapy paradigm for adults who have hearing loss (Getty & Hétu, 1991; Hétu &

Getty, 1991). Their approach (sometimes referred to as *The Montreal Method*) was based on two principles:

1. "Knowing that hearing disabilities affect not only the victims themselves, but also anyone with whom they interact, rehabilitative help must consider several levels of coordinated interventions in order to reach the target individuals, families, social networks and institutions; and

2. In order to facilitate the interaction between victims of [hearing loss] and others, a change in attitudes and behavior is required" (Hétu & Getty, 1991, p. 306).

Their objectives were threefold:

1. "To offer a psychosocial support to help affected [patients] and their [frequent communication partners] to better deal with the effects of hearing loss;

2. To allow the [patients] and their [frequent communication partners] to understand the nature and the consequences of the hearing problem; and

3. To develop new skills that will help in coping with the effects of hearing loss" (Getty & Hétu, 1991, p. 318).

Others who have built on this work include Hallberg (1996, 1999) (working in Sweden), Hogan (2001) (working in New Zealand and Australia), Stephens (1996) (working in Great Britain), and the team working at the Central Institute for the Deaf and Washington University Medical School (Heydebrand, Binzer, Mauzé, Tye-Murray, and Skinner, submitted; Binzer, Mauzé, Tye-Murray, Heydebrand, & Skinner, submitted). In common practice, psychosocial therapy is incorporated into communication strategies training. Psychosocial therapy helps patients recognize:

- The impact of hearing loss on their lives and self-image.
- How they may have internalized negative perceptions about hearing loss.
- How these negative perceptions limit their living a full and satisfying life.
- How new attitudes about themselves and others may allow them to live life in a new and proud fashion, where pride can be defined as made up of "self-confidence, ability, self-esteem, security, a sense of the future, and a sense of where I fit in the world" (Hogan, 2001, p. 18).

Psychosocial therapy is typically provided in small groups of three to eight persons. Often, the participants' frequent communication partners are encouraged to attend the sessions, as they play a profound role in shaping the participants' self-image and self-confidence. The therapy may be provided in intensive sessions over 2 or 3 days for 8 hours a day, or might be provided in shorter sessions over the course of several weeks. A sample curriculum for a 2-day program is presented in Appendix 5-1. This curriculum was adapted from Hogan (2001), which in turn drew heavily from Getty and Hétu (1991).

Problem-Solving Framework

The framework for psychosocial therapy is a problem-solving model (Figure 5-6). Through a series of activities or exercises, participants learn to identify the kinds of problems they are experiencing, understand the nature and affect of these problems, and then finally, generate effective solutions for resolving them.

PROBLEM IDENTIFICATION

During problem identification, the participants turn the spotlight on the issues. Problem identification can begin by asking the participants in a psychosocial therapy group, *What's the worst thing about living with a hearing loss?* (Hogan, 2001). Both the person with hearing loss and the person's frequent communication partner should be encouraged to respond to this question. Answers can be written on a whiteboard or a hanging easel. Figure 5-7 presents an array of responses that might be elicited during this activity. As this figure demonstrates, the worst thing might range from specific situations that might be easy to address, such as an inability to hear the doorbell, to more general and more difficult-to-address responses, such as depression, stress, anger, and feelings of stupidity. This exercise can be emotionally wrenching for some, as it may be painful for participants to verbalize their diffi-

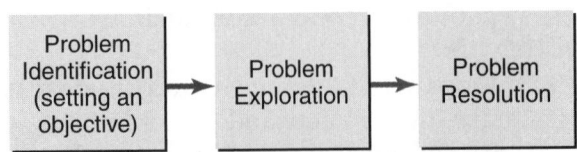

FIGURE 5-6. A problem-solving framework for psychosocial therapy.

Joe:	"I can't hear the doorbell. People come and ring the doorbell and they think we're not home or I'm rude."
Darren:	"Having to ask a couple of times what is being said. I get exasperated and frustrated."
Katie:	"Missing out and feeling isolated. I miss the social aspect of being in a group of hearing friends and understanding what they're saying. I also miss not being able to go to movies, and having to wait for the videos to come out. Feeling left out. How many times have I stayed at home because I didn't want to be bored?"
Gaylyn:	"People treat you like you're two years old or stupid. It makes me feel very, very mad."
Mary:	"I've kept it in for so long I can't get the words out. I get angry, depressed, and tongue tied."
Joan:	"Stress with my partner."
John:	"I tend to shut myself in. If we were having a class reunion tomorrow I wouldn't go because I would have to explain to fifty people about my hearing loss. It makes me uncomfortable."
Jerry:	"I miss music."
Archie:	"Having to ask for help."

FIGURE 5-7. Responses generated during an identification activity to the question, What is the worst thing about living with hearing loss? Respondents are adult cochlear implant users.

culties to others or to consider how their lives have been affected by the presence of hearing loss. In some cases, the group leader may realize that the psychosocial issues of a particular individual may require referral for more in-depth psychotherapy.

Often, the problem identification segment of the program includes establishment of objectives, which helps make a problem manageable. For example, one woman identified her problem as, "Because I have a hearing loss, my husband and I never talk any more." To tackle this issue in every conversational setting and at every time of day might be overwhelming. However, if the woman were to identify the problem, then establish a well-defined objective, problem solving could be targeted in a concrete manner. For instance, in this case, the woman was asked to identify those times when conversation was most important to her. She responded, "Before I begin to fix dinner, after I get home from work." The objective for this woman and her husband then became, "I would like to converse effectively with my husband for 30 minutes every night before I begin to fix dinner." Solutions were then generated to meet this objective (problem exploration, described next) and included, *sit together in a quiet place before dinner, turn off the television for thirty minutes*, and *refuse to take phone calls during this time.*

The difficulties identified during this stage of therapy will help guide the remainder of the program. For example, if stress seems to be a common theme in the responses, then the participants can discuss ways of managing stress and practicing relaxation techniques. If managing communication breakdowns seems to be the prevailing theme, then the group can focus on using repair strategies effectively.

Problem Exploration

Move the Flowers?

In an exploration scenario, the group leader set up the following situation:

I'm your wife/husband's cousin. I am having a pretty big dinner party. I want you to meet some of the other people at my party so I am not going to sit you next to your partner. The flowers are in the center of the table. Would you ask me to move the flowers?

Here is the dialogue that ensued:

Jim:	"I would explain the situation. I might say, 'It would help me to read lips and participate in conversation if you move the flowers.'"
Group Leader:	"Is that explaining part hard to do?"
Jim:	"Yes. Admitting a problem is hard to do."
Sue:	"It's hard. It's not fair that we always have to come up with a solution or that we have to explain things."
Mary:	"When you're a guest in someone's home, you hate to impose on them. After all, it's their house so why should you be telling them what to do?"

Notice that during this exercise, some of the emotional underpinnings that prevent people from using facilitative strategies are revealed. Jim is embarrassed to tell people that he has a hearing loss. Sue resents that the onus of managing the communication environment always falls on the person who has hearing loss. Mary feels she does not have the right to impose on others.

Once problems are identified, they can be explored in more depth. During problem exploration, the group focuses on the personal and social impact of hearing loss. In so doing, they address the social realities of hearing loss, the impact on the conversational partner of living with a hard-of-hearing person, and the difficulty of seeking accommodations to hearing loss from other persons. For example, asking a person to turn off the background music requires self-confidence and a healthy self-image (e.g., *I have the right to communicate as effectively as I am able at this gathering*), trust in the communication partner (e.g., the partner could become annoyed or the partner could develop a negative perception of the person with hearing loss as a result of the request), and a willingness to be rejected (e.g., the partner could say no). Often, during periods of exploration, participants in a group will realize they do not manage their communication problems effectively because they do not want to draw attention to their hearing loss, they are fearful of others' reactions, or they want to take the easiest course of action.

Two means of engaging in problem exploration are through creating scenarios and compiling self-profiles. In creating a scenario, the group leader might describe a hypothetical situation:

I'm inviting you to my party. There will be lots of people out there. We are going to cook hamburgers and hotdogs out on the grill. The party will be at night, so I'll have a few lanterns burning. And oh yes, I'm going to have some great music. My brother is lending me his boom box. What would keep you from joining us?

The responses to this kind of scenario might range from, "I won't be able to lipread anyone," and "The music will be too loud to hear anything," to "No one will talk to me because I'm deaf," and "Parties are boring, I just stand off by myself."

As they speak about their reasons for avoiding social situations, the group can explore why they might behave in the ways they predict (e.g., *I don't want to burden people; It's not fair to my wife to have to interpret everything for me*) and what their options are for dealing with difficulties.

In compiling a self-profile, the participants are asked to describe themselves to each other. This might entail them pairing off and taking turns talking to one another, or drawing a picture of themselves, or creating a collage using pictures torn from magazines.

For instance, in one therapy session, participants were divided into groups of three and asked to construct a collage using pictures cut out from a stack of old magazines. One group included a picture of a woman falling out of her high heel shoes and another picture of a woman with her back to the camera, holding a telephone receiver to her ear. When describing their collage to the others, the group members noted that the woman falling out of her shoes conveyed their sense of feeling off balance in a hearing world. The woman with her back to the camera conveyed their feelings of being ignored and excluded in everyday events.

PROBLEM RESOLUTION

"If a patient requests information, the response [of the audiologist or speech and hearing professional] should provide information, and if the patient expresses an emotion, the response should let the patient know that the emotion was acknowledged and respected."

—English, Mendel, Rojeski, & Hornak, 1999, p. 35

Problem resolution is the third stage of the process illustrated in Figure 5-6. Some of the techniques described in Chapter 4, "Communication Strategies Training," can be employed during this stage, particularly if managing communication problems and difficult listening situations have been cited during problem identification and exploration.

In developing ways to resolve problems, individuals may engage in self-examination and ask themselves such questions as, *What are my rights as a person with hearing loss? What are the consequences of not managing my problems effectively? How will I feel if I successfully overcome this difficulty?*

Some of the ways to identify solutions are through role playing (e.g., pretending that two participants are ordering food in a restaurant with loud background music and poor lighting), modeling (the group leader models desirable behavior), and brainstorming.

Gagné and Jennings (2000, p. 569) present a step-by-step process for problem solving. First, they suggest that the group or an individual sets an objective and defines a desired outcome. For example, an objective might be, "Mr. Smith will use repair strategies during his weekly bridge game. As a result of his participation in this class, he'll be able to understand messages intended for him after using one or two repair strategies." Step two in this problem-solving process is to identify possible solutions. For each of the solutions, the implications of using it (e.g., its feasibility, acceptability, potential advantages and disadvantages) are considered. The third step in problem solving is to select a solution and to try it out. Finally, the benefits of applying the selected solution are considered, as well as the factors that facilitate or hinder its implementation.

Example of the Problem Identification-Exploration-Resolution Framework

In an actual session, Mary, the wife of a hard-of-hearing man, said that the most difficult aspect of living with someone who has hearing loss was as follows:

I'm working in the kitchen and John is in the living room reading. It takes a very, very, very long time for him to respond to me. He hears talking but he doesn't respond.

After identifying this problem, the participants in the group explored it. They asked the couple about other times when this kind of communication difficulty occurs. They discussed who has control of the situation and who has responsibility. The group leader asked whether the situation could be changed. What core beliefs may get in the way of thinking about the possibility of change? During this discussion, Mary noted ruefully, "If you say something he wants to hear, he'll respond."

This remark prompted another member of the group to observe, "You can't jump to conclusions. I just make sure my mother hears what I say and then I wait for a response."

Later in this discussion, some of the emotional undercurrents of the couple's communication problem emerged:

Mary: "I enjoy talking and he doesn't. Finally, I have to just cut it off. There is no point aggravating myself. He doesn't talk anymore, but when I want an answer, I get it."

Ben: "This is kind of frustrating or aggravating. Hearing loss is a frustrating situation because now you cannot achieve what you would like regularly. I would love to communicate with her. I would like to talk on the phone, listen to music, and not just noise. A hearing problem is very frustrating."

During the resolution phase of this issue, the group leader asked the participants to generate a list of possible solutions. Here is what they came up with:

- Mary go over to Ben and wave.
- Mary yell.
- Mary throw something at Ben to get his attention.
- Mary repeat.
- Mary tap him.
- Ben read the paper in the kitchen.
- Ben help prepare dinner.
- The couple sit together in a quiet, well-lit room for 20 minutes every night before Mary starts to prepare dinner. Communicate then, when conditions are optimal.

The group leader suggested that the couple pick one, try it, and then review its effectiveness.

Assertiveness Training

Although some people who have hearing loss are comfortable with using communication strategies in a secure clinical setting, or even in home situations with familiar communication partners, many often have difficulty using them in other environments. These persons might benefit from assertiveness training. The goal of assertiveness training is to increase the cooperativeness between the person with hearing loss and his or her communication partners, while still maintaining equality among the participants who engage in a conversation (e.g., Trychin, 1987a, 1988; Trychin & Wright, 1989). Patients develop neutral, nonaggressive behaviors that allow them to maintain their self-esteem without encroaching on the rights of others and that allow them to engage in satisfying conversational interactions. Key elements of assertiveness training entail learning:

■ Ways to indicate a hearing loss (e.g., "I have a hearing loss. I may not understand everything you say to me.")
■ Means to request a change in the communication environment (e.g., "The light in here is dim. I'm having difficulty reading your lips. May we walk over to another room?")
■ Ways to suggest how the communication partner can facilitate the patient's understanding of spoken messages (e.g., "It helps me to understand you if I can clearly see your face.")
■ Means to provide positive feedback to communication partners to reinforce desirable behaviors (e.g., "I appreciate your coming into the room to talk to me. Thank you.").

Assertiveness training often encourages people to use language that is not accusatory. Training also focuses on a patient's right (and responsibility) to understand what is being said in a conversation.

During **assertiveness training,** emphasis is placed on choice of language and on the consequences of behaviors. For example, patients may compare the consequences of using language such as, "You never speak clearly when I try to talk to you on the phone even though you know I have a hearing loss!" to those resulting from a statement such as, "It helps me to understand what you are saying when you speak at a slow but not too slow speaking rate." Whereas the former statement is accusatory and puts the communication partner on the defensive, the latter is a neutral statement that provides explicit guidance about how the communication partner can foster understanding.

■ RELATED RESEARCH

Research suggests that these interventions are effective and that people want these services. For example, patients who do not receive counseling are less likely to use their hearing aids than patients who received counseling. Counseling reduces the amount of hearing handicap perceived by persons who have hearing loss (Brooks, 1979; Taylor & Jurma, 1999) and increases their knowledge about hearing-related issues (Borg, Danermark, & Borg, 2002). After a psychosocial-based communication training program, workers with noise-induced hearing loss were more confident in dealing with their hearing difficulties (Getty & Hétu, 1991), and persons with occupational hearing loss realized at least short-term gains (Hallberg, 1996). Adult cochlear implant users spent significantly less time in conversational breakdowns during conversations with an unfamiliar communication partner following their participation in an intensive 2-day psychosocial workshop (Binzer, Mauzé, Tye-Murray, Heydebrand, & Skinner, submitted). Moreover, 12 months following their participation, the adults identified concrete ways they managed communication difficulties that formerly seemed challenging. They also reported fewer maladapted behaviors, such as withdrawing, as measured by the CPHI.

However, Borg et al. (2002) did not note a change in measures of conversational fluency on average among their 13 subjects and their frequent communication partners, including the frequency of communication breakdowns (although two of the three subjects with the most frequent rate of breakdowns decreased the frequency postintervention), and no change in the use of specific versus nonspecific repair strategies. Their program is a departure from those described in this chapter in that the hard-of-hearing patients only participated in counseling and psychosocial therapy, and then they were responsible for addressing the communication problems of their frequent communication partners. The investigators did find, during interviews conducted 1 month following the intervention, that participants reported increased understanding and insight regarding hearing loss and felt increased self-esteem. For communication partners, irritation for the hard-of-hearing person had decreased.

Patients and their families want these services. As just one of many possible examples, Sweetow and Barrager (1980) found that 20% of parents did not feel comfortable asking their audiologists questions. Over one third of them believed their audiologist did not provide them with adequate emotional support.

CASE STUDY 1

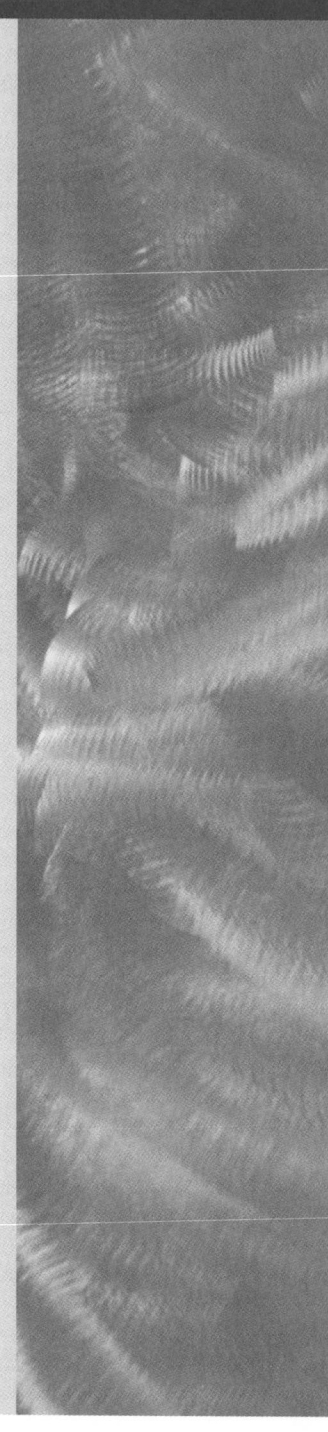

In assessing the effects of an intensive two-day psychosocial workshop for cochlear implant users and their spouses, we developed a before-and-after measure. The "Before" question asked them to described a common situation where it was difficult for them to manage hearing another person. Then in a series of "After" questionnaires, we asked them to revisit their "Before" answer (we provided them with a photocopied version of their remarks) and determine whether they were managing the situation differently. Here are the responses of Diane, a 39-year-old woman who had used a cochlear implant for 2 years. After reading each response, consider how you might lead a group of students through a discussion of her situation, at each point.

Baseline Challenging Situation

[Diane wrote,] "Conversations in groups of three or more in a dark or noisy environment are most difficult, especially if my friends are talking about something exciting. By the time I figure out who is talking, I've missed half of what was said, and then another person starts talking and I have to locate them."

Three-Month Challenging Situation

"I am more assertive in asking friends to repeat what I've missed using appropriate strategies. Sometimes if the conversation is going too fast, I will raise my hand, ask for a time-out, explain to everyone that I can understand them better if they speak slower or one at a time or raised their hand before talking—depends on if we are in a meeting or a social gathering. Occasionally, I may quietly ask someone next to me a small part of what I missed . . . rephrasing what I heard and having them fill me in to catch up on the conversation."

(continues)

Six-Month Challenging Situation

"Really no change from 3 months ago. I continue to stop and ask friends to repeat or fill me in on conversation. If I get a key word, I may paraphrase it silently to someone next to me in order to catch up. I am doing well and have made significant progress."

Twelve-Month Challenging Situation

"Managing well. I usually ask the group to speak one at a time and at a slower pace. Sometimes they forget and the topic is 'heated' or very fast paced and I will stand up and make a Big 'T' and say, 'Time out please; I'm having a hard time keeping up with the conversation, can we slow it down so I can hear and understand what is going on?' I sometimes have to do this two or three times but I've noticed over time that another member of the group will take the time to slow things down and remind others. It just takes repetition and I've gotten *much* better."

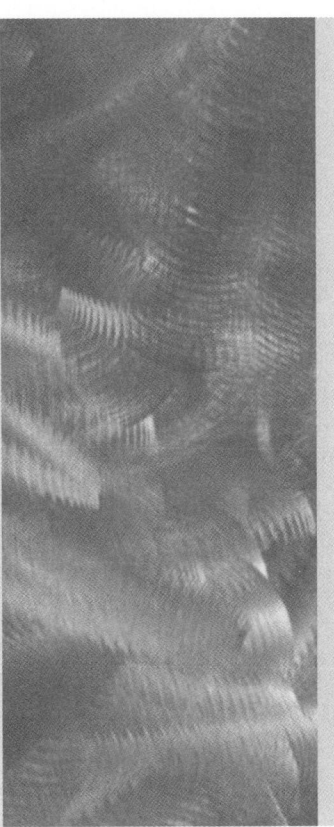

■ FINAL REMARKS

There is a tremendous need for aural rehabilitation specialists to learn how to effectively provide counseling to their patients and to ensure patients receive the kinds of support necessary so they best communicate in their everyday environments. Hearing aids and other listening devices alone are not the answer. Between the aided ears rests a feeling, thinking person who may be struggling with the changes hearing loss has wrought in his or her world. When persons experience a catastrophe in their lives, it is not unusual for the educational and health-care systems of our country to provide emotional and psychological support. Certainly, hearing loss should be afforded the same status as other negative life events.

◼ KEY CHAPTER POINTS

✔ Counseling provides many benefits to hard-of-hearing individuals and their families, including better self-acceptance and reduced stress and discouragement. A clinician might provide information counseling, rational acceptance and adjustment counseling, or emotional acceptance and adjustment counseling.

✔ Counseling approaches are often categorized as cognitive, behavioral, or emotional, or a combination of any of these three.

✔ Individuals who suffer a hearing loss, whether it is sudden or gradual, often develop a sense that they have gone from being able-bodied to being abnormal. Some of these individuals might benefit from psychosocial therapy.

✔ Psychosocial therapy aims to facilitate emotional adjustment to hearing loss. The outcome is increased self-confidence, increased self-acceptance, and more effective use of communication strategies.

✔ In a problem-solving approach, patients learn to identify the kinds of problems they are experiencing, understand the nature and effect of these problems, and generate effective solutions for resolving them.

✔ During assertiveness training, individuals learn to increase cooperativeness with their communication partners and to develop neutral nonaggressive behaviors that allow them to maintain their self-esteem without encroaching on the rights of others.

✔ During assertiveness training, emphasis is placed on choice of language and on the consequences of behaviors.

✔ Sometimes losing one's hearing constitutes a catastrophic life experience. Individuals require and deserve adequate emotional and psychological support.

◼ MULTIPLE CHOICE QUESTIONS

1. An intervention that focuses on conversational behaviors and effective means for interacting with others can best be described as:

    a. Assertiveness training

    b. Rational acceptance counseling

    c. Psychosocial therapy

    d. Empathetic understanding intervention

2. Someone who behaves in a genuine fashion and who does not assume a façade of professionalism is said to have:

    a. Unconditional positive regard

    b. Empathetic understanding

    c. Congruence

    d. Rational acceptance

3. Mrs. G. has just been told she has a hearing loss. She does not know much about the anatomy of the ear, hearing loss, hearing aids, or assistive listening devices. At this point, the clinician is most likely to provide:

    a. Informational counseling

    b. Personal adjustment counseling

    c. Rational acceptance counseling

    d. Communication strategies counseling

4. Mr. Z. has a noise-induced hearing loss, incurred after years of working in a noisy factory. Some of the feelings he might be experiencing most likely include:

    a. Ear pain

    b. Remorse

    c. Social anxiety and depression

    d. Determination to obtain optimal hearing health care

5. The stages of a problem-solving approach in psychosocial therapy are:

    a. Problem exploration, research, solution

    b. Problem identification, exploration, resolution

    c. Problem resolution, practice, review

    d. Problem exploration, identification, management

6. Psychosocial therapy typically focuses on all of the following except:

    a. The impact of hearing loss on self-image.

    b. The spouse's ability to deal with the effects of hearing loss.

    c. Understanding the time course of hearing loss over time.

    d. Negative attitudes about self and others.

7. Creating a scenario is one means of initiating:
    a. Counseling
    b. Self-profiling
    c. Exploration
    d. Problem identification

8. Patients' frequent communication partners are often encouraged to attend psychosocial therapy sessions for many reasons, but especially because:
    a. They need to understand the effects of hearing loss on speech recognition.
    b. Research suggests that patients are more likely to attend intervention sessions if they are accompanied by their spouses.
    c. They too can learn assertive conversational behaviors.
    d. They play an influential role in shaping patients' self-images and self-confidence.

KEY RESOURCES

The curriculum for the St. Louis Psychosocial Hearing Rehabilitation Workshop (Heydebrand, Binzer, Mauzé, Tye-Murray, and Skinner, submitted). Persons who use cochlear implants and their frequent communication partners attend this 2-day workshop.

Day One

9:30–9:45 Introduction

Fitting of Group FM assistive devices

Outline of group

■ About communication strategies (and why it may be hard to use them)
■ Problem identification
■ Problem exploration
■ Problem resolution

Ask group to generate rules of group communication

- Right to pass on responding to a question
- Mutual respect
- One at a time
- Confidentiality
- "I" statements
- Speak, as you want others to speak to you—"clear speech"
- When you finish speaking, signal

Goals

What do you expect from the group? What do you hope to gain by the end of this workshop? [Have participants write down individual goals.]

9:45–10:30 Ice breaker: Spondee exercise: Select one of the spondee cards (e.g., "base" or "ball") and introduce yourself to the person who has the other half of your word

- What do you expect to get from your participation in this workshop?

10:30–10:40 Break

10:40–11:15 What's the worst thing about living with a hearing loss? For example, What do you miss? If you could change something, what would you change? What frustrates you or upsets you the most?

This group workshop is designed to:

- Help you better understand the problems you face
- Identify strategies for dealing with these difficulties

11:45–12:00 Susan's dinner party (schematic of the living room where the party is being held is included in your materials folder)

- Would you come to my party? Why or why not?
- Will you have a good time? Why or why not?
- What might your partner do?
- If you don't do anything, why?
- What does it feel like?
- If you don't come, what would you say to me?

Introduction to choices, what is hard/easy about this?

Choices on a continuum, from doing nothing and being passive to being aggressive; brainstorm choices as a group.

General discussion

[Problem identification and exploration]

Which situations do you (or would your partner) find difficult?

What would you do in each situation? What might your partner do? If you don't do anything, why? If your partner would do nothing, why?

[Problem resolution]

Strategies (categories)

- Eliminate the problem
- Assert your needs
- Negotiate a better environment
- Situate yourself away from the noise
- Put up with it
- Stay home

12:00–2:00 Lunch

1:00–2:00 How do you identify yourself? Are you deaf, hard of hearing, impaired, disabled?

- How do you think of yourself?
- Are you happy with how you explain your problem to others?
- Are you comfortable with it?
- Do you see yourself in the hearing world or the deaf world?
- How do others see you?

Break into groups of four and build a collage, using pictures from magazines, to show the world who you are.

2:00–2:10 Break

2:10–3:00 Exploration of passive, assertive, and aggressive behaviors

Marian's social gathering

Identify strategies as: passive, assertive, or aggressive

3:00–3:30 The effects of deafness on the body—stress, what is the connection?

■ How do you know if you are stressed? (brainstorm)
■ What can we do about it? (brainstorm)

Relaxation exercise

3:30–4:00 Wrap-up, anticipation of possible emotional reactions to what we've done today

Day Two

9:30–10:00 Review of previous day

How was it for you?

10:00–10:30 Changing roles—participants meet with one clinician, frequent communication partners meet with the other clinician

■ How has your role changed since the onset of the hearing loss? Since the receipt of a cochlear implant?
■ How do you feel about your role?
■ What style of communication use? Why?
■ Can you help him or her become more assertive? How?

10:30–10:45 Break

10:45–12:00 Explore role changes together

■ Being helpful versus taking over
■ What it's like to be a "partner"/dependent
■ Finding the balance

Partner issues

■ Being helpful versus taking over
■ "Rescuing" and dependency
■ What it's like to be a "partner"
■ What has changed since the hearing loss?
■ Finding the balance

12:00–1:00 Lunch

1:00–2:00 How to be assertive

- Role-play difficult situations, discuss communication style and use of communication strategies within the context of each role-playing scenario. For example, at the bank; in the doctor's office. Are behaviors assertive, aggressive, or passive? Effective?

2:00–2:10 Break

2:10–2:45 Individual goals and contracts

Setting realistic goals (examples)

What do you want to change?

What are you in control of?

Step-by-step progress

Journals?

2:45–3:00 Relaxation exercises

3:00–3:45 Evaluation/debriefing

- What was the most important thing you learned?
- What was least useful?
- Will what you've learned help you in your everyday life?
- Has your partner's presence changed anything in how the workshop went for you? What made you decide to come?

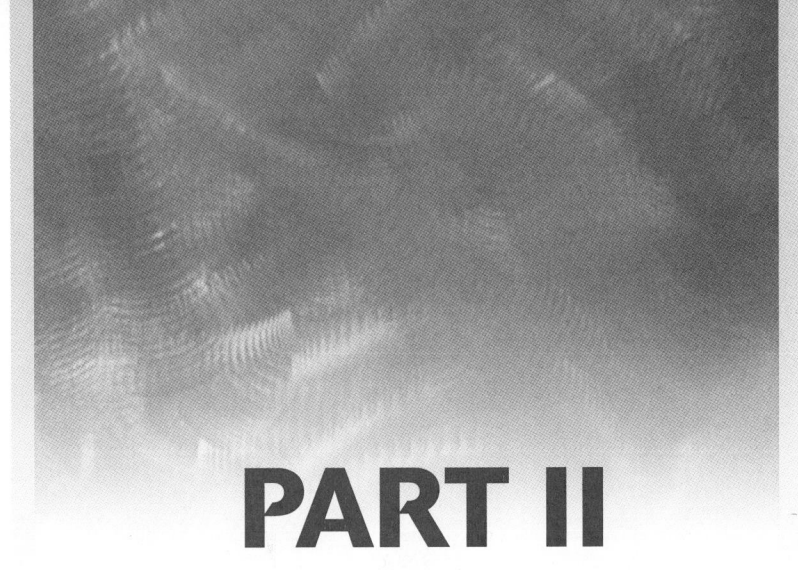

PART II
Speech Perception

CHAPTER 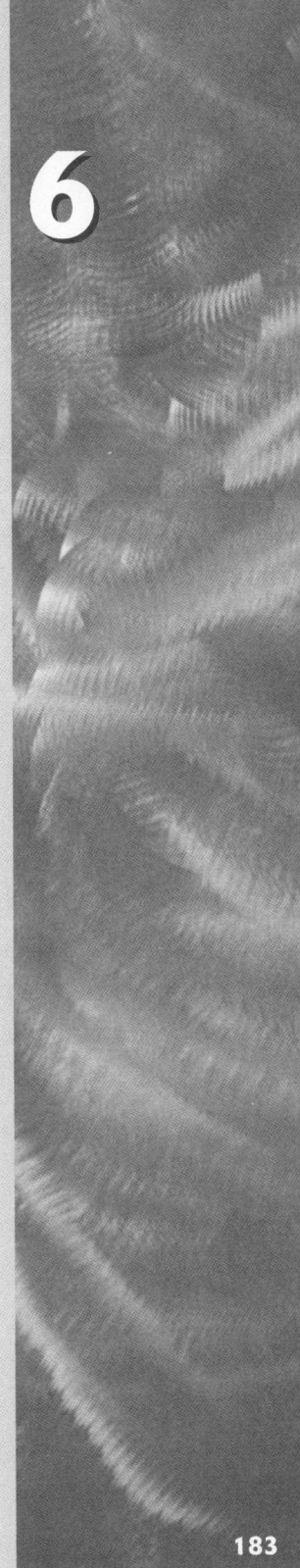 6

Assessing Hearing and Speech Recognition

TOPICS

- Review of the audiological examination and the audiogram

- Purpose of speech recognition testing

- Patient variables

- Stimulus units

- Test procedures

- Difficulties associated with speech recognition assessment

- Multicultural issues

- Case study

- Final remarks

- Key chapter points

- Multiple choice questions

- Key resources

The preceding chapters have provided a global treatment of conversational fluency, from defining it as a construct, to assessing it, to developing it as a skill set in patients and their frequent communication partners, to addressing some of the personal adjustment and psychosocial issues that might impede it. Starting with this chapter, we focus more narrowly on a specific component of conversational fluency, speech recognition. The reason that conversational fluency is often degraded is that persons with hearing loss cannot recognize the spoken messages of their communication partners. In this chapter and the four that follow, we consider issues of speech recognition, including assessment, technology that enhances performance, the contribution of visual information, and training that enhances both auditory and auditory-visual performance. There is a direct relationship between speech recognition and conversational fluency, and to the extent that the aural rehabilitation plan enhances the former, concomitant gains will be realized in the latter.

The audiogram provides a general description of the magnitude of a person's hearing loss. However, the audiogram does not always adequately portray the communication difficulties an individual may experience nor the person's aural rehabilitation needs. This is one reason why conversational fluency and communication handicap are assessed (see Chapter 3). Speech recognition measurement also is an important element in assessing how hearing loss affects an individual's life and communication interactions. The term *speech recognition* refers to the reception of *speech information* through listening, lipreading, or speechreading.

speech recognition:
The reception of speech information through listening, lipreading, or speech reading.

In this chapter, we will focus on important considerations underlying the assessment of speech recognition. These considerations are (Figure 6-1):

- Purpose
- Patient variables
- Stimuli units
- Test procedures

Before we turn to these topics, we begin with a brief review of the audiogram and other components of the audiological examination.

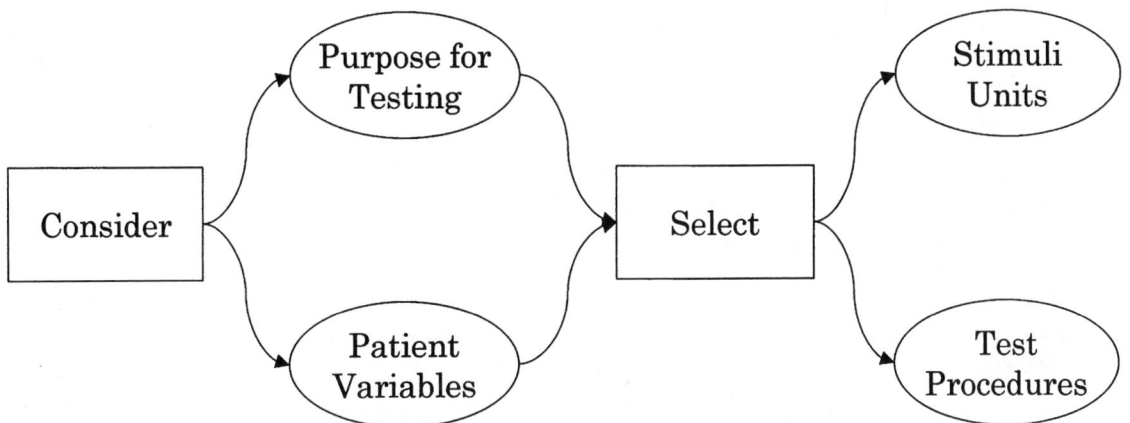

FIGURE 6-1. Assessing speech recognition.

■ REVIEW OF THE AUDIOLOGICAL EXAMINATION AND THE AUDIOGRAM

A typical audiological assessment includes an *audiogram,* a determination of speech recognition threshold, and an assessment of speech discrimination. Sometimes the examination might entail a determination of most comfortable loudness and uncomfortable loudness levels for speech as well.

The audiogram provides an objective assessment of an individual's ability to detect sounds. The test typically is performed by an audiologist, with the use of an audiometer. The audiometer presents tones, and the individual indicates when he or she hears them. The goal is to determine the softest sound level at which the tones can be detected, or the threshold. A *threshold* is defined as the level of sound so faint that it can only be detected 50% of the time.

The tones may be presented by *air conduction,* either through headphones or soundfield, or by *bone conduction,* through a vibrator placed behind the ear against the temporal bone. Air conduction test results indicate hearing losses that might be either *conductive hearing loss* (involving the outer or middle

An **audiogram** is a graphic representation of hearing thresholds as a function of stimulus frequency.

Threshold: Level at which sound can be detected only 50% of the time.

Air conduction: sound that travels through the air into the internal auditory canal and progresses through the middle ear, inner ear, and to the brain.

Bone conduction: transmission of sound through the bones in the body, particularly the skull.

Conductive hearing loss is used to describe hearing loss that stems from an impairment in the outer or middle ear.

Sensorineural hearing loss is a type of hearing loss that has a cochlear or retrocochlear origin.

Air-bone gap: the difference between air- and bone-conduction thresholds; a difference may indicate a conductive component in the hearing loss.

Sound level is the intensity of sound expressed in decibels.

Frequency: the number of regularly repeated events in a given unit of time; usually measured in cycles per second and expressed in Hertz (Hz).

Pure tone average (PTA): Average of hearing thresholds at 500, 1000, and 2000 Hz.

ear) or *sensorineural hearing loss* (involving the inner ear, eighth nerve, brain stem, midbrain, or auditory cortex) in nature. Bone conduction test results reflect only the sensorineural component. By comparing the air and bone conduction results, the audiologist can determine whether there is hearing loss stemming from a problem in either the outer or middle ear. The difference between the two sets of thresholds is termed the *air-bone gap*.

Audiological thresholds are plotted on an audiogram, where the Y-axis indicates *sound level* (loudness) and the X-axis indicates *frequency* (pitch). As shown in Figure 6-2, an X on the audiogram represents the left ear and an O represents the right ear thresholds when the test signals are presented via air conduction. A left bracket ([) indicates a bone conduction threshold for the right ear, and a right bracket (]) indicates a bone conduction threshold for the left ear. The capital letter A typically denotes an aided threshold or how the patient hears when wearing a hearing aid or cochlear implant. In this figure, the patient's audiogram indicates that her threshold for 250 Hz is 20 dB in the right ear and 60 dB in the left ear. The *pure tone average* (PTA) is a means to summarize someone's hearing status. The pure tone average is an average of the hearing thresholds for the frequencies of 500, 1000, and 2000 Hz (Figure 6-2).

The pure tone average often is used to assign a label to indicate the degree of hearing loss. The following descriptors are used to denote degree:

> **Normal:** The PTA is 25 dB HL or better.
>
> **Mild:** The PTA is between 26 and 40 dB HL.
>
> **Mild-to-moderate:** The PTA is between 41 and 55 dB HL.
>
> **Moderate:** The PTA is between 56 and 70 dB HL.
>
> **Severe:** The PTA is between 71 and 90 dB HL.
>
> **Profound:** The PTA is poorer than 90 dB HL.

Configuration refers to the extent of hearing loss at each frequency and gives an overall description to the hearing loss.

Table 6-1 indicates the relationship between degree of hearing loss and speech recognition, as a function of the descriptors outlined previously. Another class of descriptor often assigned to a patient's audiogram is the configuration of the hearing loss. As noted in Chapter 1, *configuration* refers to the extent of hearing loss at each frequency and provides an overall picture of hearing sensitivity. Four common configurations of hearing loss appear in

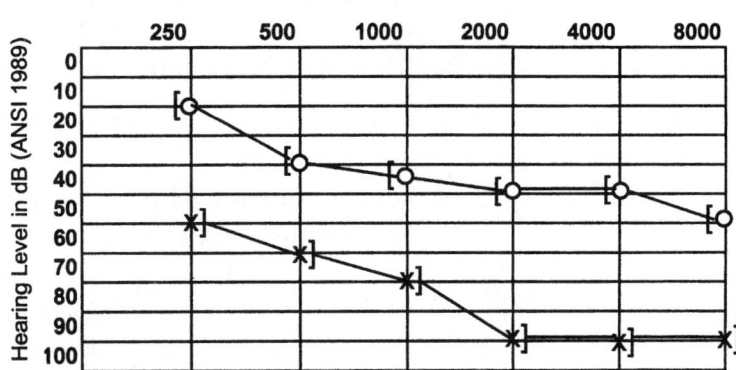

FREQUENCY IN HERTZ

o = Right ear, air conduction
x = Left ear, air conduction
[= Right ear, bone conduction
] = Left ear, bone conduction

FIGURE 6-2. Audiogram for someone who has a PTA of 35 dB in the right ear (a mild hearing loss) and 73 dB in the left ear (a severe hearing loss).

Table 6-1. How degree of hearing loss affects speech recognition.

HEARING LOSS	EFFECT ON WORD RECOGNITION
Mild (PTA = 26–40 dB HL)	In quiet situations, speech recognition will be fairly unaffected. In the presence of noise, speech recognition may decrease to 50% words correct if the PTA is 40 dB HL. Consonants are most likely to be missed, especially if the hearing loss involves primarily the high frequencies.
Mild-to-Moderate (PTA = 41–55 dB HL)	Will understand much of the speech signal if it is presented in a quiet environment face-to-face, and if the topic of conversation is known and the vocabulary is constrained. If a hearing aid is not used, the individual may miss up to 50–75% of a spoken message if the PTA is 40 dB and 80–100% if the PTA is 50 dB.
Moderate (PTA = 56–70 dB HL)	If the individual does not use a hearing aid, he or she may miss most or all of the message, even if talking face-to-face. Will have great difficulty conversing in group situations.
Severe (PTA = 71–90 dB)	May not even hear voices, unless speech is loud. Without amplification, the individual probably will not recognize any speech in an audition-only condition. With amplification, he or she may recognize some speech and detect environmental sounds.
Profound (PTA = 90 dB HL or greater)	May perceive sound as vibrations. An individual will rely on vision as the primary sense for speech recognition. May not be able to detect the presence of even loud sound without amplification.

Source: Adapted from Flexor, C. (1999). *Facilitating hearing and listening in young children.* Clifton Park, NY: Delmar Learning.

Figures 6-3, 6-4, 6-5, and 6-6, which illustrate a flat configuration of hearing loss, a high-frequency configuration, a low-frequency configuration, and a saucer-shaped configuration of hearing loss, respectively. These configurations may be defined as follows:

■ **Flat:** Thresholds are within a 20 dB range of each other across the span of frequencies tested.
■ **High-frequency:** Thresholds are within normal range for the low and mid frequencies, but decline for the higher frequen-

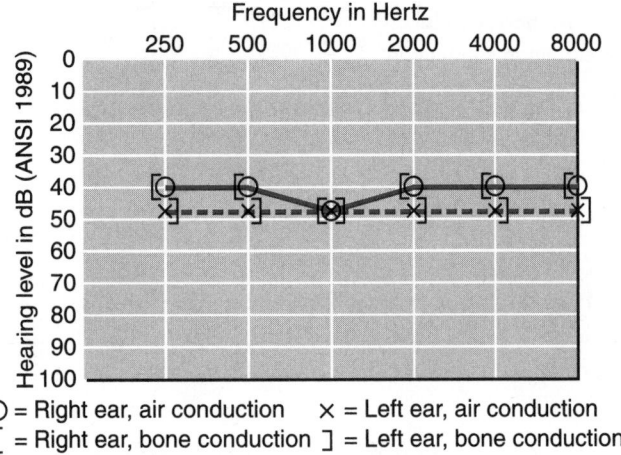

O = Right ear, air conduction   × = Left ear, air conduction
[= Right ear, bone conduction] = Left ear, bone conduction

FIGURE 6-3. Audiogram for someone who has a flat configuration of hearing loss.

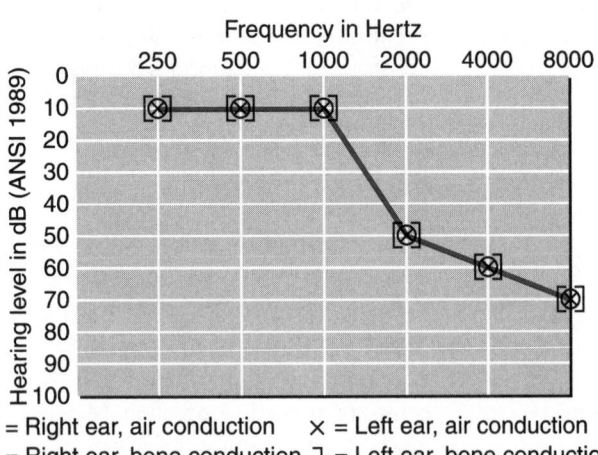

O = Right ear, air conduction   × = Left ear, air conduction
[= Right ear, bone conduction] = Left ear, bone conduction

FIGURE 6-4. Audiogram for someone who has a high frequency configuration of hearing loss.

cies. A high-frequency loss may be described as *precipitous* if the loss at each of the higher frequencies is at least 20 dB greater with each ascending frequency. It may be described as *sloping* if thresholds for the higher frequencies are 20 dB or poorer than for the lower frequencies.

■ **Low-frequency:** Thresholds are lowered for the low frequencies but are within normal range for the mid and higher frequencies.

■ **Saucer-shaped:** The loss is confined to the mid frequencies.

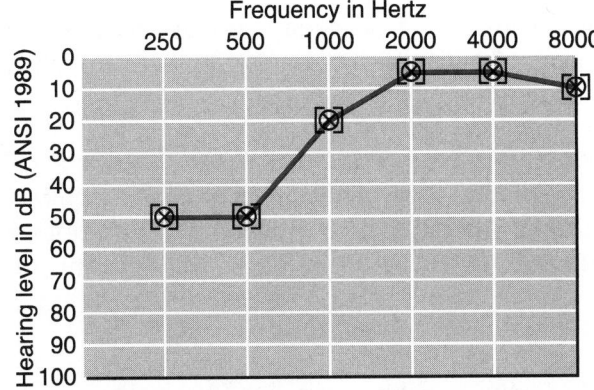

O = Right ear, air conduction   × = Left ear, air conduction
[= Right ear, bone conduction] = Left ear, bone conduction

FIGURE 6-5. Audiogram for someone who has a low-frequency configuration of hearing loss.

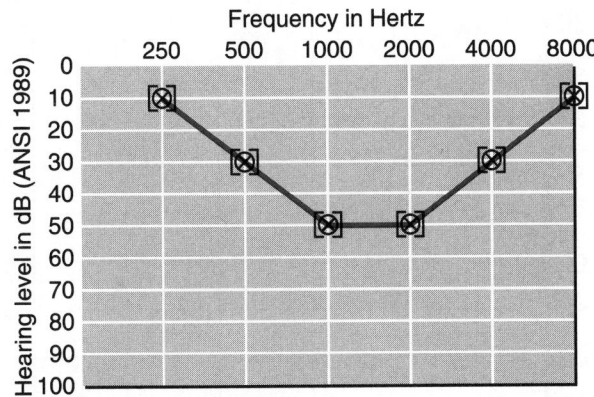

O = Right ear, air conduction   × = Left ear, air conduction
[= Right ear, bone conduction] = Left ear, bone conduction

FIGURE 6-6. Audiogram for someone who has a saucer-shaped configuration of hearing loss.

The configuration of hearing loss, as well as the degree, affects how well the patient may recognize speech. Most of the acoustic information that contributes to speech recognition lies within the frequency band of 1000 Hz to 3000 Hz, as shown in Figure 6-7, which shows the approximate intensity and frequency of the speech sounds. For this reason, someone who has a low-frequency configuration (Figure 6-5) may likely receive more speech information and hence recognize more speech than someone who has a high-frequency configuration (Figure 6-4), even if they have similar PTAs. The person with the audiogram shown in Figure 6-6 will likely not hear such high-frequency consonant sounds as [s, sh, t, p, k, f] while listening to everyday conversation, and he or she may not receive enough information to distinguish from one another consonants such as [d, b, g, v, zh, l, r, w].

Speech reception threshold (SRT): the lowest presentation level for spondee words at which 50% can be identified correctly.

When determining the ***speech reception threshold (SRT)***, the audiologist determines the softest level at which a patient can understand simple words. In one procedure, an audiologist might ask the patient to repeat *spondees*. These are bisyllabic words that

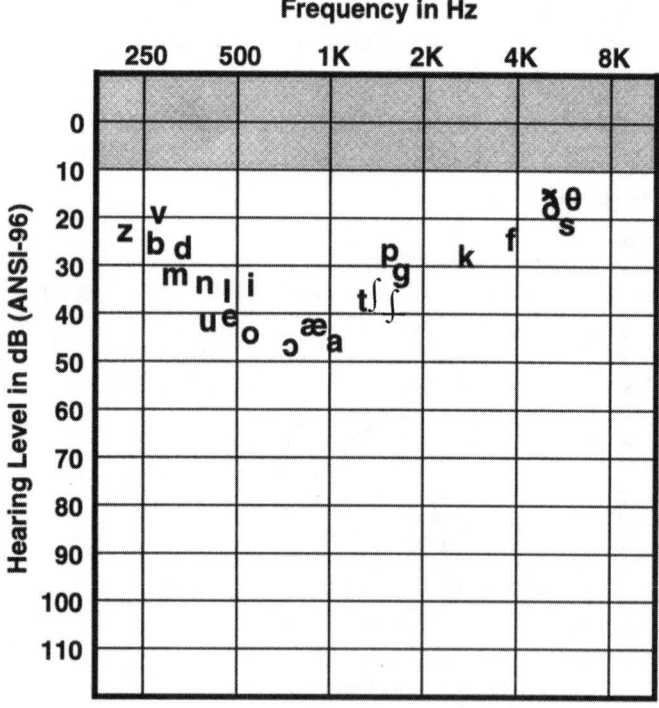

FIGURE 6-7. Generalized phonetic representations of speech sounds occurring at normal conversational levels plotted on an audiogram.

have equal stress on both words, such as *baseball, ice cream, hotdog,* and *sidewalk.* The words are presented through the audiometer, and the level is varied until the patient is able to repeat just 50% of the words correctly. This level is recorded as the SRT.

The audiological examination usually includes a test of speech recognition, in addition to the audiogram and SRT testing. For instance, the clinician might present monosyllabic words at a comfortable listening level and expect the patient to repeat each word. When word recognition scores are referred to in a clinical setting, they are often called *speech discrimination scores.* The term speech recognition is preferred in this text, to avoid confusion with the term discrimination when it is used in a training context, to indicate discriminating one stimulus from the next.

Speech discrimination score: the percentage of monosyllabic words presented at a comfortable listening level that can be correctly repeated.

Sometimes the audiologist might want to determine the hearing level at which speech is most comfortable to listen to and the level at which it becomes too loud. The *most comfortable loudness level (MCL)* typically is determined by asking the individual to listen to running speech. The initial presentation level may be just above the level of the SRT, and then it is gradually increased. The individual indicates when it is at a comfortable level, when it is too soft, and when it is too loud. The *uncomfortable loudness level (UCL)* is the threshold level at which the speech changes from being comfortably loud to being uncomfortably loud.

Most comfortable loudness (MCL): level at which sound is most comfortable for a listener.

Uncomfortable loudness level (UCL): level at which sound is uncomfortably loud for a listener.

Sound-Field Testing

Often, tests of speech recognition are presented in soundfield as opposed to under headphones. If the patient typically wears a hearing aid, he or she often wears the aid for testing. Newby and Popelka (1992) discussed the reasons for soundfield testing:

"Testing with a loudspeaker is referred to as *sound-field testing* because the sound is not confined, as it is in an earphone, but is circulated in a field about the patient's head. Unless we are talking over the telephone, or for some reason listening through earphones, all our listening throughout the day is of the sound-field type. To judge how the patient hears in a typical sound-field listening situation is the main reason that we give speech tests through a loudspeaker" (pp. 182–183).

Sound-field testing: the determination of hearing sensitivity or speech recognition ability accomplished by presenting signals in a sound field through a loudspeaker.

■ PURPOSE OF SPEECH RECOGNITION TESTING

When designing an aural rehabilitation plan for a particular patient, you will almost always want information about his or her speech recognition skills. There are many ways to use the results of this assessment. These include the following:

- **To determine need for amplification.** If a person demonstrates reduced speech recognition, then amplification might be considered.
- **To compare performance with a listening aid to performance without an aid.** This comparison can be accomplished by measuring speech recognition with and without the device.
- **To compare different listening devices.** An individual might be tested with one listening device and then another to determine the device that affords the best performance. This testing is feasible when two or three devices are being compared, but becomes problematic when many devices are under consideration. In recent practice, speech recognition testing has been used less frequently for the purpose of selecting listening devices than in former times (Mueller, 2001).
- **To demonstrate to patients that their ability to recognize speech is diminished.** Especially during counseling, information gained from speech testing can illustrate how speech understanding is impaired relative to persons who have normal hearing.
- **To demonstrate the benefits of visual speech information.** By testing in an audition-only condition and then an audition-plus-vision condition, you can gain information that helps the patient realize the importance of visual speech information and the importance of speechreading and focusing on the talker's facial movements.
- **To obtain information that might elucidate environment- related listening issues.** By performing speech testing in the presence of background noise, and comparing the results to performance in quiet, you can gain information that can be used to counsel patients about their particular listening difficulties. For instance, background noise may be more problematic for certain people, such as older persons, than for others.

■ **To assess performance longitudinally.** There may be instances when you want to monitor speech recognition over time and answer questions such as, "Is the patient's hearing deteriorating because of use of a listening device?" or "Has speech recognition changed as a result of auditory training?" Care must be taken that measurements are not affected by the learning of test materials with repeated administration or, in the case of children, by language growth or cognitive maturation.

■ **To determine need for speech perception training.** If an individual experiences difficulty in recognizing speech, even when using appropriate amplification, then the person may be a candidate for training.

■ **To determine placement within a training curriculum.** Not every individual begins a speech perception training program with the same tasks. People will enter training with different skill levels, and training objectives will need to be selected accordingly.

■ **To determine if expected benefit has been achieved.** One goal of providing a listening aid or providing speech perception training is to improve speech recognition. You may assess whether individuals obtained expected benefit by comparing their performance with that of a group of persons who have a similar hearing loss or who have received similar interventions.

The purpose may dictate the test. For instance, you may use one test to determine placement in an auditory training curriculum and another test for assessing benefit from a hearing aid. Other important variables that will influence test selection pertain to the patient.

PATIENT VARIABLES

In selecting appropriate test materials for assessing word recognition, it is important to consider variables such as cognitive/linguistic level and hearing ability, for these will affect how an individual performs on a particular test. A consideration of patient variables will help you choose between test stimuli, response format, testing conditions, and whether to use live or recorded stimuli.

The patient must have the maturity and cognitive skills to take the test. For example, it would be inappropriate to expect a

3-year-old child to repeat a seven-word sentence, as it would be to expect an elderly person with dementia to do so. If a young child takes a closed-set test, then it might be necessary that the response items can be illustrated by pictures, because the child could not read orthographic choices.

Similarly, the test must present items that are within the linguistic competency of the individual. Otherwise, you will not know whether someone performed poorly on a test because he or she did not know the vocabulary or grammatical structures or because of hearing limitations. For example, you might ask a child to repeat the sentence, *The man ate an artichoke for dinner.* If a child is unfamiliar with the word *artichoke,* it is unlikely the child will be able to repeat it during a speech recognition test, especially if he or she has a significant hearing loss.

The degree of hearing loss will affect test selection. For instance, if an adult just received a cochlear implant, it may be inappropriate to administer a monosyllabic word test in an audition-only condition, because the individual likely will exhibit a "floor" performance.

Sometimes you will need to consider communication mode and other disabilities. For example, if a child uses sign, the test instructions should be presented with sign, and provisions for recording the child's responses must be made (i.e., if the child signs responses, then someone must interpret them). If an individual has decreased speech intelligibility as well as a hearing loss, the responses may have to be written.

▆ STIMULI UNITS

Once you have identified your purpose for testing and have thought about patient variables, test selection can be made. Test stimuli that are used typically to assess speech recognition are summarized in Table 6-2. Examples of tests that correspond with each type are also listed, for both children and adults. Each kind of stimulus presents both advantages and disadvantages.

Phonemes and Phoneme Contrasts

Phoneme testing permits phonetic errors to be examined. The items may be designed to assess consonant or vowel recognition.

Table 6-2. Examples of word recognition tests that use phoneme, word, and sentence stimuli for children and adults. These tests typically are administered in an audition-only condition.

TEST	AUTHOR(S)	STIMULUS TYPE	STIMULUS UNITS	RESPONSE FORMAT	TARGET POPULATION
Speech Pattern Contrast Test (SPAC)	Boothroyd, 1994	Phoneme (also includes test of suprasegmental contrasts, such as word stress)	Words and phrases	Closed set	Children over age 10 years
Audiovisual Feature Test	Tyler, Fryauf-Bertschy, & Kelsey, 1991	Phoneme	Rhyming words, including b, c, d, key, me, knee	Closed set (10-choice)	Children
Iowa Consonant Confusion Test	Tyler, Preece, & Tye-Murray, 1986	Phoneme	Nonsense bisyllables, including eemee, eesee, eedee, eebee	Closed set (13-choice)	Adults
Iowa Vowel Confusion Test	Tyler, Preece, & Tye-Murray, 1986	Phoneme	Monosyllables with an [hVd] format, including heed, who'd, had, head	Closed set (9-choice)	Adults
Nonsense Syllable Test (NST)	Edgerton & Danhauer, 1979	Phoneme	Nonsense bisyllables	Open set	Children and adults
Minimal Pairs Test	Robbins, Renshaw, Miyamoto, Osberger, & Pope, 1988	Phoneme	Monosyllabic word pairs (e.g., pair vs. bear)	Closed set (2-choice)	Children, about age 4 years and older
Northwestern University Children's Perception of Speech (NU-CHIPS)	Elliott & Katz, 1980	Word	Monosyllables constructed with the most frequently occurring phonemes in the English language, such as fork, dog	Closed set (4-choice)	Children who have the receptive language abilities of age 2.6 years or older

(continued)

Table 6-2. (continued)

TEST	AUTHOR(S)	STIMULUS TYPE	STIMULUS UNITS	RESPONSE FORMAT	TARGET POPULATION
Word Intelligibility by Picture Identification (WIPI)	Ross & Lerman, 1971	Word	Monosyllabic words, such as *bear, pear, stair, chair, ear, hair*	Closed set (6-choice)	Children ages 5–6 years with moderate hearing loss; ages 7–8 years with severe hearing loss
Phonetically Balanced Kindergarten (PBK)	Haskins, 1949	Word	Monosyllabic words	Open set	Children, 6 years and older
Northwestern University Auditory Test No. 6 (NU-6)	Tillman & Carhart, 1966	Word	Monosyllabic words	Open set	Adults
Central Institute for the Deaf (CID) Auditory Test W-22	Hirsh et al., 1952	Word	Phonetically balanced monosyllabic word lists	Open set	Adults
Early-Speech Perception Test (ESP)	Moog & Geers, 1990	Word	Words varying in number of syllables	Closed set	Children 6 years and older (there is a version available for children as young as 2 years)
Lexical Neighborhood Test (LNT)	Kirk, Pisoni, & Osberger, 1995	Word	Words, some of which are lexically "easy" and some of which are lexically "hard," with easy words having few other word choices that are phonetically similar (e.g., *thought, live*)	Open set	Children

(continued)

Table 6-2. (continued)

TEST	AUTHOR(S)	STIMULUS TYPE	STIMULUS UNITS	RESPONSE FORMAT	TARGET POPULATION
			and hard words having many words that are similar (e.g., *mole, wed*)		
Bamford-Kowal-Bench Sentences (BKB)	Bench & Bamford, 1979	Sentence	Sentences constructed with vocabulary familiar to 8- to 16-year-old hard-of-hearing children	Open set	Older children and adults
Central Institute for the Deaf (CID) Everyday Speech Sentences	Davis & Silverman, 1978	Sentence	Sentences that vary in length and structure	Open set	Older children and adults
Revised Speech Perception in Noise (SPIN)	Bilger et al., 1984	Sentence	Sentences that have either high context for the last word in the sentence or low context	Open set, presented with a background of speech babble	Adults
CUNY Sentences	Boothroyd, Hanin, & Hnath, 1985	Sentence	Unrelated sentences	Open set	Adults
Hearing in Noise Test (HINT)	Nilsson, Soli, & Sullivan, 1994	Sentence	Unrelated sentences	Open set, presented with a background noise	13 years and up (there is a version available for children between the ages of 6–12 years)
The Connected Speech Test (CST)	Cox, Alexander, & Gilmore, 1987	Sentence	Sets of 10 related sentences pertaining to familiar topics	Open set	Adults

(continued)

Table 6-2. (continued)

TEST	AUTHOR(S)	STIMULUS TYPE	STIMULUS UNITS	RESPONSE FORMAT	TARGET POPULATION
The Synthetic Sentence Test (SSI)	Jerger, Speaks, & Trammell, 1968; Speaks & Jerger, 1965	Sentence	Synthetic sentences with minimal contextual cues and minimal redundancy	Closed set	Adults
Speech in Noise (SIN), also, the QuickSIN	Killion & Vilchur, 1993	Sentence	Sentences recorded at a variety of signal-to-noise ratios	Open set, presented with varying levels of four-talker babble	Adults, particularly new hearing aid users

Test results indicate the kinds of speech features utilized during speech recognition. For example, an individual may not have scored high on a test that presents a closed set of items such as *eemee, eenee, eesee, eebee, eepee,* and *eetee.* However, an analysis of errors may reveal that even though overall performance was poor, the individual consistently utilized the voicing feature. For instance, *eepee* may have been heard as *eetee* or *eesee,* both of which contain unvoiced elements, but never as *eebee* or *eenee,* which contain only voiced elements. Thus, in designing auditory training goals, you might aim to build on this ability to utilize the voicing feature.

Although you can evaluate subjectively an individual's errors and qualitatively assess error confusions, formal statistical and mathematical analyses can be performed on the results. These provide a quantitative indication of the kinds of information an individual utilizes during speech. Such analyses include information transmission analysis (Miller & Nicely, 1955), multidimensional scaling, and clustering.

A feature analysis of consonant phoneme confusion errors indicates which parameters of the speech signal are detected and utilized. Features that typically are included in this kind of analysis include nasality voicing, duration fication, place, and envelope. A commonly used consonant classification system appears in Table 6-3.

Table 6-3. An example of a classification system for consonants that may be used to classify consonant phonemes for a feature analysis. The numbers are arbitrary and serve only to indicate the group to which a sound belongs within a feature.

CONSONANT	VOICING	PLACE	NASALITY	DURATION	FRICATION	ENVELOPE
b	1	0	0	0	0	1
d	1	1	0	0	0	1
g	1	3	0	0	0	1
p	0	0	0	0	0	0
t	0	1	0	0	0	0
k	0	3	0	0	0	0
v	1	0	0	0	1	1
f	0	0	0	0	1	2
z	1	1	0	1	1	1
s	0	1	0	1	1	2
ʃ	0	2	0	1	1	2
m	1	0	1	0	0	3
n	1	1	1	0	0	3

For the nasality feature, consonants /m and n/ are classified as nasal consonants. A person who appears to hear the nasality feature is probably responding to the frequencies around and below 300 Hz. Consonants that are aperiodic in nature (/p, t, k, f, s, ʃ/) are grouped together for the voicing feature, whereas the relatively long duration consonants are grouped together for the duration feature (/z, s, ʃ/). The voicing and duration features probably relate to temporal cues and the voice pitch. Consonants produced with steady turbulence (/v, f, z, s, ʃ/) usually are grouped together for the frication feature. This feature relates to high-frequency turbulence. The place feature, for which consonants are categorized according to whether they are produced in the front, middle, or back of the vocal tract, is cued by spectral or frequency changes over time, particularly in the region of the second vowel formant (see Chapter 8). Finally, the envelope feature reflects time-intensity variations in the audio signal. To recognize words, persons must detect and utilize at least some of these features in the signal. A feature analysis indicates how well a patient can distinguish these cues from one another. We will revisit the topic of features in Chapters 8 and 10 when we consider designing objectives for auditory and speechreading training.

Nonsense syllables:
syllables of speech that have
no meaning.

An advantage of using phoneme stimuli is that performance is relatively independent of an individual's vocabulary level. It is not important that individuals be familiar with the test stimuli, and indeed, the stimuli are often *nonsense syllables,* such as *eesee* and *eeteee.* This same advantage can become a disadvantage if you are testing young children, who often must be tested with vocabulary they know.

A principal disadvantage of using phoneme stimuli is poor face validity. We do not communicate with these kinds of stimuli typically, and it is not straightforward how recognition relates to conversational speech understanding. For instance, nonsense syllables do not require individuals to organize streams of information into linguistically meaningful chunks, nor to process speech information with the same rapidity as ongoing speech.

Words

The most commonly used stimuli for assessing speech recognition are monosyllabic words. Many word lists are designed to be

Features and Cues

When considering speech recognition, the terms features and cues often are used. Dorman (1993) defines them as follows:

"The term 'cue' refers to a specific aspect of an acoustic signal that has been demonstrated to be important for recognition of a phonetic segment, or for distinguishing between two phonetic segments. The term 'feature' generally refers to articulation, and not to a particular acoustic cue. Thus, the feature 'place of articulation' encompasses sounds with extremely different acoustic signatures. For example, the place cues for voiced stop-consonants reside in transient bursts and formant transitions of brief duration, but the place cues for fricatives reside in long duration fricative noises which differ greatly in frequency and in amplitude. This must be kept in mind when sorting through the results of studies that report on the reception of features by . . . patients." (p. 146) *phonetically balanced,* meaning that the words include phonemes in the same proportion in which they occur in spoken English. The Phonetically Balanced Kindergarten word lists (PB-K) developed by Haskins (1949) are commonly used to assess spoken word recognition. More recently, word lists for testing purposes have been based on principles of lexical neighborhoods (Luce, 1986; Luce & Pisoni, 1998), for example, the Lexical Neighborhood Test (LNT) and the Multisyllabic Lexical Neighborhood Test (MLNT) (Kirk, 1998; Kirk et al., 1995). Words that have a similar frequency of occurrence (i.e., how often the words occur in the during every day language use) and that share similar acoustic-phonetic characteristics belong to the same neighborhood. A word that belongs to a dense neighborhood (many words that are similar, such as *cat, mat, sat, fat, pat, bat,* etc.) is typically more difficult to recognize than a word that belongs to a sparse neighborhood (few words that are similar; the words *thumb, tea,* and *lost* belong to sparse neighborhoods). Most word lists are comprised of monosyllables that have the phonemic structure of consonant-vowel-consonant (e.g., *cat* or *man*). These stimuli generally are difficult to recognize, more so than phrases or simple sentences.

Simple questions that may reveal presence of hearing loss are:

- Can you hear on the telephone?
- Do people tell you that you set the TV volume too high?
- Do you often ask people to repeat?
- Do you have problems listening in a noisy room?
- Do people seem to mumble?
- Are women and children especially difficult to hear?

One advantage in using real words is that they have somewhat higher face validity than phonemes. We communicate with words in daily conversation. The tests are also easy to score, and allow a wide range of skill levels to be assessed. Responses from a word test can be scored by percent of words repeated verbatim, or percent of phonemes correct (e.g., if the word is *bat,* and an individual responds *pat,* two of the word's three phonemes are scored as correct). The reasons that percent phoneme scores are sometimes computed are to obtain a fine-grain understanding of an individual's performance and to provide a different vehicle for comparing test results. For example, two people might achieve the following scores on the same test:

Person 1: 30% words correct, 40% phonemes correct

Person 2: 30% words correct, 65% phonemes correct

Even though the individuals erred an equal number of times in repeating the words, Person 2's errors better approximate the target than do Person 1's error responses. Thus, the second person may have better listening ability than the first person.

As with phonemes, word stimuli may not reflect adequately how an individual performs in everyday listening situations because we typically listen to connected discourse. For instance, words are presented rapidly during conversation. We do not pause to think about the identity of each word as it is spoken, as one does when taking a test of isolated word recognition. Research suggests that, during normal conversation, we might receive speech at between 140 and 180 words per minute (Miller et al., 1984). It is possible for two people to perform similarly on a word test, in which the demands of fast on-line processing are not great, and yet function differently in everyday conversation. Another problem in using words as test stimuli may arise if the test-taker has a language delay because performance on word tests may be influenced by vocabulary. A child who has a limited vocabulary may perform poorly simply because he or she is unfamiliar with the test words. As an example of a word test, lists from the lexical neighborhood test (Kirk et al., 1995) are reprinted in the Key Resources.

Phrases and Sentences

A speech recognition test may consist of a series of unrelated phrases or sentences. For instance, the test may commence with the sentence, *The cook cut the apple,* and then continue with, *The boy and girl walked to school,* which is contextually unrelated to the first sentence. Alternatively, the test may present sentences centered on a common theme. For instance, before the test begins, the individual may be informed, "The sentences you will hear concern activities to do at the lake." The first sentence may then be, *We paddled a canoe.* The second sentence may be, *We went for a swim this morning,* and so forth. Performance will be better for topic-related than unrelated sentences.

Sentence stimuli have high face validity because we typically communicate with phrases, sentences, and paragraphs. As such, performance on a sentence test may better reflect how a person performs in the real world than performance on a phoneme or isolated word test. Sentences have the following features, which are characteristic of everyday speech:

Prosodic cues are provided by intonation, rate, and duration of speech sounds.

■ *Prosodic cues:* When we listen to speech, we attend not only to individual sounds, but also to intonation, rate, and duration cues, and these help us identify words and understand meaning. For example, an individual may be presented with a complete sentence, but because of hearing loss, the person may hear only, *mmm mm-mm mmm?* Even though the individual receives a gross approximation of the message, there is still enough information to know that a question is being asked, and that the question contains four syllables, and possibly, enough information to know that it contains three words.

■ *Contextual information:* The words in a sentence provide contextual redundancy. Recognition of some words facilitates recognition of other words. If an individual hears, *Mary closed the* _____, it is possible to deduce that the final word is a noun, based on grammatical context, and that the word might be *door,* based on semantic cues.

Contextual information facilitates recognition of other words.

■ *Coarticulation:* When words are spoken in succession as in a sentence, they blend together and vary as a function of what precedes and follows. For example, the schwa sound in the word *the* will sound different if the word *blue* follows than if the word *green* follows. These coarticulation effects provide redundant cues for word recognition.

Coarticulation, the influence of one phoneme on either a preceding or succeeding phoneme.

Even though sentences have these features of everyday speech, they also pose some disadvantages for assessment. One disadvantage of using sentence-level stimuli is that performance can be influenced by linguistic knowledge and familiarity with the topic. For example, a young child with limited grammatical knowledge may not perform as well as an older child who has good language skills, even though the two children might have similar perceptual skills. Memory also may affect results. If you present a 10-word sentence to a 5-year-old child, the child may forget the beginning of the sentence by the time you present its end.

Sentence tests are usually scored by computing a percent words correct score, although sometimes they are scored for percent phonemes correct and only sometimes selected keywords are assessed. For a word to be scored as correct, it must be repeated verbatim. If the sentence is, *The girls walked to school,* and a person responds, "The girl walked to school," that sentence is scored as four out of five words correct. The omission of /s/ from *girls* makes it an incorrect repetition. As an example of a sentence test, lists from the CID everyday sentence test (Silverman & Hirsh, 1955) are reprinted in the Key Resources.

Selection of Test Stimuli

There are no cookbook procedures to follow when deciding which test stimuli to use. However, one guiding principle is that the measures chosen should inform you about how an individual performs in natural situations and should be independent of confounding factors such as vocabulary and grammatical knowledge, cognitive abilities, and memory (Boothroyd, 1991). Often, clinicians opt to use a test-battery approach, using more than one test so that the aggregate presents different kinds of speech units.

▆ TEST PROCEDURES

We have now considered tests and test selection. First, you must decide your purpose for testing, then you must consider characteristics of the test taker, and then decide on the test stimuli. Once a test has been selected, decisions must be made about the protocol that will be followed for administering the test. In this section, we turn our attention to test procedures. Considerations for assessing speech recognition include the test condition, the type of response set, and whether testing occurs with live voice or recordings.

Test Condition

Audition-only: presentation of only an auditory signal in testing.

Vision-only: presentation of only a visual stimulus in testing.

Audition-plus-vision: presentation of both auditory and visual signals simultaneously, as in speechreading.

Tests of speech recognition can be administered in one of three conditions (Figure 6-8):

- *Audition-only:* Only the auditory signal is presented, usually at a normal or moderately loud conversational level.
- *Vision-only:* Only the visual signal is presented, usually showing the head and neck of the test talker (this is a lipreading condition).
- *Audition-plus-vision:* Both the auditory and visual signals are presented (this is a speechreading condition).

AUDITION-ONLY

The audition-only condition is most frequently used for speech recognition assessment because it relates most directly to hearing

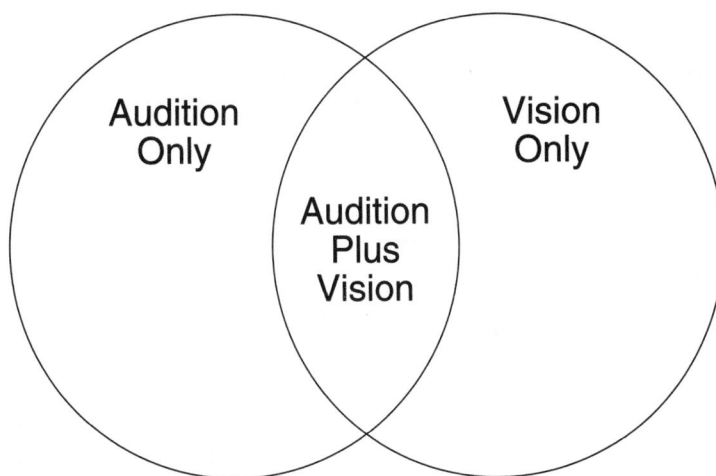

FIGURE 6-8. The test conditions used for speech-recognition testing.

ability. The signal may be presented in quiet or in the presence of noise.

The sound level for presenting the speech stimuli is often at a normal or moderately loud conversational level (60–70 dB SPL). Alternatively, the level might be set at about 30 to 40 dB above the patient's SRT. When this latter level is chosen, we say that the stimulus is 30 to 40 dB *sensational level (SL)*. The intent of using sensation levels is to liken functional listening levels across patients.

Sensational level (SL): the level of a sound in dB above a person's threshold.

Noise may be introduced to increase the difficulty of the listening task or to gain a better understanding of how the person performs in the real world. The noise signal may be talker babble (e.g., six people read text, and their speech signals are overlaid to create a signal noise source) or masking noise (which sounds like a radio off-station). Sometimes the competing noise signal is semantically meaningful. A meaningful competing signal might be used to determine how well an elderly individual can tune out distracting competitors.

When a speech recognition test is performed in the presence of noise, the audiologist records the *signal-to-noise ratio (SNR)*, which indicates the difference between the sound level of the signal and the sound level of the noise. Thus, if the signal is presented at 40 dB, and the noise is presented at 30 dB, the SNR is +10 dB.

Signal-to-noise ratio (SNR): the level of a signal relative to a background of noise.

VISION-ONLY

Sometimes a test of speech recognition is administered in a vision-only condition. The visual signal typically is comprised of the talker's head and shoulders, with the talker facing the patient head-on. The talker should be well lit, so his or her face is fully visible and not in shadows. The talker usually is placed before a plain, nondistracting background.

AUDITION-PLUS-VISION

Usually, performance for a particular individual will be optimal for an audition-plus-vision condition. This condition is used when best performance is desired or when hearing is so poor that the auditory signal provides only a supplement to lipreading.

Both the vision-only and audition-plus-vision conditions are employed when one is interested in accessing speechreading enhancement or determining goals for speechreading training. ***Speechreading enhancement*** is computed by comparing speech recognition scores in a vision-only condition to scores obtained in an audition-plus-vision condition. Two different computations may yield a speech reading enhancement score. First, A simple difference score may be computed by subtracting the percent correct score obtained in a vision-only condition (V) from the percent correct score obtained in an audition-plus-vision condition (AV): AV% correct − V% correct. The greater the difference between the two scores, the greater the amount of enhancement provided by the auditory signal.

Second, a normalized ratio score may be computed. This computation is done by first figuring out how much room for improvement there is in a vision-only condition then referencing the amount of improvement gained with the addition of the auditory signal to that amount available. The formula for computation is AV% correct − V% correct/100% − V% correct. Table 6-4 presents an example of the two computation methods. In this table, Patient A recognized 50% of the words correct when a test was presented in a vision-only condition and 75% words correct when the auditory signal was added. Patient B recognized 10% and 55% of the words in the two conditions, respectively. Note that while Patient B appears to have achieved greater speechreading enhancement than Patient A when the simple difference score is used, they appear to have equal gains with the

Speechreading enhancement: the difference or ratio between speech recognition performance in an vision-only condition and an audition-plus-vision condition.

Table 6-4. Two different formulas may be used to compute speechreading enhancement. In this example, Patient A scored 50% words correct in a vision-only condition and 75% words correct in an audition-plus-vision condition. Patient B scored 10% words correct in a vision-only condition and 55% words correct in an audition-plus-vision condition (AV = audition-plus-vision; V = vision-only).

PATIENT	DIFFERENCE SCORE COMPUTATION METHOD (AV − V)	NORMALIZED DIFFERENCE SCORE COMPUTATION METHOD (AV − V/100 − V)
A (V score = 50% AV score = 75%)	25% enhancement (75% − 50% = 25%)	50% enhancement (75% − 50% / 100% − 50% = 50%)
B (V score = 10% AV score = 55%)	55% enhancement (55% − 10% = 45%)	61% enhancement (55% − 10% / 100% − 10% = 50%)

Hearing Loss Can Be Difficult to Detect in a Good Speechreader

Sometimes mild or moderate and even severe hearing losses go undetected in children because they are proficient speechreaders. Some children may mispronounce some sounds or words, but their parents and teachers do not readily associate their articulation problems with hearing loss. Jeffers and Barley (1971) related the following incident:

"Richard, age five, was [a child whose hearing loss went undetected]. The parents suspected that his younger brother had a hearing loss, but had no idea that Richard might also be similarly involved. His speech was excellent for his age, and his comprehension and recall vocabularies, larger than average. His loss was discovered through a whim of the audiometrist who decided that she might as well check Richard's hearing at the same time that she was testing his brother. Richard was found to have a binaural hearing loss of 42 dB [for the pure tone average of 500, 1000, and 2000 Hz] . . . and to be severely hard-of-hearing (60 dB or greater) for a good part of the consonant range. A year later his first grade teacher evinced complete disbelief regarding the loss and almost convinced the parents that a misdiagnosis had been made. On a test of speech intelligibility without speechreading given at normal conversational level, he made a score of 48 percent, which would indicate great difficulty in understanding. With speechreading, his score was 84 percent, indicating good comprehension." (p. 10) addition of the auditory signal when the normalized difference score is employed.

A few tests are available for assessing speechreading and speechreading enhancement. Tests for children include the Craig Sentences, the Craig Words (Craig, 1964), and the CAVET (Tye-Murray & Geers, 2002). Tests for adults include the Iowa Sentence Test (Tyler et al., 1986) and the City University of New York (CUNY) sentences (Boothroyd et al., 1985).

The CAVET (Children's Audiovisual Enhancement Test)

Assessing speechreading enhancement can be problematic. Individuals vary widely in their vision-only word recognition. For instance, in a test comprised of sentences, one person might recognize 90% of the words using only the visual signal, and another person might not recognize any of the words. The first person has a "ceiling effect" and has little room for improvement when the auditory signal is added. The second person has a "floor effect," and may not be helped when a degraded auditory signal is added.

Another difficulty that can arise when attempting to assess speechreading enhancement, particularly with regard to children, is that the individual's linguistic skills can greatly influence performance. For instance, a child with good linguistic skills will recognize more words in a sentence than a child with poor linguistic skills, all other factors being equal.

The CAVET (Tye-Murray & Geers, 2002) is a test of speechreading enhancement for children, specifically designed to minimize ceiling and floor effects and to eliminate the effects of syntactic factors and minimize the effects of semantic factors on performance. It is comprised of 40 words. Half of the test words are highly likely to be recognized in a vision-only condition, and half are less likely to be recognized. The test affords these advantages: (1) Ceiling and floor effects are minimized and (2) it is appropriate for testing a diverse group. The complete test is presented in the Key Resources at the end of this chapter.

Response Format

Another important issue to consider when testing speech recognition is what kind of response format will be used to elicit responses. Many standardized tests have an *open-set* format. This format means that no response choices and no contextual cues are provided. The materials are not familiar to the patient, and have never been practiced, say during training.

Closed-set tests often are used with cochlear-implant users and with children. These tests provide a limited set of response choices and are easier than open-set tests. The members and the size of the response set can be selected to test features of speech recognition and to vary test difficulty. For example, if a teacher is interested in determining whether a new cochlear-implant user utilizes suprasegmental cues, the response choices when the test word *ball* is spoken might be *ball, ice cream,* and *tricycle,* words that vary in duration and stress pattern. On the other hand, if the teacher is testing an experienced cochlear-implant user, the response set might be *ball, bill, bowl,* and *bell,* which will require the child to attend to more fine-grained segmental cues. The task will be more difficult when there are four response choices as opposed to only three.

An **open-set** task or test does not provide choices.

A **closed-set:** a stimulus or response set that contains a fixed number of items known to the patient.

Live-Voice Versus Recorded Test Materials

The next issue to consider in regard to selecting speech-recognition test materials is whether testing will be performed *live-voice* or whether *recorded stimuli* will be used. As the terms imply, test items can be presented by a live talker or they can be presented via a playback system, such as a tape recorder or compact disc player. The advantages of using live voice are that no playback equipment is required, and the talker can adjust the rate of stimulus presentation to meet performance needs. Many young children are more comfortable with a live-voice test paradigm than a recorded-voice paradigm.

Live-voice testing: stimuli in a test of speech recognition are presented by a talker in real time.
Recorded stimuli: test items are presented via a tape recorder, compact disc player, or a DVD player.

Despite these advantages, there are even more disadvantages associated with using live voice rather than recorded speech. Live talkers can introduce variability from one test session to the next and from one test site to another. Talkers have different speaking styles, and they may vary in their style from one day to another. For instance, test talkers may vary on any of the following variables:

- **Voicing frequency:** Female test talkers usually have high pitches and may be more difficult to understand than male test talkers, who have characteristically low-pitched voices. Most people have better hearing in the lower frequencies than in the mid and high frequencies.
- **Intonation:** Sentences spoken with appropriate and expressive intonation are generally easier to understand than ones spoken with a monotone or inappropriate intonation. Thus, a test talker who uses more voice inflection while speaking the test sentences will be easier to understand than a test talker who uses less inflection.
- **Speech rate:** Rapidly spoken speech is more difficult to recognize than moderately slow speech. One test talker may speak slowly whereas another may speak more quickly.
- **Clarity of articulation:** Clearly articulated speech is easier to recognize than conversational or mumbled speech. Test talkers may vary in their ability to speak clearly.
- **Physical characteristics:** In an audition-plus-vision or vision-only condition, talkers who have pronounced lip and jaw displacement, no facial hair, and expressive facial movements will be relatively easier to speechread or lipread.

It is important that talker characteristics not confound test results. Otherwise, you will not be able to monitor an individual's performance over time or compare his or her performance to that of other people who have been tested in other clinics. In today's world, many audiology clinics and other hearing-related settings rely exclusively on recorded materials to assess speech recognition. Live-voice testing is becoming increasingly rare.

SYNTHESIZED AND ALTERED SPEECH

Most recorded test materials present speech spoken by an adult talker, speaking as clearly as possible. However, there are two other kinds of recorded materials that sometimes are used to assess word recognition: synthesized speech and altered speech.

Synthesized speech is created with a computer or other techno-logical apparatus and not by a human vocal tract. Synthesized speech may be used if the tester wants to determine how a patient utilizes a specific cue for speech recognition. For example, a series of acoustic waveform samples may be created so that there is a systematic variation in the voice-onset time for /b/ in the word *bat*. The tester then might determine at what step in the continu-um the patient hears the word *bat* versus *pat*.

Altered speech is human speech that is recorded and then altered in some way, usually by means of computer software. Altered speech may be time-compressed, extended, or filtered. *Time-compressed speech* has been digitized and then processed so that small seg-ments are periodically deleted from the ongoing signal waveform. When it is played back, time-compressed speech sounds like natural speech produced at a fast speaking rate. Conversely, *expanded speech* is created by duplicating small segments of the signal so that the speech sounds as if it were produced with a slow speaking rate. *Filtered speech* is created by passing the speech signal through fil-ter banks. *Low-pass filtered speech* includes the lower but not the higher frequencies, whereas *high-pass filtered speech* includes the higher but not the lower frequencies. Altered speech sometimes is used when the tester is interested in how well the patient can recog-nize speech when the auditory system is challenged.

In sum, synthesized speech and altered speech often are used to examine the effects of specific acoustic cues on speech recognition or to create a difficult speech listening condition. These stimuli might be used to address the following questions:

- Does an individual utilize the plosive burst cue when distinguishing a /t/ from a /s/?
- Even though a young and aged person have similar hearing thresholds, is the older person less able to understand time-compressed speech, which is a more taxing listening task?

▪ DIFFICULTIES ASSOCIATED WITH SPEECH RECOGNITION ASSESSMENT

There are several problematic issues that should be considered when attempting to evaluate speech recognition and the effects of

Synthesized speech is created with a computer not the human vocal tract.

Altered speech is human speech that is recorded and then altered in some way.

Time-compressed speech is speech that has been accelerated by removing segments of the waveform and then compressing the remaining segments together without changing its frequency composition.

Expanded speech is recorded speech that is altered by duplicating small segments of the signal so that it sounds like a slow speaking rate.

Filtered speech is passed through filter banks for the purpose of removing or amplifying frequency bands in the signal.

Low-pass filtered speech has been passed through filter banks that removed the higher, but not the lower, frequencies.

High-pass filtered speech has been passed through filter banks that removed the lower, but not the higher, frequencies.

training on speech recognition performance. Three of the more significant issues are:

- Learning effects
- Test-retest variability
- Clinical significance

Learning Effects

Learning effects: performance on a test improves as a function of familiarity with the test procedures or items, not as a result of a change in ability.

Montgomery and Demorest (1988), among others, noted that clients often learn the test items when they are presented more than once, even when several weeks separate the test periods. Thus, because of *learning effects,* performance improves for reasons other than an aural rehabilitation intervention, such as receipt of speech perception training. For example, suppose someone was presented with the sentence, *The boy and girl are walking to school* during a speechreading test and recognized the words, *The boy _____ _____ _____ walking _____ _____.* If the patient repeated the test 3 months later, he or she might recognize all of the words, because he or she remembered the sentence remnant and used that information as contextual cues for identifying the rest of the sentence. Even recognizing the sentence rhythm and syllabic pattern might trigger recall. You may not think it is possible to remember dialogue for that length of time, but one simply need reflect how the words of a song learned in grade school come back after many years of not hearing it, often after just hearing the first couple words.

Equivalent lists contain items that are presumed to be equally difficult to recognize.

One way in which the learning problem has been addressed is with the use of *equivalent lists,* that is, sets of sentences that are presumed to be equally difficult to recognize. Equivalency is usually established by playing the separate tests to a large group of subjects. If, on average, the subjects recognize an equal number of words on each list, then the lists are said to be equivalent.

The problem with this tactic is that the lists may be equivalent when some listening devices are used but not others. For instance, a group of hearing aid users may perform similarly on two lists of test items, whereas a group of cochlear-implant users may not. Similarly, equivalency may vary with the configuration of hearing loss, such that a group of individuals with a sloping mild-to-moderate loss will not perform like a group of individuals who have a flat severe hearing loss. List equivalency also may vary as a function of test condition. For example, two lists may be equivalent when presented in a vision-only but not in an audition-plus-vision test condition.

Some researchers have tried to minimize learning effects by constructing tests that have a large number of items, say 100 or more sentences (Tyler, Preece, & Tye-Murray, 1986). With so many test items, it is thought that patients may be less likely to remember them, even with repeated testing. However, there is little empirical data available to support this assumption.

Test-Retest Variability

Another difficulty related to assessing speechreading performance is that patients, especially children, vary in their performance from day to day. Thus, a patient may achieve a score on one day, take it on another day and achieve a different score, even though it is the same test. There may be several factors that contribute to *test-retest variability.* One reason for this relates to the individual. For example, on some days a child may be highly motivated to perform well, whereas on others, the child may be restless and uninterested. As such, scores may improve or decrease over time, not as a result of training, but as a result of fatigue, interest, and mood.

Test-retest variability is a measure of the consistency of a test from one presentation to the next.

The nature of the test also may contribute to variability. Most tests are inherently variable, such that simply taking the test two times will yield somewhat different results, even if all testing parameters are held constant. If a test presents a closed-set of choices, the patient may perform better on one day than another as a function of chance.

Test-Retest Reliability

An issue closely related to variability is *test reliability*. Reliability of a test relates to the extent that test results are repeatable, and the level of reliability is expressed in terms of a standard error of measurement. Mendel and Danhauer (1997) define reliability as follows:

> "Reliability concerns the extent to which measurements are repeatable by the same individual using

(continues)

different measures of the attribute, or by different people using the same measure of the attribute without the interference of error (Bilger, 1984). Reliability can be expressed in terms of the standard error of measurement. If a listener is given the same test many times, the score determined from an average of the test scores would approach some value (that is, the true score) more and more closely. The degree to which a single test score approximates the true score determines the reliability of the test." (pp. 10–11)

Finally, test conditions can affect variability. Changes in any of the following variables can shift test scores:

■ *Mode of presentation:* for example, changing from live-voice stimuli to recorded stimuli may result in a decline in scores.
■ *Location:* for example, changing from a sound-treated booth to a clinic office may also lead to decreased performance.
■ *Talker:* for example, someone who is familiar versus unfamiliar, and someone who is male rather than female, will typically be easier to understand.
■ *The number of times an item is repeated:* for example, presenting a test item twice, or as often as an individual requests, usually leads to better performance than presenting it only once.

Use a Conservative Interpretation

"As with auditory discrimination ability, performance on speechreading tests can vary from day to day or moment to moment depending on alertness, motivation, fatigue, and so on. If we consider that a particular speech test may have an expected reliability of ±15% when performed in the [audition-only] condition and similar reliability when

(continues)

performed as a speechreading task, then the same test as an auditory-visual task may only be reliable within a range of 40% (±20%) due to the addition of the variances in the combined condition. This will also depend on the actual scores obtained and the assumptions made about the variance in the combined condition. This suggests that caution should be exercised in assessing performance based on [audition-plus-vision] test scores. For reliable assessment, it is necessary to have a complete battery of testing and to minimize any controllable sources of variance." (Dowell, Brown, & Mecklenburg, 1990, p. 199)

Clinical Significance

Another difficulty associated with speech recognition assessment relates to clinical significance. It sometimes is difficult to determine whether a small change in performance is clinically significant. For instance, an individual might recognize 30% of the words in a sentence test prior to receiving speechreading training. Afterwards, the person might recognize 36% of the words. In this instance, the hearing professional must determine whether speechreading has improved in a meaningful way.

A within-subject statistical procedure has been used to compare posttraining performance to pretraining performance to establish whether a change is statistically significant. The number of words repeated verbatim in each sentence of a pretraining test can be compared to the number of key words repeated verbatim in the same sentence following training. A paired t-statistic can be computed using all sentences in a list. Although statistical significance does not necessarily equate with clinical significance, it does indicate whether a change is robust.

■ MULTICULTURAL ISSUES

With the U.S. population becoming increasingly diverse, multilingual testing has gained importance as an issue in aural rehabilitation. When considering multilingual testing, it is important

Monolingual: Term used to describe a person who speaks only one language.

Bilingual: Term used to describe a person who speaks two languages.

to determine whether the patient is ***monolingual*** (speaks only one language) or bilingual (speaks two languages). A ***bilingual*** individual is sometimes described as being a native speaker, such as a native Spanish speaker (e.g., Comstock & Martin, 1984; Weisleder & Hodgson, 1989), to imply proficiency comparable to that of a language speaker who originates from the country where the language is spoken. Performance on a speech recognition test may vary from one patient to another, depending on whether that person is monolingual or bilingual, and on other such language variables as language history (e.g., When did the individual begin to learn English? Which language was learned first?) and competency (e.g., the individual's proficiency in a language). There is evidence that monolingual and bilingual individuals perform differently from each other on speech-recognition tests, and Spanish tests of speech recognition yield better performance than English tests for native Spanish bilingual individuals (see von Hapsburg & Pena, 2002, for a review).

There is a demand for speech-recognition materials that are appropriate for non–English-speaking patients or patients who use English as a second language. Unfortunately, the demand at present exceeds the supply. The few examples of tests that have been developed for Spanish-speaking patients include the Spanish Bisyllables (Weisleder & Hodgson, 1989), 50-word lists of bisyllabic consonant-vowel-consonant-vowel Spanish words presented in an open-set response format, and the Synthetic Sentence Identification (SSI) test (Benitez & Speaks, 1968). The Key Resources section of this chapter presents a list of references that provide additional information on speech recognition testing of Spanish monolingual and bilingual patients.

One difficulty in assessing nonnative English speakers for clinicians is that they may not understand the language of their patients, and hence, may have difficulty in scoring responses to test materials. At least one test, The Spanish Picture-Identification Test (McCullough, Wilson, Birck, & Anderson (1995), has been modified to circumvent this problem (McCullough & Wilson, 2001). The test consists of two 50-word lists. The test words (spoken in a carrier phrase context) are common, bisyllabic nouns and verbs that can be easily pictured. The items are presented in a four-choice closed-set, with the foils (or alternative responses) rhyming with the target word. The choices are presented in picture form to patients via a computer screen monitor. The advantage of using the picture-based closed-set format is that the clinician administering the test does not need to understand Spanish to test the patient. In addition, the close-set results compare similarly to results obtained when the test is administered in an open-set format. The word lists appear in the Key Resources as an example of a Spanish language test.

Bilingualism Defined

"The broadest definition of a bilingual includes anyone who knows two languages (Baker, 1993). Yet, this definition remains too broad to be useful, because the degree to which an individual knows each language depends on many circumstances. Factors such as when the languages were learned, how the languages were learned, what language skills (reading, writing, speaking, listening) were acquired, and how the languages are used on a daily basis affect the state of bilingualism in any individual. Some consider bilinguals only those who are equally fluent in both of their languages, known as *balanced* bilinguals or *ambilinguals*. . . . A functional or wholistic view of bilingualism takes into consideration that individuals learn and use each of their languages for different purposes and in different communication contexts. Therefore, a functional view of bilingualism recognizes that a bilingual may become more competent in one language in certain communication contexts and competent in the other language for other contexts. From the functional perspective, then, it becomes important to ask why the languages were acquired, how they were acquired, when they were acquired, and how they are used." (von Hapsburg & Pena, 2002, p. 203)

CASE STUDY 1

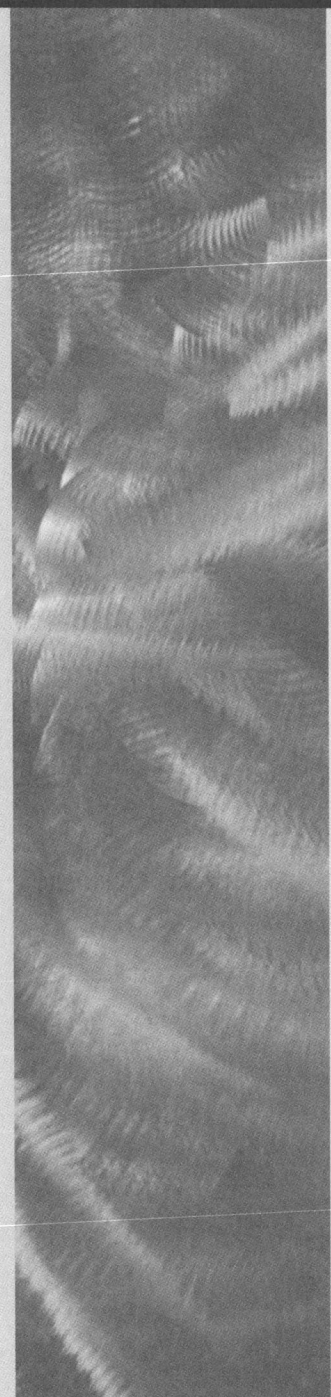

Lindsey Mooreland, an audiologist, wanted to compare the listening skills of three of her older male patients. At first, she thought she might administer only a word test, The Children's Audiovisual Enhancement Test (CAVET). Because she had extra time, she went ahead and administered a consonant test (the Iowa Consonant Test) and a sentence test (The Iowa Sentence Test), too. The results for the three true-life patients appear in Table 6-5.

Table 6-5. Percent correct scores for three patients on three different tests that each present a different stimulus type, presented in an audilion-only condition.

TEST AND STIMULUS TYPE	PATIENTS' SCORES IN %		
	Al	Tom	Bob
Iowa Consonant Test (Consonants)	55	61	87
CAVET (Words)	45	45	30
Iowa Sentence Test (Sentences)	58	38	48

If she had administered only the word test, the three men would have appeared similar in their listening skills. Scores ranged from a low of 30% words correct (Bob) to a high of 45% (Al and Tom).

The test battery approach reveals a more complex picture, and the conclusions as to which patient has the best listening skills is not as straightforward as it would have been if she had administered only a word test. In terms of consonant recognition, Bob scored the highest of the three (87% consonant correct), whereas Al scored the lowest (55% correct). For sentence recognition, Al scored the highest (58% words correct), and Tom scored the lowest (38%).

(continues)

Time available for testing and your purpose for assessment will dictate in large part which and how many tests you administer to a patient. However, if you administer only a single test, it is important to be aware that the test result may not provide a complete picture of the construct of speech recognition for a particular patient.

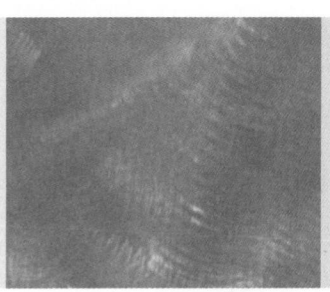

FINAL REMARKS

In this chapter, we considered in a general way how to assess individuals' ability to recognize speech. We have not focused on particular tests; rather, we have focused on the principles that must be considered when choosing a test for a particular individual. The results of speech recognition testing are invaluable when designing an aural rehabilitation plan.

KEY CHAPTER POINTS

✔ A typical audiological assessment includes an audiogram, a determination of speech recognition thresholds, and an assessment of speech discrimination/recognition. The audiogram by itself does not always adequately reflect the magnitude of a patient's communication difficulties.

✔ You might assess speech recognition abilities for any number of reasons. For instance, you might be interested in evaluating a patient's need for amplification or assessing the patient's performance over time.

✔ Patient variables, such as the cognitive/linguistic skill of the test taker, will influence selection of test materials. For example, you would not select a sentence test for evaluating a 3-year-old child.

✔ Test stimuli may be phonemes, words, phrases, unrelated sentences, or topically related sentences. Each kind of stimulus offers advantages and disadvantages.

✔ Once you have selected your test materials, you can make decisions about test procedures. For example, you might opt to present the stimuli in an audition-only condition, using live-voice and background noise.

✔ Patients may learn the items in a test with repeated testing.

✔ Test-retest variability sometimes is an important issue. Some people, especially children, may vary in their performance from day to day.

✔ Although multicultural testing is ever more commonplace, the need for speech-recognition tests in languages other than English outstrips the current supply.

✔ Bilingual individuals perform better on tests administered in their native language than on tests administered in their second language.

▬ MULTIPLE CHOICE QUESTIONS

1. Mrs. M. complains that she can hear speech with no problem, even if the talker is speaking softly, but that she cannot understand it well. Her configuration of hearing loss is most likely:
   a. Low-frequency
   b. Flat
   c. High-frequency
   d. Saucer-shaped

2. A child who has a severe hearing loss may:
   a. Recognize speech fairly well in quiet situations, but may only recognize about 50% of the words spoken in the presence of noise
   b. Not even hear voices, unless the talker is speaking loudly
   c. May perceive speech primarily as vibrations
   d. With a hearing aid, may get most of the message, unless if conversing in group situations

3. The purpose of speech recognition testing:
   a. Will dictate your choice of test
   b. May vary, but you will always present a phonetically balanced word list
   c. Is often to compare listening devices
   d. Is determined by the age of the patient

4. Stimuli such as *eepee* and *eesee* might be included in a test designed to assess a patient's:
   a. Word recognition
   b. Feature utilization
   c. Nonlinguistic sound recognition
   d. Hearing acuity

5. In speech testing, a neighborhood refers to:
   a. The group of words having similar acoustic-phonetic characteristics
   b. A battery of tests administered for a specific purpose
   c. Test stimuli included on a specific test
   d. The native language of the patient

6. A Spanish bilingual patient:
   a. Will perform the same as a monolingual patient on a speech test given in Spanish
   b. Must be tested by a clinician who speaks Spanish
   c. Cannot take a word or sentence speech-recognition test
   d. Is considered a native bilingual if he or she speaks the language like someone from the country of origin

7. The advantage afforded by adding hearing to vision is known as:
   a. Speechreading enhancement
   b. Speechreading
   c. Audition-plus-vision speech recognition
   d. A normalized ratio

8. Which is seldom true when testing speech recognition?
   a. A closed-set response mode is employed
   b. The test stimuli are presented live-voice
   c. Female talkers speak the stimuli
   d. Stimuli are isolated words

9. Equivalent lists are sometimes used to bypass the difficulties associated with:

    a. Test-retest variability

    b. Test reliability

    c. Learning effects

    d. Patient variability

KEY RESOURCES

The Lexical Neighborhood Test

(Kirk, Pisoni, & Osberger, 1995)

List 1

Easy words: juice, good, drive, time, hard, gray, foot, orange, count, brown, home, old watch, need, food, dance, live, stand, six, cold, push, stop, girl, hurt, cow.

Hard words: thumb, pie, wet, fight, toe, cut, pink, hi, song, fun, use, mine, ball, kick, tea, book, bone, work, dad, game, lost, cook, gum, cap, meat.

List 2

Easy words: down, truck, mouth, pig, give, school, boy, put, three, farm, fish, green, catch, break, house, sit, friend, jump, bird, swim, hold, want, snake, more, white.

Hard words: ear, hand, dry, zoo, goat, toy, call, sing, cut, wrong, bed, fat, man, run, hot, read, grow, bag, cake, seat, nine, sun, bath, ten, ride.

CID Everyday Sentences

(Silverman & Hirsh, 1955)

List A

1. Walking's my favorite exercise.

2. Here's a nice quiet place to rest.

3. Our janitor sweeps the floors every night.

4. It would be much easier if everyone would help.

5. Good morning.

6. Open your window before you go to bed!

7. Do you think that she should stay out so late?

8. How do you feel about changing the time when we begin work?

9. Here we go.

10. Move out of the way!

List B

1. The water's too cold for swimming.

2. Why should I get up so early in the morning?

3. Here are your shoes.

4. It's raining.

5. Where are you going?

6. Come here when I call you!

7. Don't try to get out of it this time!

8. Should we let little children go to the movies by themselves?

9. There isn't enough paint to finish the room.

10. Do you want an egg for breakfast?

List C

1. Everybody should brush his teeth after meals.

2. Everything's all right.

3. Don't use up all the paper when you write your letter.

4. That's right.

5. People ought to see a doctor once a year.

6. Those windows are so dirty I can't see anything outside.

7. Pass the bread and butter please.

8. Don't forget to pay your bill before the first of the month.

9. Don't let the dog out of the house.

10. There's a good ball game this afternoon.

List D

1. It's time to go.

2. If you don't want these old magazines, throw them out.

3. Do you want to wash up?

4. It's a real dark night so watch your driving.

5. I'll carry the package for you.

6. Did you forget to shut off the water?

7. Fishing in a mountain stream is my idea of a good time.

8. Fathers spend more time with their children than they used to.

9. Be careful not to break your glasses.

10. I'm sorry.

List E

1. You can catch the bus across the street.

2. Call her on the phone and tell her the news.

3. I'll catch up with you later.

4. I'll think it over.

5. I don't want to go to the movies tonight.

6. If your tooth hurts that much you ought to see a dentist.

7. Put the cookie back in the box!

8. Stop fooling around!

9. Time's up.

10. How do you spell your name?

List F

1. Music always cheers me up.

2. My brother's in town for a short while on business.

3. We live a few miles from the main road.

4. This suit needs to go to the cleaners.

5. They ate enough green apples to make them sick for a week.

6. Where have you been all this time?

7. Have you been working hard lately?

8. There's not enough room in the kitchen for a new table.

9. Where is he?

10. Look out!

List G

1. I'll see you right after lunch.

2. See you later.

3. White shoes are awful to keep clean.

4. Stand there and don't move until I tell you.

5. There's a big piece of cake left over from dinner.

6. Wait for me at the corner in front of the drugstore.

7. It's no trouble at all.

8. Hurry up!

9. The morning paper didn't say anything about rain this afternoon or tonight.

10. The phone call's for you.

List H

1. Believe me!

2. Let's get a cup of coffee.

3. Let's get out of here before it's too late.

4. I hate driving at night.

5. There was water in the cellar after that heavy rain yesterday.

6. She'll only be a few minutes.

7. How do you know?

8. Children like candy.

9. If we don't get rain soon, we'll have no grass.

10. They're not listed in the new phone book.

List I

1. Where can I find a place to work?

2. I like those big red apples we always get in the fall.

3. You'll get fat eating candy.

4. The show's over.

5. Why don't they paint their walls some other color?

6. What's new?

7. What are you hiding under your coat?

8. How come I should always be the one to go first?

9. I'll take sugar and cream in my coffee.

10. Wait just a minute!

List J

1. Breakfast is ready.

2. I don't know what's wrong with the car, but it won't start.

3. It sure takes a sharp knife to cut this meat.

4. I haven't read a newspaper since we bought a television set.

5. Weeds are spoiling the yard.

6. Call me a little later!

7. Do you have change for a $5 bill?

8. How are you?

9. I'd like some ice cream with my pie.

10. I don't think I'll have any dessert.

The CAVET Sentence Test

Description: The CAVET is comprised of three word lists. Each list is to be administered in a different condition. Each list contains 20 words. Experiments have determined that 10 words in each list are "easy," meaning that the majority of persons can identify them using only vision alone, and 10 words are "difficult," and only a minority of people can lipread them. The words are within the vocabulary level of 7- to 9-year-old children with profound prelingual hearing losses (Tye-Murray & Geers, 2002). Here, the words are organized by difficulty level. In practice, they are presented randomly within the list. The test is available on CD-ROM and VHS.

List A (Audition-plus-vision)

Easy:

1. telephone
2. elephant
3. mouth
4. fish
5. newspaper
6. hamburger
7. warm
8. thumb
9. chair
10. ship

Difficult:

11. ten
12. hug
13. rock
14. talk
15. sit
16. cat
17. full
18. sing
19. birthday cake
20. map

List B (Vision-only)

Easy:

1. family
2. remember
3. basketball
4. bath
5. beautiful
6. ice cream cone
7. look
8. shoe
9. light
10. cheese

Difficult:

11. line
12. neck
13. kill
14. kiss
15. dinosaur
16. sock
17. juice
18. foot
19. math
20. Mickey Mouse

List C (Audition-only)

Easy:

1. grandfather
2. fall
3. policeman
4. farm
5. ball
6. butterfly
7. push
8. love
9. hear
10. chocolate

Difficult:

11. down
12. plate
13. six
14. good
15. hill
16. tall
17. sun
18. car
19. pull
20. vegetable

KEY RESOURCES

Resources for Learning More About Spanish and Speech-Recognition Testing

Benitez, L., & Speaks, C. (1968). A test of speech intelligibility in the Spanish language. *International Audiology, 7,* 16–22.

Cokely, J. A., & Yager, C. R. (1993). Scoring Spanish word-recognition measures. *Ear and Hearing, 14,* 395–400.

Comstock, C. L., & Martin, F. N. (1984). A children's Spanish word discrimination test for non-Spanish speaking clinicians. *Ear and Hearing, 5,* 166–170.

Danhauer, J. L., Crawford, S., & Edgerton, B. (1984). English, Spanish, and bilingual speakers' performance on a nonsense syllable test (NST) of speech sound discrimination. *Journal of Speech and Hearing Disorders, 49,* 164–168.

Grosjean, F. (1989). Neurolinguists, beware! The bilingual is not two monolinguals in one person. *Brain and Language, 36,* 3–15.

Lopez, S. M., Martin, F. N., & Thibodeau, L. M. (1997). Performance of monolingual and bilingual speakers of English and Spanish on the Synthetic Sentence Identification Test. *American Journal of Audiology, 6,* 33–38.

McCullough, J., Wilson, R. H., Birck, J. D., & Anderson, L. G. (1995). A multimedia approach for estimating speech recognition of multilingual clients. *American Journal of Audiology, 3,* 19–22.

McCullough, J. A., & Wilson, R. H. (2001). Performance on a Spanish picture-identification task using a multimedia format. *Journal of the American Academy of Audiology, 12,* 254–260.

Ramos, H. S., Windham, R. A., & Katz, J. (1992). Introducing a Spanish-language version of the Staggered Spondaic Word test. *The Hearing Journal, 45*, 39–43.

Weisleder, P., & Hodgson, W. R. (1989). Evaluation of four Spanish word-recognition-ability lists. *Ear and Hearing, 10*, 387–393.

Words Comprising the Spanish Picture-Identification Task

(McCullough & Wilson, 2001)

List 1	List 2
Balón (balloon)	Ala (wing)
Barba (beard)	Balcón (balcony)
Barca (boat)	Barra (bar)
Besa (kiss)	Bastón (cane)
Boca (mouth)	Bata (robe)
Bola (ball)	Beso (kiss)
Bota (boot)	Bola (ball)
Caja (box)	Bolsa (purse)
Canta (sing)	Cabra (goat)
Capa (cape)	Cama (bed)
Cara (face)	Caña (cane)
Carne (meat)	Carga (load)
Cárcel (jail)	Carta (letter)
Coger (catch)	Casa (house)
Cono (cone)	Coca (Coke)
Corer (run)	Comer (eat)
Foto (photo)	Coser (sew)
Gorro (cap)	Dama (lady)
Hueso (bone)	Fresa (strawberry)
Jota (J)	Halcón (hawk)
Ladrón (robber)	Jamón (ham)
Llama (knock)	Llanta (tire)

Manta (blanket)	Lloro (cry)
Masa (dough)	Mala (sick-f)
Misa (mass)	Mapa (map)
Mono (monkey)	Mesa (table)
Niña (girl)	Moto (motorcycle)
Ojo (eye)	Nota (note)
Oso (bear)	Ocho (eight)
Pala (shovel)	Oro (gold)
Papa (potato)	Peso (money)
Pico (sting)	Pino (pine tree)
Pito (whistle)	Piña (pineapple)
Prisa (hurry)	Piso (floor)
Queso (cheese)	Plaza (plaza)
Rama (twig)	Riña (fight)
Ratón (rat)	Risa (laugh)
Reza (pray)	Roca (rock)
Roja (red)	Ronca (snore)
Ropa (rope)	Rosa (rose)
Rota (broken f.)	Roto (broken m.)
Sala (living room)	Saco (sack)
Salto (jump)	Sapo (frog)
Santo (Saint m.)	Santa (Saint m.)
Talon (heel)	Tapa (lid)
Tasa (cup)	Tisa (chalk)
Toca (knock)	Tono (note)
Toro (bull)	Trono (throne)
Viña (vine)	Vota (vote)
Voto (vote)	Zorro (fox)

CHAPTER **7**

Listening Devices and Related Technology

TOPICS

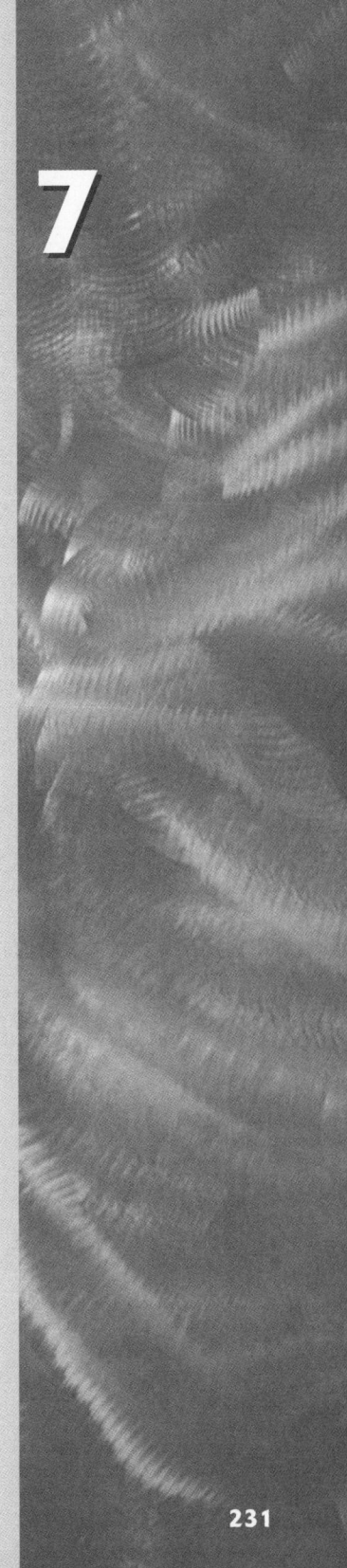

- Hearing aids
- Cochlear implants
- Assistive Listening Devices (ALDs)
- Case study
- Final remarks
- Key chapter points
- Multiple choice questions
- Key resources

After a patient receives a comprehensive audiological assessment, and before he or she receives speech perception training, appropriate listening devices must be selected and fitted. These systems may include a hearing aid or a cochlear implant, or assistive listening devices (ALDs). The provision of appropriate technical devices is an essential element in the aural rehabilitation plan, whether the patient is an adult or a child. These instruments can minimize conversational difficulties and maximize the use of residual hearing for daily functioning.

The objectives for providing an individual with a listening device are twofold:

1. **to make speech audible, without introducing distortion or discomfort, and**

2. **to restore a range of loudness experience**

In optimal circumstances, the three kinds of listening devices that we review in this chapter can be selected and fitted to achieve the two objectives just listed.

This chapter presents an introduction for readers who are unacquainted with listening devices and a key-points review for those who are familiar with them. We will discuss both related terminology and categories within device types.

■ HEARING AIDS

Prior to the 20th century, there were three ways to help a hard-of-hearing person hear better: (1) speak loudly, (2) talk right into the person's ear, or (3) provide the person with an ear horn, speaking tube, trumpet, or other similar device. The advent of electronic hearing aids revolutionized the methods available to assist hard-of-hearing persons to hear more. To appreciate the relatively rapid advances that have occurred in hearing aid technology since 1847, it is worthwhile to review Table 7-1. This table highlights some of the landmark events that have occurred in hearing aid design.

Two major trends are evident in modern hearing-aid design: miniaturization and enhanced signal processing. Over time,

Table 7-1. Some landmark events in the history of hearing-aid technology and marketing. Siemens, Oticon, Telex, Beltone, Maico, Dahlberg, Miracle-Ear, Widex, Starkey, Argosy, Microtronic, Philips, and Danavox are companies that manufacture hearing aids.

1847: Siemens is founded in Germany by Werner von Siemens. Makes many improvements in tele-graph, telephone, and electric transmission systems.

1890: National Carbon Company is founded, and later becomes Eveready Battery Co.

1904: The company that later becomes Oticon is founded by Hans Demant to import American hearing aids to Denmark.

1910: Siemens makes its first hearing aids for employees, offering them to the public in 1912. Early aids are hand-carried.

1914: Siemens introduces a small hearing aid receiver fitted close to the auditory canal, with sound carried via an animal membrane.

1919: Siemens makes the first audiometer.

1924: Siemens patents first compact carbon microphone amplifier for use in pocket hearing aids.

1929: Siemens builds first wearable tube amplifiers with improved response and loudness.

1940: Maico introduces its first wearable hearing aid (made in three parts) incorporating miniature vacuum tubes.

1941: Maico introduces tone adjustments for fitting various hearing losses.

1944: Beltone introduces first all-in-one hearing aid, the Mono-Pac.

1953: Maico markets first completely transistorized hearing aid.

1955: Dahlberg introduces the Miracle-Ear, the first electronic hearing aid designed to be worn in the ear, That some year, Dahlberg introduces innovative BTE and eyeglass instruments and begins provid-ing private-level hearing aids to Sears Roebuck. Siemens' first transistor hearing aid introduces the telecoil.

1961: Siemens introduces Auriculina, the first BTE with frontal sound pick-up.

1962: Miracle-Ear IV is first hearing aid to use integrated circuitry.

1967: Siemens develops a BTE with push-pull amplifier, and introduces the Fonator speech/auditory training instrument. Widex introduces a sound hook to reduce wind noise.

1971: Maico patents dephasing microphone that offers directional hearing.

1972: Starkey establishes right of return policy for its custom full-concha hearing aids.

1976: Danavox is first hearing aid manufacturer to launch a direct audio input system. Siemens intro-duces BTE with input compression.

1979: Oticon introduces E24V, the first hearing aid with a user-operated switch to choose between omni- and directional microphones.

1982: Argosy Electronics releases the CCA, the industry's first successful in-the-canal instrument.

1986: Beltone's new Suprimo hearing aid, offering three custom integrated circuits and eight fitting controls, is a long step toward a fully programmable instrument.

1988: Philips introduces infrared remote-controlled ITEs and ITCs.

(continued)

Table 7-1. *(continued)*

1989: Maico offers the first programmable hearing aid.

1991: Philips introduces the first very-deep-canal instrument, the XP Peritympanic.

1992: Danavox introduces DFS Genius, a digital system for suppressing feedback.

1995: Oticon announces DigiFocus, the first 100% digital ear-level hearing aid. Maico offers the first programmable CIC.

1996: Telex introduces SoftWear, a completely soft-shelled hearing aid.

1997: Argosy introduces Quadrasound, a proprietary microchip providing access to four separate signal processors within each hearing instrument. Widex introduces first digital signal processing instrument in a CIC model. Telex introduces the AcuSound, the first hearing aid to split the incoming signal into two channels based on the signal's amplitude.

2000: Songbird Medical Inc. offers a disposable hearing aid for about $40, which provides about 40 days of usage.

2001: Oticon introduces open ear acoustics, a system designed to use active feedback cancellation to allow for open ear fittings to eliminate occlusion.

Source: Adapted from the "A timeline of the hearing industry." *The Hearing Journal* (1991), 50, pp. 54–70.

hearing aids have become smaller. Early hearing aids were so large and cumbersome, they were not portable. These tabletop electrical aids often were used only in educational settings where teacher and students might sit around a shared table. The early portable aids were not much of an improvement over the tabletop devices. They were housed in large cases that had to be carried on the body or with the hand and were operated with vacuum tubes. Vacuum tubes were replaced by transistors, which made it possible for hearing aids to be worn on the head. In the last few decades, there have been rapid advances toward miniaturization so now it is possible to use a hearing aid and have it be completely invisible, unless someone looks directly into the ear. Probably the primary factor spurring this trend toward miniaturization is cosmetic concerns on the part of the users.

Along with miniaturization, there has been another trend evident in hearing-aid designs, and that is a growing sophistication in their *signal-processing* capabilities (ability to alter the signal in some way, usually according to a processing algorithm), all in virtual real time. Some of the advances related to developments in signal-processing include the following:

Signal processing involves manipulation of various parameters of a signal.

- ■ *Multiple memories,* so that a patient might adjust the hearing aid one way when listening in quiet and another way when listening in noise, to maximize sound quality and speech reception. Hearing aids that provide access to different amplification characteristics sometimes are referred to as *multiple memory hearing aids.*
- ■ *Sophisticated noise reduction circuits,* so that the hearing aid amplifies speech and not undesirable background noise.
- ■ *Acoustic feedback cancellation,* so that hearing aids will not "whistle" when sound escapes from the receiver.
- ■ *Programmability,* which allows the audiologist to set gain, frequency response, and other electroacoustic properties of the hearing aid. This feature may be especially attractive if the user is experiencing a progressive hearing loss, and the hearing aid must be altered over time to accommodate the changing listening needs.
- ■ *Digital processing,* so that the signal is converted from analog to digital form, processed to achieve a target signal, and then converted back to an analog signal.
- ■ *Multiple channels,* a signal processing technique wherein the signal is filtered into frequency bands, so that some bands (usually the high-frequency bands) receive more gain than other bands (usually the low-frequency bands).

Although these trends are indicative of evolving designs, there are some constancies in the components that make up a hearing aid, no matter what the style or special features.

Hearing-Aid Components

Figure 7-1 provides a schematic of a generic hearing aid. The *microphone* picks up the acoustic signal from the ambient environment. The microphone component converts the acoustic signal into an electrical signal. The electrical signal then passes to the *amplifier,* where the signal is selectively amplified. For example, only the high frequencies of a signal may be boosted. From the amplifier, the processed electrical signal passes onto the receiver. The receiver converts the processed electrical signal back into an acoustic signal and passes it on through any tubing and earmold.

Some hearing aids have **multiple memories** that allow the speech signal to be processed in more than one way.

Multiple memory hearing aids allow the user to select the processing strategy according to the listening environment.

Noise reduction is the difference in the sound pressure level (SPL) of a noise measured at two different locations.

Acoustic feedback cancellation is a feature that avoids the annoying squeal produced by hearing aids when the microphone picks up the amplified sound from the hearing aid and reamplifies it.

Programmability in a hearing aid means that several parameters of the instrument, such as gain, are controlled by a computer.

A hearing aid that uses **digital processing** converts the signal from analog to digital form, processes the signal to achieve a target, and then converts the signal back to an analog form.

A hearing aid that uses **multiple channels** filters the signal into frequency bands so that some bands (usually the high frequency bands) can receive more gain than others.

A **microphone** is a transducer that converts an audio signal into an electronic signal.

An **amplifier** increases the intensity of sound.

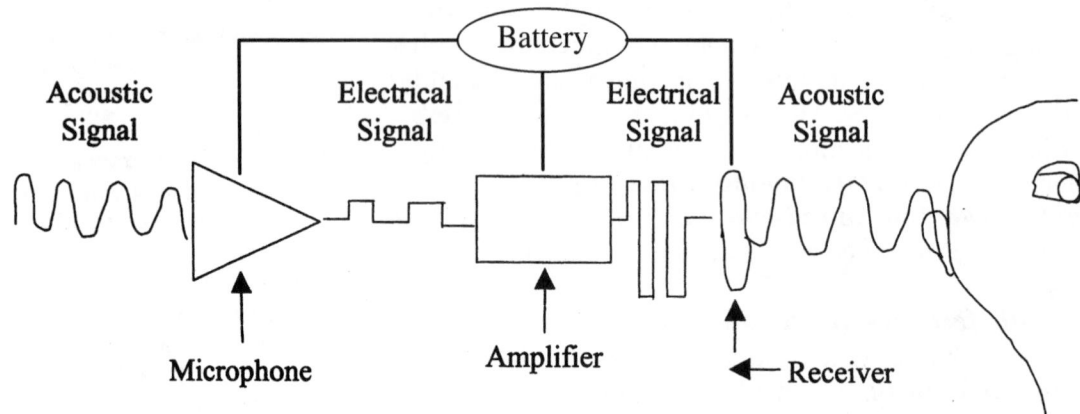

FIGURE 7-1. Schematic of a hearing aid.

A **battery** is a cell that provides electrical power.

The hearing aid also carries *batteries*, which provide power for its operation. Batteries come in at least five sizes (denoted by the following codes, from largest size to smallest: AA, 675, 312,13, 230, and 10). Batteries may be mercury or zinc, with zinc batteries lasting about twice as long as mercury. Although battery life is dependent on a number of factors, such as the kind of battery it is, the style of hearing aid in which it is used, and the volume control setting, a zinc battery will last about 1 to 4 weeks.

MICROPHONES

Microphones are designed to respond to sound, without distorting it or introducing extraneous noise. The microphone converts the audio signal into an electrical signal. The volume inside of a modern microphone case is divided into two parts by a thin polymer diaphragm. On one side is a thin metal coating that allows the diaphragm to conduct electricity. Parallel to the diaphragm is a metal backplate with an electret coating. This coated backplate can permanently store static electrical charge. The static charge on the electret causes a strong electric field to form between the diaphragm and the backplate. When the diaphragm moves from its resting position, a small voltage develops between the diaphragm and the backplate. So when a microphone is in action, sound waves travel into its front volume, causing the diaphragm to vibrate. These oscillations create an oscillating voltage signal between the diaphragm and the backplate conductor. It is this signal that is passed onto the amplifier.

There are two general types of microphones: directional and om-nidirectional. ***Directional microphones*** are designed to respond primarily to sound originating from in front of the user, and not from the back. ***Omnidirectional microphones*** respond to sound originating from all directions. Directional microphones are most common in behind-the-ear instruments, which we will consider shortly, and are meant to enhance the signal-to-noise ratio for the user. For instance, a directional microphone will pick up the speech of a talker who stands in front of the user, but not from two individuals who speak about something else in the back of the room. As such, directional microphones are often desirable for lis-tening in noisy situations.

Directional microphones are more sensitive to sound originating from in front of the user than sound coming from behind the user.

Omnidirectional microphones are sensitive to sound coming from all directions.

AMPLIFIERS

An amplifier is also a component in all hearing aids. Amplifiers increase the level of the signal. ***Gain*** describes the amount of am-plification provided by an amplifier and is defined as the differ-ence between the hearing aid's input and output. For instance, if an input signal is 30 dB SPL and the output is 60 dB SPL, the gain of the hearing aid is 30 dB.

The **gain** of a hearing aid is the difference in decibels between the input level of an acoustic signal and the output level.

The signal is selectively processed and amplified. In many hearing aids, the signal passes through three stages of the amplification process. In the ***preamplifier stage,*** the signal received from the microphone is boosted. During the ***signal processing stage,*** the signal is manipulated to enhance the quality of the sound for the patient. During the ***output stage,*** the processed signal is amplified and sent to the hearing aid receiver.

In the **preamplifier stage,** the signal from the micro-phone is amplified.

In the **signal-processing** stage, the signal is manip-ulated to enhance or extract component information.

In the **output stage,** the process signal is boosted.

Amplifiers in analog and digital hearing aids process the signal differently. In an analog hearing aid, the signal is amplified as a continuously varying amplitude over time. In contrast, in a digital hearing aid, sound is converted from an analog signal into a digi-tal representation. The processing is performed on this computer language version. The processed signal is then converted back in-to an analog signal.

Amplifiers may be classified as one of two types: peak-clipping or compression. These terms refer to their mode of limiting the out-put of the signal so that it is not so loud as to be uncomfortable to the user nor does it have the potential to cause a noise-induced hearing loss. The goal of peak-clipping or compression is to limit

Maximum power output (MPO): the maximum intensity level that a hearing aid can produce.

Peak-clipping is a method of limiting hearing aid output in which a constant or linear amount of gain is provided across a range of input levels until it reaches a saturation level, at which time the amplifier begins to "clip" off the peaks of the signal.

Saturation level: point at which an amplifier no longer provides an increase in output compared to input.

Compression is a nonlinear form of amplifier gain used to determine and limit output gain as a function of input gain.

the **maximum power output (MPO)** of the hearing aid, which is the maximum output level a hearing aid will put out in response to a very loud input signal.

An amplifier with a **peak-clipping** circuit provides a constant or linear amount of gain (or amplification) across a range of input levels. There is a one-to-one relationship between the input and output, so that the sound is amplified by a consistent amount until it reaches a saturation level. At this **saturation level,** sound coming into the amplifier is so loud that the amplifier begins to "clip" or cut off the peaks of the signal. Although this effectively limits the level of the audio signal, it also introduces distortion; therefore, sound quality decreases. Figure 7-2 presents an example of the relationship between input and output levels of the hearing aid in a peak-clipping system.

A nonlinear amplifier system usually functions with a **compression** circuitry. The use of compression has three purposes. One purpose of compression is to limit the maximum output of the hearing aid, so that sound is never so loud as to cause discomfort to the user.

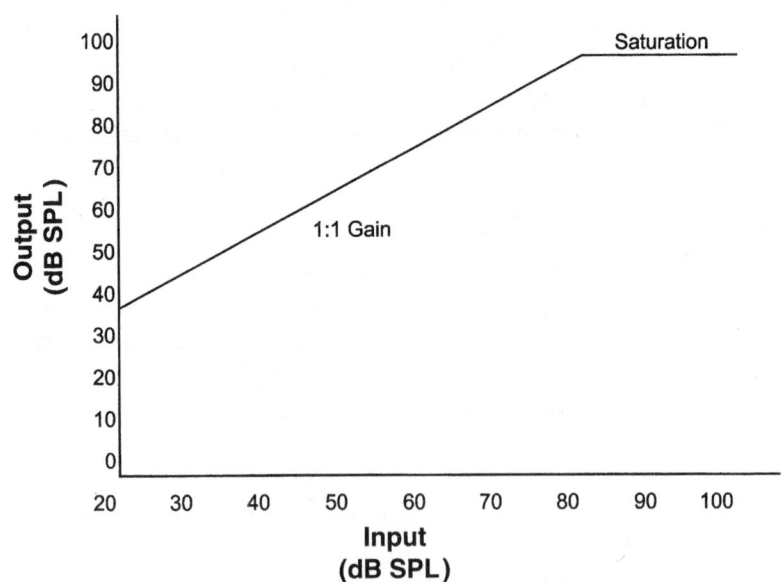

FIGURE 7-2. Input/output loudness function for a hearing aid that uses peak-clipping to limit output.

A second purpose of compression is to provide a range of sounds to the user within the person's dynamic range. ***Dynamic range*** is defined as the difference between a person's threshold for sound and the level at which the sound causes discomfort. In many persons with significant hearing loss, dynamic range is reduced and may be only 40 dB or less.

A third purpose of compression circuitry is to provide a varying amount of gain (amplification) of the speech signal as a function of the input level. Thus, soft sounds are amplified more than moderately loud sounds.

In a compression circuitry, sound may be amplified in a linear fashion until it reaches a level of incoming intensity that triggers the compression function. At this point, often referred to as the ***kneepoint,*** the signal is amplified to a lesser degree, and never amplified beyond a preselected level. This kind of output limiting is used most commonly in today's hearing aids. Figure 7-3 presents the relationship between input and output of a hearing aid that has a compression circuit and indicates the kneepoint. The relation between input and output is referred to as the ***compression ratio,*** or the ratio of the change in input SPL to the change in the output SPL. For instance, if a sound entering into the amplifier changes by 20 dB but leaves the amplifier changed by 10dB, that compression ratio is 2:1. The length of time it takes for a compression amplifier to react to a loud sound and compress it is referred to as an ***attack time.*** For example, if it takes 50 ms for a sound of 120 dB to be compressed to a level of 90 dB, than the attack time is 50 ms. Similarly, the ***release time*** is the length of time for a compression amplifier to increase its gain after a loud sound has ceased. There are different kinds of compression circuits. For example, the ***K-AMP circuit*** provides more gain for high frequencies than low frequencies at low-intensity input levels, but not for high-intensity input levels. ***Multiband compression*** permits different degrees of compression and output limiting for different frequency bands in the incoming signal, so that the growth of loudness in a signal can be controlled, and the signal can be shaped to maximize speech recognition.

RECEIVERS

The processed electrical signal enters the other energy transducer of the hearing aid, the receiver, where it is converted back to

Dynamic range is the difference in decibels between an individual's threshold of sensitivity for a sound and the level at which the sound becomes uncomfortably loud.

Kneepoint is the point on an input-output function where compression is activated.

Compression ratio is the decibel ratio of acoustic input to amplifier output.

Attack time is the time between when a signal begins to the onset of its steady-state amplified value.

Release time is the time it takes for an amplifier to return to its steady state after a loud sound ends.

K-AMP circuit is designed to provide more gain for moderate-level sound, no gain for high-intensity sound, and compression limited for the highest level sound. It often also provides more amplification for the high frequencies.

Multiband compression is a method of shaping the loudness growth of a signal to maximize speech for the listener using different degrees of compression and output limiting for different frequencies.

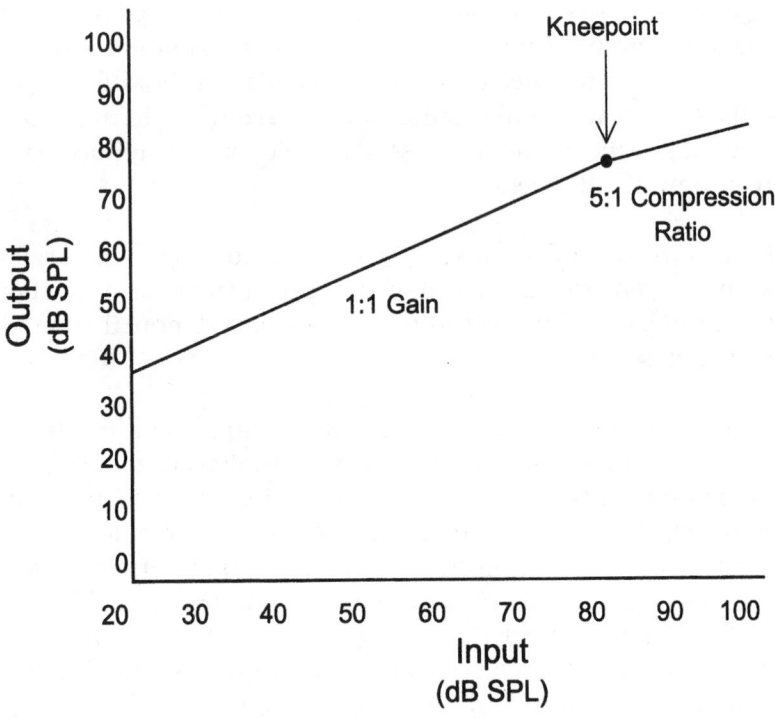

FIGURE 7-3. Input/output loudness function for a hearing aid that uses compression circuitry to limit output.

acoustic energy. In a sense, the receiver is a miniloudspeaker or a microphone in reverse (i.e., whereas the receiver converts the electrical signal into an acoustic signal, the microphone converts the acoustic signal into an electrical signal).

Why is it Called a Receiver When it's Sending Out Sound? The tradition of calling the hearing aid's miniature loudspeaker a "receiver" hails back to the telephone industry. The term comes from the speaker in the handpiece of the telephone. The receiver end of the handpiece received an electrical signal from the telephone.

EARMOLDS

In addition to a microphone, amplifier, and receiver, some hearing aids require the use of earmolds (whereas the casing actually replaces the earmold in many other kinds of hearing aids). Earmolds deliver sound from the receiver to the ear and help hold the hearing aid in place. Earmolds are custom-made to fit into the ear canal of the user. An earmold attaches to plastic tubing, which leads to the hearing-aid receiver. It can be constructed in a variety of configurations to suit the needs of the individual user. For instance, some earmolds fill the entire concha of the ear, whereas others consist only of a half-ring that anchors it within the concha. The former style of earmold might be used for a severe or profound hearing loss, and the latter for a mild loss.

Other Features of Hearing Aids

In addition to the components previously shown in Figure 7-1, some hearing aids have additional features. These include an on-off control, a volume control, a telecoil, and a remote control.

ON-OFF CONTROL

The **on-off control** may be a small switch that moves back and forth to turn the hearing aid off when not in use and on when the hearing aid is needed. The on-off control also may be incorporated into the volume control wheel. When a hearing aid does not have an on-off switch, the hearing aid is activated by inserting the battery.

On-off control: a small switch that moves back and forth to turn the hearing aid off when not in use and on when needed; may be incorporated into the volume wheel.

AUDIO INPUT

Many behind-the-ear hearing aids have an audio input that allows an audio signal to be input directly from the signal source. This direct input eliminates distortion from the surrounding environment. For example, a cable may be used to couple the hearing aid directly to a television or radio. The audio input consists of electrical contacts that accommodate a plug or an **audio boot.** It has a separate preamplifier from the microphone.

audio boot: A device that is used with a behind-the-ear hearing aid for coupling to a direct audio input cord.

TELECOIL

The **telecoil** is a special circuit that enhances telephone communication. The telephone receiver emits electromagnetic signals, which are picked up by the hearing-aid telecoil. The hearing-aid microphone thus is bypassed. The signal picked up by the telecoil is amplified and transduced to an audio signal, and then delivered to the ear. If the hearing aid has an on-off switch, it may include a *T* position for *telecoil* and an *M* position for *microphone,* so the user can switch on the telecoil before using the telephone. An

A **telecoil** is an induction coil that receives electromagnetic signals from a telephone or loop amplification system.

MT option on the on-off switch allows for simultaneous use of both the telecoil and microphone.

VOLUME CONTROL

The **volume control** on a hearing aid is used to adjust its output; may be manual or automatic.

A *volume control* allows the user to adjust the level of amplification. It usually is a rotating wheel. When a hearing aid does not have a volume control, it typically has a screw-set control that the audiologist can adjust with a screw driver.

REMOTE CONTROL

A **remote control** is a hand-held device that permits adjustments in the volume or changes in the program of a programmable hearing aid.

A *remote control* is a handheld device that can serve two purposes. First, it can be used to program the electroacoustic properties of a hearing aid. Second, a remote control can be used to switch the hearing aid from one channel to another, to adjust the volume, and to turn it off and on.

Hearing-Aid Styles

Now that we have considered the basic components of a hearing aid, let us review the ways in which the components can be packaged to function as a listening device. There are six general styles of hearing aids. These are body aids, eyeglass aids, behind-the-ear aids (BTE), in-the-ear aids (ITE), in-the-canal aids (ITC), and completely-in-the-canal aids (CIC).

BODY AIDS AND EYEGLASS HEARING AIDS

Body hearing aid: a hearing aid worn on the body and including a box worn on the torso and a cord connecting to an ear-level receiver.

The *body-aid* casement is about the size of a deck of cards and is worn on the torso. The casement leads to a custom-made earmold by means of a long cord. The body-worn casement houses the microphone, amplifier, and receiver. Body aids may provide powerful amplification and are useful for severe and profound hearing losses. They also have large controls, so they can be used by individuals who have reduced manual dexterity. Body aids are durable and can be harnessed to a young child so that the likelihood of the hearing aid being lost or damaged may be reduced.

Despite these advantages, body aids are not used often today. They are relatively bulky and highly visible. The placement of the microphone on the chest rather than near the ear also may decrease a user's ability to localize sound. They sometimes are used with children who have a pinna that cannot support a BTE hearing aid and with children who do not have an external ear canal. For these latter children, the body aid may be attached to a *bone-conductor,* which delivers sound through the skull.

A **bone-conductor** is a vibrator or oscillator used to transmit sound to the bones of the skull by means of vibration.

Like body aids, eyeglass hearing aids are rarely prescribed any more (Figure 7-4). In an *eyeglass aid,* the microphone, amplifier, and receiver are housed in the temple of the glasses. In principle, they function much like a BTE. The microphone is near the ear, and the receiver directs sound through tubing, into an earmold placed within the user's concha. Although an eyeglass aid presents the advantage of reduced hardware (i.e., the user wears only one prosthesis and not two), it also presents many disadvantages. These disadvantages include the fact that eyeglass aids are heavy, often unattractive, and a need for repair means a loss of eyeglasses.

In an **eyeglass hearing aid,** the hearing aid is housed in the temple of a pair of eyeglasses.

BEHIND-THE-EAR (BTE) HEARING AIDS

The *behind-the-ear hearing aid (BTE)* components are built into a small shell that fits behind the pinna (Figure 7-5). The hearing-aid case is connected to an earmold by a small plastic tube. This is probably the most flexible style of hearing aid because it can be fitted with many available options, such as a powerful telecoil circuit. In addition, an earmold can be constructed to accommodate the user, which may be desirable for several reasons. For instance, if a child suffers from chronic otitis media, then he or she might not be able to use a device that occludes the ear canal, as does an in-the-ear (ITE) aid. If a child is still growing, the earmold can simply be recast when the ear outgrows the existing one. With smaller

The style of hearing aid known as a **behind-the-ear (BTE)** hearing aid is worn over the pinna and coupled to the ear by means of an earmold.

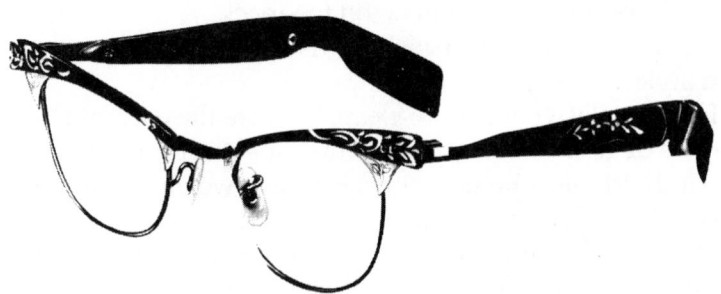

FIGURE 7-4. An eyeglass hearing aid. (Photograph courtesy of Central Institute for the Deaf)

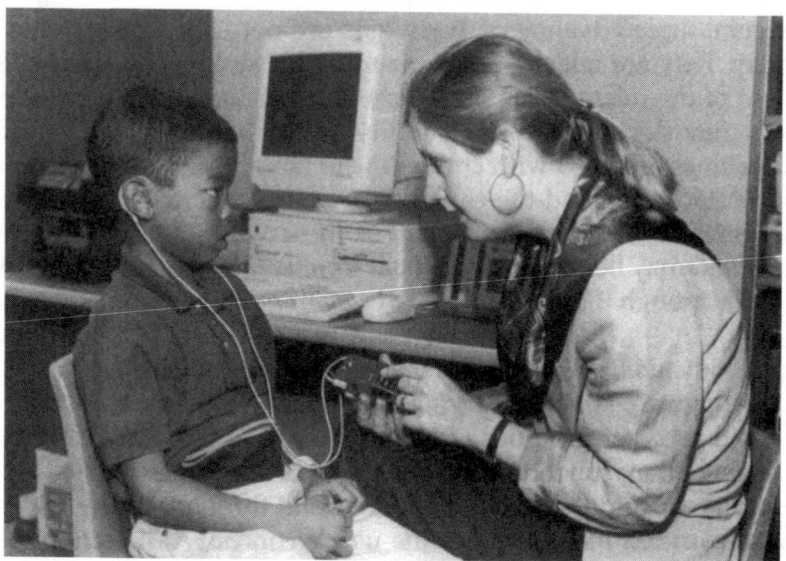

FIGURE 7-5. A behind-the-ear hearing aid. In this picture, an audiologist is fitting a personal FM trainer to the child's hearing aid. The audiologist holds the FM receiver, which connects to the child's hearing aid by a cord. (Photograph by Patti Gabriel, courtesy of the Central Institute for the Deaf)

hearing-aid styles, such as ITEs, a new hearing aid must be recast as it becomes too small to accommodate a child's growing skull. Other advantages of BTEs include the following:

- When used with a soft earmold, a BTE affords greater safety than all-in-the-ear hearing aids. This aspect is important especially for children, who may be at high risk for being hit in the ear, say, by a ball in gym class.
- A BTE has the capability of direct audio input, so it can be hardwired to an assistive listening device.
- BTEs have fewer problems with feedback.
- There are fewer repair problems than with other hearing-aid styles.
- BTEs are relatively easy to clean, because the earmold can be detached and washed. This aspect is important for individuals who perspire a lot, have wax buildup, or have chronic otitis media.
- A BTE can be used with a nonoccluding earmold, which may be important if the individual has chronic otitis media or is unable to have an occluded ear canal for other reasons.

BTEs may be undesirable if the patient is concerned about cosmetics, as they typically are visible, unless covered by long hair.

IN-THE-EAR (ITE) AND IN-THE-CANAL (ITC) HEARING AIDS

In-the-ear (ITEs) and *in-the-canal (ITCs)* hearing-aid styles fit completely in the external ear. A primary difference between the two styles is that the ITC fills less of the concha than does the ITE. The two styles of listening devices must be custom-fitted to the user's ear. The audiologist takes an earmold impression of the ear and then sends the impression to the manufacturer for construction of the aid. The casings of ITEs and ITCs house all of the hearing-aid components, and no additional tubing or earmold is necessary. These two styles are the most widely dispensed hearing aids in today's market, probably because of cosmetic reasons. Figure 7-6 presents a photograph of an ITE aid.

An **in-the-ear (ITE) hearing aid** fits into the concha of the ear.

An **in-the-canal (ITC) hearing aid** fits in the external ear canal, only partially filling the concha.

The ITC hearing aid offers at least a couple of benefits over BTE aids. The position of the microphone enhances the amplification of high-frequency sounds relative to the BTE aid, and the closeness of the receiver to the tympanic membrane means that less

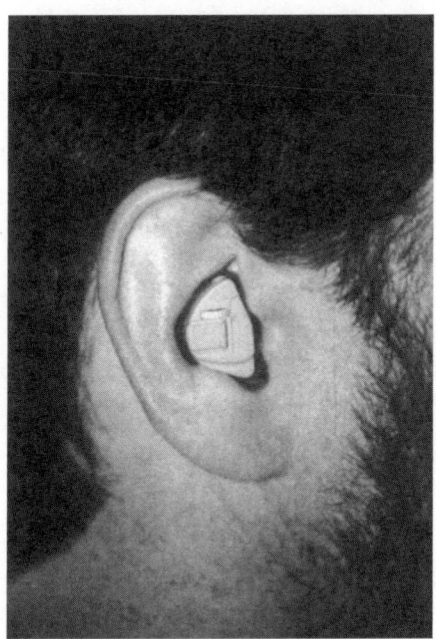

FIGURE 7-6. An ITE hearing aid. (Photograph courtesy of the Central Institute for the Deaf)

gain is required to provide adequate amplification for a particular level of hearing loss. Although at one time ITC aids did not accommodate telecoils, modern versions include them. Also, earlier versions often did not supply adequate amplification for more severe hearing losses, whereas current versions do. An ITC aid has cosmetic appeal relative to a BTE aid, but does offer some disadvantages comparatively. ITC aids are appropriate for only up to severe hearing losses, and some cannot house telecoils. In the United States, ITE aids are the most popular style of hearing aid. They comprise about 81% of the market share of different hearing aid styles. They are not quite as popular in Europe. For example, ITE aids comprise 42% of the market share in Switzerland (whereas BTE aids comprise 57% market share) and 34% of the market share in Germany (whereas BTE aids comprise 66% of the market share) (Vonlanthern, 2000).

COMPLETELY-IN-THE-CANAL (CIC) HEARING AIDS

A **completely-in-the-canal (CIC) hearing aid** fits entirely within the external ear canal.

CIC aids are worn completely inside the ear canal and do not occupy the concha. They are inserted and removed from the ear canal by means of a short clear cord attached to the hearing-aid casement. CIC aids are so small that options often are not available, such as an on-off switch, a volume control, and a telecoil. Some newer devices that use digital technology have remote controls that permit adjustments in gain and program selection. They offer many advantages. They tend to be easy to insert and remove, often more so than trying to insert an earmold, as with a BTE aid. Some people report a better sound quality with CIC aids than with other styles, which is due in part to the absence of an *occlusion effect.* An occlusion effect may occur with most other hearing aid styles. An occlusion effect, caused by plugging the ear canal, may result in speech sounding as if the individual is "listening inside of a barrel." The advantages of CIC aids can be summarized as follows:

In the **occlusion effect,** low-frequency sound in bone-conducted signals is enhanced as a result of closing of the ear canal.

- Easy to handle
- Reduction of an occlusion effect
- Reduction of feedback
- Improved sound localization
- Less electronic gain is needed than with other styles, because the volume between the end of the hearing aid and the tympanic membrane (eardrum) is minimal
- Elimination of wind noise

- Enhanced telephone use without the need for additional assistive listening devices
- Virtually invisible to others when inserted into the user's ear canal
- Greater high-frequency gain

Despite the advantages, CIC hearing aids are high-maintenance devices. Cerumen tends to build up, requiring the patient to clean the hearing aid frequently.

MIDDLE EAR IMPLANTS

Unlike conventional hearing aids that pick up sound from the environment, amplify it, and direct it to the tympanic membrane, a middle ear implant converts the sound signal into a microme-

Binaural Versus Monaural Fitting

Sometimes, the audiologist will recommend that a patient receive two hearing aids instead of one. Even though two hearing aids are more expensive than one, and may require more effort to maintain, binaural amplification fitting offers many advantages over a monaural fitting, including the following:

- **Elimination of *head shadow*:** With one hearing aid, sound coming from the unaided side of the head may be attenuated by as much as 12–16 dB, especially high frequency sounds. Use of two hearing aids allows sound to be received on both sides of the head.
- ***Loudness summation*:** When sound is received by both ears, a summing of the two signals results. Thresholds for sound may improve by 3 dB or more, as compared to monaural thresholds in either ear.
- ***Binaural squelch*:** Listening performance will be better in noise when the user wears two hearing aids instead of one. This improvement in signal-to-noise ratio may be 2 or 3 dB.
- ***Localization*:** A normally hearing person is sensitive to interaural differences in a sound's intensity and phase and this allows him or her, in part, to localize the sound source. A monaural hearing-aid fitting disrupts these cues, whereas binaural hearing aids serve to preserve this localization ability.

Attenuation of sound to one ear because of the presence of the head between the ear and the sound source is called the **head shadow** effect.

Loudness summation: a summing of the signals received by each ear, resulting in a 3-dB advantage for binaural over monaural hearing.

Binaural squelch: improvement in listening in noise when wearing two hearing aids instead of one, resulting in a 2–3 dB improvement in signal-to-noise ratio.

Localization: the ability to locate the source of a sound in space due to the normal ear's sensitivity to interaural differences in phase and intensity.

chanical vibration and transmits it directly to the ossicular chain. The ossicular chain, comprised of the malleus, incus, and stapes, spans the middle ear volume, stretching from the tympanic membrane to the oval window of the cochlea.

A middle ear implant has outer and inner components. The outer components include the power supply (battery), the microphone, and electronic components that transduce the auditory signal into an electromagnetic signal. The internal components include a receiver, a cable, and a vibrator that deliver the micromechanical vibration to the ossicular chain.

The implantable middle ear device is new and has not been widely used. Most often, it is considered to be appropriate for patients who have moderately severe to severe hearing losses (thus, about 3 to 4 million adults in the United States are appropriate candidates), although some patients who have a mild loss are also candidates (Miller & Fredrickson, 2000). The loss might be sensorineural, conductive, or mixed. The middle ear implant is purported to bypass some of the shortcomings of more traditional hearing aid styles, including problems with feedback, occlusion effects, and build up of cerumen. They may be particularly successful with patients who suffer recurrent otitis externa or chronic suppurative otitis media, both of which preclude wearing a hearing aid in the ear canal. The downside includes high cost and the necessity of undergoing anesthesia for a surgical procedure for the implant.

Selecting a Hearing-Aid Style

A consideration of hearing-aid styles leads to the question, "How do you determine which style to provide to a particular individual?" There is no pat answer to this question, but the selection of a particular style of hearing aid often is dependent on the degree of hearing loss, the patient's preference, the cost of the device, the person's age and lifestyle, and his or her physical status.

DEGREE OF HEARING LOSS

As part of a hearing-aid evaluation, an audiologist will obtain an audiogram. The magnitude and configuration of an individual's hearing loss will then help to determine the style of hearing aid selected.

Table 7-2 indicates optimum style options as a function of degree of hearing loss. For example, if an individual has a profound hearing loss, a CIC device is not appropriate because it will not provide enough amplification for the person's listening needs.

The recommendations listed in Table 7-2 are generalizations, and audiologists sometimes select these aids even if they are not optimal for the hearing loss because of other considerations, such as user preference.

USER PREFERENCE

Probably as important as the magnitude and configuration of the hearing loss in selecting a hearing-aid style is the preference of the user. The audiologist will talk with the patient, and carefully consider his or her preferences and prejudices concerning hearing-aid styles. If user preferences are not considered, the hearing aid may not be used. For example, if an audiologist provided someone

Table 7-2. Recommendations for hearing-aid style as a function of degree of hearing loss.

STYLE	HEARING LOSS FOR WHICH USE IS OPTIMAL	HEARING LOSS FOR WHICH USE IS APPROPRIATE BUT NOT OPTIMAL
Body aid	All degrees, although usually used for severe and profound losses	
Eyeglass aid	All degrees	
BTE	All degrees	
ITE	Mild through severe	Severe-to-profound; not recommended for profound
ITC	Mild through moderate	Moderate-to-severe; not recommended for severe or profound
CIC	Mild	Moderate; not recommended for severe or profound
Middle ear implant	Mild through severe	Profound

with a BTE, and the individual turned out to be too self-conscious to wear it, then the BTE probably was an inappropriate selection on the audiologist's part.

COSTS

A closely related issue to preference is cost. CIC and digital hearing aids are the most expensive hearing aids. It is important to explore an individual's financial resources to purchase certain hearing-aid styles early in the selection process. Those styles that are deemed too expensive then cannot be considered further.

LIFESTYLE

Lifestyle is also an important factor to consider during the selection process. For instance, a physician or nurse who often uses a stethoscope, and does not want to use one with a built-in amplifier, may best be served by a CIC aid, because this style can be used with a stethoscope. A person who uses the telephone for a good part of the working day may opt for a BTE hearing aid that has a powerful telecoil circuitry.

PHYSICAL STATUS

Physical status is an important consideration when selecting a hearing-aid style. Physical status includes an individual's manual dexterity and the condition of the ear. It is important to assess a person's gross and fine motor skills and to evaluate how well the individual can move his or her hands, fingers, and arms. Both fine and gross motor skills are necessary for putting on and taking off a hearing aid. In addition, fine motor control is necessary for manipulating the controls, changing batteries, and inserting and removing the hearing aid from the ear. If a person has poor skills, it might be best to consider a BTE aid, a body aid, or an assistive listening device such as a handheld amplifier. We will revisit this issue of manual dexterity in Chapter 13, when we consider older adults.

An examination of the ear will indicate whether an individual has chronic ear infections or a deformity in the ear canal. Children often have chronic otitis media. If an ITE aid is prescribed, secretions might damage the device. Hence, this is one reason a BTE aid may be more appropriate. A deformed or nonexistent ear canal also may limit (or preclude) the use of certain styles of hearing aids.

In addition to the health of the ear and physical malformations, the curve of the ear canal may influence the selection of hearing-aid style. If the individual has a straight ear canal, without a bend, then he or she probably is not a good candidate for a CIC aid. The device will not stay in place. Similarly, if the individual has a shallow concha, an ITC aid may be difficult to keep in the ear.

Electroacoustic Properties

In addition to selecting a hearing-aid style, certain decisions must be made concerning the electroacoustic properties of the hearing aid. These properties affect how the hearing aid processes the audio signal. These properties include saturation sound pressure level and gain/frequency response:

- *Saturation sound pressure level (SSPL):* This term refers to the maximum sound pressure level that can be delivered to the ear, when the volume control is tamed full on and the input signal is 90 dB SPL. This value is determined to ensure that the hearing aid's maximum power does not exceed the user's *loudness discomfort level (LDL),* also called *uncomfortable loudness level (UCL).* The LDL is the threshold at which sound becomes so loud that the hearing-aid user cannot tolerate it, even for a brief exposure. An *SSPL-90 curve* is obtained by measuring the hearing aid's output in a hearing aid test chamber called a *hearing-aid test box.* The hearing aid is connected to a 2-cc coupler that simulates the human external ear canal volume. An input signal then is presented that sweeps across frequencies, at 90 dB SPL. The output of the hearing aid is measured.
- *Gain/frequency response:* The difference between the amplitude of the input signal and the amplitude of the output signal across frequencies is referred to as the gain/frequency response of a hearing aid. Typically, a hearing aid for an individual is adjusted to deliver the greatest amount of gain for those frequencies for which the individual has the poorest thresholds.

Saturation sound pressure level (SSPL): the maximum sound pressure level that can be delivered by a hearing aid with its volume full-on.

Loudness discomfort level (LDL): the level at which sound is perceived to be uncomfortably loud.

Uncomfortable loudness level (UCL): the level at which sound is perceived to be uncomfortably loud; loudness discomfort level.

SSPL-90 curve: electroacoustic assessment of a hearing aid's maximum level of output signal, expressed as a frequency response curve to a 90 dB signal, with the hearing aid volume control set to full on.

Hearing-aid test box: an off-the-ear determination of SSPL-90 in which the hearing aid is connected to a 2-cc coupler to simulate the human ear canal; an input signal that sweeps across the frequencies at 90 dB SPL is input, and the aid's output is measured.

Gain/frequency response: the difference between the amplitude of the input signal and the amplitude of the output signal across frequencies.

Selecting the Hearing Aid and Assessing Benefits

Selection of hearing aids typically are based on the audiogram, which indicates the degree of hearing loss and the configuration. Sometimes, a formula for gain is applied, which is a formula used to compute the desired amount of amplification at each frequency This strategy is referred to as *prescription procedures.*

Prescription procedures: fitting hearing aids by using a formula to calculate the desired gain and frequency response.

Prescription procedures are often used when a hearing aid is to be ordered from a specific manufacturer. A set of optimum electroacoustic characteristics are integrated into the production of a patient's hearing aid. For example, in one procedure, the goal is to restore hearing thresholds to normal. The amount of gain prescribed at each frequency corresponds to the degree of hearing loss. In another prescriptive procedure, high frequencies are amplified more than low frequencies to maximize speech audibility. Incorporated in most prescriptive formulas is the patient's LDL, so sound is not presented at an uncomfortably loud level.

Implicit in the use of prescriptive methods of hearing aid selection is the need to verify and validate that the prescriptive targets have been met and that the fitting is appropriate for the particular patient. This verification can be done either with behavioral techniques or with probe-tube microphone measurements.

Behavioral techniques may include obtaining an aided audiogram and administering speech recognition tests (Chapter 6). Patients take a speech recognition test with and without their hearing aid, and amount of improvement in percent words correct on their performance is computed.

Probe microphone: a microphone transducer that is inserted in the external ear canal for the purpose of measuring sound near the tympanic membrane.

Real-ear measures: use of a probe microphone to measure hearing aid gain and frequency response delivered by a hearing aid at the tympanic membrane.

The second procedure for evaluating a patient's hearing aid involves *probe microphone technology.* A small flexible tube is inserted into the ear canal and positioned near the eardrum. The tube connects to a microphone, which records the decibels of power delivered at the end of the ear canal. First, sound is measured near the eardrum, so the measure is influenced by the natural resonance of the ear canal. Measurements are then repeated, but this time with the hearing aid worn by the patient. These measures are called *real-ear measures.* Although these measures do not indicate how well an individual can hear when wearing the hearing aid, results indicate whether the prescribed gain at each frequency, also called the ***target gain,*** is being delivered by the hearing aid.

A subjective procedure to assess hearing-aid benefit is the use of a questionnaire or an inventory. The patient may complete a checklist about what he or she can or cannot hear with the hearing aid, and may indicate satisfaction with the device.

Table 7-3 summarizes several self-assessment scales that may be used to assess the goodness of a hearing aid. The scales are designed to measure and validate outcomes following receipt of a hearing aid. Some instruments are geared more to gauging benefit (e.g., Profile of Aided Loudness [PAL], Mueller & Palmer, 1998), whereas others are geared more to assessing satisfaction with the device (e.g., Satisfaction with Amplification in Daily Life [SADL], Cox & Alexander, 1999). These two scales are included in the Key Resources of this chapter to provide you with comprehensive examples of the two types of self-assessment tools available for evaluating hearing aid benefit.

Target gain: the gain prescribed for each frequency of a hearing aid, against which the actual hearing aid output is compared.

Hearing-Aid Orientation

Once the audiologist receives the prescribed hearing aid from the manufacturer, the patient returns to the clinic to be fitted with the device. At this time, benefit also is assessed, and the patient receives a ***hearing-aid orientation.*** The hearing-aid orientation includes the following services:

- The audiologist describes the function of each part of the hearing aid and ensures that the patient can adjust any controls.
- The patient practices inserting and removing the hearing aid and inserting and removing batteries from the hearing-aid battery compartment.
- The audiologist reviews the limitations of amplification, and why the particular hearing aid was selected.
- The patient and audiologist determine an appropriate use pattern for the first few weeks of using the new hearing aid.
- The patient learns how to troubleshoot the device.
- The patient receives printed information about the hearing aid and warranty.

Hearing aid orientation (HAO) is the process of instructing a patient (and a family member) to handle, use, and maintain a new hearing aid.

Table 7-3. Examples of self-report measures that have been developed to assess a patient's perceived benefit from using a hearing aid.

TEST	PURPOSE	REFERENCE
Hearing Aid Performance Inventory (HAPI) ■ 64 items, based on 12 bipolar features (e.g., visual signal present/absent)	To assess the benefits of amplification in varying listening situations Example: *You are alone at home talking with a friend on the telephone.* *(5-point scale: 1 = very helpful;* *5 = hinders performance)*	Walden, Demorest, & Helper (1984)
Hearing Aid Users Questionnaire (HAPI) ■ 11-item questionnaire that assesses hearing aid use, benefit, and related problems and satisfactions	To detect problems that affect a patient's ability to use hearing aids and receive benefit Example: *How would you describe your satisfaction with hour hearing aid?* *(4-point scale: 1 = very satisfied;* *5 = very dissatisfied)*	Dillon, Birtles, & Lovegrove (1999)

Hearing Problem Inventory
 	
■ 50 items about
  emotional reaction to hearing
    hearing loss;
  effect of hearing loss on
    everyday activities;
  signal and environmental
    influences;
  use of visual cues;
  use, fit, and care of hearing aid
	To assess benefit of using a hearing aid and to identify some of the influences on a patient's perception of his or her problems and hearing aid use
	
	Example: *The telephone pick-up on my hearing aid is good.*
	(5-point scale: 1 = almost always;
	5 = almost never)
		Hutton (1980)

Profile of Aided Loudness (PAL) ■ 12 items across categories of soft, average, and loud sounds	To determine whether amplification has restored loudness Example: *You chewing soft food:* *Loudness rating (scale from 0–7:* *0 = Do not hear;* *7 = Uncomfortably loud).* *Satisfaction rating (scale from 5 to 1: 5 = just right; 1 = not good at all)*	Mueller & Palmer (1998); Palmer, Mueller, & Moriarty (1999)

(continues)

Table 7-3. *(continued)*

TEST	PURPOSE	REFERENCE
Profile of Hearing Aid Performance (PHAP) ■ 66 items in 7 subscales designedto assess the following: familiar talkers ease of communication reverberation reduced cues background noise aversiveness of sounds distortion of sounds	To generate a measure of hearing aid benefit computed from the difference between aided and unaided conditions Example: *(Answered with and without hearing aid) Women's voices sound shrill (7-point scale: A = always; G = never)*	Cox, Gilmore, & Alexander (1991); Cox & Rivera (1992)
Profile of Hearing Aid Performance (PHAP) ■ 66 items designed to measure two aspects of performance with a hearing aid, speech communication in a variety of typical workday situations, and reactions to loudness or quality of environmental sounds	To generate a measure of performance rather than benefit Example: *When I am in a quiet restaurant, I can understand conversation: (7-point scale: A = always; G = never)*	Cox & Gilmore (1990)
Satisfaction with Amplification in Daily Life (SADL) ■ 15 items in 4 subscales: positive effects service and costs negative features personal image	To quantify hearing aid satisfaction Example: *Are you convinced that obtaining your hearing aid was in your best interest? (7-point scale: A = Not at all; G = Tremendously)*	Cox & Alexander (1999)

Source: Adapted from R. A. Bentler and S. E. Kramer, 2000, "Guidelines for choosing a self-report outcome measure." *Ear and Hearing, 21,* pp. 375–495.

COCHLEAR IMPLANTS

Not all hard-of-hearing individuals have the potential to benefit from using a hearing aid. For instance, someone who has little, if any, residual hearing will probably never recognize the audio speech signal, no matter how it is processed nor how much it is amplified. Another intervention available besides a hearing aid is the cochlear implant. Cochlear implants, virtually unheard of 30 years ago, are now commonplace.

Most sensorineural hearing loss stems from a dearth or absence of hair cells (the sensory receptors of hearing) in the cochlea and not because of a damaged auditory nerve or central dysfunction. A cochlear implant is effective because it replaces the hair-cell transducer system by stimulating the auditory nerve directly, bypassing the damaged or missing hair cells. The nerve impulses are then delivered to the brain, following the route of the neural auditory pathway, as if the cochlea were stimulated in a natural way. Implants are designed to interface with the ***tonotopic organization*** of the cochlea. The implant divides sound into a series of frequency bands, and it then delivers each band to that region of the cochlea for which it is best suited. For example, high-frequency bands are delivered to the apical end of the cochlea, whereas low-frequency bands are delivered to the basil end. The level of stimulation serves to code sound intensity.

Tonotopic organization: Structures within the peripheral and central auditory nervous system are arranged topographically according to tonal frequency.

A Brief History

Although cochlear implants are a relatively new development scientists have long been tantalized by the idea of providing sound sensation by means of electrical stimulation. One of the first recorded attempts in history to stimulate the ear electrically occurred in 1790, when Volta inserted metal rods into each of his ears. The rods were connected to 30 or 40 of his newly invented electrolytic cells. With one deft move, Volta delivered approximately 50 volts to himself. The results were staggering. He perceived a sensation similar to "a blow to the head," followed by "a sound like the boiling of a viscous liquid" (Luxford & Brackmann, 1985, p. 1). The experiment was not repeated.

The more recent history of cochlear implants hails back to 1957, when two French surgeons, Djourno and Eyries, stimulated a deaf adult by placing an electrode directly on his auditory nerve. The patient reported hearing a sound like "crickets chirping," or "a roulette wheel spinning" (Luxford & Brackmann, 1985). Reports of this work filtered to the medical communities in the United States and Australia. Shortly thereafter, in the 1960s and 1970s, much activity was aimed toward the development of wearable devices. Names often associated with this work are Dr. William House of Los Angeles, California and Dr. Graham Clarke of Melbourne, Australia.

By the 1980s there was widespread use of cochlear implants among adults, and they were in exploratory use with children. The Food and Drug Administration (FDA) approved multichannel cochlear implants in 1990 for children, and now cochlear implants are considered a treatment option for both adults and children who have profound hearing loss. Increasingly, individuals who have severe hearing loss also are considered as candidates for implantation.

Overview

Cochlear implants are comprised of internal and external components (Figure 7-7). The internal components are implanted in the skull, in close proximity to the inner ear. The *internal components* typically include an internal receiver, which is placed on the mastoid bone, and an electrode array, which is inserted into the cochlea. These components are not visible after implantation, but are covered by skin and hair. The user may have a small incision scar and a slight convex protrusion behind the pinna.

In cochlear implant, the **internal components** are implanted within the skull.

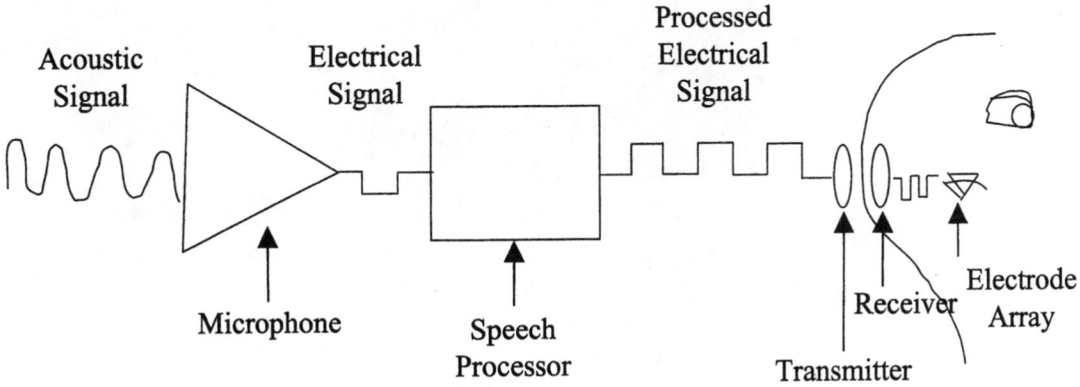

FIGURE 7-7. Schematic of a cochlear implant.

The external components include a microphone, connecting cables, a speech processor, and a transmitter. The microphone and transmitter typically are worn behind the ear. In older models, the speech processor is worn on the chest, similar to a body hearing aid. In newer cochlear implants, the speech processor can be worn behind the ear, like a BTE hearing aid. Figure 7-8 presents a picture of a young student who recently received a cochlear implant. Figure 7-9 presents a photograph of a newer cochlear implant. As can be seen, the speech processor is about the size of a behind-the-ear hearing aid.

Speech processor: the component of a cochlear implant where the input signal is modified for presentation to the electrodes in the electrode array.

The microphone of a cochlear implant picks up sound from the environment, converts it to an electrical signal, and then delivers it via connecting cables to the speech processor. The *speech processor,* as the name implies, processes the signal. Each cochlear-implant design utilizes a speech-processing strategy, or algorithm, for determining how the signal is processed. The signal may be digitized, filtered, and then segmented so that different components of the signal are presented to different electrodes in the electrode array.

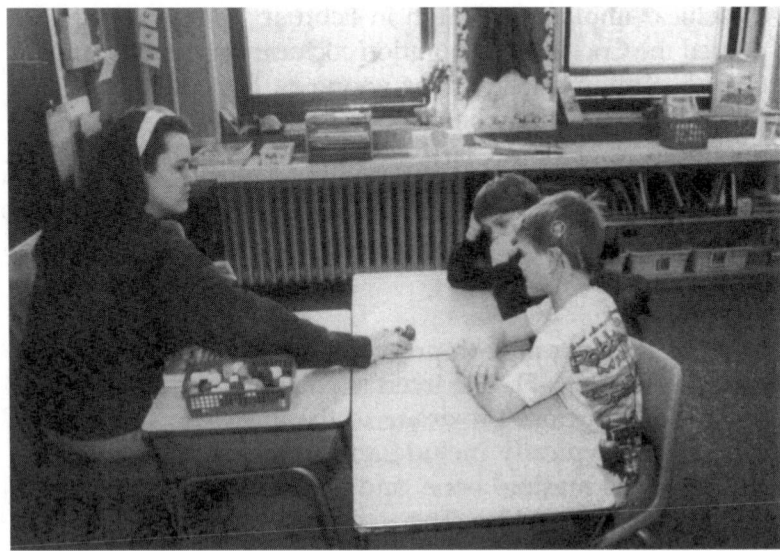

FIGURE 7-8. A young boy wearing a cochlear implant. The microphone is worn behind his ear like a behind-the-ear hearing aid. The external transmitter is held against his head by magnetic induction. This child has only been using the device for a short time, and his scar from surgery is still visible near the base of his skull. (Photograph by Kim Readmond, courtesy of the Central Institute for the Deaf)

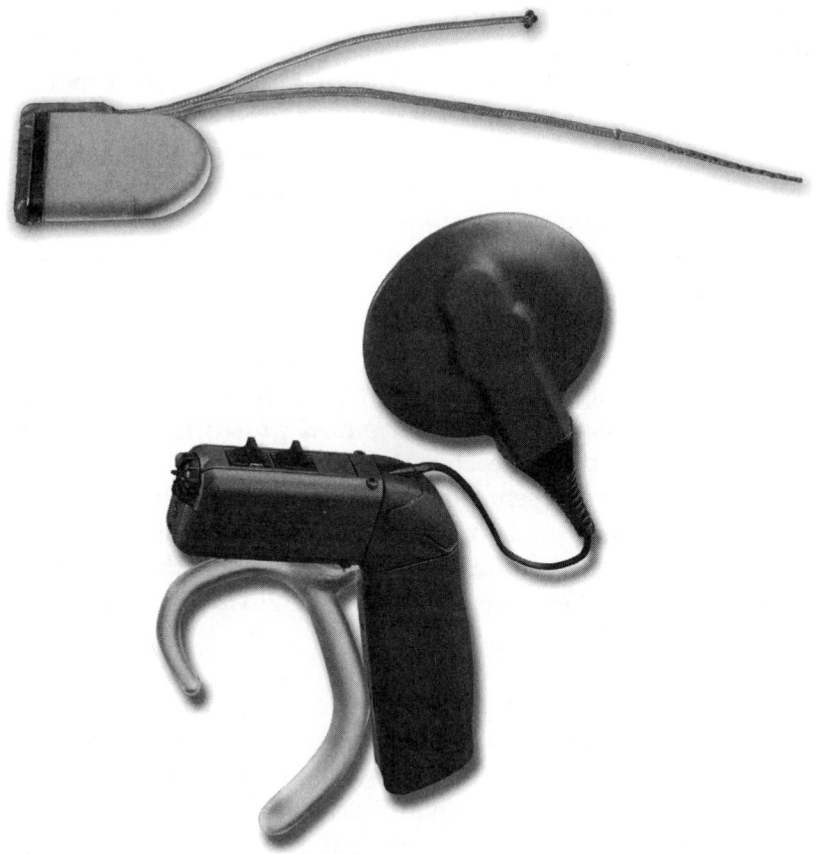

"Even after nine years, not a day passes that I don't marvel at the gift of sound and thank all those involved in providing this wondrous technology."

—Donna Sorkin, Former Executive Director for Self-Help for Hard-of-Hearing (SHHH) and a cochlear implant recipient. Hearing Loss, July/August 2002, p. 17

FIGURE 7-9. A cochlear implant. (Courtesy of Med-El, used with permission)

The processed electrical signal leaves the speech processor and is delivered to the electrode array, via a transmitter and an internal receiver. The transmitter often is worn outside of the head and delivers the signal to an internal receiver. The transmitter may be held in place by magnet. The electrical signal typically is transmitted across the skin by either electromagnetic induction or radio frequency transmission. From the internal receiver, the electrical signal passes on to the electrode array.

The *electrode array* is a small wire, inserted into the cochlea, usually through the *round window.* The electrode array carries electrode pairs. The electrode pairs, which are tiny exposed balls or rings on the wire, are comprised of positive and negative polarity contacts, between which passes current. The current stimulates the fibers of the auditory nerve.

Electrode array: inserted into the cochlea, a wire that carries the implant's electrode pairs.

Round window: membrane-covered opening between the middle ear space and the scala tympani section of the cochlea in the inner ear.

Multichannel: more than one channel. Often used to describe cochlear implants that present different channels of information to different parts of the cochlea.

Most cochlear implants in use in the United States today are ***multichannel*** devices. This means that the electrode pairs in the electrode array present different information to different regions of the cochlea. In the normal ear, different frequencies of the auditory signal excite different neurons along the cochlea. The goal of a multichannel system is to simulate the normal cochlea and present high-frequency components of the signal to the basal end of the cochlea and low-frequency components of the signal to the apical end.

Interleaved pulsatile stimulation: a cochlear implant processing strategy in which trains of pulses are delivered across electrodes in the electrode array in a nonsimultaneous fashion.

Although there are some variations in the processing strategies used by different models of cochlear implants, many current cochlear implants utilize an ***interleaved pulsatile stimulation*** algorithm. In this design, each electrode pair in the electrode array is designated to represent different frequency bands. The audio signal is processed and delivered to the electrode array by spreading pulses, in a nonsimultaneous manner (hence, they are interleaved) across the electrode pairs, from high to low or from low to high frequencies.

In the United States, three manufacturers provide most of the devices. The Cochlear Corporation developed the first multichannel cochlear implant, the Nucleus, to receive Food and Drug Administration (FDA) approval. Early models of the Nucleus cochlear implant were "feature extraction" devices because they coded first and second formant features (as we will review in Chapter 8, formants refer to vowel resonances). Today's models allow three different processing strategies: Continuous Interleaved Sampling (CIS) strategy that provides interleveaved pulsatile stimulation, one called the spectral peak (SPEAK, which is the most widely used strategy), and one called the Advanced Combined Encoder (ACE) strategy. The SPEAK strategy divides the incoming auditory signal into 20 frequency bands and cycles through the electrodes on the electrode array, stimulating an average of six electrodes on each cycle (those that correspond to the frequencies that have the most energy present in the incoming signal). The ACE strategy stimulates similarly, but uses higher rates of stimulation than the SPEAK. The Nucleus cochlear implant speech processor is available in two designs, one worn on the body trunk and one worn behind the ear.

Advanced Bionics Corporation manufactures the Clarion device. It has an eight-channel electrode array and allows two processing strategies. The first is an example of an interleaved pulsatile stimulation strategy, called CIS. The second is called the Simultaneous Analog Stimulation (SAS) strategy, and it filters the incoming auditory signal and presents it simultaneously to the corresponding bipolar electrodes.

The third manufacturer is Medical Electronic (Med-El), which developed the Combi 40+ cochlear implant (see Figure 7-9). Based in Innsbruck, Austria, its device is now available in the United States. The device has 12 electrodes and allows for a deep insertion of the electrode array into the cochlea. It uses an interleaved pulsatile stimulation strategy, and provides rapid cycling of stimulation across the electrode array.

CANDIDACY

The primary candidacy requirements for implantation are the presence of irreversible severe or profound hearing loss and good general health. There is no upper age of implantation, and adults 85 years and older have received implanted devices. The lower age of implantation for certain device types is about 12 months, although children as young as 6 months have received cochlear implants in the United States and in countries such as Australia and Austria. The cochlea is adult size at the time of birth, so implantation for babies is feasible on an anatomical basis.

Table 7-4 presents candidacy requirements for children and adults. For children, it must be demonstrated that they receive no benefit from a hearing aid. This typically requires them to undergo a 3 to 6 month trial period with a hearing aid and to receive appropriate aural rehabilitation intervention that encourages listening behaviors. Even with a trial period, determining benefit can be difficult for youngsters who do not have speech and language skills. Audiological measures and questionnaires completed by the child's parents or guardian often guide candidacy decisions.

Candidacy requirements for adults have altered since the mid-1980s, when cochlear implantation began to be performed with increased regularity. Early on, adults had to have a profound, postlingual hearing loss and could receive no measurable benefit from hearing aids. For example, if someone recognized more than 2% of the words on a monosyllabic word test while wearing a

Table 7-4. Candidacy requirements for cochlear implantation.

CHILDREN (12–24 MONTHS)	CHILDREN (25 MONTHS TO 17 YEARS, 11 MONTHS)	ADULTS
Bilateral profound sensorineural hearing loss	Bilateral severe-to-profound sensorineural hearing loss	Bilateral severe-to-profound sensorineural hearing loss
Lack of auditory skills development and minimal benefit from using a hearing aid (documented by audiological testing and parent questionnaire)	Lack of auditory skills development and minimal hearing aid benefit (word recognition scores less than 30% words correct)	Minimal benefit from wearing a hearing aid (word recognition scores less than 30% words correct)
No medical contraindications	No medical contraindications	No medical contraindications
Enrollment in an aural rehabilitation intervention that emphasizes the development of listening skills	Enrollment in an aural rehabilitation intervention that emphasizes the development of listening	

Source: Adapted from R. Miyamoto, D. Houston, and K. Kirk, 2002, "Early cochlear implantation in congenitally deaf children." *Audiology Today, Special Issue,* pp. 35–40.

hearing aid, that person was not a candidate. Today, criteria have loosened, in part because advances in speech-processing strategy design permit greater gains to be realized for persons with profound hearing loss and some speech recognition than do most hearing aids. Criteria have also loosened because more clinical research data are available about patient performance on which to make candidacy recommendations. If a patient has a severe or profound hearing loss, and modest word recognition (say, the patient is unable to recognize more than 40% of the words on an open-set sentence test or 30% on a monosyllabic word test), that individual is a candidate. Although most adult cochlear implant recipients have postlingual hearing losses, prelingual deafness no longer precludes candidacy.

We revisit the topic of cochlear implants and candidacy issues in Chapter 18, where we will consider aural rehabilitation plans for children in depth.

ASSISTIVE LISTENING DEVICES (ALDS)

Hearing aids and cochlear implants are listening devices that may be worn during almost all working hours and in almost all communication settings. ALDs usually are used in specific situations, such as when listening in a public hall or conversing in a restaurant when other kinds of listening devices are either inadequate to permit good communication or are not desirable to the patient (Table 7-5). Compton (1995) suggested that ALDs should address one or more of four communication needs. The four basic communication needs for most people are: (1) face-to-face communication, (2) broadcast and other electronic media, (3) telephone conversations, and (4) sensitivity to alerting signals and to their environmental signals. In selecting ALDs for a particular individual, you will want to consider the person's communication demands in the home, community or school environments. Table 7-6 presents a list of situations in each of these settings in which use of an ALD may be appropriate. The Key Resources section lists sources for obtaining ALDs.

ALDs are especially useful when the audio signal is presented at a distance or when the listening conditions are less than ideal. In

Table 7-5. Situations in which a person may use an assistive device.

KIND OF COMMUNICATION	POSSIBLE SITUATIONS OR PURPOSES
Live, face-to-face	Restaurants, meetings, places of worship, concerts, lectures, automobile, courtroom, classroom
Broadcast or recorded media	Radio, television, movie theaters, dictation machines
Telecommunications	Telephones, intercoms
Environment	Doorbells, smoke detectors, telephone rings, appliance timers, babies' cries, children's voices, alarm clocks

Table 7-6. Situations in which use of an assistive device might be appropriate.

Home

One-on-one conversation

Group conversation

Television reception

Radio reception

Reception of environmental signals such as the door bell

Community

Medical treatment (visiting a physician, dentist, hospital)

Working

    Office conversation

    Lectures

    Telephone communication

    Conferences and group meetings

    One-on-one meetings

Traveling and recreation

    One-on-one conversation

    Conversation in the car

    Television reception

    Reception of warning signals

Restaurants

Public spaces

School

Communication with the teacher

Communication with classmates

Speech-language therapy

---

such conditions, a hearing aid or cochlear implant may not be adequate to maximize an individual's listening potential. Because the microphone of a hearing aid or cochlear implant is at the level of the individual's ear, it may not pick up sound emanating from a distant source or may deliver not only the desired audio signal, but also any competing background noise to the listener.

Conditions that might compromise a listening environment, and where an ALD may be especially helpful, include the following (Flexor, 1997):

■ *Ambient noise:* noise that is present in a room when it is unoccupied. This noise may emanate from open windows, air handling systems, computers, fluorescent lighting systems, or piped-in music.

■ *Reverberation:* echoes caused by sound rebounding off surfaces such as walls, floors, and ceilings. Rooms that have high ceilings, hardwood floors, and plaster walls tend to be highly reverberant, whereas those that have carpet and heavy draperies tend to have less reverberation.

■ *Background noise:* is undesirable noise that masks the auditory signal of interest. For instance, in a classroom, the teacher's voice may be the target signal, and the rustling of paper and the shuffling of feet might be undesirable background noise.

In principle, ALDs work by collecting sound from the sound source (e.g., the talker's mouth) and delivering it to the user's ear. In this way, the audio signal is presented at an audible level, with a favorable signal-to-noise ratio, with minimal ambient noise, without the effects of reverberation, and with little background noise. ALDs can be categorized as one of two kinds: wireless and hardwired (Figure 7-10).

Wireless Systems

As the name implies, a wireless system does not use wire between the microphone and the unit that delivers the signal to the user's ear. Sound is transmitted from the sound source to the individual by means of radio waves or infrared signals. These kinds of systems may be used when the individual is far from the sound source, for example, in a religious service or when attending a theater play. A wireless system picks up the audio signal, either through a microphone placed near the sound source or by means of a direct electrical plug-in. The sound is then converted into an electrical signal by a transmitter and delivered through the air to a receiver worn by the user, either by means of radio waves or infrared (invisible light). The signal may be delivered to the ear either via earphones or through the individual's hearing aid, if it is a body aid or a BTE hearing aid. Delivery through the hearing aid is accomplished in one of three ways: by means of a *direct audio input (DAI)* to the individual's hearing aid, by use of the hearing aid's telecoil circuitry, or by use of the hearing-aid's microphone.

Ambient noise: noise in a listening environment.

Reverberation: prolongation of an auditory signal by multiple reflections in a closed environment, the amount of echo in a closed space.

Background noise: extraneous noise in an environment that masks the signal of interest.

Direct audio input (DAI): a hard-wired connection that leads directly from the sound source to the hearing aid or other listening device.

No ALD

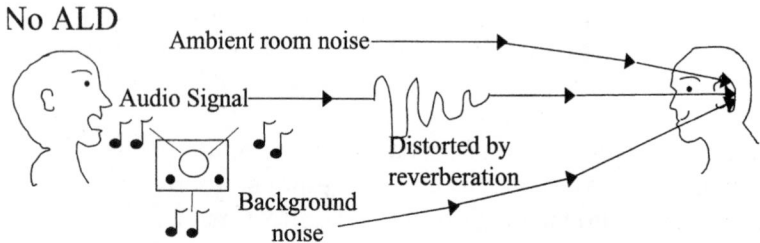

ALD, sound picked up through a microphone

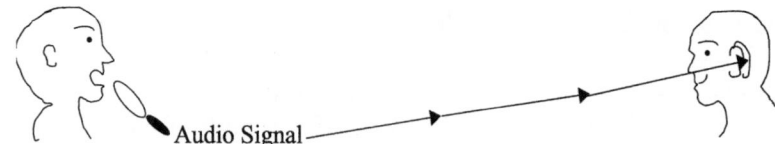

ALD, sound picked up by direct audio input (DAI)

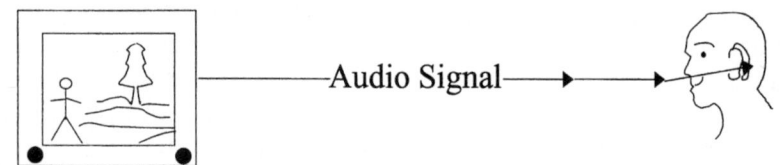

FIGURE 7-10. Schematic of an assistive listening device. In the top third of the figure, no assistive listening device is used, and the signal is distorted by reverberation and masked by background noise. In the center and bottom of the figure, sound is relayed from the source to the listener by means of an assistive listening device. In the center of the figure, sound is picked up through a microphone, whereas in the bottom of the figure, sound is picked up by direct audio input.

FM SYSTEMS

Frequency modulation (FM): the process of creating a complex signal by means of sinusoidally varying a carrier wave frequency.

Personal FM trainer: a listening device in which the speaker wears a wireless microphone and the speech is frequency modulated on radio waves transmitted through the room to the listener who wears a receiver.

Wireless systems can be further classified as FM, infrared, induction loop, or simple amplification. *FM (frequency modulation) systems* utilize radio waves to transmit sound from the source to the user.

FM systems are commonly used in classroom settings, and may be described either as a personal FM trainer or a soundfield FM system. When using a *personal FM trainer,* the teacher wears a wireless microphone (Figure 7-11), usually on a cord around her neck or clipped onto her shirt. The teacher's speech is frequency modulated on radio frequency carrier waves and transmitted through the classroom to the child, who wears a receiver. Often, the receiver connects to the child's hearing aid by a cord. If there

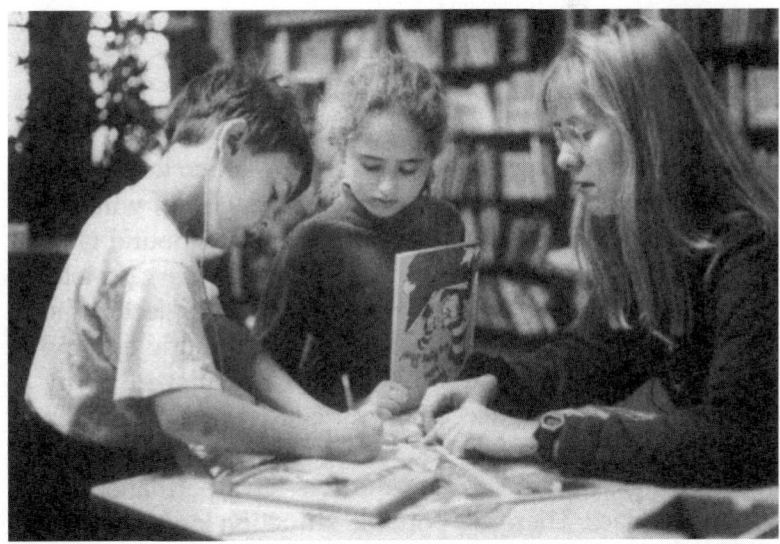

FIGURE 7-11. A teacher wearing a personal FM trainer microphone clipped to her sweater. The young boy wears an FM receiver that has a hard-wired connection to his behind-the-ear hearing aid. *(Photograph by Marcus Kosa, courtesy of the Central Institute for the Deaf.)*

is more than one hard-of-hearing child in the classroom, then each child wears a receiver and may receive the teacher's signal.

A soundfield FM system operates similarly to a personal FM trainer. A ***sound-field FM system*** differs from the personal system because the sound is transmitted to loudspeakers that are positioned throughout the room, usually two in the back of the room and one near the front. There, the signal is converted to an audio signal and played into the environment, as with a standard public address system. A child's personal hearing-aid microphone picks up the signal. Whereas a personal FM trainer offers better signal-to-noise ratios, the sound-field system is advantageous because it can be beneficial for an entire class, even for those children who do not have a hearing loss, who may have a fluctuating conductive hearing loss, who use a cochlear implant, or who have a unilateral hearing loss. FM sound-field systems also do not require a hard-of-hearing child to wear a special FM receiver. Hence, the child wears less hardware.

Sound-field FM system: a listening system, similar to the FM trainer, in which sound from a microphone is transmitted to loudspeakers that are positioned throughout the room.

Other situations in which FM systems may be used besides the classroom setting include group lectures, one-on-one communication situations, and in the car.

Question-Answer Time

Carol Flexor, a researcher who has studied sound-field FM amplification for over 10 years, fielded a series of questions about sound-field amplification. Here are a few of the questions and her responses (Flexor, C. [1997]. Sound-field FM systems: Questions most often asked about classroom amplification. *Hearsay, 11,* 5–13).

Question: What exactly is sound-field FM amplification?

Answer: "Sound-field FM technology is an exciting educational tool that allows control of the acoustic environment in a classroom, thereby facilitating acoustic accessibility of teacher instruction for all children in the room. Specifically, frequency-modulated (FM) sound-field amplification systems are similar to small, high-fidelity, wireless, public address systems that are self-contained in a classroom. The teacher wears a small, unobtrusive wireless microphone; thus, teacher mobility is not restricted. His or her speech is frequency modulated onto a carrier wave that is sent from the transmitter to the receiver where it is demodulated and delivered to the students through one to five wall-or-ceiling-mounted loudspeakers."

Question: What's its purpose?

Answer: "The purpose of sound-field FM amplification is to amplify the teacher's voice throughout the classroom, thereby providing a clear and consistent signal to all pupils in the room no matter where they or the teacher are located. The positioning of the remote microphone close to the mouth of the teacher or other desired sound source creates a favorable speech-to-noise ratio (S/N ratio)."

Question: Which populations of children would benefit from learning in a classroom that is amplified?

Answer: "Children with fluctuating conductive hearing impairments, primarily caused by ear infections or ear wax. . . . Children with unilateral hearing impairments. . . . Children with slight permanent hearing impairments (15-25 dB HL). . . . Children who have normal peripheral hearing sensitivity but who are in special education classrooms due to language, learning, attending, or behavioral problems. . . . Children with mild to moderate hearing impairments who wear hearing aids. . . . Children who have normal peripheral hearing sensitivity but who have difficulty processing, understanding or attending to classroom instruction. . . . Children with cochlear implants."

INFRARED SYSTEMS

Infrared systems operate similarly to FM units, but use infrared signals to transmit sound. A transmitter/emitter sends the signal encoded in infrared light waves to a wireless receiver, which contains a photo detector diode. A photo detector diode picks up the infrared signal and converts it back to the audio signal. An individual may either wear an infrared receiver that inputs directly into the ears or may receive the signal through a DAI or by activating the hearing-aid telecoil switch. Common situations in which infrared systems are used include television watching and movie theaters. Infrared systems are not appropriate for outdoors, as sunlight interferes with transmission. The infrared signals also cannot travel through walls.

Infrared system: an assistive listening device that broadcasts from the sound source to a receiver/amplifier by means of infrared light waves.

INDUCTION LOOP SYSTEMS

The third kind of wireless system is the induction loop system. For an *induction loop system* to operate, a loop of wire must be placed around the circumference of a room. Sound is pick up by means of a microphone or a direct input (e.g., a television direct connection). Sound is converted into electrical signals and fed through the loop. Electromagnetic energy is broadcast throughout the room and can be picked up by a hearing aid when the telecoil circuit is activated. The listener must sit either inside of the loop of wire or beside it. Some religious settings, classrooms, and theaters have permanent loop systems in place. There are portable induction loop systems so that any room can be optimized for communication. A variation of the large area loop system is the *neckloop,* which is a wire that can be worn around the neck.

Induction loop system: a system that works by running a wire around the circumference of a room or table that conducts electrical energy from an amplifier and thus creates a magnetic field, which induces the telecoil in a hearing aid to provide amplified sound to the user.

Neckloop: a transducer worn around the neck as part of an FM assistive device system, consisting of a cord from a receiver; transmits signals via magnetic induction to the telecoil of the user's hearing aid.

SIMPLE AMPLIFICATION

Simple amplification systems merely amplify the audio signal so that it may be more audible to the person with hearing loss. The most common implementation of simple amplification systems is in telephones. *Telephone amplifiers* either replace the telephone handset or clip onto existing handsets. Replacement handsets have built-in amplifiers, so that the signal is amplified before it is delivered to the user's ear. Often, these kinds of handsets have volume controls; therefore, they may also be used by persons who have normal hearing.

Simple amplification systems merely amplify the audio signal so that it is more audible to a person with hearing loss.

Telephone amplifiers amplify sound from a telephone receiver.

Hardwired Systems

Hardwired assistive listening devices: devices that are directly connected by wires.

The other kind of assistive listening device can be described as hardwired. *Hardwired assistive listening devices* connect the sound source to the listener by actual wire. A microphone may pick up the audio signal (Figure 7-12) or there may be a DAI jack that plugs into a piece of equipment, such as a television. The audio signal is converted into an electrical signal. It travels through the connecting wire, terminating at the user's hearing aid, headphones, or a neckloop. This system provides a favorable signal-to-noise ratio to the user and, usually, an adjustable amount of signal amplification. These kinds of systems are used most often for listening to television, radio, or music. However, such systems are not widely used because they require the user to be tethered to the sound source.

FIGURE 7-12. A woman and her daughter are learning to use a hard-wired assistive listening device, while a clinician (standing) provides encouragement. The daughter speaks into a microphone, while the woman listens through headphones. This kind of assistive listening device is often used in restaurants. (Photograph by Kim Readmond, courtesy of the Central Institute for the Deaf)

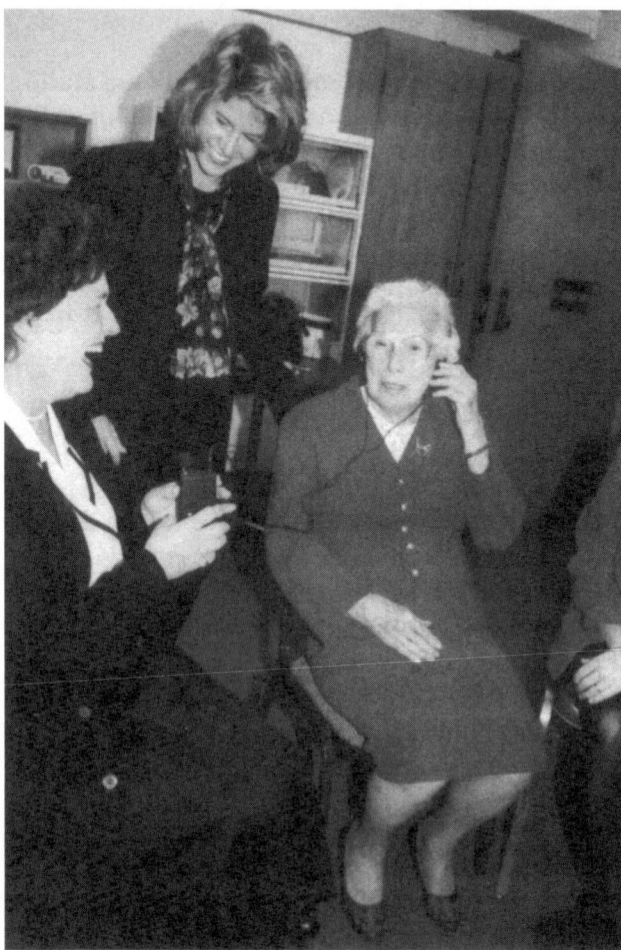

Other Kinds of Assistive Devices

Other assistive devices are available that cannot be classified as wireless or hardwired assistive listening devices per se. These devices are those that allow access to the environment and communication through modalities other than hearing. One of the most commonly used examples of assistive devices include television *closed-captioning* devices, which provide a written text to match the spoken words on a television program. Another example is a vibratory pager, which allows individuals to receive pages. Instead of emitting auditory beeps, a *vibratory pager* vibrates against the user to signal a call. Other examples include:

- Vibrating alarm clocks, where a vibrator might be placed under the user's pillow
- Flashing alarm clocks, where a flashing lamp or strobe light might signal the alarm
- A doorbell signal coupled to a lamp, which flashes when the doorbell is rung
- A smoke detector, where light flashes signal the presence of smoke
- A baby cry alert system, where a parent can be signaled if a baby begins to cry in another room

Closed captioning: Printed text or dialog that corresponds to the auditory speech signal from a television program or movie.

Vibratory pagers: instead of emitting audible beeps the pager vibrates against the user to signal a call.

I Need to Make a Call

In addition to using a telephone amplifier hard-of-hearing individuals have at least two other options available for using the telephone. These options are:

Text telephones (TTs): A telephone terminal comprised of a telephone, a keyboard, and a message display screen. The telephone handset fits into the terminal cradle. Both parties must have a terminal set. They communicate by typing their messages to one another. The messages are displayed on the message display screen. TTs are some times referred to as telecommunication devices for the Deaf (TDDs).

Relay systems: All states provide relay systems as a service for their hard-of-hearing residents. A trained operator serves as an intermediary in a telephone conversation. The hard-of-hearing person communicates with the operator via a TT (and possibly voice), while the normally hearing person communicates with the operator via voice. To place a call, the initiator contacts a relay operator, who in turn contacts the recipient of the call.

Text telephones (TTs) consist of a telephone, a keyboard, and a message display screen. The telephone handset fits into the terminal cradle. Both parties communicate by typing their messages.

Relay system: used by persons with significant hearing loss to use the telephone; individual contacts a relay operator who serves to transmit messages between the caller and person called by means of teletype or voice.

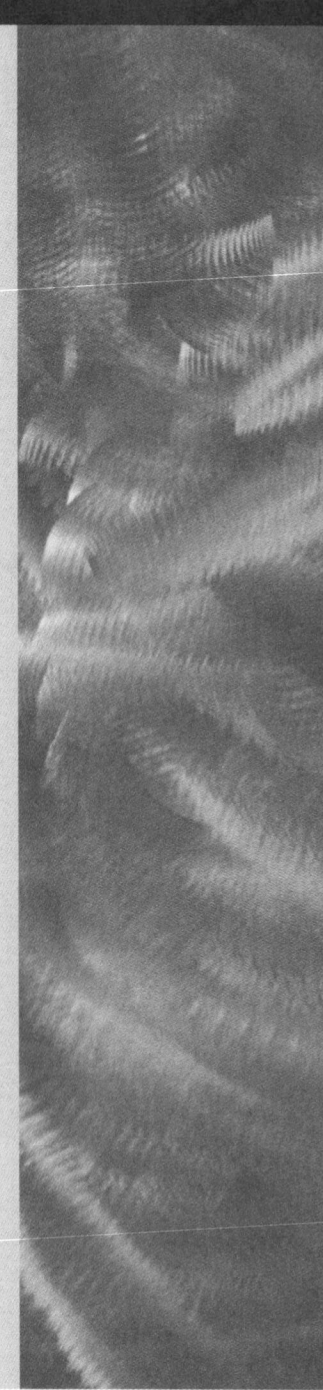

CASE STUDY 1

Sally Anderson, a former music teacher from Des Moines, Iowa, went to the opera with her husband, David, and imagined the lyrics and the music. If they went to parties, David would serve as translator and repeat everything that was said in a group conversation. Similarly, on a trip to England, he repeated the tour guides' commentaries during museum and cathedral visits.

Like her aunt, Sally began to lose her hearing in her late twenties and lost much more of it after her second pregnancy. For the next 15 years, Sally graduated to a series of increasingly powerful hearing aids. The realization of deafness occurred when she was sitting next to the telephone one evening while reading the newspaper. "Answer the phone," her teenage daughter said, poking her in the shoulder. Sally had not heard it ringing.

A year ago, her husband convinced her to contact a cochlear implant center after he read an article about cochlear implants in *Newsweek* magazine. An audiological examination revealed a bilateral profound hearing loss. After a comprehensive medical examination to ensure good health and no cochlear anomalies, Sally signed up for surgery. "It was an opportunity I couldn't pass up. They said I was a prime candidate. I'd had hearing until adulthood, I hadn't been totally deaf for a very long time, and I was highly motivated to hear." She told her audiologist that she could not wait to hear the birds sing or the radio play. The price was offsetting—$50,000 for the surgery alone, and that fee did not include follow-up aural rehabilitation—but, the clinical coordinator at the implant center helped Sally determine that her insurance company would provide coverage.

Immediately on hook-up of the instrument, Sally recognized the sound of chairs scraping against the floor, a door banging, and a telephone ringing. The audiologist adminis-

(continues)

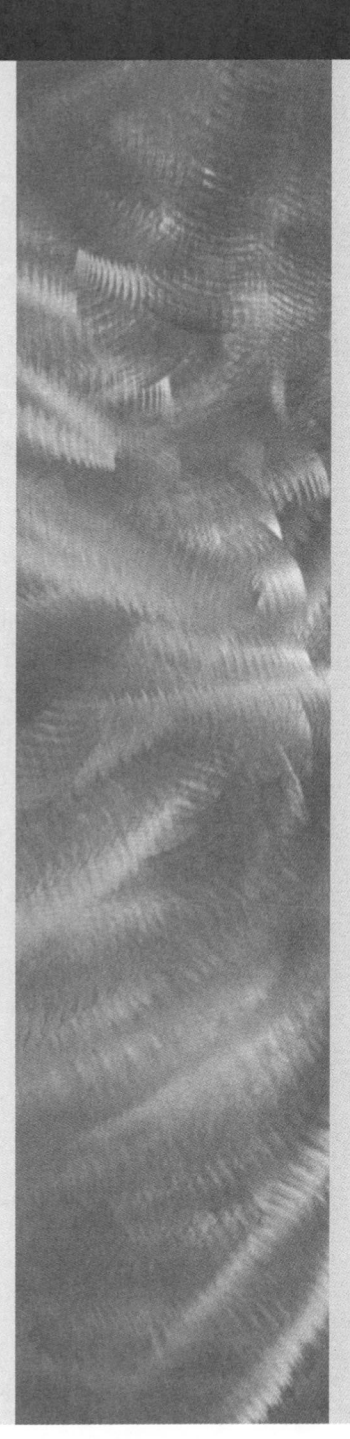

tered a sentence test in an audition-only condition, and she recognized about 20% of the words. During her first year of use, her score on the sentence test rose to almost 60% words correct. Sally discarded the hearing aid she had long worn on her un-implanted ear, saying that the little sound she received from it just made listening with the cochlear implant, "more confusing."

Her initial disappointment with the device pertained to music. It just did not sound like she remembered it. During the second week of implant use, she talked her husband into taking her to a symphony concert. The experience was so disturbing she had to turn her device off midway through the concert.

Sally enrolled in a music-based aural rehabilitation program. A music therapist with experience working with cochlear-implant users started Sally on a simple program where she listened to recorded tunes of familiar songs, such as "Twinkle, Twinkle" and "Happy Birthday to You." The renditions of the songs consisted of simple orchestrations and a male solo singer. Sally easily identified the melodies, and this success motivated her to continue with the training. During the past few months, she has graduated from familiar songs (her favorites are Beatles' tunes from the sixties), to country and western music (which, for many implant users, is pleasurable because of its rhythmicity and repetiveness), to familiar symphonic pieces.

Last week, David Anderson took his wife to a presentation of the play, "South Pacific." Following the advice of her aural rehabilitation music therapist, Sally took a score of the music with her. The couple sat in the balcony, where Sally could discretely set up the music sheets and follow along. This time, she left the auditorium with tears of joy in her eyes. Sally said she recognized every note and every lyric.

FINAL REMARKS

In this chapter, we have reviewed some of the fundamental aspects of the most widely used technology in aural rehabilitation. We concentrated on hearing aids, cochlear implants, and assistive listening devices. There is one other kind of listening device available for individuals who for some reason cannot use a hearing aid or cochlear implant, and who are not well served by assistive listening devices. This device is a tactile aid.

Tactile aids: aids that transduce sound to vibration and deliver it to the skin for the purpose of gross sound awareness and gross sound identification.

Tactile aids permit sound awareness by delivering vibrotactile sensation to the user's skin. Most devices look like a body aid, but instead of having a long cord leading to an earmold, they have a cord leading to a vibrotactile or electrotactile array.

These arrays may be placed against the chest or strapped to the wrist. When sound occurs in the environment, the device microphone picks it up. The signal is transduced into an electrical signal and then delivered to the vibrotactile or electrotactile array, where the skin is stimulated. Some of the more sophisticated devices present a spectral display to the skin, and thus may provide some information about the spectral characteristics of the signal. These devices serve primarily as a supplement to lipreading and rarely permit the user to recognize speech without the visual signal. With the advent of cochlear implants, they are not used by many people today.

KEY CHAPTER POINTS

✔ The objectives for providing an individual with a listening device are to make speech audible, without introducing distortion or discomfort, and to restore a range of loudness experience.

✔ Hearing aids, cochlear implants, and assistive listening devices are the primary listening devices available to hard-of-hearing persons. Tactile aids are used by a small number of people, primarily those who cannot benefit from the more commonly used devices.

✔ Two major trends in modern hearing-aid design are miniaturization and enhanced signal processing.

✔ Hearing aids have three fundamental components: a microphone, an amplifier, and a receiver. They also have a power source. Microphones may be directional or omnidirectional. Amplifiers may use peak-clipping for output limiting or compression.

✔ There are six general styles of hearing aids. Selection of style is dependent on the degree of hearing loss, user preference, costs, patient lifestyle, and the patient's physical status.

✔ Hearing aid benefit may be assessed with behavioral measures, probe microphone technology, and self-assessment scales.

✔ Cochlear implants provide sound sensation by means of directly stimulating the auditory nerve. Candidacy requirements for implantation include the presence of irreversible severe or profound sensorineural hearing loss and good general health.

✔ Most cochlear implants in use are multichannel devices and utilize an interleaved pulsatile stimulation algorithm.

✔ Assistive listening devices are used to address communication needs related to face-to-face communication, broadcast and other electronic media, telephone use, and sensitivity to environmental signals and stimuli. General categories of devices are wireless and hardwired.

▄▄ MULTIPLE CHOICE QUESTIONS

1. A hearing aid that permits the patient to adjust the way sound is processed, depending on the listening conditions and the sound stimuli, is said to have:

    a. A sophisticated noise reduction circuit

    b. Multiple memories

    c. Digital processing

    d. Multiple channels

2. Mrs. Cantor is a loan officer at a bank. She works at one of several desks that line the bank's main hall. She wants to be able to talk to her clients one-on-one, even though the hall is noisy. Her audiologist most likely would equip her hearing aid with:

    a. An omnidirectional microphone

    b. Peak-clipping circuitry

    c. A volume control wheel

    d. A directional microphone

3. The input SPL compared to the output SPL in a compression circuitry is know as:
   a. Attack time
   b. Compression ratio
   c. Kneepoint
   d. Peak-clipping ratio

4. The receiver of a hearing aid:
   a. Acts as a miniature loudspeaker and delivers sound to the tympanic membrane
   b. Receives signals from the environment
   c. Includes a preamplifier stage
   d. Is housed within the small shell that fits behind the pinna for BTE aids

5. The most popular style of hearing aid sold in the United States is:
   a. The body aid
   b. BTE
   c. ITE
   d. CIC

6. Which statement is true?
   a. The most appropriate style of hearing aid for a young child is an ITE.
   b. If a person has chronic otitis media, then a BTE aid with a nonoccluding earmold may be the most appropriate style of hearing aid.
   c. Most CIC aids have a volume control wheel.
   d. CIC aids create an occlusion effect.

7. An advantage of binaural amplification is:
   a. The enhancement of low-frequency sound reception
   b. Loudness multiplication
   c. Binaural squeal
   d. Elimination of head shadow

8. A middle ear implant:
   a. Directly stimulates the auditory nerve
   b. Is invisible because all of the components are worn internally
   c. Delivers micromechanical vibration
   d. Is relatively inexpensive

9. Mr. Howard has been deemed an appropriate candidate to receive a hearing aid. When considering what kind of hearing aid to prescribe, his audiologist first:
    a. Asks him about his preference
    b. Performs probe-tube measurements
    c. Presents recommendations and reasons for making them
    d. Determines his loudness discomfort level (LDL)

10. Jennifer Martin is a 12-month-old baby. She had her hearing tested 2 weeks ago. Her audiologist determined she has a bilateral sensorineural hearing loss. The audiologist would recommend that:
    a. Jennifer be scheduled for cochlear implant surgery
    b. Jennifer be fitted with an ITE aid
    c. Jennifer undergo a trial period with a hearing aid for 3 months and then be considered for cochlear implant candidacy
    d. Jennifer be fitted with amplification and then evaluated at age 2 years for cochlear implantation

11. The component of a cochlear implant that modifies the acoustic signal and separates it into frequency bands is called:
    a. The speech processor
    b. The electrode array
    c. The receiver
    d. The transmitter

12. Most manufacturers of cochlear implants today offer:
    a. Body worn devices only
    b. One processing strategy
    c. A processing strategy that utilizes interleaved pulsatile stimulation
    d. Analog processing strategies

13. Noise that is present in a room, even when it is empty, is referred to as:
    a. Background noise
    b. Reverberation
    c. Static
    d. Ambient noise

14. An example of a ALD wireless system is:
    a. DAIs
    b. Neckloops
    c. Induction loops
    d. Headphones

15. A person with profound hearing loss who wishes to make a telephone call to her insurance agent may take advantage of (choose the best option):
    a. A relay system
    b. A text telephone
    c. A telephone amplifier
    d. A telecoil

KEY RESOURCES

Self-Assessment Instruments That Can Be Used To Evaluate Hearing-Aid Use Benefits: Example of a Benefit-Assessment Scale

Profile of Aided Loudness (PAL)*

Name _____ Date _____

Status _____ Unaided _____ Previous Hearing Aids _____

Current Hearing Aids _____

INSTRUCTIONS: Please rate the following items by both the level of loudness of the sound and also by the level of satisfaction that you have for that loudness. For example, you might rate a particular sound as "Very Soft." If "Very Soft" is your preferred level for this sound, then you would rate your loudness satisfaction as "Just Right." If on the other hand, you would like the sound to be louder than "Very Soft," then your loudness satisfaction rating might be "Not Too Good" or "Not Good At All." The Loudness Satisfaction rating is not related to how "pleasing"

*Palmer, Mueller, and Moriarty, 1999. Profile of aided loudness: A validation procedure. *The Hearing Journal, 52,* 34–42.

the sound is to you, but rather, the appropriateness of the loudness. Here is an example:

The hum of a refrigerator motor:

Loudness Rating		*Loudness Satisfaction*	
0	Cannot Hear	5	Just Right
1	Very Soft	4	Pretty Good
2	Soft	3	Okay
3	Comfortable, But Slightly Soft	2	Not Too Good
4	Comfortable	1	Not Good At All
5	Comfortable, But Slightly Loud		
6	Loud, But Okay		
7	Uncomfortably Loud		

In this example, the hearing aid user rated the loudness level of a refrigerator motor running as "Comfortable, But Slightly Soft" and rated his Loudness Satisfaction for the sound as "Just Right." This satisfaction rating indicates that this person believes that it is appropriate for a refrigerator motor to sound "Comfortable, But Slightly Soft."

Circle the responses that best describe your listening experiences. If you have not experienced one of the sounds listed (or a similar sound), simply leave that question blank.

Profile of Aided Loudness (PAL)

1. An electric razor:

Loudness Rating		*Loudness Satisfaction*	
1	Cannot Hear	5	Just Right
2	Very Soft	4	Pretty Good
3	Soft	3	Okay
4	Comfortable, But Slightly Soft	2	Not Too Good
5	Comfortable	1	Not Good At All
6	Comfortable, But Slightly Loud		
7	Loud, But Okay		
8	Uncomfortably Loud		

2. A door slamming:

Loudness Rating

1   Cannot Hear
2   Very Soft
3   Soft
4   Comfortable, But Slightly Soft
5   Comfortable
6   Comfortable, But Slightly Loud
7   Loud, But Okay
8   Uncomfortably Loud

Loudness Satisfaction

5   Just Right
4   Pretty Good
3   Okay
2   Not Too Good
1   Not Good At All

3. Your own breathing:

Loudness Rating

1   Cannot Hear
2   Very Soft
3   Soft
4   Comfortable, But Slightly Soft
5   Comfortable
6   Comfortable, But Slightly Loud
7   Loud, But Okay
8   Uncomfortably Loud

Loudness Satisfaction

5   Just Right
4   Pretty Good
3   Okay
2   Not Too Good
1   Not Good At All

4. Water boiling on the stove:

Loudness Rating

1   Cannot Hear
2   Very Soft
3   Soft
4   Comfortable, But Slightly Soft
5   Comfortable
6   Comfortable, But Slightly Loud
7   Loud, But Okay
8   Uncomfortably Loud

Loudness Satisfaction

5   Just Right
4   Pretty Good
3   Okay
2   Not Too Good
1   Not Good At All

5. A car's turn signal:

Loudness Rating

1   Cannot Hear
2   Very Soft
3   Soft
4   Comfortable, But Slightly Soft
5   Comfortable
6   Comfortable, But Slightly Loud
7   Loud, But Okay
8   Uncomfortably Loud

Loudness Satisfaction

5   Just Right
4   Pretty Good
3   Okay
2   Not Too Good
1   Not Good At All

6. The religious leader during the sermon:

Loudness Rating

1   Cannot Hear
2   Very Soft
3   Soft
4   Comfortable, But Slightly Soft
5   Comfortable
6   Comfortable, But Slightly Loud
7   Loud, But Okay
8   Uncomfortably Loud

Loudness Satisfaction

5   Just Right
4   Pretty Good
3   Okay
2   Not Too Good
1   Not Good At All

7. The clothes dryer running:

Loudness Rating

1   Cannot Hear
2   Very Soft
3   Soft
4   Comfortable, But Slightly Soft
5   Comfortable
6   Comfortable, But Slightly Loud
7   Loud, But Okay
8   Uncomfortably Loud

Loudness Satisfaction

5   Just Right
4   Pretty Good
3   Okay
2   Not Too Good
1   Not Good At All

8. **You chewing soft food:**

Loudness Rating
1 Cannot Hear
2 Very Soft
3 Soft
4 Comfortable, But Slightly Soft
5 Comfortable
6 Comfortable, But Slightly Loud
7 Loud, But Okay
8 Uncomfortably Loud

Loudness Satisfaction
5 Just Right
4 Pretty Good
3 Okay
2 Not Too Good
1 Not Good At All

9. **Listening to a marching band:**

Loudness Rating
1 Cannot Hear
2 Very Soft
3 Soft
4 Comfortable, But Slightly Soft
5 Comfortable
6 Comfortable, But Slightly Loud
7 Loud, But Okay
8 Uncomfortably Loud

Loudness Satisfaction
5 Just Right
4 Pretty Good
3 Okay
2 Not Too Good
1 Not Good At All

10. **A barking dog:**

Loudness Rating
1 Cannot Hear
2 Very Soft
3 Soft
4 Comfortable, But Slightly Soft
5 Comfortable
6 Comfortable, But Slightly Loud
7 Loud, But Okay
8 Uncomfortably Loud

Loudness Satisfaction
5 Just Right
4 Pretty Good
3 Okay
2 Not Too Good
1 Not Good At All

11. **A lawn mower:**

Loudness Rating
1 Cannot Hear
2 Very Soft

Loudness Satisfaction
5 Just Right
4 Pretty Good

Loudness Rating

3 Soft

4 Comfortable, But Slightly Soft

5 Comfortable

6 Comfortable, But Slightly Loud

7 Loud, But Okay

8 Uncomfortably Loud

Loudness Satisfaction

3 Okay

2 Not Too Good

1 Not Good At All

12. **A microwave buzzer sounding:**

Loudness Rating

1 Cannot Hear

2 Very Soft

3 Soft

4 Comfortable, But Slightly Soft

5 Comfortable

6 Comfortable, But Slightly Loud

7 Loud, But Okay

8 Uncomfortably Loud

Loudness Satisfaction

5 Just Right

4 Pretty Good

3 Okay

2 Not Too Good

1 Not Good At All

Self-Assessment Instruments That Can Be Used To Evaluate Hearing-Aid Use Benefits: Example of a Satisfaction-Assessment Scale

Satisfaction with Amplification in Everyday Life (SADL)*

Name _____ D/O/B _____ Today's Date _____

INSTRUCTIONS: Listed below are questions about your experiences with obtaining and using your current hearing aid(s). For each question, please circle the letter that best corresponds to your opinion about your current hearing aid(s). Use the list of words below to determine your answer:

A. Not at all   E. Considerably

B. A little   F. Greatly

C. Somewhat   G. Tremendously

D. Medium

*Cox, R. M., and Alexander, G. C. 1999. Measuring satisfaction with amplification in daily life: The SADL scale. *Ear and Hearing, 20*, 306–320.

Keep in mind that your answers should reflect your opinions about the hearing aids that *you are currently wearing or have most recently worn.*

While we would like you to answer every question, if you feel that a question cannot apply to your experiences, please write an "x" through the number in front of the question.

1. Compared to using no hearing aid at all, does your hearing aid(s) help you understand the people you speak with most frequently?

   A B C D E F G

2. Are you frustrated when your hearing aid(s) pick up sounds that keep you from hearing what you want to hear?

   A B C D E F G

3. Are you convinced that obtaining your hearing aid(s) was in your best interest?

   A B C D E F G

4. Do people notice your hearing loss more when you wear your hearing aid(s)?

   A B C D E F G

5. Does your hearing aid(s) reduce the number of times you have to ask people to repeat?

   A B C D E F G

6. Do you think your hearing aid(s) is worth the trouble?

   A B C D E F G

7. Are you bothered by an inability to turn your hearing aid(s) up loud enough without getting feedback (whistling)?

   A B C D E F G

8. How content are you with the appearance of your hearing aid(s)?

   A B C D E F G

9. Does wearing your hearing aid(s) improve your self-confidence?

   A B C D E F G

10. How natural is the sound from your hearing aid(s)?

    A B C D E F G

11. How helpful is your hearing aid(s) on MOST telephones with NO amplifier or loudspeaker?

A B C D E F G

12. How competent was the person who provided you with your hearing aid(s)?

A B C D E F G

13. Do you think wearing your hearing aid(s) makes you seem less capable?

A B C D E F G

14. Does the cost of your hearing aid(s) seem reasonable to you?

A B C D E F G

15. How pleased are you with the dependability (how often it needs repairs) of your hearing aid(s)?

A B C D E F G

Additional Comments: _____

_____

_____

_____

_____

_____

Additional Questions

Experience With Current Hearing Aids:

       Less than 6 weeks

       6 weeks to 11 months

       1 to 10 years

       Over 10 years

Total Hearing Aid Experience:

       Less than 6 weeks

       6 weeks to 11 months

       1 to 10 years

       Over 10 years

Daily Hearing Aid Use:

    Less than 1 hour

    1 to 4 hours per day

    4 to 8 hours per day

    8 to 16 hours per day

Degrees of Hearing Difficulties:

    None

    Mild

    Moderate

    Severe

For Audiologist's Use Only

Hearing Aid Fitting:	Monaural Binaural
Right ear	Left Ear
Make _____	Make _____
Model _____	Model _____
Ser. No. _____	Ser. No. _____
Fitting date _____	Fitting date _____

Hearing Aid Type:

CIC

ITC

ITE

BTE

Hearing Aid Features (all that apply)

Directional mic	Peak clipping	Multi-program
Output limiting	Multi-channel	K-amp
T-coil	WDRC	FM
Curvilinear	DAI	BILL
	Vent	Other _____

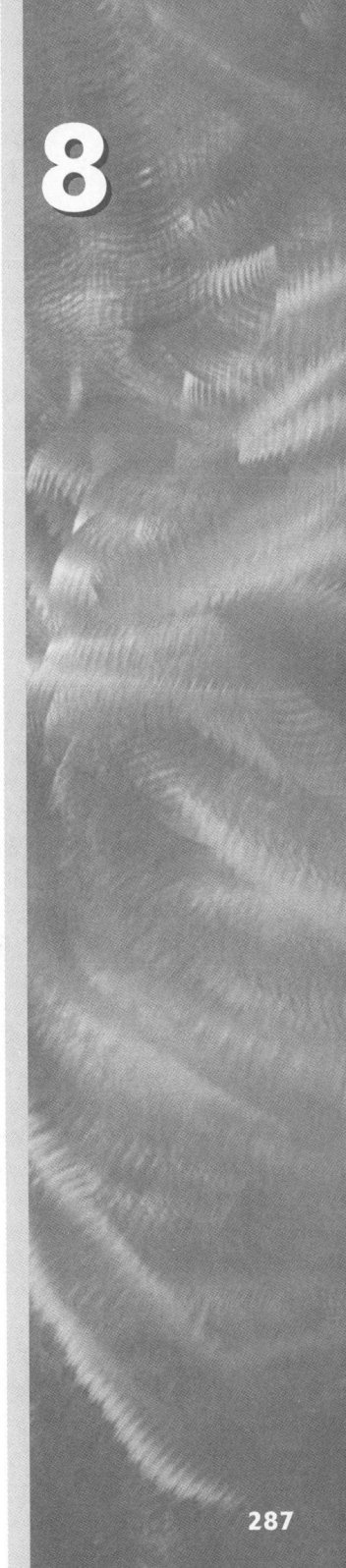

CHAPTER **8**

Auditory Training

TOPICS

- Candidacy for auditory training

- Four design principles

- Developing analytic training objectives

- Developing synthetic training objectives

- Formal and informal auditory training

- Interweaving auditory training with other components of aural rehabilitation

- Benefits of auditory training

- Case studies

- Final remarks

- Key chapter points

- Multiple choice questions

- Key resources

- Appendix 8-A

- Appendix 8-B

For further detail see, Tye-Murray and Fryauf-Bertshy (1992), Auditory training. In Nancy Tye-Murray (Ed.), *Cochlear implants and children* (pp. 91–114). Washington, DC: A. G. Bell Association.

The goal of auditory training for persons who have hearing loss is to develop their ability to recognize speech using the auditory signal and to interpret auditory experiences. Training helps them use their residual hearing to their maximum capability. During formal auditory training, you probably will not encourage individuals to watch your mouth movements as you speak. In fact, you may obscure your mouth, either by covering it or by sitting out of view (Figure 8-1).

Persons should be fitted with appropriate amplification before starting an auditory training program. A hearing aid (or cochlear implant) makes some speech sounds more audible. Auditory training will not change hearing sensitivity, but will enhance a person's ability to utilize whatever sound is available. By ensuring that individuals have the best amplification system possible, you will increase the raw material they have to work with and enhance their potential to benefit from training.

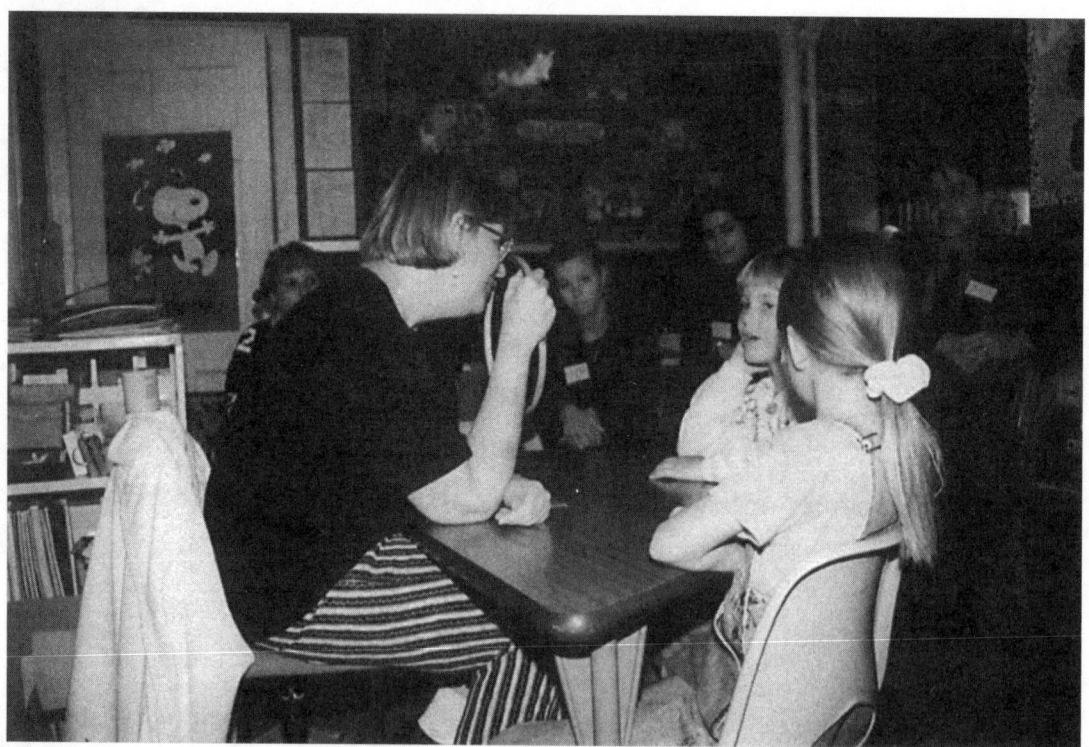

FIGURE 8-1. Formal auditory training. During a typical auditory training exercise, a teacher may cover her mouth movements with a mesh screen held within an embroidery hoop. (Photograph by Kim Readmond, Courtesy of the Central Institute for the Deaf)

Historical Notes

The procedures and techniques we use to provide auditory training have evolved gradually over time. Pollack (1970) notes that the value of using residual hearing has long been realized. Archigenes in the 1st century and Alexander in the 6th century both were know to hold ear trumpets to their ear to intensify the speech signal. Reports of analytic training exercises date back to as early as 1791, when Emaud designed analytic exercises for his deaf pupils. In 1805, Jean Marc Gaspard Itard, at the Paris Institute for the Deaf, provided drill training to children, asking them to discriminate one spoken utterance from another using only their residual hearing. Toynbee noted in 1860 that deaf individuals could learn to attend to their muted voices for the purposes of modulating speech production.

A seminal event in the history of auditory training in the United States occurred when Dr. Max Goldstein left his native St. Louis in 1893 to study with Dr. Adam Politzer, an otologist, and Professor Victor Urbantschitsch, an educator of the deaf, for 2 years in Vienna. Dr. Goldstein returned to St. Louis, convinced that children with significant hearing losses could learn to talk and to listen. He founded the Central Institute for the Deaf and promoted auditory and speech training for deaf children both nationally and internationally.

Rapid advances in technology during the 20th century increased the potential importance of residual hearing. After World War II, personal hearing aids became more effective and smaller in size so that they could actually be worn throughout the day. At this time, auditory training became a meaningful component of aural rehabilitation for a large segment of the hard-of-hearing and deaf populations. Clarence Hudgins worked with children at Clarke School for the Deaf in Northampton and conducted research that ultimately demonstrated that children who received amplification could increase their speech recognition through listening training (Erber, 1982). Raymond Carhart developed auditory training procedures for veterans returning from World War II, many of whom had incurred noise-induced hearing losses from weapons exposure.

The advent of cochlear implants in the latter part of the 20th century led to an explosion in the development of auditory training materials and methods. Computers and training packages founded on sound theoretical underpinnings have changed the complexion of auditory training.

CANDIDACY FOR AUDITORY TRAINING

Auditory training typically is provided to children who either incurred a hearing loss before acquiring speech and language (i.e., children who are prelingually deafened) or who incurred their hearing loss afterwards (i.e., children who are postlingually deafened). Children who have prelingual and profound losses may have no memory of how speech sounds and may have limited language skills and world knowledge. Thus, they cannot draw on memories of how speech should sound nor utilize acquired knowledge for interpreting the degraded auditory signal. During auditory training, these children first must learn to attend to the auditory speech signal, and eventually they must learn to relate the auditory signal to their vocabulary.

Children who have more hearing, or children who lost their hearing after acquiring some speech and language, often have a larger vocabulary and greater familiarity with grammar and may be better able to deduce meaning from the auditory speech signal, at least initially. The presence of more residual hearing, especially for the mid and high frequencies, portends good progress in auditory skill development. These children will probably begin with more difficult tasks than children who have prelingual, profound hearing losses.

It is less common for adults to receive auditory training. Adults who receive training typically are those who have experienced a recent change in hearing status. For example, someone who has just received a cochlear implant may receive auditory training to accelerate the learning process that often occurs during the first months following implantation (Figure 8-2). Someone who has incurred hearing loss following trauma or use of ototoxic drugs may receive training to adjust to his or her radically altered listening state. Speech through a listening device may sound different from how they remember it, and they must learn to interpret what they hear.

■■■ FOUR DESIGN PRINCIPLES

Many auditory training curricula are organized according to four design principles (Table 8-1). These four design principles are followed in developing and ordering training objectives. You may note that, in some ways, the principles we review in this chapter parallel the considerations for assessing speech recognition that we reviewed in Chapter 6.

Auditory Skill Level

The first consideration in designing an auditory training curriculum pertains to the person's hearing abilities. Results from an

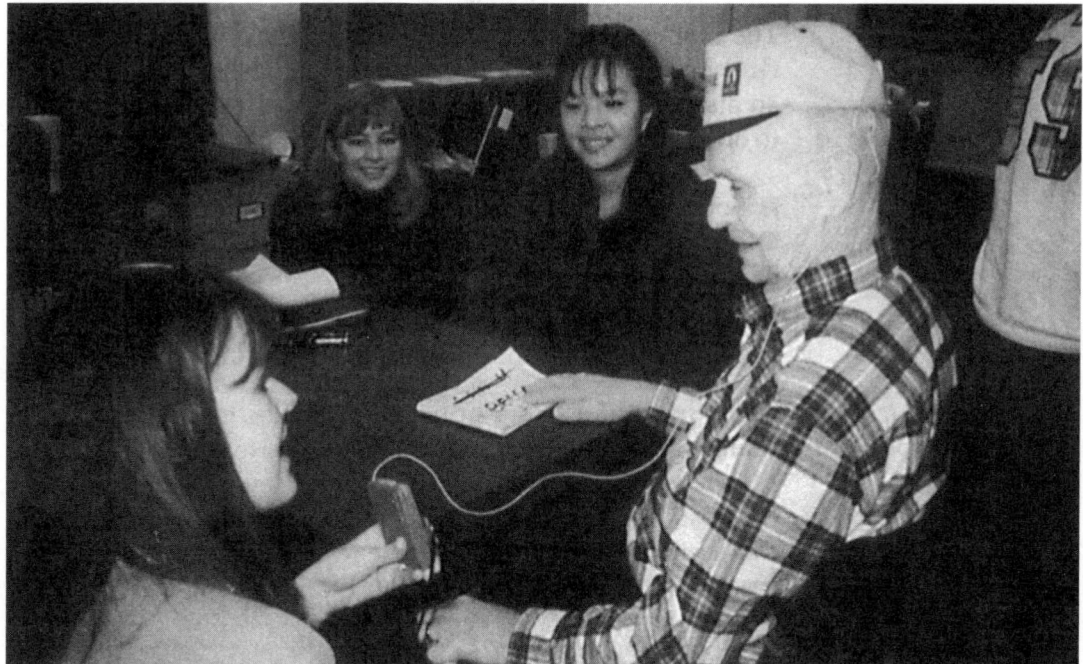

FIGURE 8-2. Auditory training for adults. Adults who may benefit from auditory training are those who have recently received a cochlear implant. (Photograph by Kim Readmond, Courtesy of the Central Institute for the Deaf)

Table 8-1. Four design principles by which activities in an auditory training curriculum may be developed and organized.

A. Auditory Skill	**D. Difficulty Level**
Sound Awareness	Response Set
Sound Discrimination	closed
Identification	limited
Comprehension	open
	Stimulus Unit
	words
B. Stimuli	phrases
Phonetic-level	sentences
Sentence-level	Stimulus Similarity
	Contextual Support
	Task Structure
C. Activity Type	highly structured
Formal	spontaneous
Informal	Listening Conditions

audiological assessment often are used to assign a student to one of four auditory skill levels (Erber, 1982):

■ Sound awareness
■ Sound discrimination
■ Identification
■ Comprehension

As Figure 8-3 indicates, these levels are not discrete benchmarks in auditory development but, rather, represent a continuum of skills. A person may be able to perform some activities associated with a sound discrimination level and some activities associated with identification at about the same time. In this section, we consider the four stages through use of a case study. Table 8-2 presents auditory training activities that may be appropriate for each stage.

Elizabeth Jenkins was born with a profound, bilateral hearing loss. Shortly after her third birthday, she received a cochlear implant. During the first few weeks of device use, Elizabeth did not respond spontaneously to sound. For instance one night her

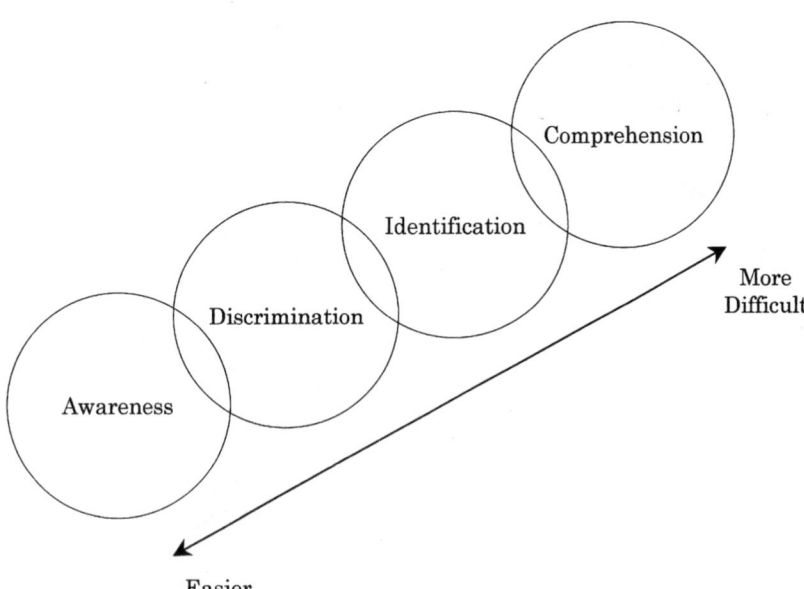

FIGURE 8-3. Four levels of auditory skill development. Auditory skill levels do not represent discrete benchmarks.

Table 8-2. Auditory training activities appropriate for each stage of auditory skill development (for children).

Sound Awareness

Play Peek-a-boo. Play musical chairs. March to the beat of a drum. Push the toy car whenever the clinician says "Vrrrrm."

Sound Discrimination

Play a game with toy animals ("The cow says 'moo', the sheep says 'baaa'").

Respond to the command ("Give me a crayon" "Draw").

Play the same or different game ("boy boy" "toy boy").

Repeat what you hear ("ma ma ma"/"pa pa pa").

Identification

Play the game Candyland and listen for the names of the colors.

Play with sets of postcards or stickers ("Show me the cat").

Play 'Go Fish' with cards ("Give me your sevens"; "Give me your twos").

Comprehension

Listen to a read-aloud story.

Play *I Spy,*

Play *20 Questions.*

---

father dropped a stack of plastic dinner plates near the room where Elizabeth was playing. Elizabeth did not turn around to see what had happened. When a telephone rang a few minutes later, she continued playing without a glance toward the sound source.

Several weeks elapsed before Elizabeth consistently demonstrated *sound awareness,* wherein she was aware when sound was present and when it was absent. Spontaneous response to sound began to occur once Elizabeth realized that sound has meaning, and that action often produces sound.

Elizabeth entered the next auditory skill level, *sound discrimination,* during the latter part of her first year of cochlear implant use. Elizabeth now could recognize when two sounds were the same and when two sounds differed, although she could not necessarily associate meaning with the two sounds or name them. For instance, she could indicate that an "Eeeeeeeeeeeeeee" spoken by her teacher was different from an "Eh."

Sound awareness is the most basic auditory skill level, awareness of when a sound is present and when it is not.

Sound discrimination is a basic auditory skill level in which the listener is able to tell whether two sounds are different or the same.

Identification is a basic auditory skill level in which the listener is able to label some auditory stimuli.

After about 9 months of cochlear implant use, Elizabeth entered into the *identification* level of auditory skills development and began to label some auditory stimuli. If her mother asked for a blue crayon, she could pick the blue crayon from a box of four other crayons. This skill relates to an awareness that objects have names, and names have auditory representations. At the identification stage, there were some occasions when Elizabeth imitated someone's utterance, but did not comprehend what the utterance meant.

Comprehension is a higher auditory skill level in which the listener is able to understand the meaning of spoken messages.

More than a year elapsed before Elizabeth begin to demonstrate some of the listening behaviors associated with the *comprehension* level of auditory skill development, in which she understood the meaning of spoken messages. This stage requires not only advanced auditory skills but some knowledge of vocabulary and grammar as well. At this time, Elizabeth's mother could ask a question with her face not visible and expect that Elizabeth might answer it appropriately, especially if the question was supported by linguistic and environmental context.

Children with significant residual hearing and adults who have had normal hearing before incurring a hearing loss may not progress through these four stages of auditory skill development in the same way as Elizabeth did. For instance, an adult cochlear-implant user will be aware of the presence or absence of sound the first time the device is turned on and likely will have some speech discrimination skills. A child who has some residual hearing, or who has incurred a hearing loss gradually over time, also will demonstrate more advanced listening skills.

DASL

Gayle Stout and Jill Van Ert Windle, authors of one of the most popular auditory training curricula in print for children (*The Developmental Approach to Successful Listening* II [DASL], 1992), have developed a placement test. This test determines whether a child should begin an auditory training program with sound awareness tasks or more advanced listening tasks. The following description summarize some initial items:

(continues)

Sound Awareness

1. The tester beats a drum while standing behind the child. The child must raise a hand when he or she hears the beats. A child who consistently responds correctly is aware of the presence of low-frequency sound.
2. The tester speaks a syllable, /ba/, with mouth covered, and the child must indicate when the syllable is spoken. A child who responds to speech consistently is aware of speech in a structured listening setting.
3. The tester familiarizes the child with several different noisemakers. The child must listen and indicate when the teacher sounds a noisemaker and when the teacher stops the sound. This task taps into the ability of the child to detect the presence and absence of environmental sound stimuli.

During the awareness phase of auditory learning, which usually will only involve infants, babies, and children, as most adults have sound awareness, you might make a point of showing a child the source and meaning of a sound, and reinforce the child when he or she responds to sound. For example, you might say:

- "I hear a loud noise. (Point upwards.) Look, it's a helicopter."
- "I'm turning on the water. (Turn the handle on a water faucet.) Listen. Now you try it."
- "I hear Janie. She must be coming. Listen."

Common auditory training activities for the second level of auditory training task, discrimination, might require a child to first make gross sound discriminations (again, children are more likely to pass through this stage before identification than adult patients). In an auditory training session, the child might be asked to discriminate between syllables, words, phrases, and sentences that are *short* and *long* (e.g., "The car goes *beep* and the cow says *mooooooooo.*") or between words that are *long* or *soft*. For example: "The baby is *sleeping*," versus, "The baby is **laughing.**" Other discriminations that might be practiced, often with supporting toys such as a stuffed cat and stuffed dog, include:

- (continuous versus interrupted) "The whistle goes *eeeeee* and the drum goes *boom-de-boom-de-boom.*"

- (one versus two) "The dog says woof and the cat says mee-ooow."
- (slow versus fast) "This car goes slow, *putt . . . putt . . . putt*, this car goes fast, *putt-putt-putt*."

In an identification task, older children might play card games like "Go Fish" and board games like "Candyland." In a comprehension task, you might read a story to the patient and then ask questions about what you read.

Stimulus Units

The second design principle of many auditory training curricula, after a consideration of auditory skills level, pertains to the stimuli used in the training activities. Although a particular program might emphasize one more than the other, most auditory training curricula include both analytic and synthetic kinds of training activities (Figure 8-4).

During an analytic training activity, students' attention is focused on segments of the speech signal, such as syllables or phonemes. More emphasis is placed on utilizing acoustic cues, such as the presence or absence of voicing in the words *coat* and *goat* than on gaining meaning from the speech signal. Presumably, one's ability to recognize these segments in isolation will carry over to real-world communication tasks, allowing students to recognize connected discourse better.

During synthetic training, individuals learn to recognize the meaning of an utterance, even if they do not recognize every sound or word. They do not perform an analysis of the signal on a sound-by-sound or syllable-by-syllable basis.

There is no clear dichotomy between analytic and synthetic training; rather, this is a continuum, and listening activities will gravitate from focusing attention on acoustic cue recognition to focusing attention on understanding the gist of a message. In the same

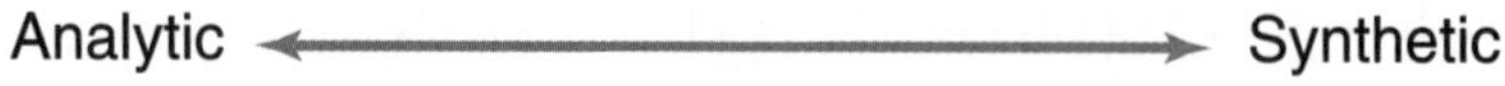

Analytic ←——————————————————→ Synthetic

FIGURE 8-4. Analytic and synthetic training. The distinction between analytic and synthetic activities is a continuum.

lesson, a student might perform analytic training activities and then switch to synthetic activities.

Activity Kind

A third design principle by which many auditory training curricula organize component activities relates to the nature of the training activity (Table 8-1), whether it is more formal or informal. Formal kinds of training activities occur during designated times of the day, usually with a one-on-one lesson between clinician and student, or in a small group of students. *Formal training* activities often are highly structured and may involve drill. Students may receive reinforcements for performing a formal training task. For instance, a clinician may speak a series of words without letting the student watch. The student then repeats each word. After every successful repetition, the student drops a coin into a bank. In this example, the speaking of a series of words represents a drill activity. The collecting of coins represents a reinforcement activity.

An *informal training* activity occurs as part of the daily routine and often is incorporated into other activities, such as conversation or academic learning. For instance, a wife may alert her husband when a horn honks or a bird sings after he receives a cochlear implant. She is using informal instruction to draw his attention toward sound and to place names on particular sound patterns.

Except when students are very young, the optimal auditory training program includes both formal and informal training activities. Children who are very young should receive primarily informal training. Programs for adults tend to include more formal than informal activities.

Difficulty Level

The final design principle of the four listed in Table 8-1 in which training programs are organized relates to the level of difficulty inherent in the training activity. There are at least six ways to vary training difficulty and to advance students from one skill level to the next (Figure 8-5).

Formal training: training that presents highly structured activities; may involve drill; usually scheduled to occur during designated times of the day, either in a one-room lesson format or in a small group.

Informal training: training activities that occur during the daily routine, often incorporated into other activities, such as conversation or academic learning.

Hierarchy of Listening Tasks

Warren Estabrooks (1994) presents an example of how training stimuli can be ordered to create a hierarchy of listening tasks, once the student (who, in his example, is a child) has readied the comprehension stage of listening. This hierarchy is listed below, beginning with the easier stimuli and ending with the more difficult stimuli.

- Familiar expressions/common phrases
- Single directions/two directions
- Classroom instructions
- Sequencing three directions
- Multielement directions
- Sequencing three events in a story
- Answering questions about a story: closed set and open set
- Comprehension activities/exercises in noisy environments
- Onomatopoeic words (p. 58).

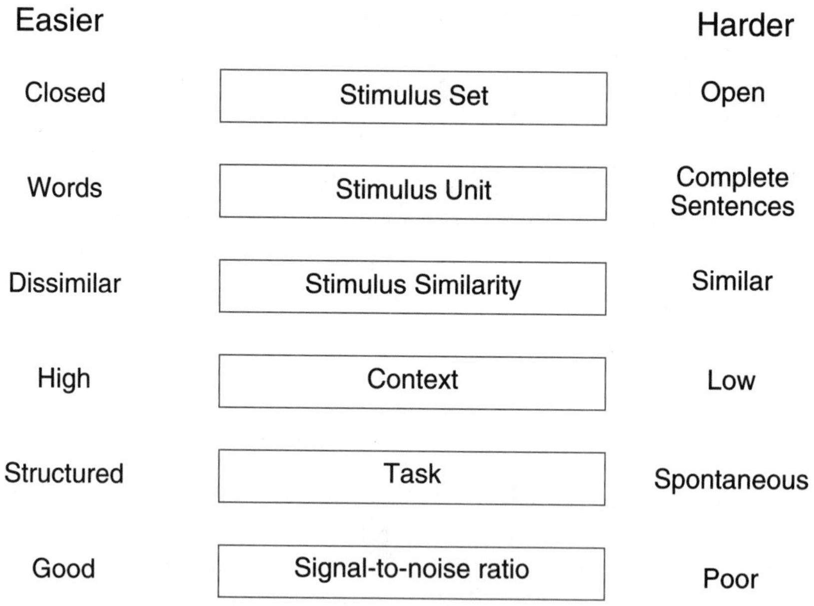

Easier		Harder
Closed	Stimulus Set	Open
Words	Stimulus Unit	Complete Sentences
Dissimilar	Stimulus Similarity	Similar
High	Context	Low
Structured	Task	Spontaneous
Good	Signal-to-noise ratio	Poor

FIGURE 8-5. Ways to vary the difficulty of the training task.

The first way to vary the level of difficulty is to vary the size of the stimuli set used for listening tasks. The size of the response set can be varied from a closed set, to a limited set, to an open set. As we noted in Chapter 6, a closed set means the student is presented with a limited set of known choices. For example, a child might be ask to recognize numbers from a closed set consisting of the numerical digits *one, two, three,* and *four.* A *limited set* is one defined by situational or contextual cues. For example, the set may include words pertaining to Halloween, but the student is not briefed about the specific words that might occur during a training exercise. An open set has few inherent constraints; a wide assortment of words are possible as response choices. As a student progresses from closed to limited to open response sets, the listening task becomes more difficult.

A second way to modulate training difficulty is to vary the stimulus unit. A clinician might employ sentences rather than words and phrases. Students typically perform training activities with words or phrases more easily than with sentences. For instance, a student more likely will identify the word *cat,* from the response set of *cat-mouse-dog* than to identify the sentence, *That's a cat over there,* from the response set of, *That's a cat over there, That's a mouse over there,* and *That's a dog over there.* When using sentences as training stimuli, those with simple syntactic structure typically are more difficult to recognize than those with complex structure.

The third way to vary difficulty relates to stimulus similarity. The similarity or dissimilarity of the stimuli can be varied to alter training difficulty. Most teachers begin with stimuli that differ acoustically and, later, present stimuli that are similar. For instance, initially, when the two items in a training stimulus pair differ, they will be quite dissimilar. For instance, a clinician may say the three syllable phrase, "How are you?" and then the single syllable, "Hi." As an individual progresses through auditory training and acquires more listening experience, the items in a stimulus pair will become more similar. The pair might represent a voicing contrast (e.g., *bee* vs. *pea*), a vowel contrast (e.g., *team* vs. *Tim*), or a stress contrast (e.g., *MY dog went home* vs. *My dog went HOME*).

The fourth way to influence difficulty level of training involves context. Speech stimuli that are supported by either linguistic or

A **limited set** of stimuli is defined by situational or contextual cues.

environmental context are relatively easy to recognize. For instance, *I had Wheaties for breakfast* is easier to recognize if the talker is standing in the kitchen holding a box of cereal than if the talker is speaking in the office lounge.

A fifth way to increase training difficulty is to move from structured listening tasks to spontaneous tasks. A student may acquire the skill to recognize a word during a structured activity, but may still not recognize it when it occurs in spontaneous conversation. If you prime a child to listen for his or her name and then speak it, the child will be more likely to respond to it than if you happen to say the name while the child is engaged in a quiet activity.

Finally, in addition to varying response set, stimulus unit, stimulus similarity, contextual support, and task structure, training difficulty also can be adjusted by altering the listening environment or the presentation of the stimuli. For instance, background noise, such as the playing of music, may be introduced to decrease the signal-to-noise ratio and increase the difficulty of the listening task. The level of the speech may be varied, either by the talker speaking more or less softly or by moving closer to or farther from the student.

You will want to adjust the level of training difficulty so that students are challenged but not frustrated. As a general rule of thumb, when providing formal auditory training, the level of difficulty should be increased if someone responds correctly to training stimuli 80% of the time or more. The difficulty level can be decreased if the person responds correctly to less than 50% of the training items.

■ DEVELOPING ANALYTIC TRAINING OBJECTIVES

At the onset of an auditory training program, a hierarchy of specific training objectives is developed. In developing a hierarchy, you will consider an individual's current skill levels, then consider in which sequence the person might best acquire more advanced listening skills and how to promote them. This process yields a well thought-out plan of action. It is not written in stone, however, and can be modified over time, according to the person's progress.

If someone has few auditory skills, training typically begins with developing an awareness of sound. If the student is very young,

Table 8-3. Objects that may teach children about the relationship between action and sound.

■ Hammer and peg toy	■ Computerized game
■ Toy drum	■ Water faucet
■ Piano	■ Hair dryer
■ Vacuum cleaner	■ Whistle

the child may have to learn that sound has meaning and that it is often the byproduct of an action. Children who have just acquired listening potential, such as a child who has received a cochlear implant, may not realize this important relationship between sound and activity. Nonspeech stimuli may be used to teach these concepts, such as those listed in Table 8-3. A young child who has had little experience with the auditory signal may need to develop these concepts before moving on to more challenging auditory tasks.

Once sound awareness has been established, early auditory training activities may involve gross discrimination of loudness, pitch, and rate, as in the following examples performed with a xylophone:

- **Loudness:** Strike a xylophone softly, and ask the student whether the sound is "soft" or "loud."
- **Pitch:** Play a rising octave, and ask whether the sound is going "up" or going "down."
- **Rate:** Strike a rapid series of notes, and ask whether the pattern is "slow" or "fast."

Once these kinds of tasks are mastered, then analytic and synthetic training activities might be introduced.

Two kinds of training objectives often are targeted with analytic training: vowels and consonants. Vowels usually are more intense than consonants and have more energy in the low frequencies, so are perceived more readily. For this reason, training for vowel recognition usually begins before training for consonant recognition. It is helpful to review the acoustic properties of vowels and consonants before attempting to design specific training objectives and lesson materials.

Vowel Auditory Training Objectives

Vowel formants are resonances in the vocal tract that cause some frequencies to have more energy than other frequencies.

Vowel auditory training objectives typically are designed to contrast vowels that have different formants. ***Vowel formants*** are the result of resonances in the vocal tract that cause some frequencies to have more energy than other frequencies. For instance, if you blow into a long, rounded bottle, you will produce a low-pitched sound because the bottle's shape enhances the resonance of sound waves associated with low pitches. On the other hand, blowing into a short, tubular bottle will produce a high-pitched sound. This bottle's shape enhances the resonance of sound waves associated with high pitches. In a similar fashion, the way you shape your mouth when you speak a vowel determines the vowel formants.

Each vowel can be distinguished by at least two characteristic formants. These are called the first and second formants. The combination of these two formants causes each vowel to sound different from every other vowel.

How wide you open your mouth determines the first formant. If you vocalize with your mouth relatively opened, you will produce a vowel that has a high-frequency first format. The vowel /a/ in *sod* is associated with an open mouth position and also has a high first formant compared to most other vowels. More closed mouth openings, such as that associated with the vowel /u/ in *blue*, produce low-frequency first formants.

Whether the tongue body is more forward or backward in the mouth greatly determines the frequency of the second formant. Moving your tongue more forward, as when saying /i/ in *seed*, will result in a higher frequency second formant. Moving your tongue body back towards the throat, as when saying /u/, will produce a lower second formant. Approximate first and second formant values for the vowels of English appear in Table 8-4 (Peterson & Barney, 1952).

Training may begin with developing vowel awareness, especially if the student is a very young child, and has little experience with the auditory signal. Toys such as farm animals may be used. The child listens as the cow makes a *moooo* sound, the lamb makes a *baaah* sound, and the chick says *cheeeep*.

Table 8-4. Typical first and second formant frequency values for the vowels of English, spoken by an adult male talker.

VOWEL	EXAMPLE	FIRST FORMANT (HZ)	SECOND FORMANT (HZ)
/i/	heat	270	2290
/ɪ/	hit	390	1990
/ɛ/	head	530	1840
/æ/	hat	660	1720
/a/	hot	730	1090
/ɔ/	hall	570	840
/ʊ/	hook	440	1020
/u/	who	300	870
/ʌ/	hut	640	1190
/ɚ/	hurt	490	1350

Once the student demonstrates vowel awareness, vowel training objectives might require students to discriminate between vowel stimuli and then to identify them. Initially, contrasts will concern vowels that differ in first formant information. For instance, a student might determine whether the words *meet* and *mat* are the same or different. Most persons with hearing loss are more likely to have residual hearing in the low frequencies than the high frequencies; therefore, first formant contrasts may be more perceptually salient than contrasts which include vowels differing in their second formants. As training progresses, students can discriminate and identify vowel stimuli that differ on the basis of second formant information, such as *bee* and *boo*. Table 8-5 presents a sample hierarchy of vowel auditory training objectives (Stout & Windle, 1992; Tye-Murray & Fryauf-Bertschy, 1992). These objectives were developed for a child who uses a cochlear implant and who has demonstrated consistent sound awareness.

Table 8-6 presents examples of word pairs that might be used for achieving the first three objectives. In typical discrimination exercises, like those required for the first three objectives, a student may sit before two pictures, for example, one of a key and one of

Table 8-5. A sample hierarchy of vowel training objectives.

The student:

1. Will discriminate vowels that differ in first formant information, using a two-item response set; for example, *meat* from *mat.*

2. Will discriminate vowels that differ in second formant information, using a two-item response set; for example, *bee* from *boo.*

3. Will discriminate words that have vowels with similar first and second formant information, using a two-item response set; for example, *mate* from *mit.*

4. Will identify words with different vowels, using a four-item response set; for example, *beet* from the response set of *beet, boot, bat,* and *bet.*

5. Will identify words with different vowels, from an open set of vocabulary.

---

a bee. The clinician might say one of the words, and the student is to point to the correct word. If the student is younger, he or she may place a coin or a piece of cereal on the picture. This provides visible reinforcement, and student and clinician can count the number of markers placed, once the task is completed.

If the student has difficulty in discriminating a stimuli pair, he or she can first practice speechreading (i.e., watching and listening both) the items using a *same/different* task. Figure 8-6 presents a response illustration that can be photocopied. It has a picture indicating *same* and one indicating *different.* The instructor can speak two words or phrases, such as *That's a pop/That's a peep,* or *That's a pop/That's a pop.* The student then indicates whether the stimuli are the same or different by touching the appropriate picture or by placing a coin on it.

Ideally the words used in a discrimination task should be alike except for the contrasting sounds; for example, the student might discriminate *beet* from *bat,* where the two vowels are contrasting. Such word pairs are relatively easy to construct when the student can read and has an extensive vocabulary. However, when the student cannot read, pictures or objects must be available so that he or she can respond by touching a representation of the word. A list of common one-syllable words that can be illustrated and used for vowel auditory training appears in the Key Resources at the end of this chapter.

Table 8-6. Vowel and word pairs that can be used for achieving the first three analytic auditory training objectives for vowels.

Objective 1: The student will discriminate vowels that differ in first formant information, using a two-response set.

Vowel pairs:

/u/ versus /ɜ/, /æ/, /ʌ/, or /a/   /ɪ/ versus /ɛ/, /æ/, /ʌ/, or /a/
/ʊ/ versus /ɛ/, /æ/, or /a/   /ɪ/ versus /ɛ/, /æ/, /ʌ/, or /a/

Word pairs:

shoe/shop	tune/ten	pin/pig
bee/bat	tooth/tap	moon/men
boot/bat	shoe/shut	put/pet
book/back	put/pot	bead/bed

Objective 2: The student will discriminate vowels that differ in second formant information.

Vowel pairs:

/ɪ/ versus /u/   /c/ versus /e, ɚ/
/o/ versus /e, ɚ/   /a/ versus /æ/
/e/ versus /ɚ/   /ʊ/ versus /ɪ/

Word pairs:

bee/boo	low/lay	low/learn
fawn/fern	hot/hat	book/bit
me/moo	shock/shake	lock/lake
coat/cake	beet/boot	pot/pat

Objective 3: The student will discriminate vowels with similar first and second formant information.

Vowel pairs:

/o/ versus /ɔ/   /ɛ/ versus /e/
/aɪ/ versus /ɪ/   /a/ versus /ʌ/
/e/ versus /ɪ/

Word pairs:

pen/pain	hot/hut	ship/sheep
get/gate	hog/hug	fit/feet
ship/sheep	show/shawl	chip/cheap
tin/teen	wet/wait	net/knit

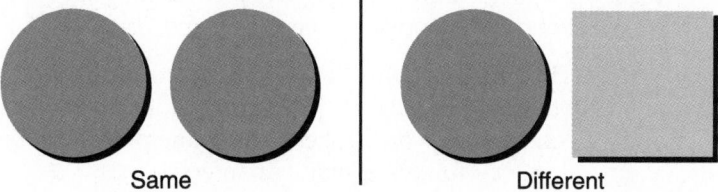

Same   Different

FIGURE 8-6. A response picture that can be used during a "same or different" auditory training exercise.

For the fourth objective listed in Table 8-5 (i.e., *The student will identify words with different vowels, using a four-item response set*), the response sets increase from two to four choices, for example, the instructor might say the word *beet*. The student's task is to touch one of four pictures: a beet, a boot, a bat, or a bed. For young children, toys or objects may be used in place of pictures.

For the fifth objective, the student must identify words using an open-set format, that is, without a set of response choices. In one exercise, the student might identify words whose vowels have a high-frequency second formant. For example, the instructor might say, "That's a bat," and ask the student to repeat the word without providing a group of words or pictures from which to choose.

General Procedures of Auditory Training With Minimal Pair Words

Here are steps you might follow when providing auditory training with minimal pairs (from Ertmer, Leonard, & Pachuilo, 2002).

Introduce minimal pair words by saying each word several times as you place pictures or printed words in front of the child. Encourage the child to pay attention to auditory and speechreading cues by holding the cards/objects close to your face as you name them. Discuss any unfamiliar words. Objects, rather than pictures, should be used whenever possible to hold the interest of toddlers and preschoolers.

After introduction, place picture or word cards representing two minimal pair words in front of the child. Present one of the words without speechreading cues by covering your mouth with a screen (a needlepoint hoop with two layers of loosely knit cloth). For example, say "Show me cat" while covering your mouth as the child chooses between "cat" and "rat."

The child repeats the target word aloud and then points to the picture, printed word, or object that represents that word. Tokens and game pieces can be given as reinforcers to maintain interest.

The target word can be repeated with or without speechreading cues as a prompt whenever an incorrect choice is made. If speechreading cues are provided, allow the child to see you say the word and then say the word again while covering your mouth with a screen.

Randomize the order of the words as you say them. Work at a steady, brisk pace to present 10 trials for each pair of words. Three to five word pairs can be presented in 10 minutes, depending on the child's concentration. Keep a tally of correct and incorrect responses to determine when criterion has been reached. (p. 217)

Designing Consonant Auditory Training Objectives

Consonant auditory training objectives often are designed to contrast three features of articulation: place, voicing, and manner (see also Chapter 6). Table 8-7 presents a list of consonants grouped together according to these features.

Place of articulation refers to where in the mouth the primary constriction occurs for the particular sound. Traditional place classifications include:

Place of articulation: classification of a speech sound according to where in the vocal tract it is produced (e.g., bilabial).

- **Bilabial,** such as /m/ in *man,* wherein the two lips meet to produce the sound
- **Labiodental,** such as /v/ in *van,* wherein the lower lip and upper teeth contact
- **Linguadental,** such as /θ/ in *thumb,* wherein the tongue tip contacts the upper teeth
- **Alveolar,** such as /d/ in *dot,* wherein the tongue tip approximates or contacts the roof of the mouth just behind the front teeth
- **Palatal,** such as /ʃ/ in *ship,* wherein the midsection of the tongue body approximates or touches the roof of the mouth
- **Velar,** such as /g/ in *glove,* wherein the back of the tongue approximates or touches the roof of the mouth

Table 8-7. A listing of consonants grouped together according to the features of place of articulation, voicing, and manner of articulation.

A. Consonants classified by manner of articulation

Stops: /p, t, k, b, d, g/

Fricatives and affricatives: /f, v, σ, h, s, ʃ, z, dʒ, tʃ/

Nasals: /n, m/

Glides and liquids: /w, j, r, l/

B. Consonants classified by voicing

Voiced: /b, d, g, v, z, m, n, l, w, j, r/

Unvoiced: /p, t, k, t ʃ, f, θ, h, s, ʃ/

C. Consonants classified by place of articulation

Bilabial: /m, p, b, w/

Labiodental: /f, v/

Linguadental: /θ/

Alveolar: /t, d, s, z, n, l/

Velar and palatal: /k, g, ʃ, j, tʃ, h/

Voicing: classification of a speech sound according to whether it is produced with or without voice (e.g., /b/ vs. /p/).

For training purposes, consonants that traditionally are considered palatal may be grouped together with velar consonants.

The ***voicing feature*** is used to classify sounds according to whether the vocal folds vibrate during the constriction phase of production. For example, /p/ is classified as an unvoiced sound whereas its cognate /b/ is classified as a voiced sound.

Manner of articulation: classification of a speech sound as a function of how it is produced in the oral cavity (e.g., glide).

Manner of articulation is used to classify consonants by the kind of articulatory movements required to produce the particular sound. Consonants can belong to one of five manner groups:

- **Stops,** such as /p/ and /d/. Stops are produced by completely closing the vocal tract at some point, and allowing pressure to build up behind the constriction. The constriction is released quickly, resulting in a burst of air. Stops are soft sounds and can be produced with or without voicing.
- **Nasals,** such as /m, n/. They are produced by lowering the velum and allowing air to flow through the nasal cavities. The nasal consonants tend to have high energy in the low frequencies, and they are louder than stops or fricatives.

- **Fricatives,** such as /f, s/. These sounds are produced by forcing the breath stream through a small constriction in the mouth, which results in a turbulent airflow. Fricatives tend to have a hissing sound. They are louder than stop consonants and longer in duration. They may be produced with or without voicing.
- **Affricatives,** such as /tʃ/. They are produced by combining a fricative with a stop, as in *chop*. For training purposes, fricatives and affricatives are sometimes grouped together.
- **Glides,** such as /w, j, l/. Glides are produced with slow, opening articulatory gestures. For instance, notice that when you say the word *lot*, your mouth opens more slowly than when you say the word *tot*. The first word begins with a glide whereas the second word begins with a stop consonant. Glides also are louder than either stops and fricatives and are always produced with voicing.

The easiest features to distinguish for most hard-of-hearing persons, even those with significant hearing loss, are voicing cues, and manner cues that signal whether a consonant is a nasal. Many individuals can distinguish *bat* from *pat* (a voicing distinction) and *bat* from *mat* (a manner distinction signaling nasality). These distinctions are easiest to hear because voiced sounds and nasals are comparatively loud, and they have energy in the low frequencies.

The most difficult cues to hear are those that relate to the place feature. This difficulty occurs because these cues are conveyed by mid- and high-frequency information, and many hard-of-hearing individuals have their greatest hearing loss for these frequencies. Many students will not be able to distinguish *pea* from *tea* from *key* through listening alone.

Knowledge of articulatory features, and how easily they can be heard, will help you to order your auditory training objectives. Early auditory training exercises might include consonant stimuli that differ in manner and voice and/or place of production, such as *tap* and *map*. The sounds /t/ and /m/ differ in terms of manner of articulation, place of articulation, and voicing. Later exercises might require students to identify consonants that differ in place of production but share voice and manner. For instance, they might distinguish between words such as *bag, tag,* and *gag*. These words are similar in their acoustic properties.

Table 8-8 presents a sample hierarchy of consonant auditory training objectives for young cochlear implant users.

Table 8-9 presents consonant and word pairs that exemplify the kinds of contrasts and words that might be utilized in achieving the first four objectives. When possible, at least five different sets of words should be presented for each consonant pair when using a discrimination task, although the student's vocabulary may limit the number of stimuli pairs that can be used for training. The Key Resources section presents a list of common one-syllable words that can be illustrated, which can be used in auditory training activities for very young children who cannot read.

After the objectives have been achieved with consonants in the initial position, exercises can include them in the final position of words. A carrier phrase such as, *That's a* _____ , can be used for presenting noun stimuli.

Table 8-8. A sample hierarchy of consonant auditory training objectives.

The Student:

1. Will discriminate nasal versus non-nasal unvoiced consonants that differ in place of production; for example, *mean* from *teen*.

2. Will discriminate nasal versus non-nasal voiced consonants that differ in place of production; for example, *map* from *gap*.

3. Will discriminate unvoiced fricatives versus voiced stops that differ in place of production; for example, *son* from *gun*.

4. Will discriminate unvoiced fricatives versus unvoiced stops that differ in place of production; for example, *sea* from *key*.

5. Will identify words in which the consonants share manner of production from a four-item and then six-item response set; for example, *sat* from the response set of *sat, fat, shot,* and *van*.

6. Will identify words in which the consonants are all either voiced or unvoiced from a four-item and then six-item response set; for example, *cat* from the response set of *cat, pat, tap,* and *sack*.

7. Will identify words in which the consonants share place of production from a four-item and then six-item response set; for example, *pat* from the response set of *pat, mat, bat,* and *fat*.

8. Will identify words in an open-set format, where the words are familiar vocabulary words.

Table 8-9. Consonant and word pairs that can be used for achieving the first four analytic auditory training objectives.

Objective 1: The student will discriminate nasal versus nonnasal unvoiced consonants that differ in place of production.

Consonant pairs:
/m/ versus /ʃ, s, t, k, tʃ, h f/
/n/ versus /p, k, f, h, ʃ/

Word pairs:

meat/seat	milk/silk	near/fear
net/pet	news/shoes	no/so
man/fan	neat/feet	might/fight
may/say	no/toe	nap/top

Objective 2: The student will discriminate nasal versus nonnasal voiced consonants that differ in place of production.

Consonant pairs:
/m/ versus /d, g, l, w, r/
/n/ versus /b, g, w, r/

Word pairs:

nail/rail	nine/wine	note/goat
mail/whale	mice/dice	kneel/deal
make/rake	knot/dot	make/lake
nail/bail	mow/dough	nap/lap

Objective 3: The student will discriminate unvoiced fricatives versus voiced stops that differ in place of production.

Consonant pairs:
/f/ versus /d, g/
/s/ versus /b, g/
/h/ versus /b, d/
/ʃ/ versus /b, d/

Word pairs:

fun/gun	sell/bell	same/game
shoe/do	heart/dart	shed/bed
she/bee	hay/day	hat/bat
sack/back	song/gone	fall/doll

Objective 4: The student will discriminate unvoiced fricatives versus unvoiced stops that differ in place of production.

Consonant pairs:
/f/ versus /t, k/
/s/ versus /p, t/
/h/ versus /p, t/
/ʃ/ versus /p, t/

Word pairs:

fall/tall	shell/tell	sing/king
fan/tan	sand/can	fat/cat
some/came	show/toe	shine/pine
fin/tin	phone/cone	soil/coil

Cycling

A student does not necessarily have to meet one training objective before progressing to the next one. Vergara, Miskiel, and Oller (1994) described an auditory training program that utilizes cycling. "*Cycling* involves presenting a skill within a specified time period and then moving on to another objective . . . For example, after targeting one objective for two weeks, the teacher may choose to move on to another objective returning to the original objective at a later date . . . Cycling provides the opportunity for students to process new concepts. For example, after an initial introduction, children are provided with opportunities to experiment with a particular task so that at the time of the second presentation, they may experience a higher level of success" (p. 58). Cycling is a potent means to build listening skills and is effective in helping students overcome a plateau in their listening performance.

Cycling: coming back to a training objective that has been achieved with some success in order to provide reinforcement and additional learning.

▨ DEVELOPING SYNTHETIC TRAINING OBJECTIVES

Suprosegmentals are prosodic aspects of speech, including variations in pitch, rate, intensity, and duration, that are superimposed on phonemes and words.

In this section, we consider synthetic training objectives. Depending on the student's skill level, synthetic training objectives might begin with simple discrimination activities that involve suprasegmental aspects of speech. *Suprasegmental* aspects, sometimes referred to as prosodic features, include intonation, stress, duration, and loudness (see Chapter 16). During training, you might ask a child to move a toy car at a fast or slow pace, depending on whether you quickly bark, *go-go-go-go* or leisurely intone, *Gooo—Gooo—Gooo.* You might speak one of two student's names with a conversationally loud voice or a whisper, and ask that the named student imitate your production.

Once these kinds of tasks are mastered, the program can address objectives like those listed in Table 8-10. Students can discriminate and later identify multiword utterances such as *I'm going home* from single word utterances, such as *home.* This will require them to attend to information about the number of syllables in the phrase. Table 8-11 presents long and short training pairs that can

Table 8-10. A sample hierarchy of synthetic auditory training.

The Student:

1. Will discriminate multiword utterances from single-word utterances, using a closed response set; for example, *How ore you today?* from *Hi!* Later, he or she can be asked to discriminate long words from short words; for example, *Halloween* from *cat*.

2. Will discriminate a spondee from a one-syllable word; for example, *ice cream* from *shoe*. Later, he or she can be asked to discriminate a spondee from a two-syllable word; for example, *There's a toothbrush* from *There's a pony*.

3. Will discriminate between words having the same number of syllables; for example, *That's my cat* from *That's my dog*.

4. Will identify simple words from a four-item and then a six-item response set, for example, *cat* from the response set of *cat, dog, elephant,* and *camel*.

5. Will identify picture illustrations from a closed-set, after hearing one-sentence descriptions.

6. Will follow simple directions and answer simple questions, using a closed response set.

7. Will listen to two related sentences, and then draw a picture about them, for example, he or she might draw a picture after hearing, *The boy is playing. He has a ball*.

---

be used for achieving the first objective listed in Table 8-10, and Table 8-12 presents two-syllable spondees that can be used for achieving the second objective listed in Table 8-10.

The next step may be for students to identify simple words from a closed set of choices; for instance, the word *Tom* from the response set of *Tim, John, Don,* and *Tom*. As skills progress, the size of the response set can be increased from four to six choices.

Comprehension activities can begin with a closed-set format and move to a more open-set format. Young students might be asked to, *Show me your nose, Show me your ears, Show me your mouth,* and *Show me your hair*. Later, they may be asked to draw a picture, step by step, without knowing what directions might occur, for example, *Pick up a blue crayon* (the student demonstrates comprehension by picking it up), *Draw a circle* (the student demonstrates comprehension by drawing the circle), *Put a fish in the circle* (the student draws a fish), and so forth.

Table 8-11. Long and short training pairs that can be used for achieving the first synthetic auditory training objective listed in Table 8-10.

The student will discriminate multiword utterances from single-word utterances:

■ How are you/Hi   ■ Beat the drum/clap

■ See you later/Bye   ■ The cat in the hat/dog

■ Santa Claus/tree   ■ Give me the crayon/draw

■ Motorcycle/car   ■ A box of cookies/milk

Table 8-12. Examples of word pairs that can be used for the second objective listed in Table 8-10 for synthetic auditory training.

The student will discriminate a two-syllable from a one-syllable word:

Airplane/pop   Snowball/ice

Milkshake/cup   Toothbrush/teeth

Flashlight/cake   Popcorn/bowl

Hotdog/bun   Sandwich/gum

Pancake/plate

If students are adults, a comprehension task might be to listen to a recorded passage and then to answer written questions. Afterwards, they listen to the passage a second time, reading a transcript of the passage while listening. The second presentation provides additional listening practice and allows them to check the accuracy of their answers to the questions.

■■ FORMAL AND INFORMAL AUDITORY TRAINING

Once training objectives have been formulated, they can be pursued with formal and informal instruction.

Formal Auditory Training

General guidelines for conducting formal auditory training are presented in Table 8-13. Training activities and materials should be appropriate for students' age, gender, language

Table 8-13. Guidelines for conducting formal auditory training.

A. **Training stimuli should become more challenging to discriminate over time.**
  Many hard-of-hearing individuals can determine whether a sound is nasalized or voiced and, less often, whether the sound has frication. They have difficulty in distinguishing place of articulation. In initial training, students may be asked to discriminate between sounds that differ in manner and voice. In late training, they can discriminate between sounds that differ only in place.

B. **A variety of talkers should speak training items.**
  Students learn that the same sounds or words can be acoustically different when repeated or when spoken by different talkers. This realization allows them to generalize what they learn in training to a variety of talkers. Tape recorders, VHS tapes, and digitized speech samples can be used to present stimuli.

C. **Many, many training items should be presented during a relatively short period of time.**
  Concentrated training focuses students' attention on listening and maintains their interest, leading to fast learning. Adherence to this guideline means that training reinforcements are provided sparingly, since they may be time consuming and distracting.

D. **Nonspeech training stimuli should be used only with young students who are prelingually deaf, and only for a short period.**
  Nonspeech stimuli develop two important concepts: First, sound conveys meaning and second, action often produces sound. The child might turn on and off a water faucet or clap hands. The exception to this guideline is the student who is interested in developing his or her ability to appreciate music.

E. **An auditory training exercise can include both analytic and synthetic level stimuli.**
  Occasionally the student's attention is focused on recognizing speech sounds and single words or phrases, and occasionally on recognizing words in a meaningful context.

F. **Training progresses from closed-set to open-set response modes.**
  Early in training a young student might be asked to color a shape red and need to choose between a red or blue crayon (closed-set). Later, the student might be asked to select the red crayon, when crayons from an entire box are available as options (open-set).

G. **Ten to 15 minutes a day should be devoted to formal auditory training, preferably at the same time everyday.**
  Training thus becomes a part of the daily routine.

H. **Formal training objectives should be pursued informally throughout the day.**
  When opportunity arises during conversation or academic instruction, the student can be presented with listening tasks that reinforce the formal auditory training objectives.

I. **Training activities must be engaging and interesting.**
  Otherwise, the adult may simply pass through the motions of training without receiving benefit; the child may not cooperate.

---

skills, and everyday experiences. For instance, a young boy might respond to materials that concern soccer. An adult might enjoy materials about current news events. If possible, auditory training should occur with no more than one to three students at time, in a quiet room that offers minimal distractions. The optimal distance between the teacher and student is 6 to 12 inches. A sample lesson plan for an auditory training session is presented in Table 8-14.

To make formal auditory training stimulating for children, *reinforcements* are often essential. After students complete a set number of items or perform so many activities, they receive something desirable, such as a sticker or special privilege. The

Reinforcement: something desirable provided to a student after he or she performs a training activity or performs in a desired manner.

Table 8-14. An example lesson plan for an auditory training session.

Title:

Snake and Ice Cream Game

Objective:

The student will discriminate a nasal consonant versus non-nasal unvoiced consonant that differs in place of production.

Materials:

1. a picture of a snake to represent the /s/ sound
2. a picture of a boy about to eat an ice cream sundae to represent the /m/ sound.
3. a stack of 26 pennies for reinforcements

Procedures:

1. Introduce the picture of the snake by pointing to it and saying "sssssssss . . ." Ask the child to imitate your production. Similarly, introduce the picture of the sundae, and say "mmmmmm . . .," Ask the child to imitate your production.
2. Say each sound with your face visible. After each utterance, ask the child to point to the corresponding picture.
3. Place 13 pennies on each picture. Cover your mouth. Randomly say one sound after another. After each production, the child may pick up a penny from one of the two pictures. If the child removes a penny from the correct picture, he or she can keep it. If incorrect, the penny must be placed back on the picture.
4. Continue until all pennies are spent.

following are general principals to follow when choosing and providing reinforcements:

A. The child should be able to perform a reinforcement activity quickly; he [she] should not spend more time with the reinforcement activity than with the training activity.

B. Reinforcement activities should not be too challenging or too absorbing; otherwise the child will not attend closely to the training task.

C. Activities must be varied; drawing lines on a paper may hold a child's interest for a few minutes, but the activity quickly wears thin.

D. Activities should interest the child; for example, if the child enjoys playing with money, he or she might drop coins into a bank.

E. The child should perform the reinforcement activity immediately after responding to a training item correctly.

F. Activities should be appropriate for the child's age and gender.

Reinforcements

Reinforcements are often utilized during formal training activities. Reinforcements must be appropriate for the age and interests of the students. The following two lists present reinforcements that might be appropriate for young children and adolescents:

List 1: Young children
- Collecting stickers in a sticker book
- Putting features onto a Mr. Potato Head
- Placing puzzle pieces one at a time into a puzzle board
- Blowing soap bubbles
- Playing a card game or board game
- Stringing beads onto a bead necklace

List 2. Adolescents
- Earning tokens that can be used to purchase desirable privileges, such as time with a computer game
- Earning tokens that can be used to buy school supplies, such as pencils and notepads
- Earning tokens that can be used to buy extracurricular rewards, such as a gift certificate to a fast food restaurant

---

Special Considerations for Adults

Many adults will be reluctant to participate in an auditory training class. Hectic schedules, a long workday, and transportation difficulties are possible obstacles to participation. This state of affairs has resulted in some attempts to develop home training and programmed self-instruction procedures. Students may receive exercises they complete at home. They may listen to audiotaped cassettes or perform a listening activity with a family member or friend. They inform the teacher about their progress, perhaps by mailing a record-keeping schedule or workbook pages on a regular basis. The clinician stays in contact with the adult student, by making telephone calls or sending e-mail messages on at least a weekly basis throughout the course of the home training program.

Informal Auditory Training

"Once I got my cochlear implant, I went to the bookstore and bought several mystery books on audiotape. I also bought the printed versions. At night, I listened to the tapes, while following along with the printed text. It was great. I practiced listening and caught up on my reading, both at the same time."

—Ralph, adult cochlear implant user.

Informal auditory training is a powerful means of fostering listening skills because listening practice occurs in the context of meaningful communication and is not removed from situational context. Informal auditory training can enhance students' confidence in their abilities to engage in conversation and also increase their motivation to rely on hearing for communication.

When students are children, classroom teachers can incorporate informal listening practice into the academic curriculum. For example, a classroom teacher might expect students to comprehend familiar phrases associated with the calendar. The teacher might query, with mouth hidden, "Tell me what today is," "Tell me what day it was yesterday," and "Tell me what will tomorrow be." The teacher may instruct, with face clearly visible, "Go to the chalkboard. I will say a number between 1 and 10." These instructions establish a context for recognizing her next instruction, which will be spoken while the student faces the chalkboard: "Write the number seven."

Auditory Training at Home

You might recommend informal auditory training activities to perform in the home. For example, parents can play musical chairs with their child to promote sound awareness. In making recommendations, you might also stress the importance of "fun time," and the need for a parent to be a parent rather than a teacher and the need for the child to have time to be a child.

INTERWEAVING AUDITORY TRAINING WITH OTHER COMPONENTS OF AURAL REHABILITATION

Commonly, auditory training is provided in conjunction with speechreading training and, if the student is a child, speech therapy. By interweaving auditory and speechreading training, you will build a student's associations between corresponding auditory and audiovisual representations of speech. It is common for training stimuli to be presented in the audiovisual condition before being presented in an audition-only condition. Students will recognize considerably more stimuli when they can both see and hear the talker rather than only hear the talker.

There are at least two reasons to incorporate speech production practice into auditory training. First, a child's awareness of oral representations of words may relate closely to the child's ability to identify the words auditorily. For instance, there appears to be an underlying linguistic structure that links speech perception and speech production. This structure reflects a child's knowledge of phonology, as well as grammar (Lachs, Pisoni, & Kirk, 2001). Thus, the gains that children make in their abilities to perceive the sounds of speech develop and fine-tune their phonological representations of words cognitively. In turn, these phonological representations affect the child's ability to produce them. This process likely is a two-way street. As a child's ability to produce sounds improves, the phonological representations of words become more developed and refined, which, in turn, may affect speech perception.

The second reason to link speaking and listening practice together is that by doing so, the child may realize that one purpose of learning to listen is to learn how to utilize auditory information to enhance speech production. Children must get in the habit of monitoring their own speech as they talk. Through auditory training and speech therapy, they can learn to attend to the suprasegmental qualities of their speech outputs (e.g., *Am I talking too loudly? Too softly? Is my voice conveying the nuances of meaning that I intend?*) and attend to the clarity and accuracy of their sound production.

■ BENEFITS OF AUDITORY TRAINING

Some researchers have shown that auditory training improves the listening performance of adults (Alcantara, Cowan, Blarney, & Clark, 1990; Lansing & Davis, 1988; Walden, Erdman, Montgomery, Schwartz, & Prosek, 1981); other studies have not (Rubinstein & Boothroyd, 1987). Blarney and Alcantara (1994) suggested that the contradictory results may relate to different types of practice that were provided to the research subjects in the different experiments, the different kinds of listening skills that were evaluated, and, finally, to the varying level of performance of the subjects at their entry into a training program. An interesting line of work has emerged in the past decade that hints at the effectiveness of auditory training. Brain activity has been shown to change as a result of auditory training (e.g., Kraus et al., 1995; Tremblay & Kraus, 2002; Trembly, Kraus, Carell, & McGee, 1997). With electrodes glued to subjects' scalps, researchers have demonstrated that the shapes of the waveforms evoked as a result of brain activity (evoked potentials) change following training. If the training stimuli are speech sounds, the change in activity is greater over the left hemisphere (known as the language hemisphere) than the right hemisphere. These changes in neural activity are usually accompanied by behavioral changes, that is, subjects who demonstrate a change in neural activity also demonstrate a new ability to distinguish two sounds that they were unable to discriminate prior to receiving training.

Little research has been performed on the benefits of auditory training per se for children. However, there is evidence that children who use aural-oral communication and rely on listening and speechreading for recognizing messages tend to perform better on tests of speech recognition than children who use simultaneous communication and rely on speech and sign language (Geers & Moog, 1992). Children in an aural/oral educational program often receive more auditory training than children in a simultaneous communication program, so one interpretation is that aural/oral children perform better on speech recognition tests because of the increased amount of auditory training they receive.

The benefit accrued from auditory training will vary greatly from one student to the next. For some students, benefits accumulate gradually over time, whereas others receive little or no benefit throughout the course of training. Often, young students progress in spurts. Listening skills improve, then plateau, and then improve more. The rate and extent of benefit may be influenced by at least two factors, the characteristics of the student and the program content.

Characteristics of the Students

Students who have more residual hearing, or who receive a significant amount of information through their listening devices, likely will achieve higher levels of auditory performance than students who have less hearing or who receive less information. The kind of listening aid that the student uses is important. Current cochlear implants allow many users to hear mid- and high-frequency components of the speech signal. They may hear more information about place and frication, as well as other parameters of speech, than individuals who have similar hearing loss and use hearing aids.

Progress also may be influenced by the student's age, motivation to receive training, age at which the hearing loss was incurred, duration of hearing loss, family situation, and the student's personality. For example, an elderly individual who has had a hearing loss for many years probably will receive less benefit from auditory training than a recently deafened adolescent. An outgoing, extroverted child who frequently interacts with children who have normal hearing might have a greater intrinsic desire to develop listening skills than an introverted child who prefers solitary activities.

Program Content

Program content also interacts with training gains. Issues related to program content include the appropriateness of the training activities, that is, whether the activities are enjoyable and motivating for the student and whether they are appropriate for helping the student meet the training objectives (Figure 8-7). The consistency with which teachers and other significant individuals in a student's life provide auditory stimulation and reinforce training objectives informally throughout the day, also will affect the amount of benefit received.

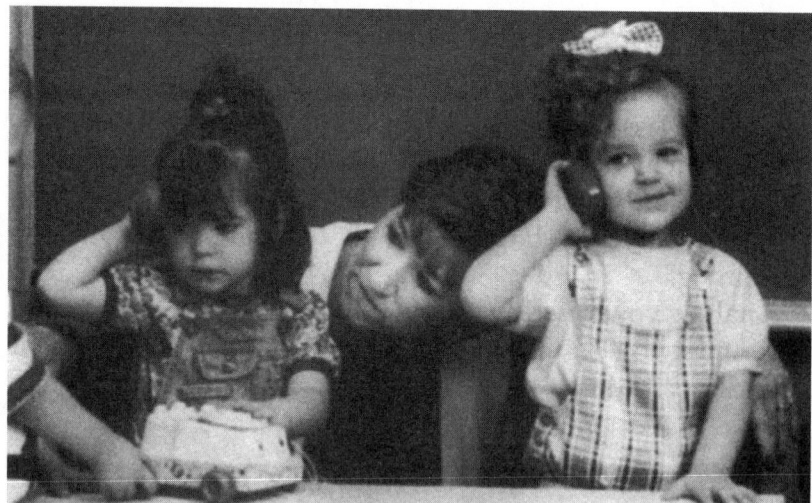

FIGURE 8-7. The success of an auditory training program depends in part on whether the training activities are enjoyable and motivating for the students. Activities should be age appropriate. (Photograph by Marcus Kosa, courtesy of the Central Institute for the Deaf)

In this section, we summarize two case studies. These two children were described by Ertmer, Leonard, and Pachuilo (2002). At the onset of the description, both children had received cochlear implants. These two examples demonstrate how an auditory training program might be implemented and adjusted to meet the specific needs of the individual. The first child, Drew, had experience with normal hearing and then usable residual hearing for many years before incurring a profound hearing loss. His preimplant experiences with hearing allowed him to quickly associate the electrical signal with his memories of how speech used to sound. In contrast, the second child, Bobby, suffered a hearing loss much earlier in life than did Drew, and his auditory skills emerged more slowly.

Case Study 1: A Child with Prelingual Onset of Deafness

Drew had normal hearing until shortly after his third birthday, when he contracted pneumoccal meningitis. He suffered a moderate sensorineural hearing loss in his right ear and a severe loss in his left ear. He received binaural hearing aids and joined a preschool for children who have hearing impairments. His family and teachers used simultaneous communication with him (i.e., communicated using both spoken language and sign language that has English syntax), although he expressed himself only with speech.

At the age of 7 years, Drew lost his hearing completely and thereafter received a cochlear implant. He began individualized intervention sessions with a speech and hearing professional, twice weekly for 1-hour periods. This intervention lasted 20 months.

(continues)

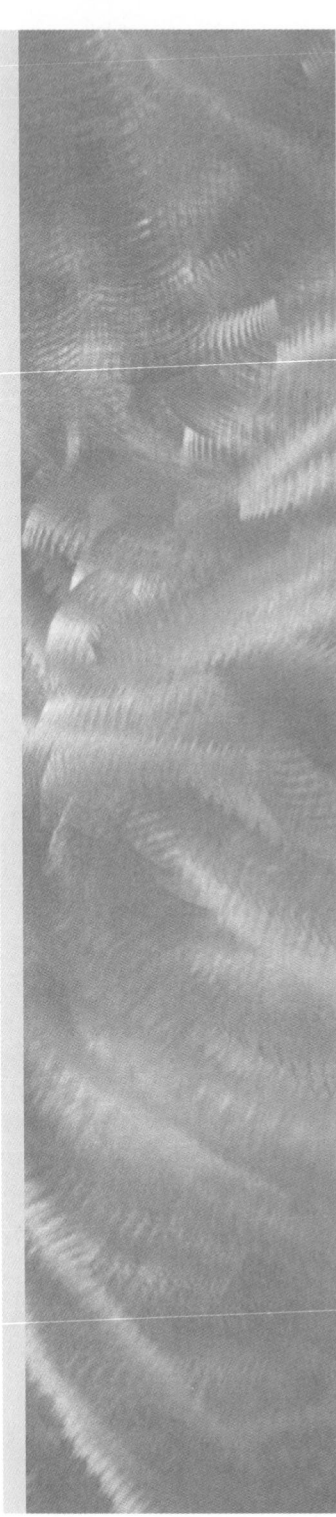

Speech sounded qualitatively different to Drew through a cochlear implant than through the hearing aids he had used prior to his complete loss of hearing. Thus, the primary goals of intervention were to "help Drew make sense of the new signal" (p. 206) and to increase his hearing performance so as to improve speech and language skills. His intervention integrated activities in auditory training and speech and language therapy.

For auditory training, Drew participated in both analytic and synthetic listening activities. The analytic auditory training focused on the parts of speech so to enhance Drew's ability to distinguish between vowel and consonant features. The program objectives were similar to those presented in this chapter, in Tables 8-5 and 8-8. Speech sound contrasts progressed from requiring Drew to make gross distinctions to fine distinctions, and the number of choices in a response set increased as Drew became more proficient in his listening skills. He had to meet a criterion of 80% accuracy for two consecutive intervention sessions initially for a contrast (e.g., distinguishing pair /t/ words from /d/ words). As his skills developed, this criterion level was raised to 90% accuracy for a single session. This upgrade was done to allow Drew to spend the majority of his time working on difficult contrasts and less time on those that were perceptually salient for him already.

Drew's progress for analytic listening tasks concerning consonants is plotted in Figure 8-8. Similar progress was noted for vowel discriminations. The light bars indicate his average score for a specific consonant contrast prior to training, and the darker bars indicate his performance following training. The number of sessions devoted to establishing the contrasts is denoted in parentheses above the bars.

Drew's initial scores ranged from 70% to almost 90% correct after just one training session. He received training only for those items that did not meet the 90% criterion level. Some of the contrasts that needed three or more sessions to establish included the following contrasts: /e/ versus /æ/ and stops versus fricatives.

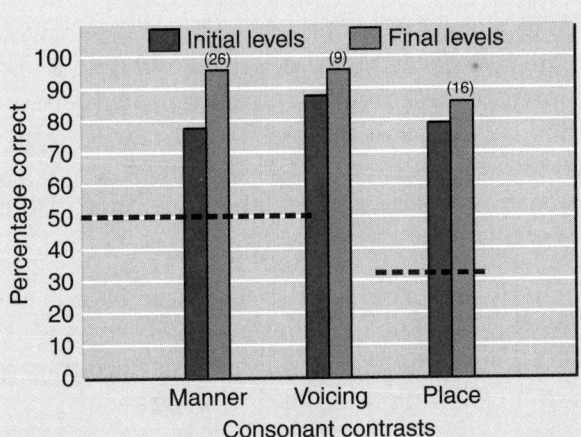

FIGURE 8-8. Drew's scores for percent correct consonant features at the onset and the termination of auditory training intervention for each contrast. (Dashed lines = chance-level performance; numbers in parentheses = number of sessions devoted to the contrast). (Adapted from Ertmer, D. J. Leonard, J. S. and Pachulio, M. L. 2002, Communication intervention for children with cochlear implants: Two case studies. *Language, Speech, and Hearing Services in Schools, 33,* pp. 207.

For synthetic auditory training, an emphasis was placed on comprehension of meaningful speech. Training tasks included repeating and completing sentences and answering questions about spoken material, which allowed Drew to utilize contextual and syntactic cues.

SYNTHETIC AUDITORY TRAINING PROCEDURES

In an auditory training program for Drew, one of their students, Ertmer, Leonard, and Pachuilo (2002) implemented the four procedures described next:

> Picture [vocabulary] books . . . were particularly useful during the first months after implantation because they contained abundant vocabulary words for everyday situations and allowed auditory training to be game-like. For example, after reviewing the vocabulary words on a given page, . . . Drew and the clinician took turns making up sentences such

(continues)

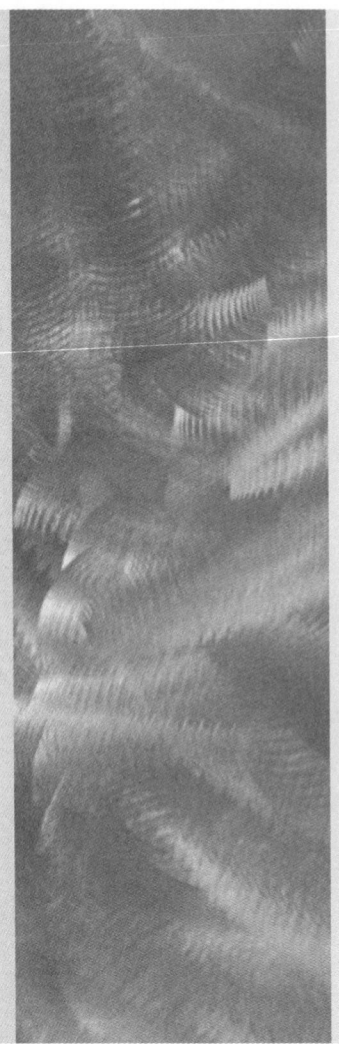

as, "I see a red hat on the table." The listener would then find the corresponding picture. At first, a short, simple sentence format was used repeatedly (e.g., "I see X." or "Can you find X?"). As Drew's auditory, syntactic, and semantic skills improved, more complex and varied sentences were introduced.

Conversations about selected topics (e.g., basketball, vacation plans, school) also provided practice in auditory comprehension. . . . A topic was selected and then discussed for a few minutes. Drew was encouraged to guess if he did not understand what was said.

A [continuous discourse] tracking procedure . . . was used with high-interest stories to improve sentence comprehension and syntax skills. During this activity, Drew was asked to repeat sentences exactly as they were read to him. He was also encouraged to ask for repetitions and clarifications. This task was often difficult when Drew was unfamiliar with the story. He was most successful when the page had been read with the clinician before the sentence repetition task.

Riddles and jokes provided challenging material for synthetic auditory training during the second year of intervention. The clinician would read a riddle or joke and then Drew would repeat what he heard before guessing the answer. (p. 208)

CASE STUDY 2

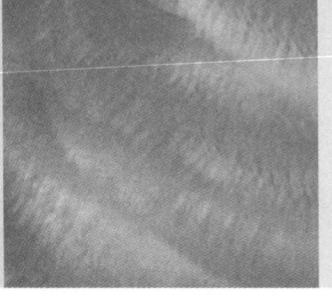

A Child with Prelingual Onset of Deafness

Bobby lost his hearing when he was 5 months of age, after a bout of spinal meningitis. He received a cochlear implant at the age of 3 years, and in the interim received approximately a year of family-centered speech and language intervention. Those around him used manual sign language to communicate with him, and he mainly expressed himself through gesturing and pointing. He wore a hearing aid for only a few weeks following his illness. He was described as shy and reluctant to try new tasks.

At the onset of intervention (which did not start until about a year following implantation), Bobby demonstrated some sound awareness. For example, he alerted to the ring of the telephone and the sound of water running. However, he did not respond to sound in a meaningful way and he did not respond to his spoken name.

The initial auditory training goals were designed to teach Bobby to identify nonspeech sounds, such as a drumbeat or a bell ring. Training with speech stimuli began with asking Bobby to identify words that differed in syllable number and to recognize frequently occurring words, including his name, the clinician's name, and the names of familiar toys. He worked on recognizing familiar phrases, such as *Sit down*.

During the analytic segments of training, Bobby initially could not perform a two-choice listening task. The clinician used praise, encouragement and reinforcers (e.g., puzzle pieces) to maintain Bobby's attention and to motivate him. When he misidentified items, the clinician presented the items audiovisually and then presented an auditory-only model again to reinforce contrasts between phonemes.

Word pairs that differed in number of syllables (e.g., *orange* vs. *strawberry*) were first presented and practiced for about 10 to 15 of the 22 intervention sessions. By the end of the intervention, he identified syllables differing by number of syllables with about a 75–81% accuracy. Once this milestone was achieved, Bobby began to focus on discriminating between phonemically dissimilar words that have the same number of syllables (e.g., *car* vs. *sheep*).

His auditory training program also focused on enhancing auditory comprehension in meaningful contexts. His synthetic training activities included practice in recognizing

(continues)

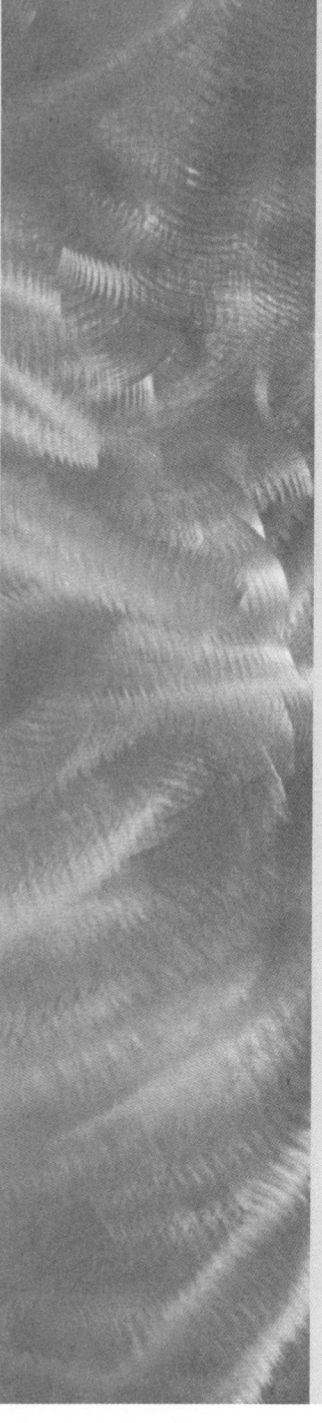

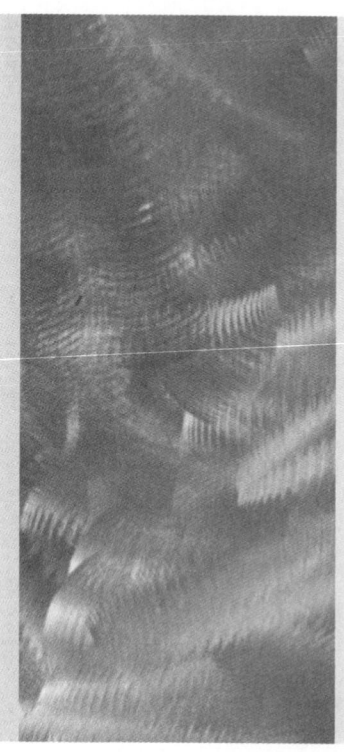

names, phrases, and statements and questions. He listened to simple books, where the clinician and his mother took turns reading pages. The readings were recorded, and Bobby took home the audiocassette for home practice.

After 2 years of experience with his cochlear implant, Bobby was just beginning to discriminate between gross acoustic patterns consistently. He demonstrated improved awareness of speech and environmental sounds, but he still had only emerging abilities in associating speech with meaning.

Comments About the Case Studies

Drew and Bobby present different challenges for auditory training intervention. Whereas with a child like Drew, you will be hard-pressed to keep up with his rapidly emerging listening skills, a child like Bobby will progress slowly and may require you to develop novel ways of motivating and keeping him interested in intervention.

■ FINAL REMARKS

When individuals have hearing loss, listening skills often do not emerge spontaneously. Deliberate and systematic auditory training is required to foster listening potential. We have considered basic principles of auditory training in this chapter. Other resources for training curricula and activities appear in the Key Resources section.

Auditory training need not be confined to speech and environmental stimuli. Some individuals with hearing loss may desire instruction that will enhance their recognition and appreciation of music. For instance, adult cochlear implant users who enjoyed music before losing their hearing often wish to begin listening again once they have received their implants. Work is currently under-way in some cochlear implant programs to develop music training programs and to evaluate the efficacy of this kind of program for enhancing music enjoyment (Gfeller and Witt, 1999).

KEY CHAPTER POINTS

✔ Usually, children with significant hearing losses receive auditory training. Adults are less likely to receive training.

✔ Most auditory training curricula are designed to progress a student from one auditory skill level to the next. The four skill levels underlying most programs are sound awareness, sound discrimination, identification, and comprehension.

✔ Many auditory training curricula include both analytic and synthetic kinds of training activities, and formal and informal activities.

✔ Difficulty of training can be adjusted by varying the size of the stimuli set used for listening tasks, the stimulus unit, stimulus similarity, context, structure, and the listening environment. As a general rule of thumb, you will want to alter the level of difficulty if a person response correctly to training stimuli 80% of the time or more, or responds correctly to less than 50%.

✔ A hierarchy of specific training objectives typically is developed at the onset of a patient's auditory training program. The objectives are targeted with both analytic and synthetic training.

✔ Analytic vowel auditory training objectives are designed to contrast vowels with different vowel formants. Consonant auditory training objectives are designed to contrast features of articulation, such as place, voice, and manner.

✔ Brain activity appears to change as a result of auditory learning.

✔ Students may vary widely in how quickly they progress, in part as a function of their hearing history, their personalities, and their listening environments.

▬ MULTIPLE CHOICE QUESTIONS

1. Which modification would make an auditory training activity more difficult?
   a. Switching from an open response set to a limited response set
   b. Switching from a spontaneous activity to a highly structured activity

c. Contrasting words beginning with /m/ and /n/ rather than words beginning with /d/ and /sh/

d. Asking a child to determine whether two phrases are the same or different rather than asking the child to answer questions presented auditorally

2. Janice is a 20-year-old female who lost her hearing a year ago after head trauma experienced during a car accident. She received a cochlear implant 6 months after the accident. She is now seeking auditory training. The highest level of auditory skill she will demonstrate at this point in time is most likely to be:

a. Identification

b. Awareness

c. Discrimination

d. Recognition

3. Saundra dropped the lid to a pan onto the tile kitchen floor. Her daughter, playing in the room next to the kitchen, turned her head. The daughter's response is best described as:

a. Sound awareness

b. Sound identification

c. Sound discrimination

d. Analytic listening

4. An activity where a student is asked to discriminate word pairs is best described as:

a. Introductory

b. Analytic training

c. Synthetic training

d. Phonemic training

5. You can decrease the level of training difficulty in an auditory training intervention session:

a. By increasing the signal-to-noise ratio

b. By decreasing the task structure

c. By increasing stimulus similarity

d. By changing the number of items in the stimulus set

6. Which of the following tasks is likely to be included later rather than earlier in an auditory training intervention?
   a. Discriminating vowels that differ in first formant information
   b. Discriminating vowels that differ in second formant information
   c. Discriminating monosyllables from bisyllables
   d. Discriminating vowels with similar first and second formant information

7. The consonant feature that is typically most difficult for persons with hearing loss to hear is:
   a. Manner of articulation
   b. Place of articulation
   c. Voicing
   d. Nasality

8. The activity that a beginning student most likely will perform early on in auditory training is the following:
   a. Discriminate nasal versus nonnasal unvoiced consonants
   b. Discriminate unvoiced fricatives from unvoiced stops that differ in place
   c. Identify words in which the consonants are all either voiced or unvoiced, from a four-item response set
   d. Discriminate words varying in place of production

9. Ms. Hoffman has prepared a reinforcement for her 5-year-old student. Every time little Jean recognizes a word correctly, she will get to make an animal out of clay. This activity is:
   a. Not an optimal reinforcement activity because it is not age-appropriate
   b. Not an optimal reinforcement activity because it is too time consuming
   c. An optimal reinforcement activity because it is challenging
   d. An optimal reinforcement activity because it takes no advanced preparation on Ms. Hoffman's part

KEY RESOURCES

Auditory Training Curricula

The Developmental Approach to Successful Listening II (DASL), 2nd Edition

Authors: G. G. Stout and J. V. Ert Windle

Available from:
Resource Point, Inc.
61 Inverness Drive East, Suite 100
Englewood, CO 80112

CHATS: The Miami Cochlear Implant Auditory and Tactile Skills Curriculum

Editors: K. C. Vergara and L. W. Miskiel

Available from:
Intelligent Hearing Systems
10689 North Kendall Drive
Miami, FL 33176

Auditory Enhancement Guide

Authors: Personnel of the Clarke School for the Deaf

Available from:
Clarke School for the Deaf
Center for Oral Education
47 Round Hill Road
Northampton, MA 01060-2199

Communication Training for Hearing-Impaired Children and Teenagers: Speechreading, Listening and Using Repair Strategies

Author: N. Tye-Murray

Available from:
PRO-ED
8700 Shoal Creek Boulevard
Austin, TX 78758-6897

Cochlear Implant Auditory Training Guidebook

Author: D. Sindrey

Available from:
A. G. Bell Association for the Deaf and Hard-of-Hearing
3417 Volta Place NW
Washington, DC 20007-2778

Listening Games for Littles

Author: D. Sindrey

Available from
B. G. Bell Association for the Deaf and Hard-of-Hearing
3417 Volta Place NW
Washington, DC 20007-2778

Ski-HI Model: A Resource Manual for Family-Centered Home-Based Programming for Infants, Toddlers, and Preschool-Aged Children with Hearing Impairments

Authors: S. Watkins and T. Clark

Available from:
Hope Publishing Inc.
1856 North 1200 East
North Logan, UT 84321

Conversation Made Easy

Author: Nancy Tye-Murray

Available from:
Central Institute for the Deaf
4560 Clayton Ave.
St. Louis, MO 63110

Bringing Sound to Live: Principles and Practices of Cochlear Implant Rehabilitation.

Authors: M. Koch

Available from:
York Press
P.O. Box 504
Timonium, MD 21094

Speech Perception Instructional Curriculum and Evaluation

Authors: J. Moog, J. Biedenstein, and L. Davidson

Available from:
Central Institute for the Deaf
4560 Clayton Ave.
St. Louis, MO 63110

Communication Training for Hard-of-Hearing Adults and Older Teenagers: Speechreading, Listening, and Using Repair Strategies, 1997.

Author: N. Tye-Murray

Available from:
PRO-ED
8700 Shoal Creek Boulevard
Austin, TX 78758-6897

Guide for Optimizing Auditory Learning Skills (GOALS), 1996.

Authors: J. Firszt and R. Reeder

Available from:
Alexander Graham Bell Association for the Deaf and Hard of Hearing
3417 Volta Place, N.W.
Washington, DC 20007

APPENDIX 8-A

Words That Can Be Illustrated and Used for Vowel Auditory Training Exercises

/u/	/ʊ/	/i/
soup goose	book hood	beak geese
boot tool	hook wood	wheat feet
food moon	foot pull	beat peel
suit pool	full shook	seat sheet
shoe fool	bull cook	bean meat

/ɪ/	/ɛ/	/æ/
bit men	net head	bat fat
sit mitt	bell men	bag gas
lid pill	wet red	man hat
pin kick	bed pet	mat pan

/ʌ/	/a/	/ɚ/
gun up	shot doll	bird turn
pup one	top sock	shirt girl
cut bun	rock knot	burn curve
run gun	hot hop	pearl purse

/e/	/o/	/s/
rake cake	bow coat	shawl lawn
eight rain	note bone	long fawn
lake cave	pole boat	dawn ball
tape bait	hose goat	walk chalk

APPENDIX 8-B

Words That Can Be Illustrated and Used For Consonant Auditory Training Exercises

/p/	/b/	/t/
pan pea	bee boot	tea tool
peach pick	ball bell	top team
pool pill	bat boat	tooth top
pop pin	beet bed	tack toad

/d/	/k/	/g/
dog dock	K can	gas gum
dad dough	cop cap	goose game
dot ditch	cook keys	geese girl
doll D	cat cob	gun goat

/tç/	/dʒ/	/f/
church cheer	jar J	fat fall
chair chew	jump jack	foot feet
chick chain	jeep jeans	fan fox
chin cheek	jet juice	fish face

/v/	/ζ/	/l/
vase vault	thumb three	leg lamp
van vane	thigh thick	loop leaf
veil vest	thin thorn	lamb light
vine valve	thread thief	lock lime

/h/	/s/	/s/
hot hay	seat sail	sheep shorts
hit house	suit sock	shoes shirt
ham hip	sack sew	sheet shack
heel hand	seed soup	shell ship

/m/

mouse   moon

men   mat

man   mice

mail   match

/r/

red   rice

rain   rose

rake   wrap

run   rock

/n/

nail   net

knot   nap

knees   neck

kneel   nose

/w/

wet   web

wig   witch

wave   wire

wine   wood

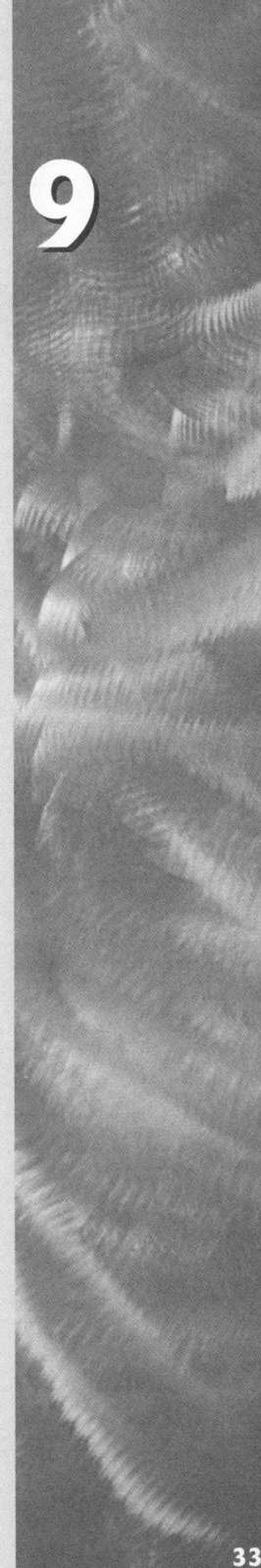

CHAPTER 9

Speechreading

TOPICS

Lipreading is the process of recognizing speech using only the visual speech signal and other visual cues, such as facial expression.

Speechreading is speech recognition using both auditory and visual cues.

Before we consider speechreading training, which we will do in the next chapter, it is important to review the general topics of lipreading and speechreading. The two terms often are used interchangeably. In our discussion, we follow the conventions of Thorn and Thorn (1989), Walden, Prosek, Montgomery, Scherr, and Jones (1977), and Lansing and Helgeson (1995). When *lipreading,* a person relies only on the visual signal provided by the talker's face for recognizing speech (Thorn & Thorn, 1989). When *speechreading,* the person attends to both the talker's auditory and visual signals, as well as the talker's facial expressions and gestures, and any other available cues. These clues include the setting in which the conversation is occurring or what has been discussed beforehand (Walden et al., 1977).

■ SPEECHREADING FOR COMMUNICATION

Persons with normal hearing routinely rely on speechreading. Consider these examples: When we are at a noisy restaurant, we understand more if we watch the talker's face while we listen. We may feel unsettled when we view dubbed foreign films, because the words we hear do not match those we see. A raised eyebrow imparts additional meaning to the question, "You're not working today?" A number of experimental paradigms have been developed that demonstrate that even if you have normal hearing, you rely on visual speech information to recognize and comprehend a message. If someone reads aloud Kant's *Critique of Pure Reason,* which is difficult-to-grasp philosophy, you will better understand the content if you see and hear the reader than if you only hear the person's voice (Arnold & Hill, 2001; Reisberg, McLean, & Goldfield, 1987). If you "shadow" someone who is reading a passage, that is, attempt to repeat each word the reader speaks as quickly as you can, you will do so at a faster rate if you see and hear the reader than if you are only listening (Reisberg et al., 1987). Evidence that visual information is used routinely for speech recognition also comes from studies employing functional magnetic resonance imaging (fMRI), a noninvasive means of mapping brain activity. When you try to recognize speech using the visual signal only, the auditory cortex (i.e., the superior temporo-parietal area) becomes activated. Activation will not occur if you simply watch a face make rhythmic movements of the jaw and mouth without opening the lips (see Campbell, 1998, for a review). Even infants engage in speechreading. If a 5-month-old baby hears someone phonate "eeeeeee," and simultaneously views a side-by-side projection of the same talker, on one side saying "eeeeeeee" and the other side saying "aaahhhh," the baby most likely will fixate on the visual signal that corresponds to the acoustic signal (Kuhl & Meltzoff, 1982).

A person with hearing loss will depend more on the visual signal for speech recognition than will individuals who have normal hearing. Whereas most persons can converse on the telephone with ease, or follow a news broadcast on the radio, a person with hearing loss will experience decreased speech recognition when only the auditory signal is presented. The greater the hearing impairment, the more an individual will rely on visual information for communication.

■ CHARACTERISTICS OF A GOOD LIPREADER

An audiologist arrives at the office on Monday morning and finds two persons waiting in the clinic area, Dr. Kevin Evans and Mr. Peter Climpton. The audiologist reads their charts and learns that Dr. Evans is a 42-year-old pharmaceutical executive who holds a doctorate degree in organic chemistry. He has had a moderate bilateral hearing impairment since the age of 16 years. Mr. Climpton is a 17-year-old male who has always had normal hearing. He recently applied for a position to work on an assembly line in a noisy factory and is required to undergo a comprehensive audiological workup. With only this information, can the audiologist accurately predict which individual will perform better on tests on lipreading?

The answer to this question is *no*. A plethora of research has revealed it is difficult to predict lipreading performance. Performance cannot be predicted by an individual's intelligence, educational achievement, duration of deafness (and hence, practice with the lipreading and speechreading tasks), age at hearing-loss onset, nor socioeconomic status. As such, Dr. Evans is as likely to be a better or poorer lipreader than Mr. Climpton, as vice versa. Even with additional information about their verbal abilities, cognitive skills such as visual memory, and personality, the audiologist could not make an infallible prediction (see Summerfield, 1989, for a review), although some research suggests that particular cognitive skills might correlate with lipreading. These skills include visual word decoding, lexical identification speed (e.g., how quickly you can determine whether a string of letters constitutes a word), phonological processing (e.g., how quickly you can decide whether two words rhyme), and verbal inference-making (e.g., how well you can complete sentences that have missing words) (Andersson, Lyxell, Rönnberg, & Spens, 2001).

A handful of other variables may be somewhat predictive. Some data suggest that women may lipread better than men, on average (Dancer, Krain, Thompson, Davis, & Gentry, 1994), although recent work suggests otherwise. As shown in Figure 9-1 (Tye-Murray, Sommers, & Spehar, submitted), women and men perform about the same on tests that present consonant, word, and sentence stimuli. This study included both young adults and individuals over the age of 65.

Young adults lipread better than elderly adults (Farrimond, 1959; Honnell, Dancer, & Gentry, 1991). Figure 9-2 shows the difference between how well young and old adults lipread consonants, words, and sentences. These individuals have normal hearing and no visual impairment. As the figure suggests, the younger adults can lipread all three types of speech stimuli better than the older adults. There is some evidence that age yields influence on lipreading performance on the other end of the lifespan as well. Younger children do not recognize some phonological contrasts as well as older children (Hnath-Chisolm, Laipply, & Boothroyd,

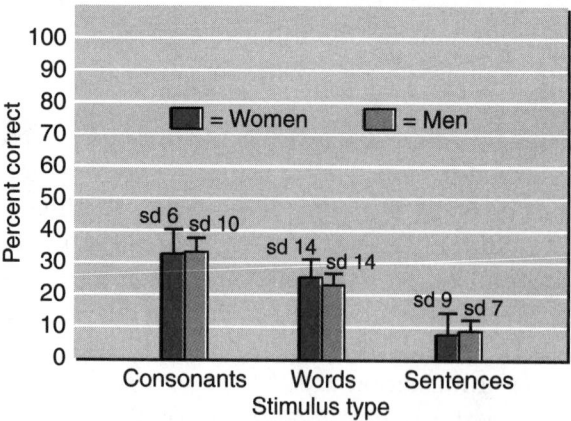

FIGURE 9-1. Results from a lipreading test comparing gender performance (32 men, 68 women).

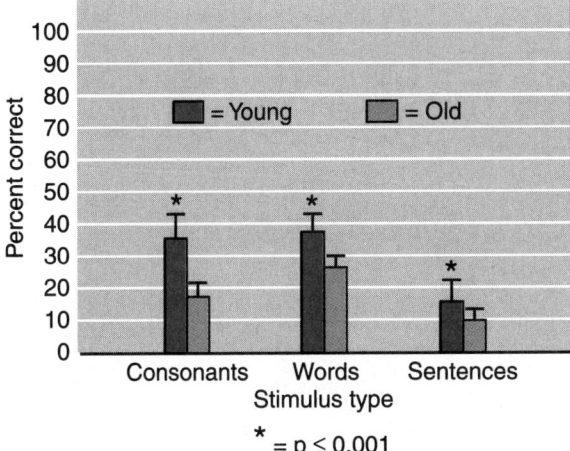

FIGURE 9-2. Percent correct scores for a group of 45 young lipreads (ages 18–24 years) and a group of 45 older lipreaders (ages 65 years and older) (Adapted from Sommers, Tye-Murray, and Spehar, 2002.)

1998; Kishon-Rabin & Henkin, 2000). For instance, children between the ages of 5 and 7 years appear not to recognize the place of production of final consonants as well as children between the ages of 9 and 11 years do.

There is also some evidence, albeit conflicting, that neurophysiological measures relate to performance. The latencies of recorded electrical potentials made at the cortex following stimulation of the eye by a flash of light may correlate with lipreading performance (Shepherd, 1982; Shepherd, DeLavergne, Frueh, & Colbridge, 1977; but see Samar & Sims, 1983; Summerfield, 1992), with shorter latencies being characteristic of good lipreaders. Shorter latencies indicate more rapid transmission of neural impulses from the eye to the brain and are unlikely to be affected by an individual's experiences, personality, or circumstances.

Some speech and hearing professionals have cited more nebulous characteristics that may relate to lipreading performance, including individuals' ability to capitalize on contextual cues, their willingness to guess, their mental agility, and their willingness to revise interpretations of a partially recognized message (e.g., Jeffers & Barley, 1971). Especially in children, linguistic and world knowledge can constrain proficiency. Someone who has a limited vocabulary, limited knowledge of grammar, and limited world knowledge will likely experience lipreading difficulties. For instance, if a child has a limited knowledge of geography, the child will not readily recover the word missed when lipreading the sentence, "_____ *is the capital of the United States.*"

Predicting Lipreading Performance

People vary widely in their lipreading performance. Some individuals can score 80% words correct or better on a vision-only test condition, as measured by verbatim repetition of test words, whereas others score 5% or worse on the same stimuli (Bernstein, Demorest, Coulter, & O'Connell, 1991). The amount of practice in lipreading does not account for variability. Some college students who have normal hearing and who have never received lipreading training perform better on a sentence recognition test presented in a vision-only condition than adults who have an acquired hearing loss, and who have been deaf (and hence, speechreading for communicative purposes) for many years (Hanin, 1988).

■ WHAT HAPPENS WHEN YOU LIPREAD?

A talker's face presents salient cues for recognizing the sounds of speech and the prosodic patterns of sentences. For instance, when a talker speaks the sound /m/, the lips press together. When the talker makes the /u/ sound, the lips pucker slightly. The eyebrows rise when the talker asks an incredulous question (e.g., *You did what?*). When you lipread, your eyes scan the talker's face, seeking both phonetic and prosodic cues as to what is being said. Eyes may stabilize, for an eye fixation, or rotate in quick, high-velocity shifts.

Researchers have studied eye movement behavior during lipreading using equipment that tracks the center of the pupil. In one study, it was found that lipreaders monitor different regions of the face, according to the kind of information they seek (Lansing & McConkie, 1999). Subjects were asked to discriminate either phonetic contrasts, (e.g., *Ron ran,* vs. *We won*) or to discriminate between questions and statements (e.g., *Ron ran?* vs. *Ron ran.*). In general, subjects tended to direct their eye gaze toward the talker's eyes, nose, and mouth, with occasion shifts to the regions of the forehead, cheeks, and chin. When seeking prosodic information about questions versus statements, they focused more on the upper face (most likely monitoring events such as forehead wrinkling, eyebrows raising, and eye widening), and when making phonetic judgments, they focused more on the lower face, monitoring lip and jaw movement. Eye gaze tended to shift to the talker's eyes at the end of an utterance, regardless of what the subjects' lipreading task happened to be.

■ THE DIFFICULTY OF THE LIPREADING TASK

If someone were to talk to you through a closed window, so you could see but not hear the person, you might recognize less than 20% of the words. (Look back at figure 9-2 and examine the percent correct scores for words in a sentence context.) Why is lipreading so difficult? The answer to this question relates to the variables listed in Table 9-1. In this section we consider five variables that compound the difficulty of the lipreading task: visibility of sounds, rapidity of speech, coarticulation and stress effects, visemes and homophenes, and talker effects.

Table 9-1. Factors that influence the difficulty of the lipreading task.

FACTOR	EFFECT
Visibility of sounds	Many sounds are not associated with visible mouth movement.
Rapidity of speech	Often, sounds occur in sequence faster than the eye can resolve them.
Coarticulation and stress effects	The appearance of words vary as a function of how they are spoken.
Visemes and homophenes	Many sounds and words appear alike on the face.
Talker effects	Talkers speak sounds and words with different mouth movements.

Visibility of Sounds

The first variable that affects the difficulty of the lipreading task that we shall consider is the visibility of sounds. Many sounds entail minimal visible mouth movement. Woodward and Barber (1960) estimated that 60% of speech sounds are not visible on the mouth or cannot be seen readily.

Words that are more visible on the face tend to begin with consonants that are made with bilabial closure (/p, b, m, w/), the lower teeth pressing the upper lip (/f, v/), or the tongue tip contacting the upper teeth (/θ/). Consonants with limited visibility include sounds that are produced within the mouth, such as /k, g, t, n/. Some features of phonemes are simply not visible at all. For instance, there is no visible evidence indicating that a phoneme is either voiced (e.g., /b, d, g/) or unvoiced (e.g., /p, t, k/). Figure 9-3 presents the consonants (excluding /h/) according to the activity of the lips and tongue. Those consonants that have lips closing during production tend to be more distinctive than those that do not; the consonants that are produced with tongue activity toward the front of the mouth tend to be more distinctive than those produced at the back of the mouth.

Vowels are considered not to be highly visible. They may or may not be distinguished by lip spreading (e.g., *beak* vs. *book*, where

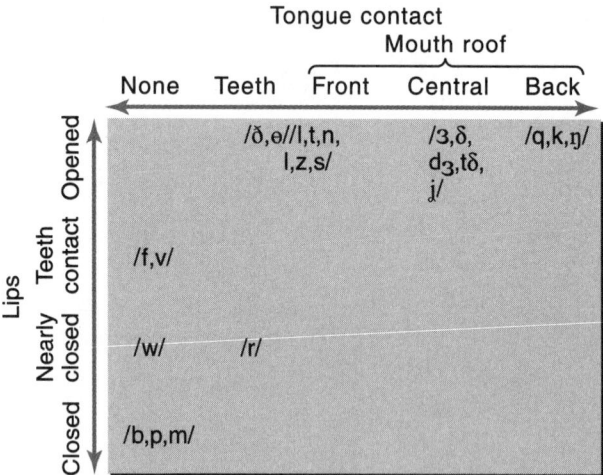

FIGURE 9-3. Consonant production as a function of tongue and lip activity.

/i/ involves more lip spreading than /ʊ/), tongue and jaw height (e.g., *bit* vs. *bought*, where /I/ is associated with greater tongue and jaw height than /ɔ/), and lip rounding (*boot* vs. *bet*, where /u/ is associated with more lip rounding than /ɜ/) (see Figure 9-3). Fortunately, even though vowels are not associated with distinctive mouth movements, they tend to be acoustically salient to individuals who have hearing loss. Vowels are relatively intense, change slowly over time in their frequency composition, and are relatively long in duration (see Figure 9-4).

Rapidity of Speech

The second factor that contributes to the difficulty of the lipreading task is the rapidity with which words are spoken. When speaking conversationally, a talker may speak anywhere from 150 to 250 words per minute, or roughly 4–7 syllables per second, excluding time spent pausing. Whereas a typical talker may produce an average of 15 phonemes per second, the human eye may be capable of registering only about 9 or 10 discrete mouth movements in this time interval. Thus, the lipreader (speechreader) has little time to ponder the identity of a particular word and even may not realize the occurrence of every word.

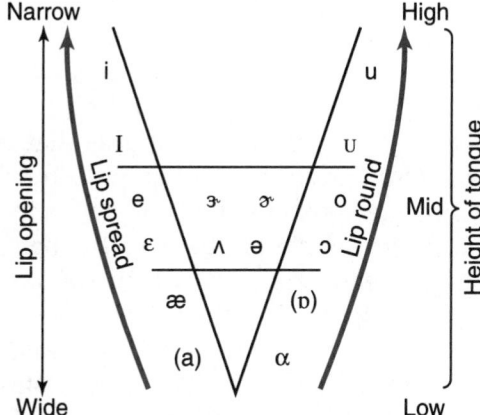

FIGURE 9-4. Vowel production as a function of lip opening, lip spreading, and tongue height. (Adapted from Berger, K. W. 1972, *Speechreading: Principles and Methods.* Baltimore, MD: National Education Press.)

Coarticulation and Stress Effects

The third factor that contributes to the difficulty of the lipreading task is coarticulation and stress effects, which may result in the same sound looking different depending on its phonetic and linguistic context. For example, the sound /b/ looks different in the word *boot* versus *beet*. The lips begin to round in anticipation of the following /u/ in the first case; the lips begin to spread in anticipation of the following /i/ in the second case. If an alveolar consonant follows a rounded vowel such as /u/ in the word *hoot,* the lip rounding may hide the tongue and the teeth.

Stress can also affect the appearance of a word. The word *you* looks different in the following question, depending on the talker's stress pattern:

> *What did ya do yesterday?*
>
> *What did YOU do yesterday?*

Visemes and Homophenes

After being introduced to a visiting professor, an academician launched into a lively discussion of current topics in theology. Only after several minutes had elapsed, with just lukewarm interest expressed by the visiting professor, did the academician realize that his hostess had introduced him to a *geologist,* not a *theologist.*

Visemes are groups of speech sounds that appear identical on the lips (e.g., /p, m, b/).

The fact that sounds belong to viseme groups and many words are homophenous increases lipreading and speechreading difficulty. ***Visemes*** are groups of speech sounds that look alike on the face (Fisher, 1968). The sounds /b, m, p/ comprise a viseme. When these sounds are spoken without voice, as in *bat, mat,* and *pat,* they are indistinguishable on the mouth. There is some disagreement among researchers as to which sounds constitute a viseme, although all agree that there are fewer visemes than phonemes (e.g., Binnie, Montgomery, & Jackson, 1974; Erber, 1974; Lesner, Sandridge, & Kricos, 1987). Two listings of consonants grouped as visemes as compiled by two different sources appear in Table 9-2.

Homophenes are words that look identical on the mouth.

Homophenes are words that look the same on the mouth. In the previous example, *theology* looked like *geology* to the academician who was talking to the visiting professor. It is not always intu-

Table 9-2. Consonants grouped as sets of visemes. Reports from two different research groups.

ERBER (1974)	LESNER, SANDRIDGE, AND KRICOS (1987)
/p, b, m/	/p, b, m/
/f, v/	/f, v/
/θ, ð/	/θ, ð/
/ð, ʒ/	/ð , ʒ, dʒ, tʃ/
/w, r/	/w, r/
/l/	/l/
/n, d, t, s, z/	/t, d, s, z, n, k, g, j/
/k, g/	
/h/	

Source: Adapted from Lesner, K., Sandridge, S., and Kricos, P. (1987). Training influences on visual consonant and sentence recognition. *Ear and Hearing, 8,* 283–287; and Erber, N. P. (1974). Visual perception of speech by deaf children: Recent developments and continuing needs. *Journal of Speech and Hearing Disorders, 39,* 178–185.

itively clear which words are homophenous and which words are not. For example, as different as the words *grade* and *yes* sound, they are nonetheless homophenous. When only the visual signal of the talker is presented, you likely cannot discriminate one word from the other. On the other hand, even though the words *boon* and *doom* sound similar, and might be confused with one another if the listening environment is noisy, you will have no problem in distinguishing one from the other if you can see the talker's face.

Table 9-3 presents a list of other homophenous word pairs. If you wanted to sensitize your patient to the existence of homophenous words, you might use these word pairs to perform an exercise like this (Kaplan et al., 1985, p. 100):

- I say, *rise.* The word that is a homophenous to this word is (circle one on your answer sheet):

  a. pies

  b. mine

  c. rice (*correct answer*)

  d. lice

Table 9-3. Examples of homophenous word pairs.

Homophenous Word Pairs (words that look alike on the face)	
Rise	Rice
Perch	Merge
Marry	Bury
Mat	Man
Bind	Mite
Aunt	Hand
Van	Fat
Pass	Ban
Down	Bout

■ I say, *merge.* The word that is homophenous to this word is (circle one on your answer sheet):

   a. lunch

   b. perch (*correct answer*)

   c. worst

   d. burn

Somewhere between 40 and 60% of words in English are homophenous (Berger, 1972). Grammatical sentence cues and other linguistic and situational cues can decrease the confusion about word identity, and some talkers will better distinguish words on the basis of the visual signal than other talkers. Nonetheless, the existence of homophenous words often makes lipreading difficult. Often, the word choices that a lipreader must consider are numerous, as illustrated in the following example. Suppose someone says, "Pat sat by a log." Table 9-4 is a matrix of possible confusions that could be made for each word.

Table 9-4. Confusions Matrix.

PAT	SAT	BY	A	LOG.
mat	sad	my		dog
bat	tanned	pie		sock
bad	sad	buy		dock
pad	dad			lock

The lipreader might come away with any number of meanings after lipreading this simple sentence, including:

- Mat sat by a dog.
- Mat tanned by a dock.
- Mad dad buy a dog.
- Pat sat by a dock.

Talker Effects

Talker effects may confound lipreading efforts because the same sound may look different when spoken by two different people. For instance, two talkers may differ in the degree of mouth opening used for speaking the vowels in the sentence, *"That is Pat's."* A person who has a pronounced accent may appear different when talking than a person who has the same regional accent as the lipreader. For instance, a native of Minnesota may not recognize visually the word, *rice* when it is spoken by a Texan.

Facial Expressions and Situational Cues

The poem below, written by a young man with significant hearing loss, underscores how facial expressions and situational cues can facilitate the speechreading task.

"I looked with longing at her lips,
To scan the words appearing.
I could not make out what she said;
Alas, I have no hearing.

But how I hoped to read those lips,
To know what she was saying;
To guess that enigmatic smile
Around the corners playing.

And as I gazed upon her face
It seemed I saw a pleading.
And then I knew, the words came through;
'Lips are not *just* for reading.'" (Berger, 1972, pp. 61–62)

■ WHAT HAPPENS WHEN YOU SPEECHREAD?

When you speechread, you must integrate what you hear with what you see. For instance, if you hear a burst of air followed by an audible low-pitched sound, and you see the lips press together and then release, you most likely will experience the percept of a /b/ sound. Your brain combines the sounds you hear with the facial movements you see.

How does this integration happen? We don't know, although many research teams have devoted a good deal of effort trying to sort out this issue. One widely explored puzzle is, at what point do we integrate auditory and visual information? Do we process the two signals independently and then combine them, or do we process them interactively? For instance, it may be that visual and auditory information are mapped onto some kind of "phonetic prototype" at the same time, or it may be that vision biases phonetic decisions about the auditory signal before a decision is made about what is being heard. Green (1998) reviews a plethora of data that address how integration proceeds and concludes that much evidence suggests that integration of auditory and visual information occurs before phonetic categorization, although there remain some contrary results to this conclusion (pp. 12–13).

What we do know unequivocally is that what we hear influences what we see, and what we see influences what we hear. Sometimes, the whole is difficult to predict from the parts. One of the most influential experimental paradigms that illustrates this assertion is the "McGurk Effect," so called because it was discovered in an experiment reported by McGurk and MacDonald (1976). McGurk and MacDonald presented discrepant auditory and visual speech stimuli to a group of normal-hearing subjects. The stimuli were consonant-vowel monosyllables. For example, a subject may have heard the syllable *ba* while simultaneously seeing someone speak *da*. For some combinations of consonants, subjects perceived a third consonant that differed from the two syllables. When they heard *ba* and saw *ga,* they typically perceived the syllable *da.* These results suggest that, when we recognize speech, we integrate auditory and visual speech information as we decode the signal and that this integration is obligatory (i.e., we can not help but do it).

IMPORTANCE OF RESIDUAL HEARING

Persons who are most dependent on the visual signal for speech communication are those who have only a minimum of residual hearing. Even a little hearing can be helpful.

Many individuals with a severe or profound hearing loss hear only low-frequency information, even when wearing a hearing aid, and receive information only about changes in voice pitch when they listen to speech. To approximate what this might sound like, clamp your hand over your mouth and recite "Humpty Dumpty Sat on the Wall." The signal you hear as you speak does not provide enough information to allow anyone to recognize your speech in an audition-only condition. However, if someone were to hear this degraded signal and have a clear view of your mouth while you spoke, this information might dramatically improve his or her speechreading performance. An experiment by Rosen, Fourcin, and Moore (1981) demonstrated this phenomenon.

Rosen et al. (1981) asked a test talker to produce a series of nonsense syllables with varying medial consonants, such as /apa/, /ama/, /ada/, and /asa/. A laryngograph was placed on his throat, which reflected vocal fold vibration, and the output was used to develop an auditory signal that reflected the changes over time in the talker's fundamental frequency (voice pitch). When the test subjects (who had normal hearing) saw but did not hear the talker, they identified 44% of the consonants correctly. When they saw the talker speak and heard the concomitant changes in fundamental frequency, their performance improved to 72% consonants correct.

The results of this experiment help to explain why so many people with profound hearing losses are dependent on their hearing aids for successful communication. Even though they receive minimal auditory information, their ability to speechread is enhanced greatly by the amplified signal.

FACTORS THAT AFFECT THE SPEECHREADING PROCESS

How well someone speechreads in a particular situation is influenced by at least four factors. As Table 9-5 indicates, these factors

Table 9-5. Factors that influence the speechreading task.

TALKER	MESSAGE	ENVIRONMENT	SPEECHREADER
Facial expressions	Length	Viewing angle	Lipreading skill
Diction	Syntactic complexity	Distance	Residual hearing
Body language	Frequency of word usage	Background noise	Use of appropriate amplification
Speech rate	Shared homophenes	Room acoustics	Stress profile
Familiarity to the speechreader	Context	Distractions	Attentiveness
Accent			Fatigue
Facial characteristics			Motivation to understand
Speech prosody (intonation, stress, and rhythm)			Language skills
Objects in or over the mouth			

are the talker, the message, the speechreading environment and communication situation, and the speechreader.

The Talker

The talker can increase or decrease the difficulty of the speechreading task (Table 9-6). For instance, many audiologists and speech-language pathologists have learned to speak with clearly articulated speech and ample, albeit not exaggerated, mouth movements. Their professional training and experience has taught them to face a person with hearing loss head-on when speaking, and to speak with supporting facial expressions and hand gestures. Patients sometimes complain to their clinician, "I can speechread you just fine. It's when I get out in the real world, talking to people that I don't know, and who don't move their lips, that I get into trouble with my speech understanding."

The talker's behaviors, familiarity to the patient, and gender may all affect speechreading performance.

Table 9-6. Speaking behaviors that impede the speechreading task. This list was generated during a group discussion with adults who are hard-of-hearing.

I have a difficult time speechreading when the talker:

- mumbles
- doesn't look at me when talking
- chews gum
- has an unusual accent
- has a speech impediment
- smiles too much
- moves around while talking
- uses no facial expressions
- shouts
- has a high pitched voice
- talks too fast
- uses long, complicated sentences and obscure vocabulary words
- has a beard and/or mustache
- wears dark glasses

TALKER BEHAVIORS

A talker who uses appropriate but not exaggerated facial expressions, who speaks with clear and not mumbled speech, and who uses body language is relatively easy to speechread. The following behaviors make a talker difficult to speechread:

- Shouting
- Mumbling
- Turning away
- Speaking rapidly
- Covering the mouth with a hand
- Smiling simultaneously while talking

FAMILIARITY

Hard-of-hearing persons will have an easier time recognizing the speech of someone who is familiar, such as a family member, than someone who is unfamiliar, because they are accustomed to the talker's mouth movements and speech patterns. There is some evidence that thin lips are easier to speechread than thick or immobile lips and that a foreign accent increases difficulty (Berger, 1972).

GENDER

Talker gender influences the difficulty of the task. Females are easier to lipread than males (Daly, Bench, & Chappell, 1996). However, even though females' speech may be more recognizable when it is presented in a vision-only condition, it may not necessarily be easier to recognize in an audition-plus-vision condition, as the higher fundamental frequency of the female voice is harder for most hard-of-hearing persons to hear than the lower fundamental frequencies associated with male voices. For male talkers, the presence of facial hair, as with a mustache or beard, can impede speechreading by obscuring lip and jaw movement.

How Something Is Said Will Affect How One Speechreads It

Try this experiment. Say to a friend, without using your voice, "Oh my aching back." As you speak, use minimal facial expression and body movements. Ask your friend to guess what you have said. Chances are, the guess will be incorrect. Now mouth the phrase again, but this time, assume a pained expression and rub your back with your hand. The odds are high that the friend will quickly recognize your utterance this second time around. This experiment reveals an important principle in speechreading: *Context cues can dramatically affect an individual's ability to speechread.*

The Message

The second factor that can influence speechreading performance is the message that a talker presents. The structure and the component words affect recognition. For example, if you were to say, "The elephant is big," a person with hearing loss would likely recognize what you said, especially if you were standing in a zoo next to an elephant cage when you said it. The word *elephant* is highly visible on the face, and has few words that look similar to it. The sentence is short and syntactically simple, and the adjective, *big*, begins with the highly visible phoneme, /b/. The setting of the zoo certainly provides situational clues for understanding the sentence. On the other hand, if out of the blue, you were to say, "The hen sat on the cart," most persons with hearing loss would be at a loss. The component words do not entail many highly visible mouth movements. For example, production of the /h/ in *hen* is invisible, and the tongue humping associated with production of /k/ in *cart* cannot be seen. The words are also one-syllabic, and most have other words that look similar on the face and are acoustically similar. For instance, words that look like and sound like the word *cart* include, among others, *kit, heart, cot,* and *hot*. The message's structure, frequency of use of the component words, the number of similar looking words, and the supporting context all affect speechreading performance.

STRUCTURE

Some messages are easier to speechread than others, depending on their length, syntactic complexity, frequency of use, similarity to other words, and linguistic context. As a general rule, the longer the sentence and the greater its syntactic complexity, the more difficult it will be to speechread. Words that have two syllables tend to be easier to recognize than monosyllables spoken in isolation.

FREQUENCY OF USAGE

Commonplace words, such as the word *sweater*, have a higher probability of being recognized than words that are used less frequently, such as the word *cardigan*. We say that the word *sweater* has a greater ***frequency of usage*** than *cardigan*, because it is more likely to be spoken in everyday conversation.

Frequency of usage is a measure indicating how often a particular word occurs during everyday conversation.

NEIGHBORHOODS

Words that have fewer response possibilities are also easier to recognize. For example, the word *bat* may be difficult to recognize, even though it begins with a highly visible mouth movement, because many other words are similar both visually (e.g., *bad, bet, mat, met, pat*) and acoustically (e.g., *cap, cat, scat, bad*). On the other hand, the word *telephone* is easier to recognize, even though it is less commonplace than the word *bat*, because not many words look or sound similar to *telephone*. We say that

Lexical neighbors are words that are phonemically (or visually) similar.

lexically easy-to-recognize words have few *lexical neighbors,* or few words that are phonemically (or visually) similar, whereas lexically difficult-to-recognize words have many neighbors (Greenburg & Jenkins, 1964; Kirk, Pisoni, & Osberger,1995).

CONTEXT

Words that are specified by context typically are easiest to recognize. For example, the word *table* is harder to identify when embedded in the sentence *Candace will buy the* _____, than in the sentence, *Candace will set the* _____ *and chairs in the kitchen.* Context cues provide cues for a word missed. Although *table* and *sable* are homophenes, and are acoustically similar, you probably would not mistake one word for the other because *table* makes more sense in this second sentence context. Grammatical structure also provides contextual cues. For instance, in the sentence, *The* _____ *read the book,* grammatical sentence structure specifies that the missing word is a common noun.

Topical Cues Can Help

Simply knowing the topic of conversation can enhance a speechreader's performance. For example, if you allow someone to read the word *homes* before asking the person to speechread the sentence, *She just moved into a three-bedroom apartment,* the person will speechread more words correctly than if no topical word is presented beforehand (Hanin, 1988). The sentence, *I cut my finger with a knife,* will be easier to speechread if it is preceded with a related sentence such as, *I was careless with a sharp blade,* than if it is preceded by an unrelated sentence such as, *You need special watering tools* (Gagné, Tugby, & Michaud, 1991).

The Speechreading Environment and Communication Situation

The third factor that can affect speechreading performance is the environment. Patients often avoid social situations because they cannot hear in certain environments. "I hate parties," a patient may complain. "The lighting is always dim and the music is too loud."

Another may say, "I bought a round dining table. With our old rectangular one, I could never read anyone's lips."

The viewing angle, the distance from the talker, room conditions, and the presence or absence of background noise may all affect how well patients speechread in any given environment or communication situation.

VIEWING ANGLE

If the speechreader sees the talker full-face, rather than in profile or turned at an angle, the speechreader will recognize more words (Figure 9-5). If a conversation is occurring in a group setting, as in a conference held around a rectangular table, the speechreader may miss the beginnings of many utterances, as one person and then another interjects comments in the discussion, because the speechreader must locate the talker first. The individual often may not have an advantageous viewing angle of the talker, particularly if the talkers turn their heads toward various participants as they speak.

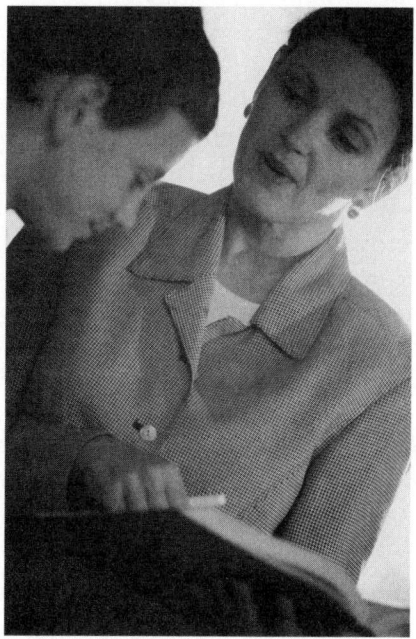

FIGURE 9-5. Talkers seen head-on are easier to speechread than talkers viewed in profile.

FIGURE 9-6. Distance from the talker will affect a person's speechreading performance. This aspect is one reason why a child should have favorable seating in the classroom.

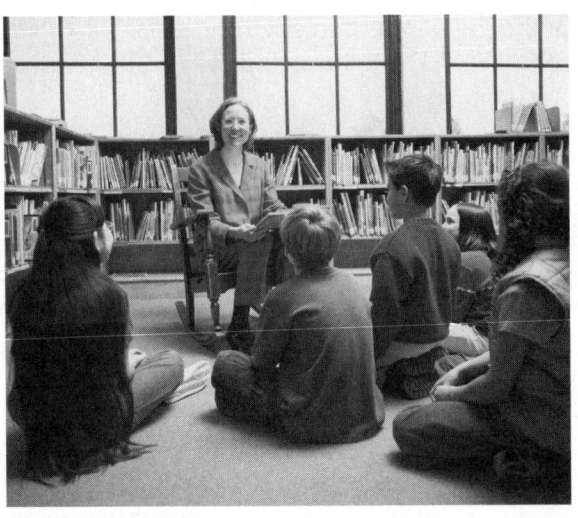

DISTANCE FROM THE TALKER

Distance from the talker also can affect performance, particularly if the speechreader is too far away to view the talker's mouth movements (Figure 9-6). A child speechreading from the back row of a classroom will not recognize as much of the teacher's spoken message as one who sits in the front row, and who has *favorable seating.* A good distance for speechreading is approximately 3 to 6 feet from the talker.

Favorable seating for speechreading includes being close enough to see the talker's lip movements, being able to see the talker full-face rather than in profile, and having the talker's face well lit.

ROOM CONDITIONS

A poorly lit talker, who speaks in front of a light source so that shadows appear on the face, will be relatively difficult to speechread (Figure 9-7) and so will one who stands before a bright window in a room with no overhead lights. Light shining in the eyes of the speechreader can impair performance. Other factors that exert an effect include room reverberation, the availability of assistive devices, interfering objects such as a support beam extending from a room's floor to ceiling, visual distractions, and room noise.

BACKGROUND NOISE

Just as with listening performance, the presence of background noise can impair someone's speechreading performance. Table 9-7 lists common sources of room noise that can interfere with the

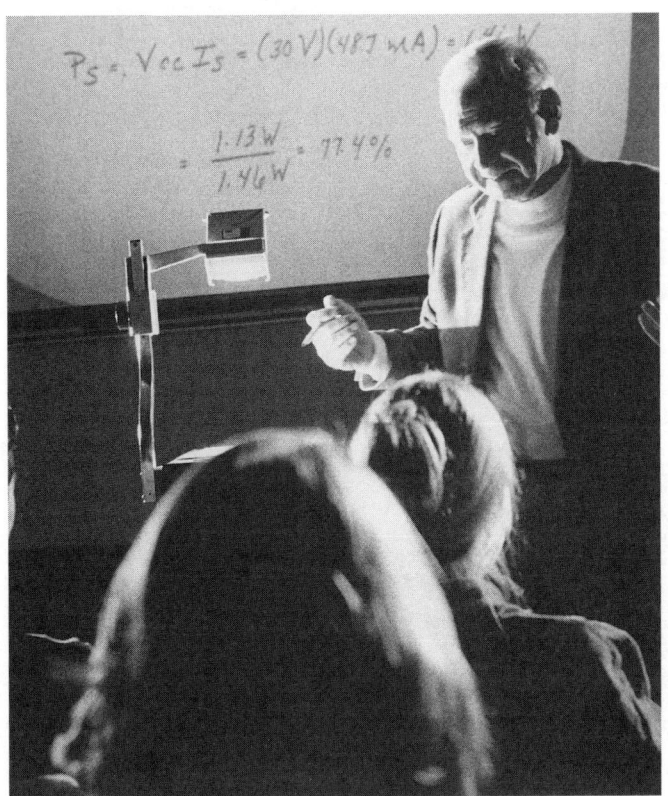

FIGURE 9-7. Poorly lit talkers are difficult to speechread.

Table 9-7. Examples of noise sources common to various communication settings.

HOME	RESTAURANTS	WORKPLACE	CLASSROOM
Kitchen sink/running water	Dishes/silverware	Computers	Children talking
Washer/dryer	Music	Printers	Paper rustling
Air conditioner	Guests talking	Machinery	Shoes scuffling
Furnace			Chairs moving
Vacuum cleaner			Projectors
Television			Fans, ventilators, furnace, air conditioner
Radio			Hall noise
Family members talking			
Open window/door (lawn mower, leaf blower, traffic)			
Refrigerator			

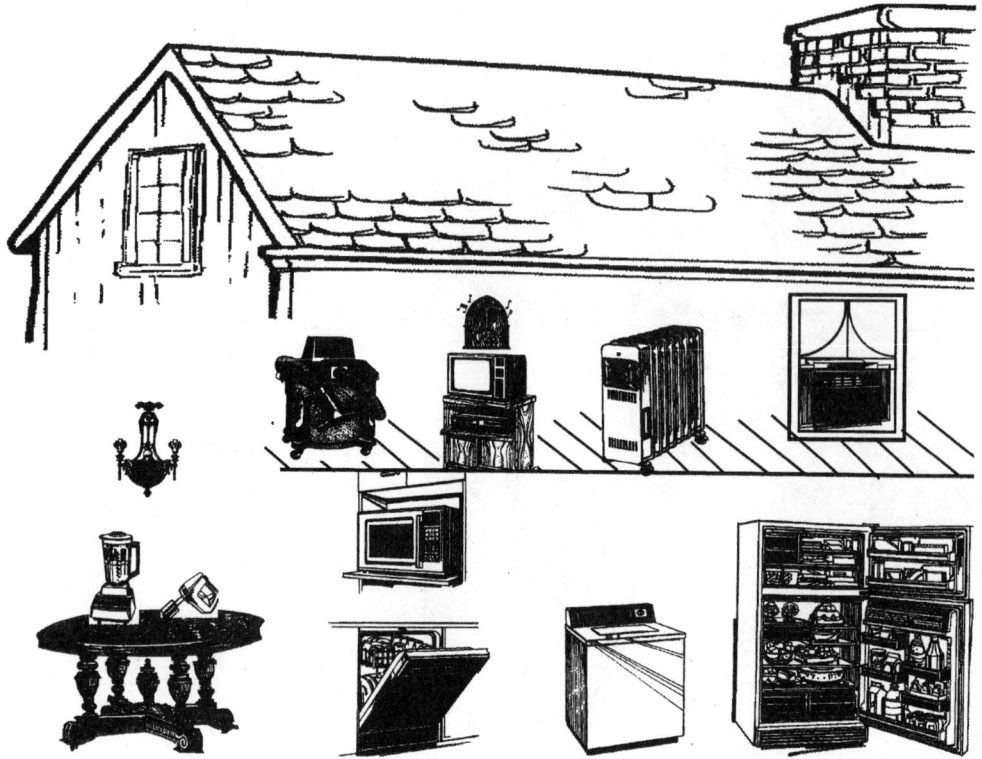

FIGURE 9-8. A sample of noise sources that may be present in the home environment.

speechreading task. A noisy environment can mask speech and decrease the speechreading enhancement effect afforded by residual hearing, as well as distract the speechreader from the speech-recognition task (Figure 9-8). The presence of visible movement, such as movement by others in the room or activity seen from a window, also can be distracting.

Talking With a Guy Named Baldy

A psychologist at the University of California, Santa Cruz, Dominic Massaro, Ph.D., has spearheaded the development of a computerized talking head. He calls his creation "Baldy," most likely because his creation looks like a flat-cheeked Yul Brynner. The three-dimensional head floats on the computer screen. When he talks, his lips move and pucker, his eyebrows raise, and his chin and facial features vary, depending on what he is saying. Baldy can be made to look like he's made of a scaffolding of triangles or a flesh-covered face that looks like its been covered in shrink-wrap. The latter result looks fairly human, almost like an animated store-front mannequin, and it is possible to lipread the head's words. The program user can change Baldy's mood (he can smile, he can frown, he can looked surprised, he can look angry), his skin coloring, and, in a recent incarnation of the program, his ethnic identity and even species (it's possible to convert Baldy into a talking monkey). The user can type in a word or sentence, and Baldy will speak it.

There are several possible uses for animated synthetic speech such as Baldy. The most obvious is for speechreading practice using a computer. The Baldy system has also been used to study the basic process of audiovisual speech perception and audiovisual integration. For instance, it is possible to make Baldy's lip appear to say one thing and the accompanying sound to say another (as when performing a McGurk Effect experiment). It has also been used to teach speech production and speechreading to children at an oral school for the deaf, Tucker Maxon Oral School in Portland, Oregon. The version of Baldy used at the school for the deaf allows the user to remove the skin off the head and thereby view the activity of the tongue body, either head-on or in a half-sagittal view. By watching the movement of the lips, lower jaw, and tongue, children learn to place their articulators during speech production.

The Speechreader

Finally, variables related to the individual can affect the person's speechreading performance.

INNATE SKILL AND HEARING ACUITY

Speechreading performance relates to lipreading skill, as well as to an individual's hearing acuity. Generally, the better the lipreading skill and the greater the amount of residual hearing, the better the speechreading performance. However, the nature of the hearing loss also affects performance. For example, two persons may have severe hearing losses. If one has a conductive loss and the other has a sensorineural loss, the latter individual may have poorer speech discrimination and therefore may perform more poorly on a speechreading task.

Speechreading performance also is influenced by individuals' use of appropriate amplification and use of eyeglasses when needed. Poor visual acuity, such as that stemming from cataracts, will of course hinder performance.

Apart from hearing skills per se, how well an individual can combine what is seen with what is heard also affects performance. For instance, two people might recognize 25% of the words on a test presented in an auditory-only condition and 25% of the words when the same test is presented in a vision-only condition. However, one might outperform the other person in an audition-plus-vision condition because the former is better at *audiovisual integration.* There is some evidence that people become less adept at combining visual and auditory speech signals as they age (Sommers, Tye-Murray, & Spehar, 2002, but see Cienkowski & Carney, 2002).

Audiovisual integration:
Combining information from the auditory and the visual signal to form a uniform precept.

EMOTIONAL AND PHYSICAL STATE

An individual's level of stress, fatigue, and attentiveness can affect performance. For example, if the speechreader is engaged in a job interview, anxiety may impair his or her speechreading performance. A businessman may not speechread family members well at home because he is fatigued from a long day of concentrating on co-workers' auditory and visual signals.

"I work so hard to understand what people are saying that my mind can't focus on what to say when they quit talking. Sometimes people must think I'm stupid because I just look at them blankly instead of answering them."

—*Judy, a hard-of-hearing woman.*

Speechreading as an Art Form

Evelyn Glennie is a classical percussionist who has a profound hearing loss. In a 1995 radio interview (KMOX, St. Louis), she was asked why she speechreads so well. Ms. Glennie replied that she approaches speechreading in the same way many people with normal hearing listen to music. At a symphony, audience members do not necessarily attend to every note, but rather, attend to the structure of the music and the interplay of the various instruments. Similarly, Ms. Glennie explained, she does not try to speechread every word. She follows the message as it is conveyed by the words she recognizes; by what has been said beforehand; and by the talker's facial expressions, head nods, body posture; and hand gestures.

![] ORAL INTERPRETERS

The final topic to be considered in this chapter concerning speechreading is the oral interpreter. Because many hard-of-hearing persons rely on the visual speech signal, occasions arise when an oral interpreter is helpful or even essential. An *oral interpreter* is someone who sits in clear view of the hard-of-hearing individual and silently repeats a talker's message as it is spoken, often lagging behind by only one or two words. An oral interpreter attempts to convey a talker's mood and intent. They must adhere to a Code of Ethics (1984), which dictates their professional code of behavior. This code includes the following guidelines:

An **oral interpreter** sits in clear view of a hard-of-hearing person and silently repeats a talker's message as it is spoken.

- They cannot share with other individuals information they learn during an interpreting assignment.
- They cannot change the meaning of a message as they interpret it for the hard-of-hearing person.
- They cannot add their opinions or personal commentary to a message.

Situations where an oral interpreter may be required include meetings, lectures, churches or synagogues, and courts of law. Castle (1988) notes that group situations, panels of talkers, and question-and-answer periods may often be difficult for those with hearing loss. In these situations, speechreaders may not know where to look as speaking turns shift rapidly, and the talkers turn this way or that way as they speak. An oral interpreter in these situations can alleviate communication difficulties.

As a speech and hearing professional, you may be asked on occasion to help locate an oral interpreter for a hard-of-hearing person.

CASE STUDY 1

A few studies have focused on exceptionally good lipreaders (e.g., Lyxell, 1994; Rönnberg et al., 1999) in an effort to understand what makes some people particularly facile at deciphering the visual speech signal.

(continues)

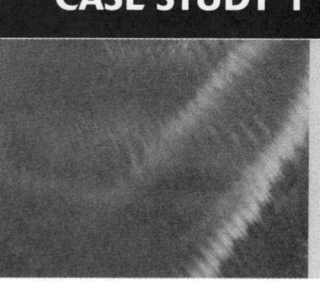

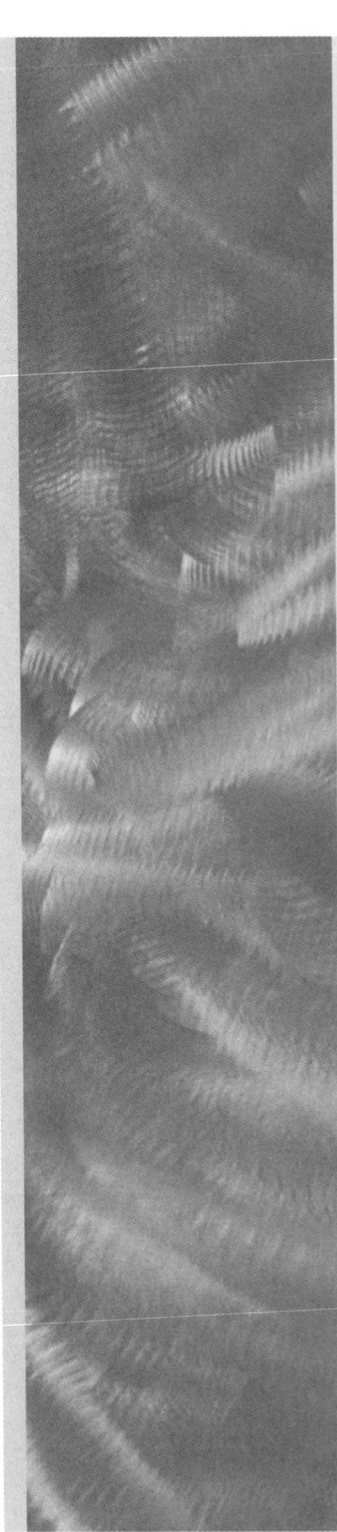

Lyxell (1994) studied a 56-year-old woman, SJ, who lost her hearing at the age of 16, following a bout with meningitis. On a sentence test administered in a vision-only condition, SJ scored 57% words correct. By comparison, the average performance of a control group of 119 subjects (49 who had hearing loss and 70 who had normal hearing) scored 24% words correct. They identified roughly half as many words as SJ. Interestingly, her ability to decode words, which means her ability to indicate whether two words spoken in a pair are the same or different, was no better than the average control subject. Thus, even though she is skilled at lipreading sentences, this skill does not transfer to word discrimination.

SJ has developed a specific strategy for lipreading. She reported that when she lipreads, she tries to repeat each spoken word as soon as she can after it is spoken. When possible, she tries to summarize the words into meaningful units, for instance, during pauses in the talker's speech. She purposefully fills in missing pieces of information and updates misperceived words.

A cognitive test battery revealed that SJ has a better than average ability to comprehend read sentences and to recall the last words of a series of sentences presented in text format. This performance suggests that she has a good short-term working memory for complex tasks. For more simple tasks, such as repeating back strings of digits presented sequentially on a computer screen, her performance was unremarkable. She was also found to have an excellent ability to fill in missing words in printed sentences, although she did not exhibit extraordinary skill in filling in letters in words.

The results from the cognitive tests mesh well with her reported strategy for lipreading. She has a large working memory that allows her to buffer up information as she lipreads. She can use this stored information to catch up on what she missed and to correct what later turns out to be a misperception. The author notes that she deviates from the general case, where working memory tends not to be predictive of lipreading performance.

◼️ FINAL REMARKS

Intuitively we associate speech recognition with the sense of hearing. However, as we have learned in this chapter, the sense of sight also can be an important component in our everyday communication. In fact, persons with hearing loss may be reliant on their vision for recognizing spoken messages. A topic that currently is receiving much attention in the research literature pertains to auditory-vision integration; that is, how we combine the disparate auditory and visual signal of a talker into a unified percept. The answer to this question may have important theoretical implications for models of speech perception. For our present purposes, this is an interesting question because exploring the answer may help us design more effective speech perception training protocols.

◼️ KEY CHAPTER POINTS

✔ Even persons with normal hearing rely on speechreading to some degree.

✔ Some people are better speechreaders than others. The reasons for this are unclear. Performance cannot be predicted by such factors as intelligence or practice with the speechreading task.

✔ When we lipread, our eyes both fixate and perform quick shifts. They often focus on talker's eyes, nose, and mouth.

✔ Lipreading is difficult. Some of the factors that may compound the lipreading task include the partial visibility or nonvisibility of many speech sounds on the face, the rapidity of speech, coarticulation, the visual similarity of many sound groups, and talker eccentricities. For instance, the words *Bob* and *Mom* are indistinguishable on the lips. The word *hick* requires minimal visible mouth movement.

✔ Although models of audiovisual integration remain nebulous, it may be that the ability to integrate is distinct from the abilities to recognize speech auditorally or to recognize speech visually.

✔ A little residual hearing can increase markedly one's ability to recognize speech when looking and listening simultaneously.

✔ The talker, message, environment, and state of the person affect how well the individual will recognize a spoken message. For instance, a talker who mumbles will be difficult to understand.

▰ MULTIPLE CHOICE QUESTIONS

1. Which statement below is false?
    a. Older adults tend to be poorer lipreaders than younger adults.
    b. If you have normal hearing, you will probably comprehend more if you hear and see a talker who is reading aloud than if you only hear the reader.
    c. Intelligence quotient correlates positively with lipreading ability.
    d. Infants have been shown to engage in speechreading.

2. When you lipread, your eyes:
    a. Fixate on the talker's mouth
    b. Scan the entire face in rhythmic saccades
    c. Focus primarily on the mouth, nose, and eye regions
    d. Focus on the eyes for phonetic content and the mouth for prosodic nuances

3. Mr. Simmons is taking a lipreading test. Which word is he most likely to identify incorrectly?
    a. Hornet
    b. Elephant
    c. Bath
    d. Thumb

4. One reason lipreading is so difficult is because:
    a. People rarely pause between sentences.
    b. Sounds look different on the mouth depending on the phonetic context of a word.
    c. Residual hearing does not supplement the visual signal.
    d. The visual signal doesn't convey place of articulation information.

5. Which two sounds are examples of a viseme?
    a. /l, w/
    b. /f, θ/
    c. /m, n/
    d. /p, b/

6. The McGurk Effect is an example of:
   a. Audiovisual integration
   b. Lipreading
   c. Viseme confusion
   d. The benefits of residual hearing for lipreading

7. Who would be the most difficult person to speechread?
   a. A woman
   b. A spouse
   c. A store clerk with a European accent
   d. A speech-language pathologist

8. Typically, a word that has a great frequency of usage is easier to identify on the face than a word that has infrequent usage. An exception to this rule of thumb is:
   a. The word has more than one syllable.
   b. The word has few lexical neighbors.
   c. The word begins with a visible sound.
   d. The word is spoken in a sentence context.

9. An oral interpreter:
   a. Signs and speaks the message
   b. Mouths the message of a talker so that a hard-of-hearing person can lipread it
   c. Quietly repeats the message so the hard-of-hearing person can speechread it
   d. Acts as an intermediary between a hearing person and a person with significant hearing loss

CHAPTER 10

Speechreading Training

TOPICS

- Candidacy
- Traditional methods of speechreading training
- Developing speechreading skills
- Analytic speechreading training objectives
- Synthetic speechreading training objectives
- Computerized Instruction
- Efficacy of speechreading training
- Case study
- Final remarks
- Key chapter points
- Multiple choice questions

In this chapter, we will consider speechreading training, including candidacy issues, training philosophies, training techniques, and training efficacy. At the beginning of the 20th century, speechreading training was a principal component of most aural rehabilitation programs, in large part because there were few alternative means for alleviating communication problems experienced by persons with hearing loss. We simply did not have the technology to reduce hearing difficulties. In those times, persons would attend speechreading classes and perform drill activities at home.

With the advent of hearing aids, cochlear implants, and assistive listening devices, individuals are better able to use their residual hearing. Concomitantly, the popularity of speechreading training has waned, so that now it rarely is found as the sole element of an aural rehabilitation program.

CANDIDACY

Who is a candidate for speechreading training? The answer to this question depends in part on who you ask. In this text, it is suggested that children may benefit from training, especially if they use simultaneous communication (Chapter 15) and do not rely solely on speechreading for everyday communication (i.e., children who use both speech and manually coded English to communicate). Adults who have recently lost their hearing also may be candidates for training. In addition to improving their speechreading skills, they may receive psychological benefits from participating in a program, feeling they have taken constructive action to deal with their hearing losses. Adults who have a hearing loss that is long-standing may benefit more from other types of aural rehabilitation intervention than speechreading training, interventions such as communication strategies training.

TRADITIONAL METHODS OF SPEECHREADING TRAINING

In the twentieth century, four speechreading training methods were popular in the United States (Berger, 1972; Jeffers & Barley, 1971). These methods were advocated originally by Bruhn, the Nitchies, the Kinzes, and Bunger.

About 1912, Martha Emma Bruhn introduced the Mueller-Walle method, a method that originated in Germany. The hallmark feature of this program was an emphasis on rapid syllable drill, such as *she-ma-flea* and *she-may-free*. Students also practiced recognizing homophenous words, using sentence context cues to distinguish between possible meanings.

Edward B. Nitchie, who published his first book, *Lip-reading Principles and Practices* in 1912, rarely employed syllable drill. Instead, he emphasized the importance of psychological processes of speechreading. Practice usually centered on sentence materials and the identification of homophenous words through contextual cues. Students sometimes practiced speechreading themselves by talking before a mirror. Training materials were presented without voice. Nitchie's text was updated by his wife Elizabeth in 1940, and it was one of the most widely read texts on the subject in the 20th century.

Cora Kinze studied with both Bruhn and Nitchie before establishing her own school for speechreading training with her sister Rose in 1917. Not surprisingly, the sisters developed an eclectic method, combining the analytic syllable drill of Bruhn with the more synthetic exercises of Nitchie.

The Jena Method was developed by Karl Brauckmann who lived in the city of Jena, Germany and published two brief textbooks in 1925. The Jena method was introduced to the United States by Anna Bunger. A hallmark of Brauckmann's approach was its emphasis on **mimetic** and **kinesthetic** forms and sensations, and the recognition that our ability to produce speech relates to our ability to perceive it. In this method, students focus on the mouth movements of the instructor, while simultaneously speaking the training materials. Training materials include repeated syllables and then words derived from the syllables.

Mimetic means imitating or copying movements.

Kinesthetic relates to the perception of movement, position, and tension of body parts.

Some of the fundamental principles underlying these seminal training programs are evident in more modern training curricula. Students' attention typically is focused on sound identification (as in the Mueller-Walle method), as well as on recognizing the gist of a sentence (following Nitchie). Most contemporary programs recommend that training items be presented with both auditory and visual signals. The notions of kinesthetic awareness of one's own speech production and of lipreading one's own speech either via a mirror or videotape has enjoyed recent attention (as with the Jena method), as investigators have attempted to show that production practice enhances perception performance, with modest success (De Filippo, Sims, & Gottermeier, 1995).

A Look Back to 1942

In discussing basic principles of learning how to lipread and speechread, a U.S. government handbook[1] offered this advice:

"Under all systems of [lipreading/speechreading] instruction the student spends much time in observing and interpreting syllables or monosyllabic words containing the sounds being studied. Although systems vary in the degree of emphasis placed on various factors in the training, the leading teachers agree that, in order to become a proficient lipreader, one must not only train the eye for accuracy, quickness, and visual memory, but also must train the mind to understand, by the context, those words which cannot be recognized by the movements of the mouth. Finally, the student must be fortified by courage, patience, and a determination to learn. He must practice his new art interminably, with his friends in conversation, in the church or lecture hall, and watching strangers on the street."

DEVELOPING SPEECHREADING SKILLS

The first class of a communication strategies training program often is informational in nature and includes a consideration of the speechreading process. A handout like the one reprinted in Table 10-1 might be used to guide discussion among adult clients. This handout reviews factors that affect the speechreading process and the importance of using speechreading cues maximally.

In addition to considering the principles outlined in Table 10-1, class participants also might be asked to reflect on their

[1] From *Rehabilitation of the deaf and the hard of hearing: A manual for rehabilitation case workers*. Vocational Rehabilitation Series, Bulletin No. 26, U.S. Government Printing Office, 1942, p. 47.

Table 10-1. A handout that might be distributed at an adult rehabilitation class to stimulate discussion about the speechreading process.

Speechreading is a process of attending to auditory and visual information to recognize a spoken message. Speechreading is not just watching others' lips to identify the words they are saying. It also consists of making the most of your hearing, and using your mind to collect all the information available to make a "best guess." Speechreading includes the following:

1. **Lipreading.** Watch the mouth movements of the talker, including the lips, jaw, and tongue tip. It is impossible to identify every word, but you can identify some words and sounds that will help you ascertain what is being said.

2. **Facial expression.** It is possible to identify people's moods or how they feel by the expression on their faces. You can also glean subtle nuances of meaning in their messages by attending to facial expressions.

3. **Gesture, posture, and movement.** What people are doing, how they are sitting, and the gestures they make give clues to what they are thinking about and what they might say.

4. **Situational cues.** You can anticipate what a person is going to talk about by the situation or place they are in and the relationships of the people present.

5. **Knowing the topic.** It is easier to follow conversation when you know what the talker is talking about. The easiest way to find out is to ask someone else who is listening. You might say, "What are we discussing?"

6. **Knowledge of language.** You might be able to make educated guesses about a particular word missed on the basis of sentence structure.

7. **Keeping informed.** Knowing what news items or subjects are of current interest to people may help you to anticipate what will be talked about. Read newspapers and magazines and watch the news on television.

8. **Emotional factors.** Keep motivated and develop self-confidence even though there will be times that you make errors.

9. **Use your hearing.** Although you have a hearing loss, you may be able to hear sounds and words that help you to identify the message or idea.

Until now, you *have* been taking advantage of these clues to some extent. One goal of this class is to make you more conscious of them so you use them maximally. Using these clues, much of the message can be predicted. Some parts of the message are less predictable (e.g., hearing a new name), making them more difficult. Therefore, you must use two kinds of information: (a) the part of the message you did understand and (b) any additional knowledge that can help you to fill in the gaps in order to figure out the whole message.

Source: Adapted from "Speechreading instruction for adults: Issues and practices," by R. Cherry & A. Rubinstein, 1988, p. 302. *Volta Review, 90.*

Table 10-2. Rules to follow when speechreading. A handout like this might be discussed during a group class.

---

1. **Watch the talker's lips.**
   This seems obvious, but often, a speechreader can be distracted by other events in the room, or the talker's hand gestures. Also, there may be a tendency to watch the talker's eyes instead of the mouth.

2. **Provide information to the talker about how to communicate with you.**
   This may include asking the talker to speak clearly and at a slightly louder than normal conversational level. The talker should not shout or exaggerate lip movements. The talker should face you when speaking, and should not chew or cover the mouth, such as with a hand.

3. **Try to ensure that the room is well-lit and that your position in the room allows for optimal speechreading performance.**
   You will want to find a seat where light does not shine in your eyes and adjust light sources so they do not cast shadows on the talker's face. Position yourself near enough to the talker so you can clearly see the talker's mouth and facial expressions.

4. **Try to minimize background noise.**
   Background noise might be minimized by ensuring that radios and televisions are turned down or off. Favorable seating, say at a table away from the kitchen in a restaurant, may also minimize background noise.

5. **Know the topic of conversation.**
   During a conversation, ask someone the topic of conversation. It is much easier to recognize a message if you know what is being discussed. If you know in advance that a specific topic will be discussed, try to learn something about it beforehand.

6. **Pay attention to context cues.**
   The situation in which the conversation occurs may provide information about what is being said. The talker's facial expressions and what has been discussed beforehand may also be informative.

7. **Keep a positive attitude.**
   Speechreading can be tiring. Stay motivated, and do not be distracted by your own anxiety and self-doubts.

---

speechreading habits and listening difficulties. They often review rules to follow when speechreading, such as those listed in Table 10-2. For instance, although *Watch the talker's lips,* the first rule presented in Table 10-2, seems like an obvious recommendation, some people become distracted by watching the talker's hand gestures or they have a habit of listening with lowered eye gaze, instead of concentrating on the talker's mouth movements. As a result, their speechreading performance is not as good as it could be.

Finally, during an introduction to speechreading, class participants might review charts like the one presented in Figure 10-1 to identify difficult listening situations and to formulate solutions for rectifying the difficulties. They might be asked to identify which seats in Figure 10-1 present the most favorable circumstances for lipreading and speechreading, and which seats present the least favorable. This kind of activity sensitizes students to the concept of favorable speechreading conditions.

Following this kind of introduction, the class may (or may not) receive formal speechreading training. In today's world, rarely if ever do participants in an aural rehabilitation class practice lipreading (vision-only speech recognition). Rather, they practice recognizing speech using both auditory and visual signals. As noted, children are more likely to receive formal speechreading training than adults. This is especially true for those who have received a cochlear implant. As with formal auditory training, formal speechreading training objectives can be divided into two categories: analytic and synthetic.

◼ ANALYTIC SPEECHREADING TRAINING OBJECTIVES

Analytic speechreading training objectives are directed toward developing vowel recognition and consonant recognition skills. The logic underlying many speechreading curricula is gradually to increase patients' reliance on the auditory signal for discriminating phonemic contrasts while they speechread (Figure 10-2).

Vowel Speechreading Training Objectives

In Chapter 8, Auditory Training, the term *vowel formant* was defined. To review, vowel formants are resonances in the mouth, which cause some frequencies of the speech signal to have more energy than other frequencies. Every vowel can be distinguished by its formant patterns.

Table 10-3 presents one possible hierarchy of analytic vowel speechreading training objectives. If a person has only rudimentary speech recognition skills, initial speechreading training objectives should focus his or her attention on distinguishing /i/,

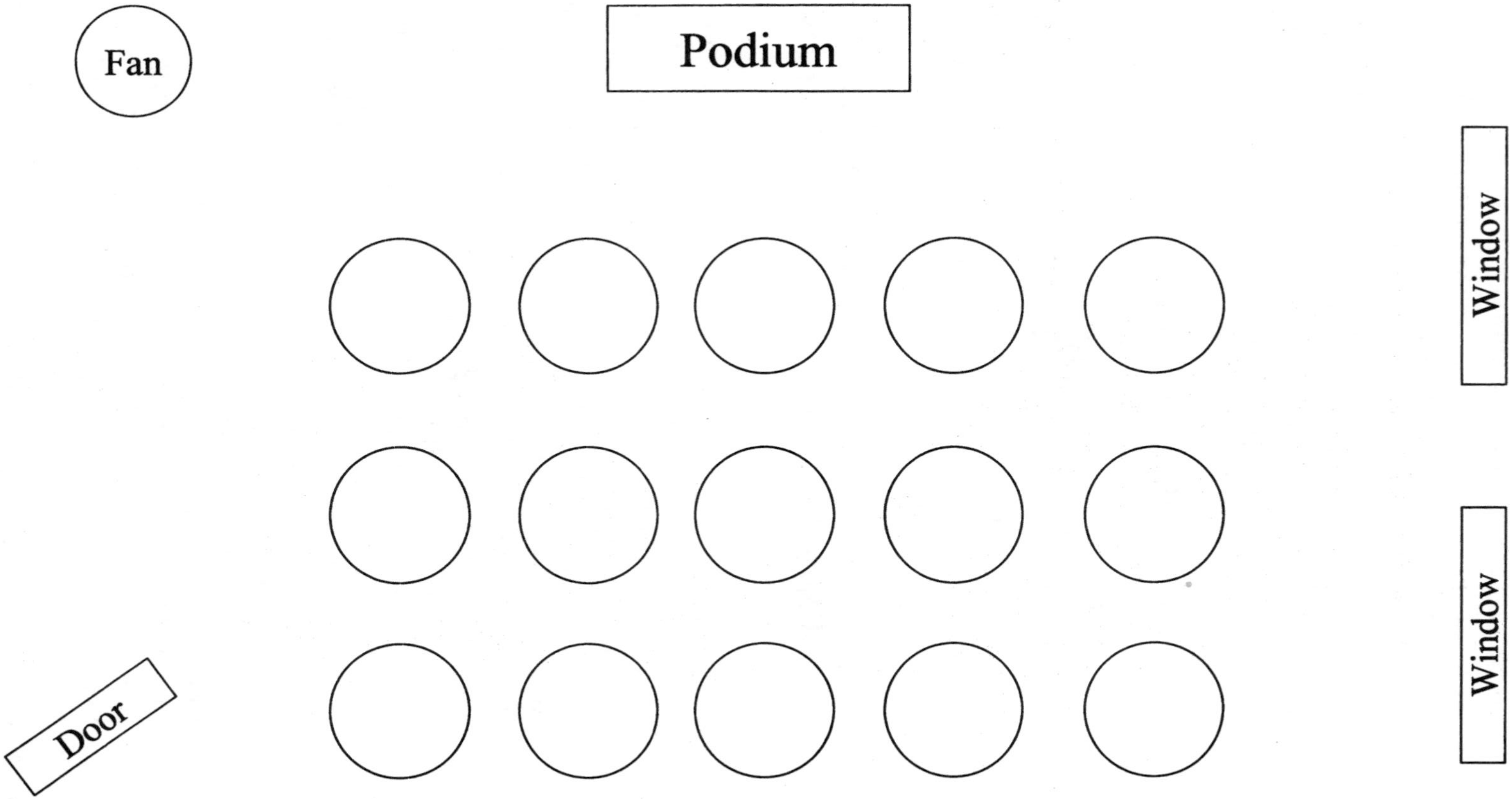

FIGURE 10-1. A chart that can be used when discussing listening environments and ways to minimize speech reading difficulties. Students might be asked to identify where they might sit to optimize speechreading performance.

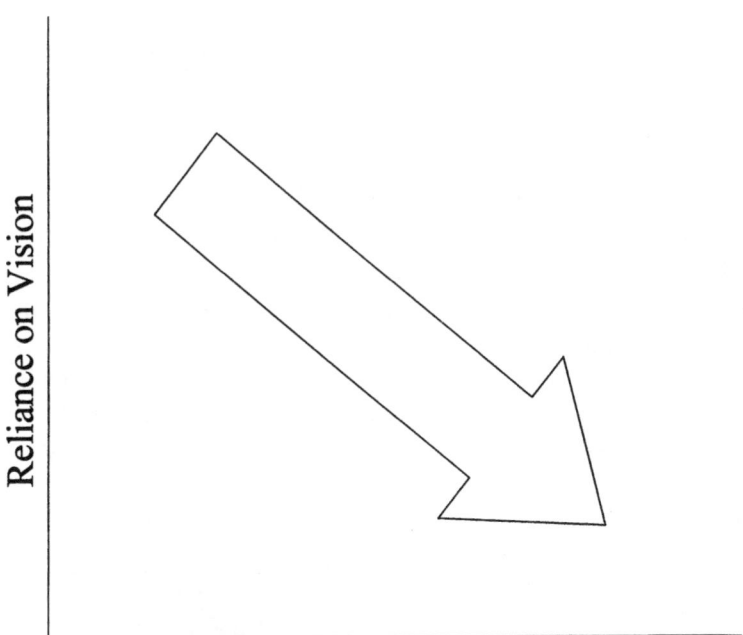

FIGURE 10-2. During speechreading training, patients become increasingly reliant on the auditory signal for speech recognition.

/u/, and /a/. These sounds differ both in their formant structure and in how they appear on the mouth. The /i/ is produced with a narrow mouth opening, with some spreading of the mouth corners. It has a first formant of low frequency, and a second formant of high frequency. Typically, the lips pucker and form a narrow opening when you phonate /u/, and both first and second formants have a relatively low frequency value. For /a/, the lips form a moderate opening and appear relaxed; the formants have mid-range values. Table 10-4 presents examples of word pairs that can be used in achieving the first three vowel speechreading training objectives listed in Table 10-3.

Consonant Speechreading Training Objectives

In our previous discussion concerning auditory training (Chapter 8), we considered three different types of speech features: manner, voice, and place of articulation, and noted that consonants can be characterized in terms of these three features. To review, manner denotes the type of articulatory gestures that

Table 10-3. Vowel analytic training objectives that were designed for young cochlear-implant users. These objectives are also appropriate for adults who have significant hearing loss.

The student:

1. Will discriminate words with /i/ and /u/; for example, *me* from *moo.*
2. Will discriminate words with /i/ and /a/; for example, *keep* from *cop.*
3. Will discriminate words with /u/ and /a/; for example, *coop* from *cop.*
4. Will identify words with /i/, /u/, and /a/, using a four-item and then six-item response set; for example, *bean* from the response set of: *bean, pot, pit,* and *pool.* The vowels in the response set may include vowels other than /i, u, a/.
5. Will identify words with /u/, /i/, and /a/ from an open set of familiar vocabulary.

Subsequent training that contrasts other vowels can be incorporated into consonant training activities.

Table 10-4. Examples of word pairs that can be used in achieving the first three analytic vowel speechreading training objectives listed in Table 10-3.

Objective 1: The student will discriminate words with /i/ and /u/.

Word pairs:

beet/boot	see/soup	she/shoe
heat/hoot	leap/loop	peel/pool
read/root	jeep/jewel	sheet/shot
keep/coop	knee/new	geese/goose

Objective 2: The student will discriminate words with /i/ and /a/.

Word pairs:

heat/hot	keep/cop	cheap/chop
peak/pop	fear/far	deal/doll
see/sod	pea/pod	seed/sock
team/top	read/rod	jeep/job

Objective 3: The student will discriminate words with /u/ and /a/.

Word pairs:

two/top	clue/clock	goose/got
who/hot	pool/pot	suit/sock
juice/job	dew/dog	clue/clock
boot/box	room/rot	moose/moss

you use to produce a particular sound. Manner categories include glides (e.g., /l/ as in *lip*), stops (such as /t/ in *top*), fricatives and affricatives (such as /f/ in *fruit*), and nasals (such as /n/ in *new*). The voicing feature indicates whether the vocal folds vibrate during the consonantal constriction, for example, /b/ is voiced whereas /p/ is not. The place of articulation feature indicates where in the mouth that the primary constriction occurs. Place designations include bilabial (such as /b/ as in *boy*), labiodental (/θ/ as in *thick*), linguadental (/f/), alveolar (e.g., /t/), palatal (e.g., /δ/) and velar (e.g., /g/).

It is fortuitous that the visual signal associated with consonant production ideally complements the auditory signal. Cues that signal manner and voice often are easier for hard-of-hearing persons to hear than are cues that signal place of articulation. For instance, someone with a severe hearing loss who uses amplification is likely to hear the difference between the words *bat* and *pat*. However, if presented with only the visual signal, these two words will be indistinguishable. In contrast, cues about place of articulation tend to be somewhat visible, but place of articulation is difficult to determine through listening alone for persons who have significant hearing loss. A hard-of-hearing individual might discriminate the words *pat* and *sat* if he or she can see the talker, but may not be able to discriminate them if the individual only hears the talker.

A list of consonant speechreading training objectives appears in Table 10-5. The first speechreading consonant training objectives may involve discriminating consonants that differ in place of production, and that share either voice or manner (Table 10-5). For example, a student may be asked to discriminate between the /p/ in *pay* and the /s/ in *say*. The clinician speaks the two items and the student then indicates whether they are the *same* or *different*. The clinician attempts to speak with constant loudness and intonation. The next two objectives require students to discriminate between consonants that share place, but that differ on other signal parameters (Objectives 2 and 3 in Table 10-5).

Table 10-6 presents examples of consonant pairs and words pairs that might be used for achieving the first three consonant speechreading training objectives presented in Table 10-5.

Table 10-5. Consonant analytic speechreading training designed for young cochlear-implant users. These objectives also are appropriate for adults who have significant hearing loss.

The student:

1. Will discriminate consonant pairs that differ in place of production and share either voice or manner, for example, *tag* from *bag.*
2. Will discriminate consonant pairs that share similar place of production but differ in manner and voice, for example, *pan* from *man.*
3. Will discriminate consonant pairs that share place and manner or voice, for example, *park* from *bark.*
4. Will identify consonants that share manner of production, using a four-item and then a six-item response set; for example, *tag* from the response set of: *tag, bag, back,* and *gas.*
5. Will identify consonants from a four-item and then a six-item response set of voiced or voiceless consonants; for example, *pop* from the response set of: *pop, cop, cap,* and *top.*
6. Will identify consonants that share place of production, using a four-item and then a six-item response set: for example, *pan* from the response set of: *pan, man, bat,* and *mat.*
7. Will identify words from an open set of familiar vocabulary.

After a student achieves the first three consonant speechreading training objectives, intermediate objectives in a speechreading curriculum (Objectives 4 and 5 in Table 10-5) might focus attention on identifying consonants that share manner or voice. The student will progress from performing a discrimination task, as in the first three speechreading training objectives, to performing a closed-set identification task. For example, individuals might identify the word *cat* from the response set of *cat, pat, pet,* and *kit,* words that all begin with voiceless consonants. Following a discrimination activity, they then may perform an identification activity, using a closed-set response format. For this kind of training activity, the clinician might set before the individual a set of five or six picture cards, such as the set shown in Figure 10-3. The clinician then speaks one of the items, and the student indicates which item was spoken. This kind of task is a precursor to open-set word recognition. Table 10-7 presents stimuli that might be appropriate when the goal is to identify words beginning with the /p/ and /b/ phonemes. (Figure 10-3 presents a corresponding picture set.)

Table 10-6. Examples of consonant and word pairs that can be used in achieving the first three consonant speechreading training objectives listed in Table 10-5.

Objective 1: The student will discriminate consonant pairs that differ in place of production and share either voice or manner.

Consonant pairs:

/m/ versus /d, dʒ, g, j, l/
/p/ versus /d, tʃ, g, ʃ, h, s/
/b/ versus /t, dʒ, n, k, j, l/
/d/ versus /k, j, dʒ/

Word pairs:

meat/geese	pill/chill	top/chop
moose/goose	pot/hot	boat/coat
bit/knit	dog/jog	peal/heal
make/lake	tear/chair	pin/chin

Objective 2: The student will discriminate consonant pairs that share similar place of production but differ in manner and voice.

Consonant pairs:

/p/ versus /m, w/
/d/ versus /s/
/t/ versus /l, n/
/k/ versus /j, dʒ/
/g/ versus /ʃðdʒ, tʃ/

Word pairs:

pan/man	tip/lip	geese/cheese
toe/low	day/say	deal/seal
dip/sip	pen/men	game/chain
tan/land	car/jar	tail/nail

Objective 3: The student will discriminate consonant pairs that share place and manner and/or voice.

Consonant pairs:

/b/ versus /m, p, w/
/d/ versus /n, t, l/
/v/ versus /f/
/t/ versus /s/
/k/ versus /g, ʃ, tʃ/

Word pairs:

bat/mat	keep/cheek	van/fan
dog/log	beak/week	cap/gap
bun/one	tail/sail	doe/no
cat/gas	two/sue	curl/girl

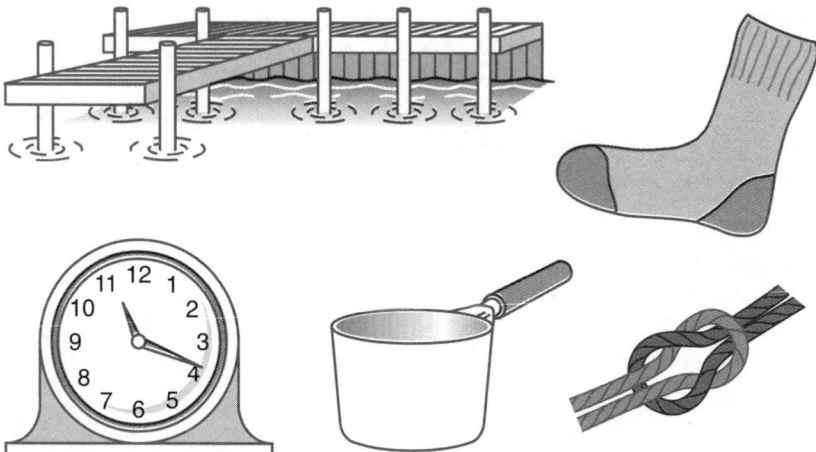

FIGURE 10-3. Illustrations that can be used with a closed-set identification task.

Advanced objectives for consonant speechreading training (Objectives 6 and 7 in Table 10-5) often focus attention on identifying consonants that share place and manner, place and voice, or place, manner and voice in a closed-set and then an open-set format. For example, students may be asked to identify /p/ as in *pole* when one of the foils is *bowl*. The /p/ and /b/ sounds are visually and acoustically similar.

Table 10-7. Stimuli used for an identification activity when the target phonemes are /p/ and /b/. A clinician might present each item five or more times during the training session. When the student can read and has fairly good listening skills, the target items can be more similar (i.e., they might rhyme), and the response choices can be presented orthographically.

That's the dock.

That's the sock.

That's the clock.

That's the pot.

That's the knot.

■ SYNTHETIC SPEECHREADING TRAINING OBJECTIVES

In comparison with sentence-level auditory training objectives, sentence-level speechreading training objectives will begin with more challenging tasks (Figure 10-4). This is because most people can recognize more speech when they can both see and hear rather than only hear a talker. For example, if the student is a child, the first task in a speechreading training curriculum may be to practice recognizing simple directions. Such a task would occur much later in an auditory training curriculum.

Table 10-8 presents a sample hierarchy of synthetic speechreading training objectives. The first objective requires students to follow simple directions, in a closed-set format. Initially, the set should be small. For example, two crayons, blue and orange, might be placed before a young child. The clinician asks the child to draw a blue beach ball. As the youth advances, the set is enlarged, and the directions become more complex. In more

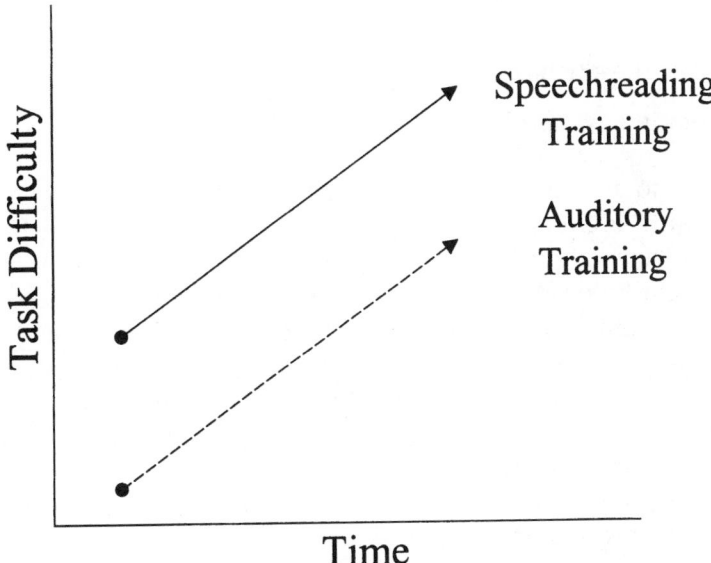

FIGURE 10-4. Initial synthetic speechreading tasks typically are more difficult than those for auditory training.

Table 10-8. Synthetic speechreading training objectives designed for young cochlear-implant users. These objectives can be modified to meet the maturity and cognitive levels of adults who have significant hearing loss.

The student:

1. Will follow simple directions using a closed response set.
2. Will identify a sentence illustration from a set of four dissimilar pictures.
3. Will identify a sentence illustration from a set of four similar pictures.
4. Will listen to topic-related sentences, and repeat or paraphrase them.
5. Will listen to two related sentences, and then draw a picture about them or paraphrase them.
6. Will speechread a paragraph-long narrative and then answer questions about it.

---

advanced exercises, the clinician might present the following directions:

1. Color the ball orange
2. Color the sand yellow
3. Color the shovel purple
4. Color the sky blue
5. Color the water blue

The second and third objectives listed in Table 10-8 require the individual to identify sentence illustrations from a set of pictures. The clinician might lay a set of pictures on a table (Figure 10-5) that might be used in a sentence recognition exercise. These are placed in front of the individual, and then the clinician speaks sentences that correspond to each picture. The student's task is to speechread the clinician and then touch the picture that illustrates the sentence. Postcards, snapshots, or magazine pictures can be used to construct picture sets. Several sentences can be developed for each picture so that a single set can provide practice for speechreading a large number of sentences.

The fourth objective for synthetic level training requires the student to recognize topic-related sentences. These are sentences that concern a common theme. A set of topic-related sentences appears in Table 10-9 as an example.

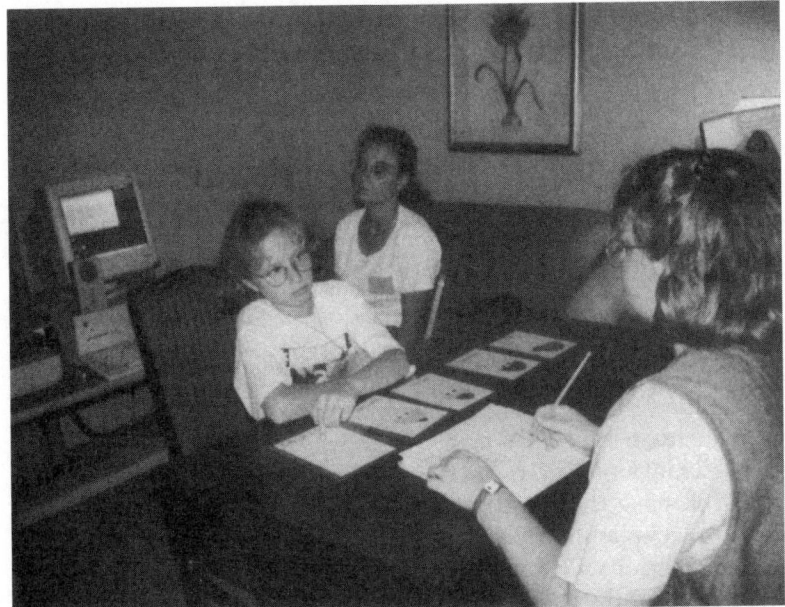

FIGURE 10-5. A clinician and child perform a sentence-recognition task using picture cards. (Photograph by Kim Readmond, courtesy of the Central Institute for the Deaf.)

Table 10-9. Example of a set of topic-related sentences that can be utilized in achieving the fourth objective for synthetic speechreading training: The student will listen to topic-related sentences, and repeat or paraphrase them.

Sentences Concerning Cooking

1. I added a cup of flour.
2. The bread is in the oven.
3. Will you hand me the measuring cup?
4. I need the box of sugar.
5. The mixer is in the cabinet.
6. The oven is set to 300 degrees.
7. Put the bowl in the sink, please.
8. The pan is filled with batter.
9. I will beat the eggs.
10. Please pour a cup of milk.

The final objectives for formal synthetic speechreading training require students to speechread paragraphs. The clinician might present a picture that provides contextual cues for recognizing the passage. As in a continuous discourse tracking task (Chapter 3), the patient must repeat (or in this task, paraphrasing is also permitted) each sentence after speechreading the clinician speak sentences one at a time from a paragraph.

A **holistic** approach to speechreading incorporates several methods and includes the child in setting goals.

A Holistic Approach to Speechreading Training for Children

Yoshinaga-Itano (1988) describes a **holistic** approach that can be used to teach children speechreading. The training goals of this approach can be summarized as follows (Yoshinaga-Itano, 1988):

- "Increase the child's knowledge of the speechreading process.
- Increase the child's ability to generate strategies to facilitate more successful communication.
- Increase the child's ability to generate strategies to facilitate more successful communication.
- Increase the child's confidence in the efficacy of speechreading by providing situations that ensure a high probability of success.
- Increase the child's tolerance for communicative situations that have a higher degree of frustration.
- Increase the child's ability to generate personal goals for improving speechreading.
- Increase the child's motivation to improve speechreading abilities" (p. 244).

In implementing a holistic approach, Yoshinaga-Itano suggests that children should participate in setting goals and should make a commitment to accomplish them. The holistic program should allow for both self-evaluation and clinician-evaluation, and speechreading practice should be provided in real-life versus drill situations.

◼ COMPUTERIZED INSTRUCTION

Several computerized speechreading training programs exist and are available for purchase. The ubiquity of home-based and laptop computers, as well as the capability of today's computer technology to accommodate massive amounts of audiovisual speech materials, have rendered computerized instruction possible. The clinician may work with the patient, or a small group of patients, in the clinical setting (see Figure 10-6). Alternatively, the patient may take the program home or may use it in a school or work setting.

Two examples of computerized programs are the *Dynamic Audio Vision Interactive Device (DAVID)* developed at National Technical Institute for the Deaf at Rochester Institute of Technology (Sims & Gottermeier, 2000; Sims, Dorn, Clark, Bryant, & Mumford, 2002) and *Conversation Made Easy*, developed in part at University of Iowa Hospitals and available through Central Institute for the Deaf in St. Louis (Tye-Murray, 2002b). DAVID presents sentences

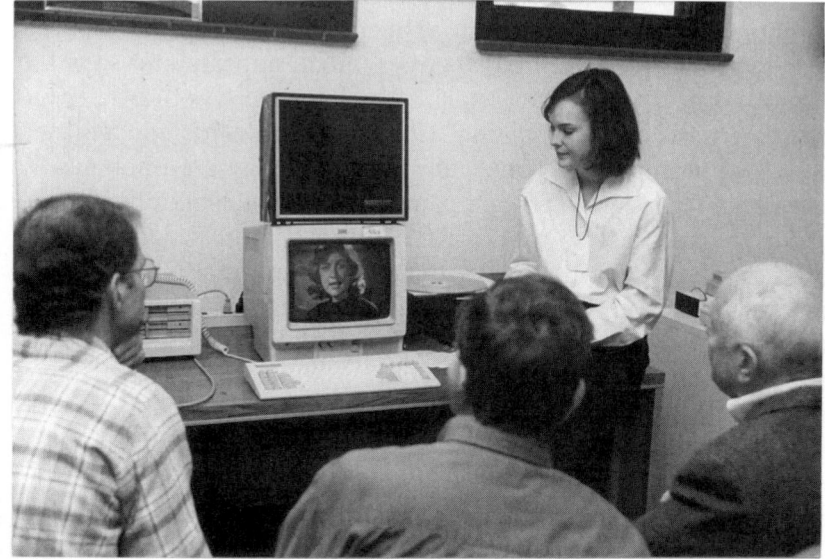

FIGURE 10-6. A clinician uses a computer-based program to provide speechreading instruction to a small group of adult patients. *(Photograph by Kim Readmond, courtesy of the Central Institute for the Deaf.)*

centered around everyday topics, such as going shopping or going to the bank. The student watches a sentence and then types a response into a keyboard. Depending on the level of difficulty, the student either selects a response from a closed set of choices (easy level of difficulty), types in content words (intermediate level of difficulty), or types in the complete sentence (challenging level of difficulty). The program provides "help" alternatives, such as the option to have a sentence repeated, to have a word spoken in isolation in clear speech, or spoken with the talker seen at a 45° azimuth view. A student's performance on the program may be documented in terms of how long it takes in seconds (i.e., response time) to get the item 100% correct.

Three versions of *Conversation Made Easy* are available: one for adults and teenagers, one for children who have low-level language skills, and one for children who have high-level language skills. In this program, students need not know how to type or spell, which makes use by children and aging adults who have dexterity problems possible. Students can enter their responses either by clicking on a picture response with the mouse or by typing a single key on the keyboard. Three kinds of exercises are provided in each version. First, students receive analytic practice, where they learn to identify sounds, words, and simple phrases. For example, in one analytic activity, a man appears on the computer monitor and says the word, *cat*, and then a woman appears and says the same word. The student's task is to indicate whether the two words are the *same* or *different*. (Even though words spoken by a man and woman are acoustically different, they are phonetically the same. This is an important concept to realize, especially if training is to generalize to real-world contexts.) In the second kind of exercise, which is called unrelated sentence practice, students recognize unrelated sentences. A talker appears on the computer monitor and speaks a sentence. Afterwards, four pictures appear, one of which illustrates the sentence. The student clicks on an alternative. If the response is correct, the text of the sentence appears on the screen, and the talker reappears and speaks the sentence. If the response is incorrect, five repair strategies are offered: repeat the original sentence, rephrase it, simplify if, elaborate it, or provide a keyword (topic word). Whichever option the student selects, it happens right away. The talker reappears on the monitor and performs the selected option. This continues for a particular sentence until the student selects the correct alternative or until no picture alternatives remain. As with the second program in *Conversation*

Made Easy, the third program provides synthetic speechreading practice. However, the sentences are related by context (e.g., for children, one exercise concerns a math class, another a science class, another lunch in the school cafeteria; for adults, one exercise concerns a visit to the physician, another a visit to the bank, another ordering in a restaurant). The materials were shot on location (e.g., a school classroom or a hospital) and provide a simulation of real-world listening environments. In addition to using the repair strategies described for the second program, the student may also use facilitative strategies. For example, if the teacher is filmed from the back of the classroom, the student can request to "move to the front of the classroom." If this option is selected, the "teacher" reappears on the computer monitor and repeats the sentence, this time filmed at a closer range. These latter two programs in *Conversation Made Easy* thereby provided practice in using both repair strategies and facilitative strategies, in addition to speechreading.

There are several advantages to using computerized instruction to supplement other aural rehabilitation efforts. These advantages include the following:

- Many items can be presented in a short period of time. For example, we found that in 3 days, adult patients working on program one of *Conversation Made Easy* completed an average of 1,800 training items. Concentrated training leads to faster learning and maintains a student's interest.
- For most available programs, the computer keeps a record of the student's response during training. Thus, even though the student may perform the training exercises at home, the clinician can still monitor training progress.
- The student can practice speechreading many people without leaving the clinic or home. For example, in the program for children in *Conversation Made Easy*, 16 different people in the second program alone speak training sentences. In the third program, many of the talkers are children, because children need practice in speechreading other children.
- For most programs, training is interactive, which is not always possible with standard audiovisual recorded materials. This interaction means that a student's response to one training item determines what will happen next. Response-contingency is an important element in any instructional design.

- Instruction is self-paced. Students can proceed through an exercise as slowly or as quickly as they choose.
- Training can occur at the student's convenience. For many people, such as those who work during the day or those who do not have transportation, coming to a speech and hearing clinic for speechreading training poses logistical problems. By using a computerized program, students can choose where and when to receive practice.

The aural rehabilitation specialist need not be present in the room while the student performs the training activities. Because aural rehabilitation is often labor-intensive and expensive, the use of computerized instruction may be one means of establishing better cost-benefit ratios. The aural rehabilitation specialist might be available to discuss the training goals and training results with the student and might role-play and practice some of the training activities with the student.

▇ EFFICACY OF SPEECHREADING TRAINING

Many researchers have considered whether speechreading skills can be developed through training and practice. At present, this issue has not been resolved clearly; some investigators report that training improves performance (e.g., Walden et al., 1981; Walden et al., 1977; Bernstein, Auer, & Tucker, 2001; Sims et al., 2002), whereas others report that speechreading training provides little measurable benefit (e.g., Heider & Heider, 1940; Lesner et al., 1987). When improvements do occur, they appear to be modest. For instance, investigators have demonstrated that adults with hearing impairment show only small improvement following training, typically improving by 10–15% in their ability to recognize speech stimuli (e.g., Alcantara et al., 1990; Gagné, Dinon, & Parsons, 1991; Walden et al., 1981).

"Before I walked into his office, I told myself, 'I can do this! I've been doing it on the computer all week.'"

—*Bonnie, recounting her visit to her doctor, after taking a situation-specific computerized speech reading training program*

Often, results are inconclusive or present contradictory findings. Some people may not show improvement in their performance on a test of audiovisual speech recognition. However, if you ask them whether they feel they benefited from speechreading training, they may provide an ardent testimonial in support of training. Some individuals may become better test takers, so their speechreading skills only appear to improve, rather than actually improving. For instance, Gagné et al. (1991) evaluated the effectiveness of a computerized speechreading training program in which participants received speechreading practice by using a modified continuous discourse tracking procedure. Changes in speechreading performance were determined by comparing scores on standard speech recognition tests obtained prior to the training program to scores obtained after training. The participants did not improve on most of the standard tests. However, they were able to repeat more words verbatim per minute during the continuous discourse tracking task posttraining than pretraining. The researchers cautioned that the improved tracking rates might have resulted from 25–30 hours of practice with the tracking procedure during training, rather than from improved visual speech recognition skills.

Few investigators have examined the extent to which children improve following training. It is possible that they have more potential to benefit from this kind of training than do adults.

CASE STUDY 1

A case study presented by Witt (1997) tells an unusual story about a man (JT) who had used a cochlear implant for 9 years. He was considered by his audiologist to be neither a "star" user, nor a "poor" user, but reflective of the average adult who uses a cochlear implant. What makes the case study unusual is that JT had used his implant for 9 years prior to entering an intensive 10-day aural rehabilitation program, where he received approximately 40 hours of aural rehabilitation therapy. It is more common for adult cochlear implant users to engage in aural rehabilitation immediately following implantation.

At the time of the study, JT was 51 years old. Although he was diagnosed with a mild hearing loss at the age of 5 years, his hearing did not worsen until he was 28 years old. He had lost his hearing completely by the time he was 41 years old.

The aural rehabilitation program included auditory training, speechreading training, assertiveness training, and telephone training (i.e., how to converse effectively on the telephone

(continues)

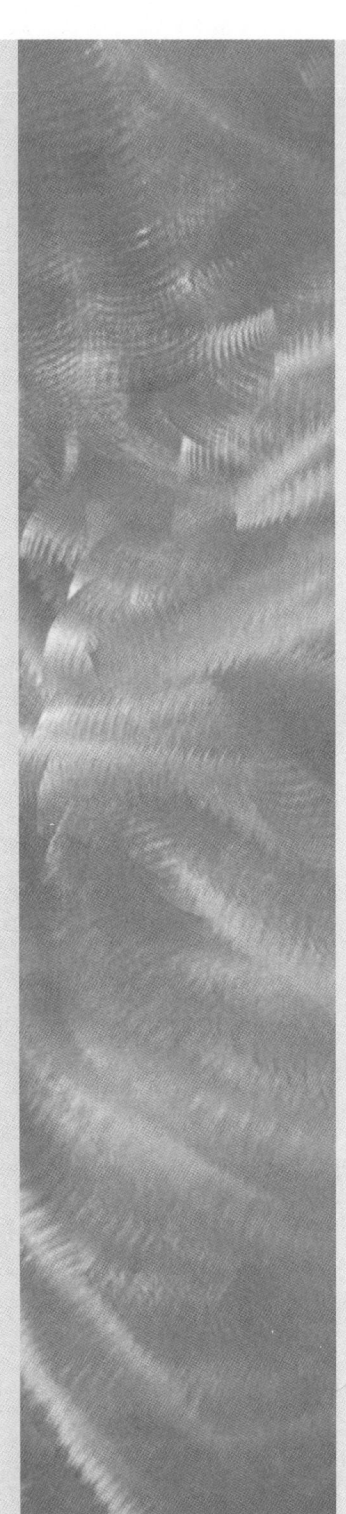

using conversational strategies). For the speechreading component, the audiologist identified those sounds that JT had the most difficulty recognizing auditorally (e.g., /k, g/). Those sounds were targeted during analytic speechreading training. In addition, the synthetic training materials were heavily weighted with these target sounds. JT practiced speechreading both with a clinician and with computerized materials (at the time, available in laser video disc format and now available in CD-ROM format, Tye-Murray, 2002c).

At the beginning of training, JT appeared intent on recognizing every sound in a message. For instance, the following exchange occurred between JT and his clinician (pp. 37–38):

Clinician: "I said, 'Is he ill?' You thought I said, 'Is she Gill?'"

JT: "I know."

Clinician: "Okay, maybe Gill is a female name, I thought it was a male name."

JT: "I knew I had it wrong when I said it, but the /s/ and the /h/ kind of all merge together here and I just said what I heard."

Clinician: "Okay, and now that you think about it and look at it, well, Gill is an odd name. If I would have said, 'Is he Bob?', you probably would not have said, 'Is she Bob?'"

JT: "I might have because I'm not thinking of the meaning in this exercise."

Clinician: "Okay."

JT: "I'm just repeating what I heard."

Clinician: "Okay, you're just repeating what you heard."

JT: "Yeah."

Clinician: "Okay, so you're not necessarily comprehending."

JT: "Right."

At the end of training, JT engaged in a synthetic training exercise that required him to answer questions. He responded

(continues)

correctly to all of the questions, demonstrating that he both recognized the speech and comprehended the message. Afterwards, he commented, "The hearing part wasn't the effort, the effort was the explaining. As we got into it I kind of relaxed and had fun."

Two measures suggest that his ability to comprehend speech in an audiovisual condition improved as a result of training (a standard test of speechreading was not administered before and after intervention). First, a test accessing how well JT could speechread and simultaneously perform a hand task *(Color Change-Dual Task)* demonstrated that he did not have to devote as much attention to recognizing utterances following training. He showed improvement on this test both immediately after training and 2 months later. Hence, he could devote greater mental energy to comprehending what he was speechreading and formulating an appropriate response. Similarly, his performance increased on a short term memory test following training, suggesting that he maintained more of what he speechread. Apparently, he was able to allocate more mental energy to storing information and less mental energy to recognizing the message on the face and with his residual hearing. At the end of training, JT recorded in his diary, "I try listening to my wife and kids. . . . My confidence is much higher. . . . I have confidence that I will recognize sounds and that recognition provides useful information to me. I think that before rehab I lacked confidence."

This case study demonstrates one of the more subtle benefits of speechreading training. With some patients, the speechreading task becomes less effortful following training, allowing them to devote more mental energy to comprehending the message and less energy to identifying sounds and words. In part, this gain may relate to an increase in confidence and, in part, to an increased facility to recognize speech audiovisually. This study also demonstrates how a clinician has the opportunity to tailor the aural rehabilitation program to meet the individual needs of the patient. JT had expressed frustration with using the telephone, so his program included telephone training. He had difficulty recognizing specific speech sounds, so his program included a preponderance of these sounds during speechreading training.

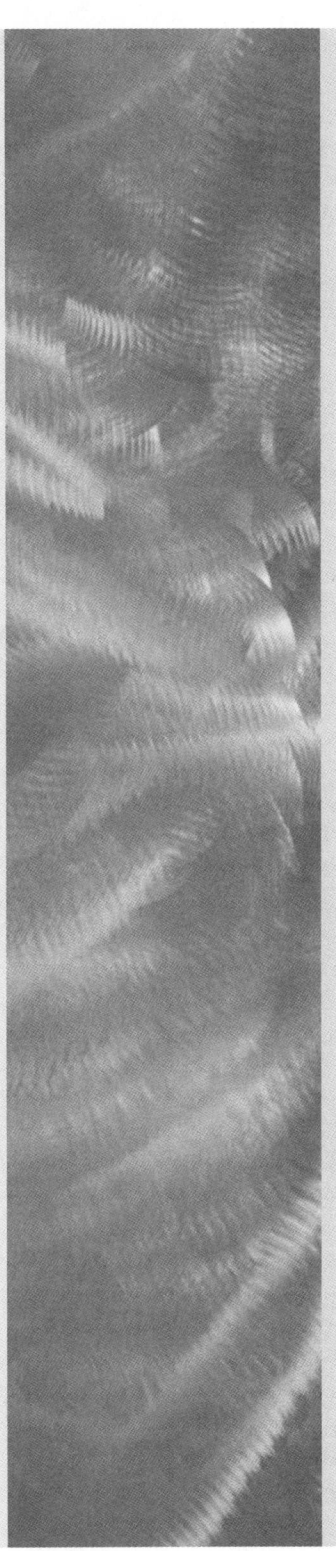

◼◼ FINAL REMARKS

At one time, many adults received aural rehabilitation that was comprised primarily of speechreading training. With the advent of sophisticated listening devices, and the increase of communication strategies training, few adults receive a great deal of speechreading training, and rarely is it provided in the absence of other aural rehabilitation services. Nonetheless, it is important for persons with hearing impairment to understand why speechreading is so difficult. The emphasis of speechreading training may be on ways to minimize the difficulty of the task, such as ways to manage the environment or ways to encourage appropriate speaking behaviors on the part of their communication partners.

◼◼ KEY CHAPTER POINTS

- ✔ Speechreading training was popular in the first half of the 20th century. The advent of more sophisticated listening devices, and questions about the benefits of training, have led to a reduced emphasis on speechreading training in an aural rehabilitation program.
- ✔ As with auditory training, a speechreading training program typically includes both analytic and synthetic training objectives.
- ✔ The logic underlying many speechreading curricula is gradually to increase students' reliance on the auditory signal for recognizing phonemic contrasts.
- ✔ Computerized speechreading training offer many benefits, including intensive practice and schedule flexibility.
- ✔ Research suggests that speechreading training provides perhaps modest benefit for adults. Little research has been performed with children.

■ MULTIPLE CHOICE QUESTIONS

1. If a person is a candidate for intensive speechreading training, this person is most likely to be:
   a. A new recipient of a cochlear implant
   b. An experienced hearing-aid user
   c. A younger adult
   d. A graduate of an oral school

2. Which of the following statements is false?
   a. The visual speech signal complements the auditory signal.
   b. The visual speech signal is redundant with the information provided by residual hearing.
   c. The visual signal presents a good deal of information about place of production.
   d. The visual signal presents information that helps the speechreader distinguish /i/ from /u/ from /a/.

3. Which exercise might appear later during a speechreading training curriculum rather than earlier?
   a. The student will discriminate consonant pairs that differ in place of production.
   b. The student will discriminate consonant pairs that share place of production, but that differ in voice and manner.
   c. The student will identify words that begin with consonants that share place of production, from a six-item response set.
   d. The student will identify words that begin with consonants that do not share place of production, from a six-item response set.

4. Asking a child to color in the states of a map of the United States (e.g., *Color Maine with the color red.*) is an example of what kind of training activity?
   a. Synthetic
   b. Analytic
   c. Identification
   d. Discrimination

5. The advantages of computerized instruction include:
    a. Patients can become familiar with a talker's facial movements.
    b. Patients can forego interactions with an aural rehabilitation specialist.
    c. Training can occur outside of the clinical setting.
    d. Patients can design their own exercises.

6. The best way to describe the data about the efficacy of traditional analytical and synthetic speechreading training is:
    a. Most data are supportive.
    b. Most data are nonsupportive.
    c. Analytic training is superior to synthetic training.
    d. The results are equivocal.

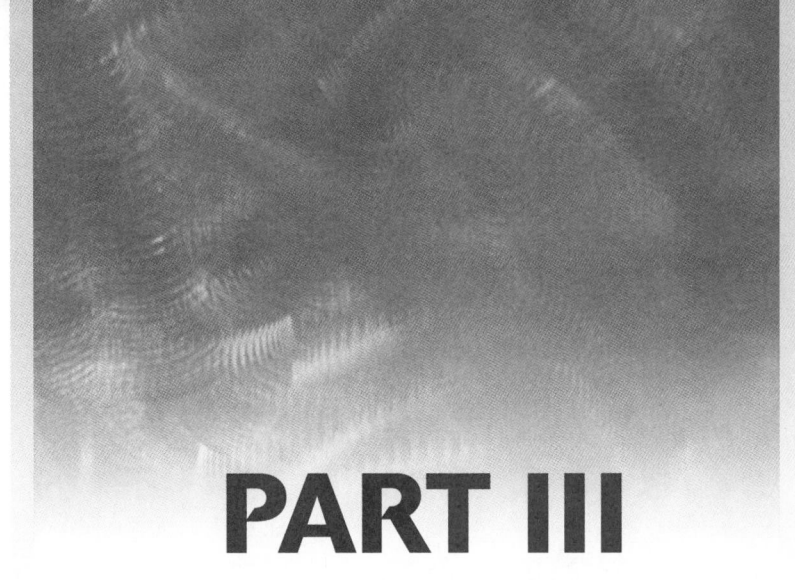

PART III

Aural Rehabilitation for Adults

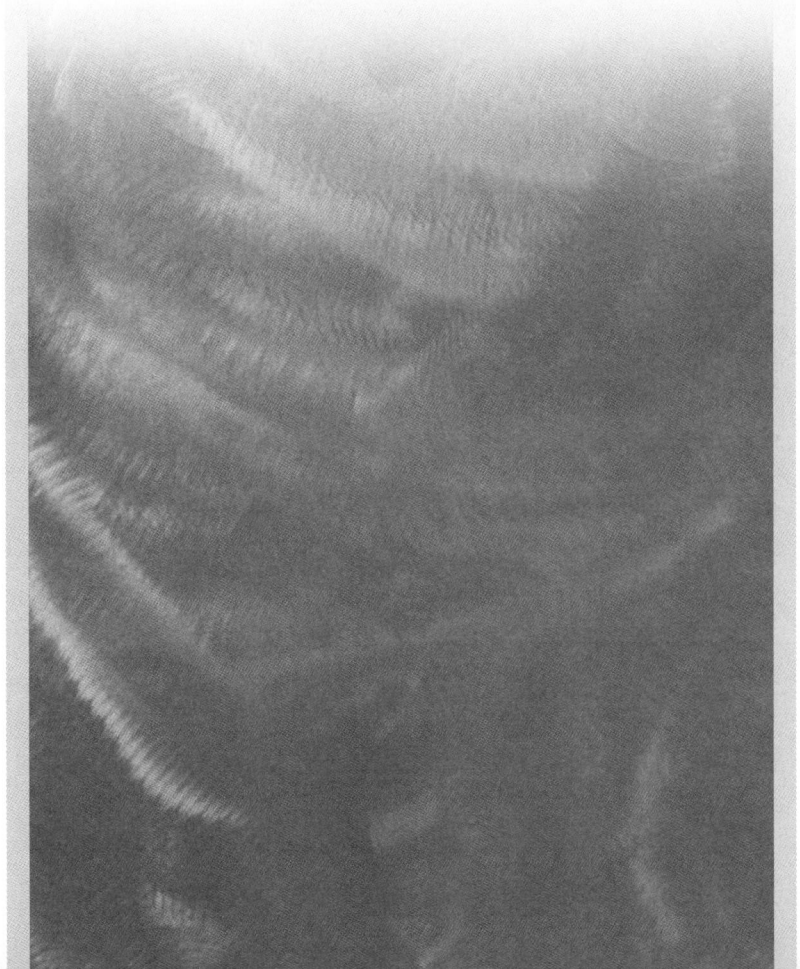

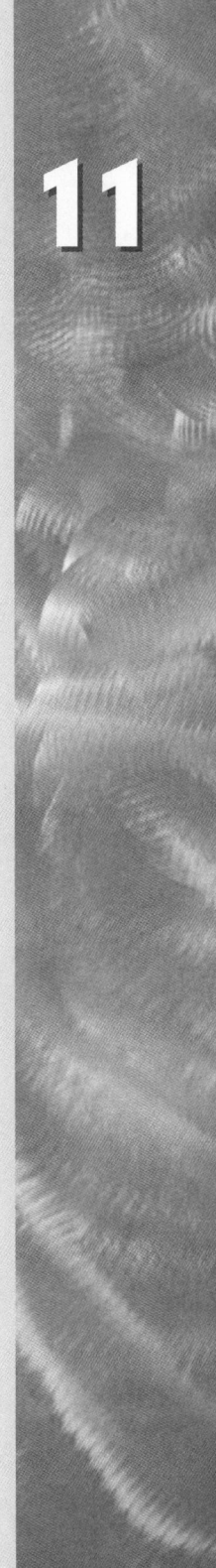

CHAPTER 11

Adults Who Have Hearing Loss

TOPICS

One of the major forces shaping American society in the first decades of the third millennium is the aging of our population. As the baby boom generation matures, an increasing number of adults are seeking hearing-related services. In this chapter, we are concerned with persons who are over the age of 16 years. Although much of what we review will be applicable to the entire adult population, Chapter 13 is devoted to special considerations for older adults, individuals who are over the age of 55 years.

It is important to develop a good sense of who the patient is and where the person is in terms of adjusting to hearing loss. We will consider first the "who" issue, and then the "where-in-terms-of-adjustment." Our guiding theme is as follows:

Any successful aural rehabilitation plan must be founded on a patient orientation.

A **patient orientation** to rehabilitation designs and delivers rehabilitation services based on the patient's background, current status, needs, and wants.

A **sales orientation** to rehabilitation emphasizes persuading the patient to pursue and procure services, interventions, and listening devices.

This is a simple idea that is the essence of a service practice. A *patient orientation* holds that the most successful aural rehabilitation program is one that best determines individuals' backgrounds, current status, needs, and wants and then accommodates them through the design and delivery of appropriate interventions. This is in contrast to a *sales orientation,* in which the emphasis is on telling or persuading people that they need certain aural rehabilitation services or listening devices and that your practice is better than the competition at providing them.

As we shall see, this philosophic orientation does not mean that we must begin with a blank slate with every new patient. Rather, certain aural rehabilitation offerings may be more appropriate for some persons than for others, and variable parameters of those services can be adjusted to meet a targeted individual need. A person who has minimal residual hearing may not receive auditory training, but rather, communication strategies and speechreading training. An individual with a mild hearing loss may receive only a hearing aid and counseling.

An important outcome of this philosophy is a high level of patient satisfaction with the aural rehabilitation plan. Individuals who receive services based on a patient orientation model usually report improved adjustment to hearing loss. They may remark, "The communication strategies program was great—I feel more in control of my hearing problems now," or "My audiologist took the time to listen, and the hearing aid she gave me made a big difference in my ability to perform at work." Such satisfaction ensures continued compliance with the plan, as well as positive word-of-mouth publicity for your service. This, in turn, will allow you to attract and serve even more people.

WHO KNOWS BEST?

In an article about why 21 million people in the United States do nothing about their hearing loss (roughly, 80% of persons with hearing loss), Taylor and Hansen (2002) suggest that professionals in the hearing health-care field might change the way they counsel potential patients. Instead of focusing on the selling of products and services, we should instead focus on the patient: What triggered his or her visit to the clinic and what is the best way to move the patient toward taking ownership of the hearing difficulties? In discussing this premise, Taylor and Hansen note:

> "We have been taught that we 'know what is best for the patient.' Unfortunately, reluctant patients are not 'getting' our message. It is even more unfortunate that hearing care professionals aren't getting the message either. *The answer to reluctance resides in the patient, not in the hearing professionals.* One cannot tell, advise, or cajole the reluctant patient into understanding and accepting their disability. If telling, advising, or complaining about the patient's hearing impairment worked consistently, the 'nagging' spouse, friends, and loved ones would have succeeded years ago in persuading throngs of people to positively address their disability. . . .

> So often in the hearing health care field, professionals are consumed with 'The Close.' This is not to imply that we're obsessed with selling products or services; rather, there is a tendency to jump forward to the conclusion before allowing the patient to come to that conclusion for him/herself. In short, we need to see our role as a hearing care professional differently. We need to become more interested in the *opening* of the patient. Nothing can be closed if it is not opened first. *It is a monumental occurrence that the reluctant, frightened, anxious, nervous, angry patient that you regularly see has come to the office*

Ownership: Feeling of responsibility and need to manage or oversee.

in the first place. We need to find out what trigger has finally caused the person to come in after putting off the visit for 7–10 years. There is a great need to move the patient toward ***ownership*** of their visit to the clinic, and not allow the patient to delude him/herself by blaming their visit on some external force like their spouse." (pp. 32–33)

▆ HEARING LOSS AMONG ADULTS

Most adults lose their hearing gradually over time. The largest segment of the hard-of-hearing adult population has mild or moderate sensorineural hearing loss. Typically, thresholds for the mid and high frequencies are poorer than those for the lower frequencies, regardless of the patient's age. The magnitude of hearing loss tends to progress with advancing age.

Hard-of-hearing adults may perceive conversational speech as too soft and as sounding mumbled. The greater loss of sensitivity in the higher frequencies compared to the milder loss in the lower frequencies often results in reception of the low-pitched acoustic segments associated with vowel sounds but not the high-pitched segments associated with consonant sounds. Hence, a commonly heard complaint among hard-of-hearing adults is, "I can hear people talk but I can't understand what they say." The presence of background noise exacerbates this problem because it can further mask the high-pitched consonant sounds that are difficult to discriminate even in quiet. Similarly, females or children may be more difficult to understand than males, due to their characteristically high-pitched voices and softer speaking levels.

▆ WHO IS THIS PERSON?

In addressing the question, "Who is my patient?" you will consider a number of variables, including a patient's stage of life, life factors, socioeconomic status, race and ethnicity, gender, psychological adjustment, type of communication difficulties, other hearing-related complaints, and onset of loss (Figure 11-1) You will also consider the patient's age, a variable we review in the next chapter.

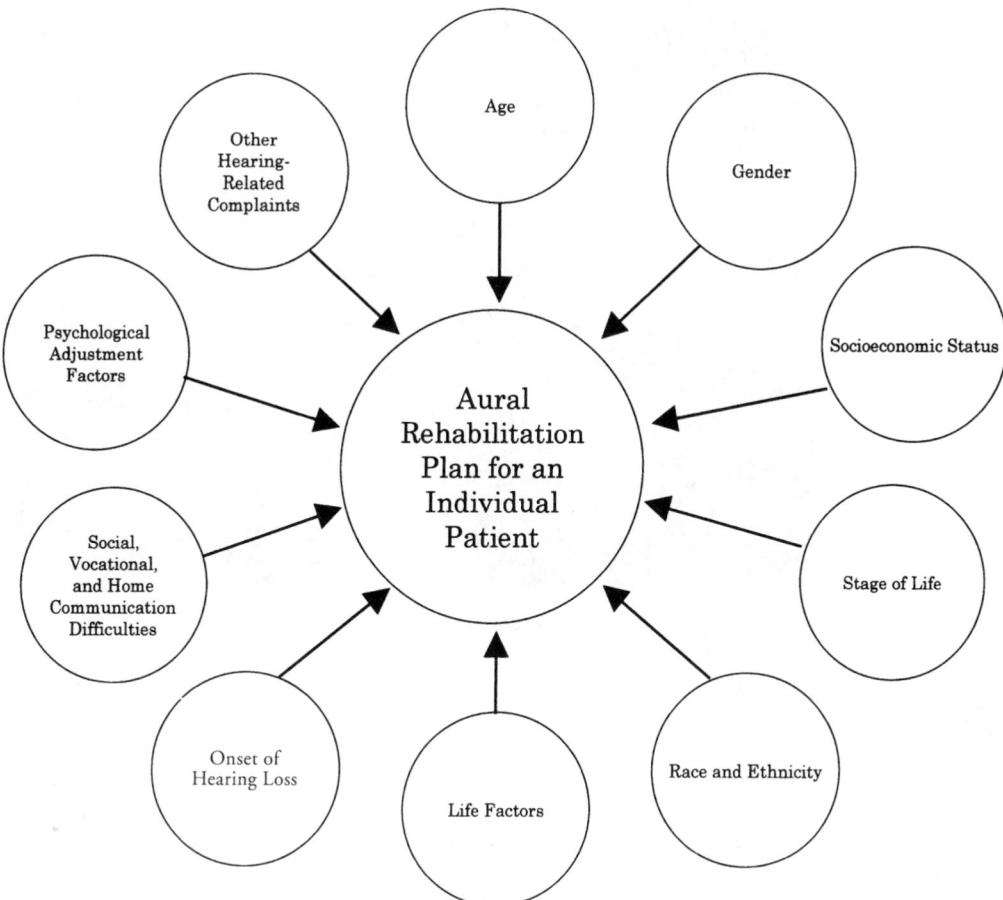

FIGURE 11-1. Variables that influence the design of a patient's aural rehabilitation plan.

Stage of Life

Jim Lawson and his 20-year-old son Kevin were in a car accident. Both received head trauma and, as a result, incurred irreversible bilateral hearing losses (Figure 11-2).

For both Lawsons, life with hearing loss will never be like it was before the accident. However, the impact differs somewhat because the two men are in different stages of life.

Jim Lawson owns a small advertising firm, which he started after college graduation. After many years of long hours and hard work, the firm is well-established and successful.

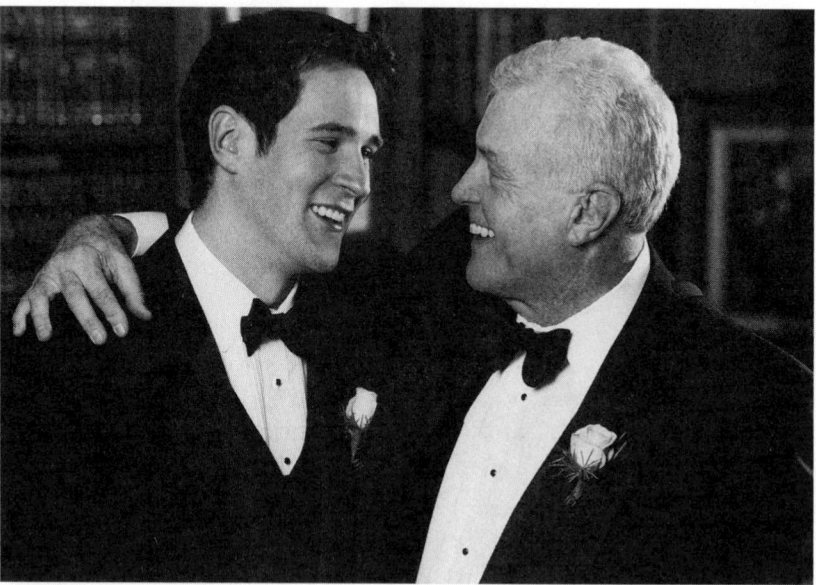

FIGURE 11-2. An aural rehabilitation plan may vary as a function of a patient's stage of life.

The accident has left Jim filled with bitterness. He believes life has dealt him a blow just when he was experiencing decreased responsibilities and more freedom to pursue leisure activities. He now contemplates early retirement because his hearing loss interferes with his ability to interact with clients, but also has misgivings because he had hoped to have a larger savings account before retiring. Jim no longer socializes at executive meetings and plays less tennis because he cannot converse easily with his friends on the court. He feels old and frequently is saddened by passing thoughts, such as the fact that he will never hear the voices of his grandchildren. Increasingly, he depends on his wife for communication with the outside world.

Jim's son is a junior in college with a major in public relations. Prior to the accident, Kevin Lawson participated in several extracurricular activities and dreamed of creating a public relations empire.

The hearing loss has left Kevin deflated. Because public relations entails communication, he wonders whether he should complete his college program. He feels embarrassed by the use of a professional notetaker in class, but fears that asking classmates to share notes might elicit pity. Kevin spends hours alone in the gym lifting weights, bedeviled by concerns for his future.

Table 11-1 summarizes *life stages* and indicates how hearing loss may have an impact (Van Hecke, 1994). Hard-of-hearing persons often experience similar emotions such as frustration, and they experience common difficulties such as communication breakdown. However, as the example of the Lawson family illustrates, the impact of hearing loss relates to an individual's *stage of life,* that is, whether the individual is in young adulthood, in the 30s, 40s, 50s, or in the later years. Depending on their life stage, patients will confront different issues. By being sensitive to where they are in the life span, you will gain additional insight into their concerns and aural rehabilitation needs.

Life stages are ranges in which a hearing loss may have a different impact.

Life Factors

By adulthood, most people have achieved socialization. They have established relationships with others, embarked on a vocation, and developed a personality and a personal view of the world. *Life factors* are in place. These factors may be socially and culturally determined, controlled by the individual, fixed, determined by the environment, or influenced by other qualities of the individual and his or her life situation. As with demographic factors, life factors influence the ways in which people cope with the advent of hearing loss. For instance, an individual with a heart problem and an extended family may not be as concerned about a subsequent mild or moderate hearing loss than someone who has been taking antidepressants and who has recently lost a job. Someone who holds prejudices about hearing loss beforehand may suffer from a negative self-image and self-stigmatization afterwards.

Life factors are conditions that help define one's life, such as relationships, family, and vocation.

Figure 11-3 presents a model of the life factor influences that have an impact on how a male patient might view hearing loss, factors that also have an impact on the patient's aural rehabilitation needs. The figure is comprised of concentric circles corresponding to self, home, work, recreation, and community. First, there is the innermost circle of self. Prior to hearing loss onset, this person viewed himself as competent and independent. Hearing loss may have at least one of two effects on his perceived role and self. He may either come away with the belief of,

Table 11-1. Life stages and the impact of hearing loss (see Van Hecke, 1994).

STAGE	EVENTS ASSOCIATED WITH STAGE	IMPACT OF HEARING LOSS
Young adulthood	Develop intimate relationships with others	Begin to reassess dreams
	Develop a vision of one's future life and begin to pursue dreams	Experience self-doubt about finding life partner
The thirties	Reassess life decisions (e.g., Is this the right job?)	Energy is not invested in reassessment
	Modify life structures or reverse decisions that now seem inappropriate	Hesitation about change arises
	Invest self in job, family, and friends	
Middle adulthood	Begin to consider own mortality	Upward mobility may cease
	Note clear signs of physical aging in self	Uncertainty about goals and ability to achieve them may increase
	May feel that this is last chance to make life changes	
The fifties	Children may have left home	May consider early retirement
	Career may be well-established	Fears of aging intensify
	Time is available to pursue leisure activities	Withdrawal from leisure activities may occur
Late adulthood	Deterioration occurs in health, physical attractiveness, and strength	Other problems related to aging are intensified (e.g., loneliness)
	Friends and family are lost through death or relocation as a result of retirement	Overall sense of loss is exacerbated
	One begins to review one's life and reflect on its meaning	

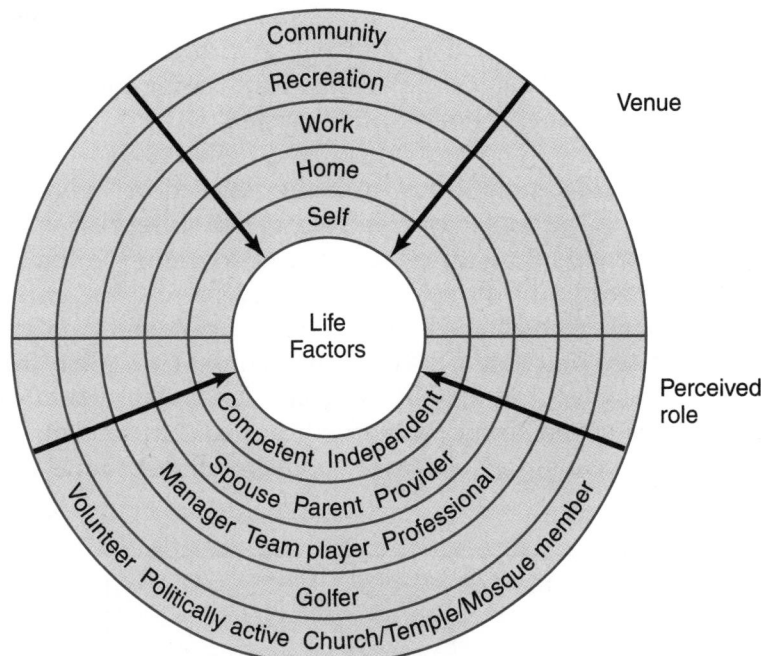

FIGURE 11-3. Life factors influence how a patient will react to the onset of hearing loss and will affect the content of an aural rehabilitation intervention plan.

"I can handle my hearing difficulties, I've tackled tougher obstacles before." Alternatively, the onset of hearing loss may pull the rug out from under who he thinks he is and fill him with a sense of loss of self. The next ring of influence is the home. In this venue, the patient may fill the roles of husband, father, and principal wage-earner. He may believe that hearing loss undermines his ability to fulfill these roles, especially if his wife and children believe likewise and hold negative stereotyped images of persons who have hearing loss. At work, the hearing loss may hamper the person's ability to manage employees and interact with colleagues during group meetings. This scenario may be especially true if he is the first person in his company to present significant hearing loss and if his workplace is unfamiliar with accommodating his listening needs. On the golf course, he may become the object of subtle teasing from his golf partners, whereas in the community, he might encounter ignorance and prejudice about disabilities. Such reactions from the community, recreational venues, and even the workplace, may result in the patient withdrawing into himself and succumbing to feelings of uncertainty and isolation. The constricting arrows in Figure 11-3 reflect a common tendency of persons with hearing loss to withdraw and to cope ineffectively with hearing loss.

The influence of community is furthered detailed in Figure 11-4 (see Hogan, 2001, Chapter 1). Here, our patient is represented as a jigsaw puzzle who might be rearranged according to the surrounding community norms, services, and mores. The patient will live in a world that has definite notions about who is an ideal citizen and to what extent a disability removes a person from achieving this ideal. He may live in community that views deafness as a tragedy, a social problem, or a medical problem. The community, and its prevailing viewpoints, will determine what

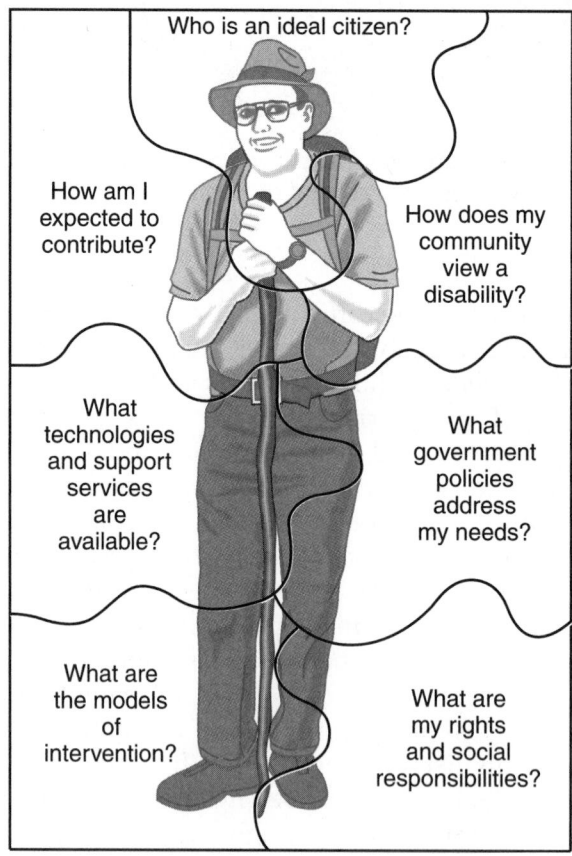

FIGURE 11-4. The community will affect how well a patient functions with hearing loss.

support services and technologies are available, and what expectations are placed on the patient about how he or she should lead his/her life. The community will help the patient answer such questions as, *What kind of help do I need and where will I get it? How am I to live my life as a person with hearing loss? What kind of financial and technical support might I expect?* and *How am I to contribute to the world around me and live my life?*

Socioeconomic Status

In addition to stage of life and life factors, one's socioeconomic status can affect the impact of hearing loss and the design of an aural rehabilitation plan. Social scientists have defined at least six socioeconomic classes in American society. One's classification within this schema is based on a consideration of income, occupation, educational level, and dwelling type. These six classes are:

- high uppers
- low uppers
- high middles
- low middles
- high lowers
- low lowers

In general, you will find that persons with lower incomes (below $20,000 per year) and less education (no high school diploma) are more likely to have hearing loss than persons with higher income (over $50,000 per year) and a high school diploma (National Council on Aging, 1999).

Ways in which socioeconomic status may affect the management of hearing loss are illustrated in the following examples:

- Financial status may relate to whether an individual can afford binaural hearing aids or assistive devices.
- Educational history may determine how much background knowledge someone has about the anatomy of the ear and its possible disorders and may dictate how the problem is discussed.
- Work schedule and level of employment may determine whether someone is able to attend aural rehabilitation classes scheduled during a weekday.

Race and Ethnicity

Health researchers tell us that socioeconomic status is closely linked with racial/ethnic status. African Americans, Hispanics, and Native Americans tend to have lower levels of income, education, wealth, and occupational status than do Whites. Their poverty rates are on average three times higher. Not only will their lower socioeconomic status affect the management of hearing loss, as just suggested, but it will have other ramifications as well. For instance, many adults of a minority may have experienced economic hardship and inadequate medical care growing up. Some may be inexperienced with interacting with health-care professionals or may be distrustful of them. Some members of minority groups may hold jobs that do not offer health-care benefits or they may be unemployed, so they may not have access to the best health care possible. They may live in poorer, less sought after neighborhoods (even if they share the same level of income as their White counterparts), and the health-care services may not match the quality, availability, and affordability of those available in more affluent neighborhoods. For instance, closures of hospitals and health clinics happen more often in low-income and minority neighborhoods (Caesar & Williams, 2002).

The last U.S. census revealed that our diversity has increased significantly during the past 10 years and will continue to do so (Figure 11-5). If current trends continue, by the year 2050, 50% of the population will be ethnically or racially diverse. About 30 years ago, the United States Bureau of the Census identified standardized categories for identifying race or ethnicity. These categories included:

- White
- African American
- Native American
- Eskimo
- Aleut
- Asian-Pacific Islander
- Hispanic American

Almost as soon as they were described, these categories proved inadequate. For instance, within the Hispanic American category alone, there are at least four discrete subcultures:

- Puerto Rican
- Mexican

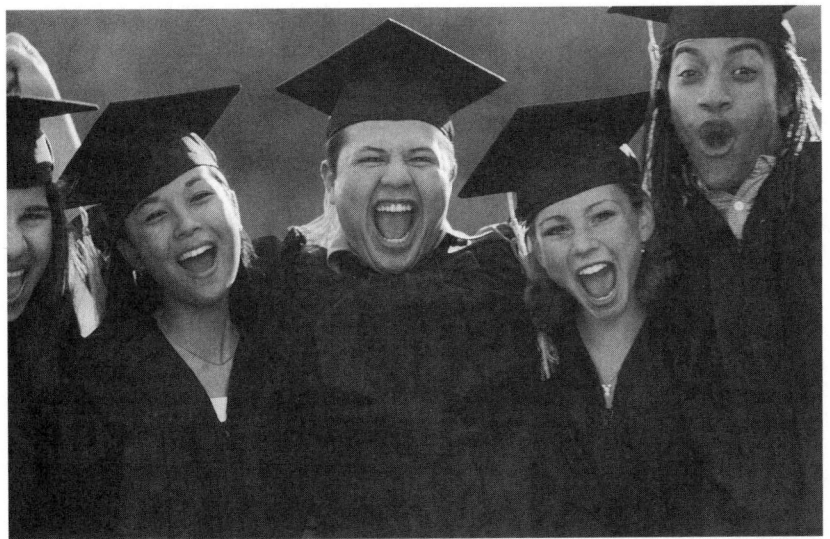

FIGURE 11-5. We are a world of cultural and ethnic diversity. Speech and hearing professionals should try to be sensitive to this diversity, and tailor their aural rehabilitation plans accordingly.

■ Cuban
■ Central American

With this shortcoming in mind, it is still valuable to consider the general make-up of the U.S. population according to broad categories so as to gain an appreciation of the diversity of the patients we will be serving. The U.S. Census Bureau's 1999 Current Population Report (*ASHA Leader*, 2002) revealed that:

■ 35.3 million respondents described themselves as Hispanic.
■ 34.6 million respondents described themselves as African American or black.
■ 10.2 million respondents described themselves as Asian.
■ 2.4 million described themselves as Native American or Alaskan native.
■ 15.3 described themselves as "some other race," but not "White."

Hearing loss is more prevalent in Whites than either African American or Hispanic populations. For example, almost 5% of Whites between the ages of 18 and 44 years have hearing loss. In contrast, only 1% of young African American adults and 3% of

Mexican Americans: Largest subgroup of Hispanics in the United States. The majority of Mexican Americans live in the Southwest: Texas, New Mexico, Arizona, and California.

Puerto Ricans: Second largest subgroup of Hispanics. The majority live in northern cities, such as New York and Chicago. In part because of Puerto Rico's commonwealth status, many move back and forth between the two countries.

Cuban Americans: The majority live in Florida, their families having arrived in the United States following Castro's formation of a communist government in 1959.

Central Americans: Persons from Central and South America have increasingly arrived in the United States, many as a result of political and social upheavals in such countries as Nicaragua, El Salvador, and Chile.

young Hispanics have hearing loss. About 30% of White adults aged 65 years or older have hearing loss, whereas only 7% of both older African American and Hispanic adults have hearing loss (Figure 11-6) (National Center for Health Statistics, 1994).

Unfortunately, despite the increasing diversity (and the complexity of that diversity) of our patient population, and the relatively high rate of occurrence of hearing loss, many speech and hearing professionals feel unprepared to serve multicultural populations. An ASHA 2001 Omnibus Survey showed that 31% of its members felt only "Slightly qualified" to provide services to multicultural populations, whereas 14% felt "Not at all qualified." Only 10% considered themselves to be "Very qualified" (*ASHA Leader*, 2002, p. 32). There is a great need for speech and hearing professionals to learn more about the people they serve, through developing relationships with people who can serve as cultural informants, by attending cultural events in their communities, and by learning how a patient's linguistic and cultural background might influence the clinical decision-making process (Tomoeda & Bayles, 2002, p. 17). For instance, racial or ethnic groups often have distinctive customs, beliefs, and service preferences, and these must be considered when customizing an aural rehabilitation program. For example, hearing loss may have greater impact on self-concepts of masculinity and femininity within a subcul-

FIGURE 11-6. African Americans are less likely to experience hearing loss than whites. Men are more likely to incur a loss than are women.

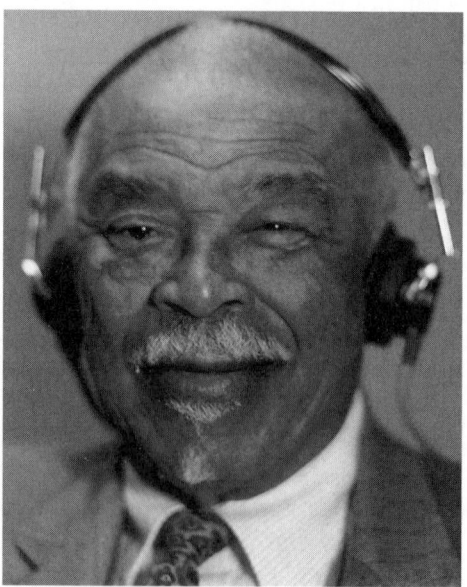

ture described as Mexican than within a subculture described as second-generation Japanese American, so counseling may be different for the two groups. The content of a communication strategies training program may be appropriate for some groups but not for others. For instance, a member of an Aleut culture may feel uncomfortable in asking a conversational partner to repeat a message following a communication breakdown, as this may be interpreted as a sign of rudeness within his or her social milieu. Thus, it might be inappropriate for the hearing professional to encourage use of the repeat repair strategy during the course of a communication strategies training program.

Sensitivity to Cultural Issues

CalOptima is an HMO in Orange, California that provides training to health-care workers who provide services to Latino, Vietnamese, and Cambodian patients. They offer these tips (Anders, 1997)

- Seek eye contact with Latino patients.
- Forgo eye contact with some Asian patients.
- Avoid using patients' children as interpreters; family dynamics may make it difficult to get candid answers.
- Address older patients in most nonwhite groups by surname and Mr. or Mrs. (p. B1).

Gender

Prevalence of hearing loss varies by gender, with men having an 11% overall prevalence and women having a 7% overall prevalence. Patients' gender may influence the content of their aural rehabilitation program (Figure 11-7). For example, in a traditional family structure, an adult female may fear that hearing loss decreases her ability to nurture her children, and she may experience a loss of self-esteem and sense of desirability. A hard-of-hearing male adult may worry that he has lost his means to provide financially for his offspring and believe that he has become less manly or less vigorous in the eyes of his friends. In these two examples, counseling will have to be tailored to suit individual concerns.

FIGURE 11-7. Gender may influence the design of an aural rehabilitation plan. Women and men may vary in their financial resources, their physiological responses to hearing loss, and their everyday listening demands.

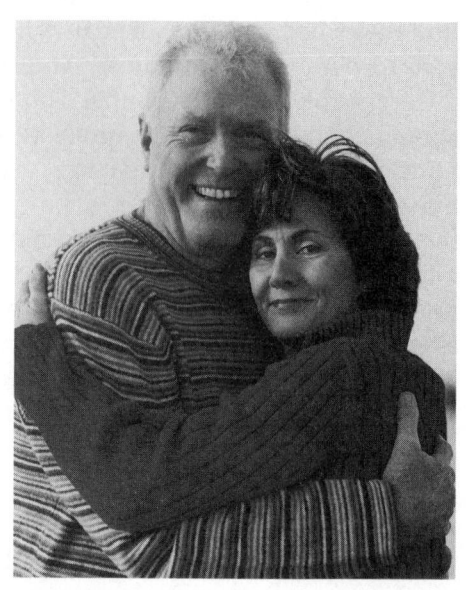

Gender effects on the aural rehabilitation needs of patients have not been well studied by researchers, although a few investigators have tackled the issue, especially with regard to the older population. Garstecki and Erler (1999) found that older females are more reliant on nonverbal repair strategies than are older males (as determined by the CPHI, see Chapter 3), and that women place a greater importance on being able to communicate in social situations. Older women also appear to be more likely to experience negative feelings (such as annoyance, anger, and aggravation) and stress during everyday communication and are more sensitive to the negative reactions of families and friends. In this study, females were more likely to report acknowledging a hearing loss than were males, and they were more likely to report actively reducing their communication difficulties (e.g., seeking favorable seating at a lecture hall). Both behaviors bode well for a successful aural rehabilitation intervention.

As is the case with race and ethnicity, gender can be divided into subcategories. For instance, females can be divided into subsegments of "homemakers" and "workers." The latter group can be distinguished further, for example, two categories are clinical-technical and management professionals. As a function of their subsegment, individuals will require different aural rehabilitation interventions. For example, a homemaker may be interested in obtaining a baby-cry alerting assistive device, whereas a business executive may inquire about group amplification systems.

The age of female patients may also affect the aural rehabilitation intervention. For example, Erler and Garstecki (in press) found that younger women (those between the ages of 35 and 45 years) viewed hearing loss and the use of hearing aids more negatively than did older women (those between the ages of 75 and 85 years). One reason is that hearing loss may pose a greater communication handicap for younger women. They tend to be engaged in child-rearing, work, and situations that require effective communication. Another reason is that older women usually have more friends and relatives who have hearing loss and who use hearing aids, and thus, hearing loss and the use of amplification are not as foreign to them as they might be to younger women.

Psychological Adjustment Factors

Psychological reactions that some hard-of-hearing individuals experience when learning of and adapting to a hearing loss may correspond to those experienced by terminally ill patients, although their emotions may be muted by comparison with sick persons. Where they are in terms of psychological adjustment will influence the kinds of aural rehabilitation services that are appropriate at any point in time.

Psychological responses to hearing loss may begin as shock and disbelief, followed by depression, then anger and guilt, and finally, acceptance. Some feel numb or disorganized when the audiologist describes their test results. They then may deny a problem exists and may blame their listening problems on other factors.

A milder version of shock and disbelief relates to *dissonance theory.* Most people do not want to receive messages that run counter to their own self-perception and self-image. They may object to audiological findings that do not fit well with their own cognitions. "Hey, I can't have a hearing loss," a young person may think, "I run marathons—my body is in great shape." Some individuals may attempt to reassert their views of the world either by searching for a disconfirmation of the diagnosis or by minimizing the importance of it. For instance, one woman made a point of telling a family member whenever she heard a noise in the next room, "See, I heard that!" Others may dismiss the hearing loss as being insignificant. "Yes," someone might say, "I miss some things, but most of what I miss isn't worth hearing anyway."

Dissonance theory concerns situations in which one's self-perception does not coincide with reality.

Depression often follows denial in reaching acceptance of a hearing loss.

Depression may follow denial, or a mourning for what has been lost (e.g., the loss of hearing, the loss of effortless conversation) and for what may lie ahead (e.g., a continued decrease in hearing, an increase in feelings of powerlessness). Persons may feel isolated from friends and family as they miss out on casual conversational exchanges. They may need to depend more on others for navigating communication with the outside world, and they may experience a concomitant decrease in self-esteem. An inability to hear environmental and body sounds, such as leaves rustling or their footsteps on the pavement, may intensify feelings of loss, as may a decreased ability to enjoy music. One woman reported, "For a while I felt tired and disinterested all the time. My daughter would ask me to go shopping and I'd say 'no.' Someone would say the sun was going to shine that day and I'd say 'so what?' I had a weight in my heart. I never felt elation and I never felt disappointment. It took me months to realize that I was depressed, and that the depression was related to my hearing loss."

Anger and **guilt** are stages that sometimes follow depression in adjusting to a hearing loss.

Anger and *guilt* may bubble up after depression, as patients realize that their lives have been inalterably changed . "Why me?" they may ask, or "What did I do to deserve this?" There may be a perception of unfairness, and a person may protest, "But I am too young to be going deaf!"

Acceptance: the final stage of adjustment to a hearing loss in which the patient realizes that life goes on, albeit differently.

Over time, *acceptance* of the hearing loss occurs. The intensity of feeling stemming from depression, anger, and anxiety cannot be maintained, and a sense of normalcy returns. The realization emerges that life goes on, albeit differently than before. As one man said, "I'm not too happy about my hearing, but I figure no one's going to take me out behind the barn and shoot me!"

Other Hearing-Related Complaints

Tinnitus is the sensation of noise in the head without an external cause.

Some patients will experience other impairments related to their hearing loss, the most common of which is tinnitus. *Tinnitus* is noise that is perceived in the ear or head and has no external physical source. The word is a derivative of the Latin word *tinnire*, which means to ring or tinkle. Tinnitus often accompanies adult hearing loss, although individuals with normal hearing also experience it. The prevalence of tinnitus in the general population may be 35%, with 17% of the population reporting that it is continuously or frequently present. This means that about

40 to 50 million people in the United States suffer from tinnitus (Davis & Refaie, 2000). The incidence of tinnitus in Europe is similarly high. British epidemiologists suggest that 0.5% of the general United Kingdom's population experience tinnitus that can be described as a "problem" (Coles, 1984). In Sweden, 2.6% of the population describe tinnitus as a "severe problem" (Axelsson & Ringdahl, 1989). About 85% of individuals who have ear problems report tinnitus (McFadden, 1982). Tinnitus is correlated with degree of hearing loss, with those who have greater hearing loss also having a greater subjective complaint of tinnitus. It is not correlated with age (Hazell, 1990). The presence of tinnitis may greatly influence, and even determine, the aural rehabilitation intervention.

Common descriptors of tinnitus include leaves rustling, the ocean roaring, crickets chirping, a radio playing off-station, a siren blasting, or a telephone ringing. The quality of sound might be crackling, pulsing, pounding, hissing, humming, musical, throbbing, whistling, popping, or whooshing. A person might perceive sound in the right ear, left ear, both ears, or inside or outside of the head.

As Table 11-2 indicates, etiologies of tinnitus relate to every level of the auditory system, although there is no clear understanding of the neuronal mechanisms that underlie it. Tinnitus can be triggered by factors associated with the external ear, middle ear, central nervous system, and especially, factors associated with the inner ear. Most tinnitus problems likely emerge from an interplay of peripheral and central factors. For instance, an abnormality at the level of the cochlea may lead to the generation of a weak neuronal signal. The signal may be detected on the conscious level as sound and, with continued occurrences, may become irritating to the patient and lead to a heightened cognitive awareness of the phantom signal. Subsequently, greater negative emotional reactions may result when the signal is detected, which may in turn lead to even greater awareness (Jastreboff, 1990).

Certain conditions or medications can exacerbate a tinnitus problem. For instance, some patients report that tinnitus worsens following stress or after taking aspirin. Table 11-2 presents a list of possible causes.

For some people, tinnitus is a minor annoyance that is bothersome only in quiet situations, such as when trying to go to sleep.

"Tinnitus puts an additional amount of stress on someone who is very often struggling to keep up with conversation anyway. An overlay of noise ranging from 'buzzing noises' to a 'full scale band playing' . . . can be the final stress factor which makes it impossible to cope. But it can be inconjunction with other factors that tinnitus is problematic, Not being able to sleep, as a result of tinnitus, causes fatigue, irritability during the day, disrupts the rest of the family, and may cause marital problems."

—Jones, Kyle, and Wood, 1987, Pg. 87.

Table 11-2. Examples of causes of tinnitus.

LOCUS/SOURCE	CAUSE
External ear	Impacted cerumen
Middle ear	Otitis media, otosclerosis, vascular anomalies, middle ear tumors
Inner ear	Ménières disease, presbycusis, ototoxicity, circulation problems, noise-induced hearing loss
Central nervous system	Migraine, acoustic neuroma, epilepsy, tumors
Other	Allergies, emotional or mental stress, medication (e.g., aminoglycoside antibiotics, indomethacin, quinine, salicylates), noise exposure, use of a hearing aid, physical work, lack of sleep, heavy smoking, alcohol

Source: Adapted from Stouffer, J. L., and Tyler, R. S. (1990). Characterization of tinnitus patients. *Journal of Speech and Hearing Disorders, 55,* 439–453.

For a significant number, however, tinnitus is debilitating, the cause of frustration, depression, hopelessness, and even thoughts of suicide. Tinnitus can result in an inability to concentrate, increased difficulty in listening because it can mask the speech signal, and loss of sleep.

Because tinnitus cannot be measured objectively, it often is difficult to quantify its degree or to understand the magnitude of disability it presents. Some ways to obtain information include patient interviews and questionnaires. Some existing questionnaires include open-ended questions (Tyler & Baker, 1983). Some include quantifiable items such as those listed below (e.g., Stouffer & Tyler, 1990), presented here with example kinds of questions:

- **Location:** Is it in the left ear, right ear, or both ears?
- **Pitch:** On a continuum corresponding to pitch, is it high pitched or low pitched?
- **Constancy:** Is the tinnitus always present? Is it intermittent? Do you tend to notice it at a particular time of day?
- **Composition:** Do you hear one sound or more than one sound?
- **Fluctuations:** Does the tinnitus change from one sound to another? Does it change in pitch?

- **Loudness:** On a continuum corresponding to loudness, is it loud or soft?
- **Conditions that exacerbate the tinnitus:** What conditions exacerbate the tinnitus (e.g., drinking coffee, smoking)?
- **Annoyance:** On a continuum corresponding to annoyance, can the tinnitus be described as not at all annoying, extremely annoying, or somewhere in between?
- **Effects on concentration and sleep:** Does it have a slight effect? Extreme effect?
- **Depression:** Does it cause minimal depression? Extreme depression?

Tinnitus Can Be Terrifying

Few people realize how debilitating tinnitus can be. Actor William Shatner, star of the Star Trek television series and movies, has experienced tinnitus for almost a decade. As the following excerpt demonstrates, he experienced desperate moments before finding some relief through a therapy offered by Dr. Pawel Jastreboff (Shatner, 1997):

"Over the years I tried herbal remedies. I tried eardrops. I bought masking devices to avoid the silence, and tapes and records of soothing sounds—Japanese music, running water. And inside my house is a little waterfall. The sound of the water is very soothing.

Getting through the nights—that was always the worst. Sometimes I paced the halls. I often turned to writing and exercise, and fatigued myself to sleep. I'd have the television on all night. It affected my marriage; if one person needs noise and the other person is sensitive to it, it can lead to separation . . . I could not sleep without sound. In my darkest moments I thought to myself, 'Will it be this way for the rest of my life, the way I am tormented by it now?' I began to think, 'What are the ways to take my life? How does one kill oneself?' I went so far as to start making plans." (pp. 154–155)

Mr. Shatner's essay ended on a somber note. He related, "Recently I made a call to somebody in California who had promised Dr. Jasterboff money, and when I called, his wife answered and said he was dead. He had committed suicide because of tinnitus" (p. 155).

Age at Onset of Hearing Loss

Heretofore, we have considered adults who are hard-of-hearing: adults who lost their hearing after acquiring speech and language. Now we will consider adults who acquired their losses before learning language and speech. Onset of hearing loss will greatly influence the nature and extent of aural rehabilitation intervention.

Deafness: Disability or Culture?

"Hearing people are always surprised to learn that deaf parents in neonatal wards cheer when they are told their babies cannot hear. Deaf Culture families see any effort to teach the deaf to speak as repugnant: The ASL sign for cochlear implant is a two-fingered stab to the back of the neck. 'Let me put it this way,' says Judith Coryell, head of Western Maryland's deaf education program and the mother of two deaf children. 'Say you were black. Do you think you'd be considering surgery to make yourself white?'" (Arana-Ward, 1997, p. 21).

DEAF CULTURE

Deaf Culture: a subculture that shares a common language (American Sign Language), beliefs, customs, arts, history, and folklore, primarily composed of individuals who have prelingual deafness.

Adult members of the ***Deaf Culture*** are individuals who lost their hearing early in life. They rely on sign language for face-to-face communication, and many believe they are culturally and linguistically distinct from hearing society. Members of the Deaf Culture use a capital D in the term "Deaf" to distinguish themselves from the audiologic condition of hearing loss. Membership in the Deaf Culture is not determined by one's degree of hearing loss, but rather, by one's identification with Deaf people. For example, two individuals may have identical severe bilateral hearing losses. One of them may use powerful hearing aids and feel a part of the hearing world, whereas the other may socialize primarily with Deaf people (Giolas & Kaplan, 1997).

Deaf individuals become acculturated by means of educational experiences and social interactions. They usually have attended schools or classrooms for the Deaf and, as adults, they interact with Deaf groups, such as those centered around religious gatherings or sports. Most Deaf individuals marry a Deaf spouse.[1]

RECENT HISTORY

Table 11-3 presents a chronology of significant events in the recent history of the Deaf Culture. The past four decades have brought about an increased visibility of the Deaf culture. Two landmark events in more recent history are the appointment of I. King Jordan as president of Gallaudet College in 1988 (now Gallaudet University) and the approval of multichannel cochlear implants for use in children by the Food and Drug Administration in 1990. These two events signify two major forces affecting Deaf adults: the growth and expression of Deaf pride and advances in medical technology.

Unfortunately, these two forces often collide in purpose. Many Deaf adults reject the infirmity model of deafness implied by the use of cochlear implants (i.e., "there's a deficit here so let's fix it with surgery"). Some Deaf adults fear that use of cochlear implants may erase their culture, especially because postimplant rehabilitation for children often includes an emphasis on speech and listening skills and a de-emphasis on the use of American Sign Language (ASL). Deaf pride, personified by the 1988 protests at Gallaudet, leads to a celebration of cultural difference in which significant hearing loss is an entryway into a minority community with shared mores, language (ASL, art forms, and traditions).

DEAF AND HARD-OF-HEARING ADULTS

In some ways, members of the Deaf Culture have different problems than hard-of-hearing individuals. For instance, unlike many adventitiously hearing-impaired adults, many members of the Deaf Culture have limited or nonexistent speech production skills, and their voices may sound strained and harsh. They may be academically delayed (many Deaf individuals never achieve more than a fourth grade reading level), and they may gravitate

---

[1] Not all Deaf individuals agree with the isolationist segment of the Deaf Culture. Some believe that deafness is a disability and that self-segregation is counterproductive. Although they still consider themselves to belong to Deaf society, these Deaf adults may not object to efforts to identify treatments, such as cochlear implants.

Table 11-3. Some significant events in the Deaf Culture movement since the 1960s.

1960s	Civil rights movement becomes visible in mainstream America: Deaf people became aware of their own ethnic possibilities.
	The largest worldwide rubella epidemic in recorded history results in a great influx of deaf children into the public school systems from 1964 to 1965, while there is a concurrent decline in the number of children with normal hearing.
1970s	Congress passes Public Law 94-142, the Education for All Handicapped Children Act, in 1975, which mandates public education of children with handicaps within the public school system, and subsequently contributes to declining enrollments in public residential schools and increasing enrollments in public day classes.
	A general consensus emerges among linguists that ASL is an official language.
	Congress passes the Rehabilitation Act of 1973 (Section 504), which prohibits federally supported programs or activities from discriminating against qualified handicapped people.
1980s	A "Deaf Pride" movement grows rapidly among young deaf adults.
	In 1988, I. King Jordan becomes the first deaf president of the country's oldest institute of higher learning for the deaf, Gallaudet University, after students stage a demonstration protesting the appointment of a hearing president.
	Harlan Lane, a professor of psychology at Northeastern University in Boston, publishes *When the Mind Hears: A History of the Deaf,* a book condemning the history of oral communication in America.
1990s	Schools for Deaf children increasingly hire Deaf teachers and administrators.
	The Food and Drug Administration (FDA) approves multichannel cochlear implants for use in children in 1990.
	The Americans with Disabilities Act (ADA) (P.L. 101-336) is passed into law in 1990 and extends civil rights protection to people with disabilities in private and federal sectors.
	The National Association of the Deaf (NAD) presents a position paper, stating that "The NAD deplores the decision of the Food and Drug Administration (to permit cochlear implantation of children) which was unsound scientifically, procedurally, and ethically" (*Broadcaster,* 1991).
	In 1994, some members of the Deaf Culture accuse Heather Whitestone, the country's first Deaf Miss America, of being an impostor because she primarily uses oral communication.
	In 2000s, NAD revises position paper, stating that cochlear implants are an acceptable listening technology, but should not preclude the use of sign language.

towards certain professions that offer limited opportunity for professional growth. However, unlike hard-of-hearing adults, many Deaf adults do not experience being cut off from the life they have known as a result of hearing loss. They can communicate with fellow signers, they have comfortable companionship with their family and require no extraordinary patience or accommodation, and they are free of many of the anxieties associated with attempts to function in a hearing world.

PSYCHOLOGICAL PROFILE

Some adults who incurred a significant hearing loss early in life present a shared psychological profile. They may be immature and may demonstrate a lack of social judgment. Some may be less flexible than adults who have normal hearing, and they may be more likely to adhere to a set routine. Other tendencies include irresponsibility, impulsivity, passivity, overacceptance, and a failure to appreciate the feelings or opinions of others (Jackson, 1992). Of course, no general description such as this can characterize an entire group of people, and you must take the time and make the effort necessary to know the individual.

PROFESSIONAL SERVICES FOR DEAF ADULTS

Deaf adults often do not solicit the kinds of services from hearing professionals that are sought by hard-of-hearing persons. For example, they may not seek hearing tests, they may not use hearing aids, and they may not be interested in communication training. Some of the professional services they may utilize include the following:

- Sign interpreting
- Notetaking
- Provision of assistive devices
- Academic and vocational counseling

Deaf persons who use speech may desire additional services as well. These include:

- **Speech and voice training:** Individuals may want to polish their speaking skills, especially if they have not received speech training for many years. They also may want an assessment of their speech, so they can better anticipate communication difficulties.
- **Communication strategies training:** Some individuals may desire training in the use of expressive and receptive communication strategies.

Professionals who interact with Deaf persons, even if only occasionally, should have some knowledge of sign language. In the best of circumstances, they should have enough skill in the use of sign to allow functional communication interactions. Kinsella-Meier (1996) notes:

> "If the language, cultural values, and beliefs held by Deaf persons are respected and understood by the clinician, then services can be provided more successfully . . . The Deaf person is likely to accommodate the hearing person by code switching to approximate English word order more closely if the hearing person is perceived to be willing to modify her own communication style." (pp. 9–10)

Sign interpreter: a professional who translates the spoken signal into a form of signed English or ASL, or vice versa.

Sign Interpreters

A *sign interpreter* is a professional who translates the spoken signal into a form of signed English or ASL, or vice versa. The interpreter does not participate in the dialogue, but simply conveys messages from one communication partner to the next. Examples of occasions in which a sign language interpreter might be utilized include one-on-one communication situations between a Deaf individual and an individual who does not know sign language, meetings, and lectures. Interpreters often accompany Deaf persons to medical, legal, and educational settings.

Professional interpreters may receive certification from the Registry of Interpreters for the Deaf (RID) or through other statewide screening programs. They are expected to adhere to a set of professional guidelines established by the RID. Scheetz (1993) summarizes the RID code of ethics:

- Interpreters shall keep all assignment-related information strictly confidential.
- Interpreters shall render the message faithfully, always conveying the content of the message and the spirit of the speaker, using language most readily understood by the person(s) whom they serve.
- Interpreters shall not counsel or advise those whom they serve, or interject personal opinions.
- Interpreters shall accept assignments using discretion with regard to skill, setting, and the consumers involved.
- Interpreters shall request compensation for services in a professional and judicious manner. (p. 274)

▰ WHERE IS THE PERSON IN TERMS OF ADJUSTMENT TO HEARING LOSS?

Now that we have considered the question of who is the patient, let us now address the question, *Where is the person in the adjustment process?* In this section, we will consider the time course of hearing loss, and where in the process the aural rehabilitation plan begins to be implemented. During your first interaction with an individual, you probably will ask questions about the progression of hearing loss. Questions may include the following:

- **When do you think your hearing loss began?**
- **How did you know you had a problem?**
- **What brought you here today?**

In recent years, much research has focused on the time course of hearing loss in hard-of-hearing adults, and how the quality of life alters throughout. Familiarity with this research will prove helpful as you ask these kinds of questions and as you consider the implications that the responses have for a person's aural rehabilitation plan.

The work of Jones, Kyle, and Wood (1987) provides a useful framework for considering adjustment to hearing loss. They identified four phases in the time course of acquired hearing loss. These four phases are summarized in Figure 11-8.

Phase 1: Pre-hearing Loss

As we have just learned, prior to incurring hearing loss, patients will have achieved a certain socioeconomic status, personality, and world view. Life factors are in place. With few exceptions, as

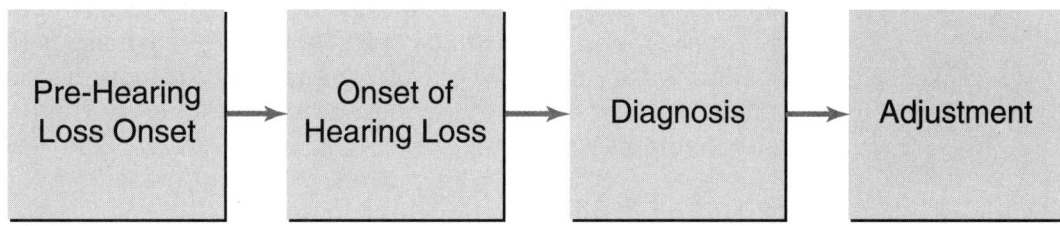

FIGURE 11-8. Four phases in the time course of acquired hearing loss.

in the case of adults who have a family history of hearing loss, few individuals ever anticipate they will suffer from hearing loss, especially while still younger than 65 years of age. Thus, when hearing loss begins, it usually takes a person by surprise.

Phase 2: Onset of Hearing Loss

Phase 2 is the time span stretching between the onset of hearing loss and diagnosis. Often, onset of hearing loss goes undetected. If asked when the loss began, a person may not know. As Hétu (1996) noted:

> "It takes a rather striking invalidation of one's percep- tual experience to start suspecting that one's sense organs no longer work properly. When hearing loss is progressive and symmetrical, there is no internal refer- ence by which to measure the decrease in one's hearing capabilities. Furthermore, a comparison with others' hearing capabilities is very limited." (p. 17)

The advance from mild loss to awareness might last anywhere from a few days to many years. Situations that often alert people to a problem include having to turn up the television or radio volume, having to ask people to repeat their messages, not hear- ing a doorbell or someone calling their name, and missing out on conversations that occur in the home. One man, reflecting on this phase, noted ruefully, "For about two years, I was snapping at my wife for talking too soft. Then I began to think that other people were mumbling too. It wasn't until my little grandson accused me of not paying attention that I thought to myself, maybe it's my hearing."

Other, less frequently cited indicants include complaining about bad telephone connections, believing that people mumble, and not knowing where sounds are coming from. Family members and others may remark about a patient's coping behaviors and rationalizations. In an initial interview, when a person may be exploring the possibility of hearing loss, the hearing professional might ask any of the following questions (based on Wayner & Abrahamson, 1996):

■ **Do you frequently ask people to repeat?**
■ **Do you feel that most people mumble?**

- Do you sometimes hear sound, but can't understand what is being said?
- Do you have to work hard to hear?
- Are you tired after you have listened for a lengthy period of time?
- Do people comment on the volume setting of your television programs?
- Has someone said that you speak too loudly in conversation?
- Has someone said that you missed what was said or did not react to speech?

When people begin to realize they have hearing loss, they often discuss the issue with family members before seeking formal diagnosis. However, they may not mention the problem at work. Many try not to disclose the presence of hearing loss to those outside the home, often for fear of stigmatization and discrimination.

Phase 3: Diagnosis

Phase 3 is a time when the hearing loss is identified by a professional and the extent of the problem is revealed. An individual may seek out the family doctor first, an otolaryngologist, or go directly to an audiologist. At this point, the individual might expect the hearing professional to provide a rapid solution, and he or she may expect a treatment and complete cure. Susan Jacobs was one such example. After her audiologist diagnosed a moderate bilateral sensorineural hearing loss, Susan responded, "My son had a hearing loss when he was 2 years old and the ear doctor gave him tubes. Now he's fine. You think surgery can help me?"

On realizing that hearing loss is here to stay, many people succumb to anxiety. They may worry about possible outcomes, such as decreased professional options, loss of independence, rejection by friends or family members, and altered social status. The magnitude of a person's anxiety may be mollified by what has occurred in Phase 2. For example, if someone has long suspected a hearing loss, then diagnosis may be less traumatic.

During the diagnostic process, the person's type and degree of hearing loss are determined, and the extent to which social, vocational, and educational activities are affected is explored.

Typically, you will obtain a pure-tone audiogram and administer speech-recognition tests. You probably will administer a self-report survey or questionnaire aimed at assessing communication handicap andor conduct an interview. The results will indicate how hearing loss interferes with everyday communication in the home, work, and social environments, and reveal related psychological difficulties. Answers to your questions will provide information about the need for amplification and assistive listening devices and the need for communication strategies training and psychological counseling.

THE INTERVIEW

When asking about the home environment, you will want to gain an idea of with whom an individual communicates, what his or her specific communication problems are, and whether assistive listening devices might be appropriate. Example questions concerning the home environment include:

- **Do you live alone? With a spouse? With children?**
- **What are your communication demands in the home?**
- **Do you watch television? Is hearing a problem?**
- **Do you have difficulty in detecting or identifying warning signals (e.g., telephone ringing, doorbell, alarm clock, a baby's cry)?**

When exploring the work environment, questions are asked about the physical environment of the workplace, specific work tasks performed by the individual, and current hearing-related problems. This information will be important as you consider appropriate listening devices, the need for noise protection, and the need for employer/employee education. Example questions about the work environment include:

- **Where do you work (e.g., a factory, an office, construction, in sales)?**
- **What is your physical work environment like (e.g., noisy, open space, quiet, small office)?**
- **Do you use or do you think you need protection for your ears against noise?**
- **Do you need to use the telephone? Is hearing a problem?**
- **Do you have to attend lectures or seminars?**

■ Do you need to recognize speech on a Dictaphone or a telephone answering machine?
■ Does your employer know about the Americans with Disabilities Act?

As with any group of adults, persons with hearing loss vary greatly in their predilections for social activities. Some people engage only in quiet, one-on-one activities; others interact in groups and attend social events such as concerts or lectures. For those who are more reclusive, you may explore whether they avoid social activities because they do not enjoy them or because they experience so many communication difficulties that the activities are unsatisfying. If the latter is the case, then you have specific direction to target your aural rehabilitation efforts. Example questions concerning the social environment include:

■ What do you do in your free time (e.g., go to movies, attend dinner parties, play bridge)?
■ What kinds of social situations do you avoid because of your hearing loss?
■ Have you ever used an assistive device in public?

Phase 4: Adjustment

In the final phase, adjustment to hearing loss, Phase 4, individuals begin to adapt to hearing loss. During Phase 4, a person may receive any or all of the following rehabilitation services: Counseling, psychosocial therapy, assertiveness training, hearing aid(s), assistive devices, and formal speechreading, listening, or communication strategies training. Aural rehabilitation is focused on minimizing or solving the communication problems identified in Phase 3.

A study conducted by Kerr and Cowie (1997) provides a general statement about the adjustment, or equilibrium state, that many people achieve. These researchers administered a questionnaire to and interviewed a group of deaf and hard-of-hearing adults who were under the age of 70 years old and who lived in the Belfast, Ireland, vicinity. In terms of the overall effect of hearing loss, almost 40% of the subjects reported that hearing loss had restricted their life at least badly, and 10% of these people felt that the hearing loss had almost destroyed their lives. These results are summarized in Figure 11-9. Factors that contributed to the experiential

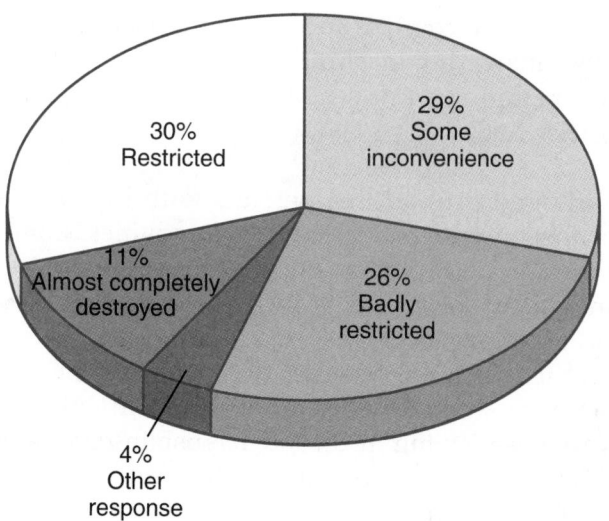

FIGURE 11-9. General effects of hearing loss on subjects' lives: Results reported by Kerr and Cowie. (Based on data presented in Kerr and Cowie, 1997)

dimensions of deafness were communicative deprivation and a sense of restriction. Those who believed that their lives were either badly or very badly affected by hearing reported that (p. 181):

- They long to hear particular sounds.
- Hearing people speak to them through someone else.
- Someone in the family, or a close friend takes over things they would do if they could hear properly.
- They find themselves spending more time at home because of their deafness.
- Hearing people ignore them in conversation.
- Someone goes with them to a medical or business appointment to help out in case their hearing makes things difficult.
- Their hearing loss holds them back from the kind of work they would like to do.
- They feel that their deafness places a strain on relationships with their family.
- They feel as if their deafness is like a glass case separating them from the world.

As this study by Kerr and Cowie (1997) implies, during adjustment to hearing loss, the patient might discover that his or her psychosocial well-being has been affected, in the home, social, and work environments. In addition, some individuals may incur negative experiences in the workplace.

PSYCHOSOCIAL WELL-BEING

As noted in Chapter 5, hard-of-hearing adults may be more likely to suffer from feelings of loneliness than their normal-hearing counterparts and more likely to experience decreased self-esteem and other emotional difficulties, including embarrassment, shame, and uncertainty about one's social identity (Hétu, 1996; Jones et al., 1987). They may feel isolated both socially and emotionally. Outside the home, adults with hearing loss may be restricted in their ability to develop and sustain relationships and may feel disconnected from their community. As their hearing losses progress, they may begin to perceive that acquaintances avoid them. For instance, one person noticed that acquaintances gradually quit talking to her at the swimming pool and other community gathering places.

At home, individuals may believe that those closest to them do not understand the ramifications of hearing loss, nor do they adequately accommodate their listening needs. Anger, frustration, and resentment directed toward one's spouse or children may be commonplace.

VOCATIONAL STATUS

Hard-of-hearing individuals may be more unhappy at work than the general population and have fewer vocational opportunities. Some people may experience a sense of being removed from the workplace mainstream, as they miss out on informal conversations and gossip. Professional growth and advancement also may be limited. For example, hard-of-hearing males between the ages of 45 and 61 years leave the workforce in higher numbers than males who have normal hearing (Armstrong, 1991). Some workers may find themselves the subject of disparaging remarks by their colleagues. A hard-of-hearing secretary once walked into the office lounge and found a co-worker entertaining others with an impersonation of her. The man perched reading glasses on the end of his nose (worn in a similar fashion as the secretary) and repeatedly bellowed "Huh?" into an imaginary telephone receiver. The secretary reported to her audiologists that she had felt mortified and hurt, and thereafter she began to eat lunch alone.

Adjustments by Family Members

Not only must patients adjust to hearing loss, but so too must their family members. Social and emotional issues that may arise include frustration over communication difficulties, impatience over the difficulties of communication (e.g., "Forget it, it's not worth repeating"), anger (e.g., "What am I supposed to do about your problem?"), guilt, and a sense of incompetence for not knowing how to minimize the listening problems for the hard-of-hearing person, pity, and anxiety (Wayner & Abrahamson, 1996).

We once posed the following question to a group of persons married to persons with significant hearing losses: "What are some of the most difficult aspects of living with a deaf family member?" Here are some of the responses:

Rhonda: "I'll list some of them: (1) Anger—communication is often difficult that he's 'not the same'; (2) concession—everyone has to change what it is he or she is doing or the way they do them (i.e., talking, listening to the TV); and (3) frustration—things have to be done his way to accommodate his hearing loss. It is just simply a whole new way of life. He has to deal with the fact that he is hearing impaired and being his family and loving him as we do, we deal (well or not) with all of the changes too."

Gerald: "I cannot communicate with her by phone when she is alone. I once called a next-door neighbor to tell her of a tornado warning—she is so damn independent she was upset about my doing that."

Mike: "Communication with a hearing impaired family member requires patience and determination. I'm sure the frustration is equally disturbing to my wife. Tempers sometimes flare as one or both attempt communication and fail. Often times communication is abandoned by one or both parties, leaving both equally frustrated."

Jan: "We have a captioning device on the TV and the kids sometimes get mad when he wants to see the news captioned and they may go to another TV—poor kids, hah!"

Anna: "I have to move and make sure he can see my face when I speak to him. And we less and less enjoy 'small talk' together. Hearing aids have helped but we have finally readied the point where we cannot talk to each other without extra effort."

Pam: "Trying to do business and explain to him what's going on. Especially if someone else is around, he gets real rude and frustrated at me because he can't hear or understand."

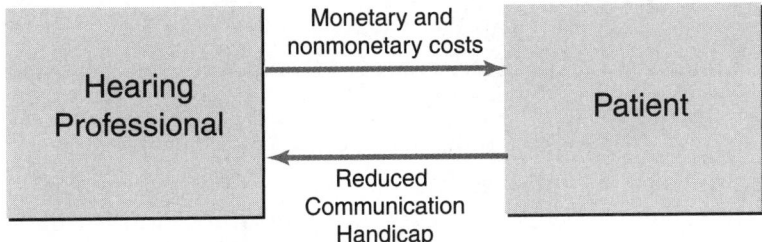

FIGURE 11-10. Monetary and nonmonetary costs associated with seeking aural rehabilitation services.

COSTS

It is important to realize that the adjustment phase extracts numerous costs from patients, both monetary and nonmonetary (Figure 11-10). For example, in the course of pursuing an audiological appointment, an individual may lay out money for transportation, the appointment itself, lost wages for the time spent during the appointment, payment for a babysitter if he or she has young children, parking fees, hearing aid molds, hearing aids, and so forth.

Perhaps less obvious and often overlooked are the nonmonetary or *psychic costs* of seeking services and adjusting to hearing loss. Such costs for people may include any of the following:

Psychic costs are nonmonetary costs that relate to a person's psychological well-being.

- **Acceptance** within themselves that they have a hearing problem
- **Anxiety** that they may be getting old
- **Awkwardness** for having to ask for time away from work and having to explain the reason for the request
- **Worry** that the hearing aid may cost too much or that the audiologist will take advantage of them
- **Fear** that nothing can be done to alleviate the communication difficulties
- **Embarrassment** for entering a hearing clinic

Often, a primary goal of the experienced hearing professional is to maximize the benefits in exchange for real and perceived monetary and nonmonetary costs.

CASE STUDY 1

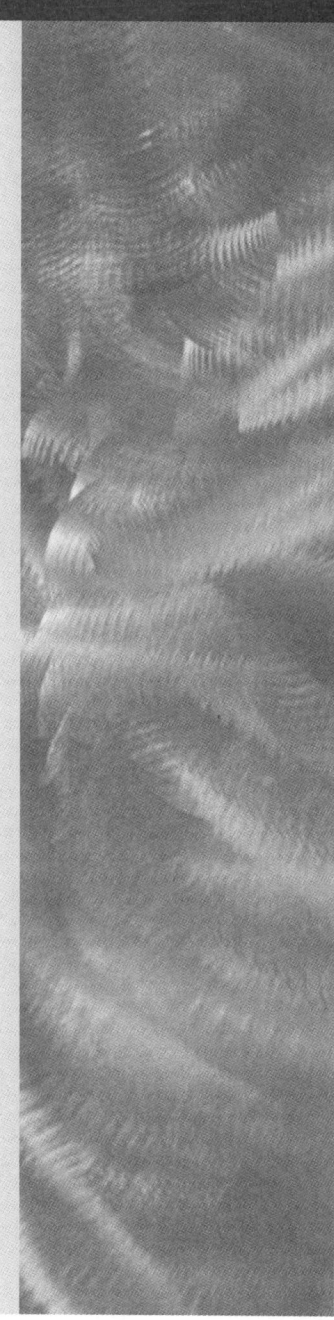

Many persons who seek the services of a speech and hearing professional will benefit from the use of a hearing aid or other listening aid. However, aural rehabilitation is not a profession of "one size fits all." Patients will vary greatly in the services and support they need before and after they receive a listening device. For example, Doug Kammer has just lost his job as a middle manager because his company merged with another. He is preoccupied with anxieties over his future: Will he get a new job? Does he no longer have the youthful look that employers are looking for? Will his savings tide him over during the interim period of unemployment? He knows at some level that he has a hearing loss and that if he is to be an effective member of a work team, he must be able to communicate effectively. Even so, accepting his hearing loss, taking ownership of his hearing problems, and pursuing a comprehensive aural rehabilitation plan are foreign ideas at this point in his personal turmoil.

Every morning, Mary Saunders starts her day with a flurry of activity—getting children ready for school, making lunches, driving carpool, and cleaning breakfast dishes. All this happens before she heads off to work as an office manager for a small law firm. Life as a single mother and sole breadwinner of two girls seems to be whizzing by her at 100 miles per hour. Some days, she feels like the day has turned into night, without ever providing her with a moment to herself. Lately, she has seemed detached from her surroundings. Her children accuse her of not listening and her co-workers tease her for being absent minded. Is she just over-stressed or is something else going on? A few days ago, she realized that she could not hear the high-pitched beeping tone of the office fax machine.

(continues)

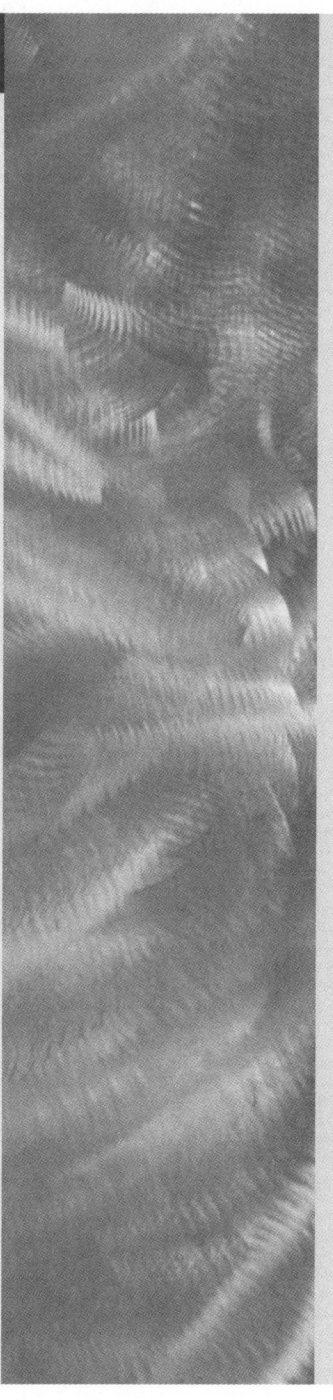

Carl King lost his wife last year. Since then, the new retiree has been struggling to get on with his life. His grown children come by his house several times a week, concerned about his psychological well-being and determined not to let him isolate himself inside his house. His daughter has talked him into going for a hearing test. She thinks one reason her father is withdrawing into himself is that he cannot hear in groups, and he cannot follow family conversations at the dinner table. Carl figures he will go to the hearing clinic to appease his daughter, but that is all he will do. Why get a hearing aid, he asks himself, when he lives alone with no one to talk to?

All these people could benefit from using a hearing aid and from receiving aural rehabilitation services before and after receiving one. Doug, Mary, and Carl live different lives, experience different demands, and harbor different hopes and expectations. Their aural rehabilitation plans must accommodate their differences. Doug needs to come to grips with the presence of his hearing loss and what having a hearing loss means in terms of his self-image. He needs to develop strategies for managing his hearing loss, both during his search for a new job and then in adjusting and accommodating to a new work setting. Mary will need to educate her children and co-workers about her communication difficulties and find time in her busy schedule to receive adequate hearing health care. Carl will have to develop the motivation to participate in everyday conversations, which may require him to expand his social network and to take a greater interest in the comings and goings of his children and grandchildren. These people will require many of the same aural rehabilitation services, but these services must be adjusted to accommodate who they are and where they are in terms of adjustment to hearing loss.

■ FINAL REMARKS

Aural rehabilitation begins with a solid understanding of the patient population. In this chapter, we have considered how adults with hearing loss differ in their cultural orientation, their demographics, their reactions to hearing loss, their communication needs and problems, and many other factors. We also have considered the four phases of adjustment to hearing loss. This information lays the groundwork for providing aural rehabilitation services to adults. In the next chapter, we consider the development of aural rehabilitation plans.

■ KEY CHAPTER POINTS

✔ A patient orientation holds that the most successful aural rehabilitation plan is one that best determines a patient's background, current status, needs, and wants and then accommodates these through the design and delivery of appropriate interventions.

✔ Most adults lose their hearing gradually over time. Typically, the loss is greatest in the high frequencies and least in the low frequencies.

✔ In following a patient orientation, you will determine "who the patient is." You will consider non-hearing-related variables such as stage of life, socioeconomic status, and psychological adjustment. These variables may affect the aural rehabilitation plan.

✔ Life factor influences pertain to self, home, work, recreation, and community. For instance, the norms, services, and morés that are present in the surrounding community will help the patient answer such questions as, *What kind of help do I need and where will I get it?* and *How am I to contribute to the world around me and live my life?*

✔ Socioeconomic status is related to racial/ethnic status. Some members of minority groups may be inexperienced with interacting with health-care professionals and some may be distrustful of them. Some minority members may not have access to quality care due to financial limitations or their location.

✔ Women are more likely to acknowledge a hearing loss than are men, and women are more likely to actively reduce their communication difficulties. Women are also less likely to incur a loss.

✔ Psychological responses to hearing loss may include the following stages: shock and disbelief, depression, anger and guilt, and, finally, acceptance. A milder form of shock and disbelief relates to dissonance theory ("this diagnosis runs counter to my self-image").

✔ Tinnitus can be debilitating.

✔ Adult members of the Deaf Culture lost their hearing early in life. They rely primarily on ASL for communication.

✔ There are four phases in an adult's adjustment to hearing loss: prehearing loss, onset of hearing loss, diagnosis, and adjustment. Aural rehabilitation often starts in the third phase. During this phase, you will want to identify a patient's particular communication problems at home, socially, and vocationally and begin to formulate solutions.

✔ Hard-of-hearing people may have more psychosocial and vocational difficulties than normally-hearing adults. They may suffer from feelings of loneliness and decreased self-esteem. They may have a sense of being removed from the workplace mainstream.

✔ Adjustment to hearing loss extracts both monetary and non-monetary costs. Psychic costs include acceptance within one's self that there is a hearing problem and anxiety of aging.

■ MULTIPLE CHOICE QUESTIONS

1. A patient orientation means that:
    a. The most successful program is one that best determines a patient's background, current status, needs, and wants and then accommodates them through the delivery of a customized aural rehabilitation plan.
    b. The most successful program is one that persuades patients to procure services.
    c. The most successful program is the one designed to accommodate the background, current status, needs, and wants of the typical patient and packages this program in a financially economical fashion.
    d. The most successful program assumes that every patient is unique, and that every plan must be from a blank slate.

2. A 50-year-old man arrives at an audiological clinic. He is most likely to have what configuration of hearing loss?

   a. Noise-induced hearing loss with the characteristic 4000 Hz "notch," so that hearing is poorer at 4000 Hz than at either 2000 Hz or 8000 Hz

   b. A sloping mild to moderate hearing loss

   c. A flat hearing loss

   d. An asymmetrical hearing loss

3. Which of the following is most likely to have an effect on the aural rehabilitation plan?

   a. The patient's religious affiliation

   b. The patient's membership in community organizations

   c. The patient's extended family

   d. The patient's stage of life

4. In the population of persons who have hearing loss, who is most likely to experience negative feelings and stress during everyday communication?

   a. Women

   b. Men

   c. Hispanics

   d. Native Americans

5. Which individual is most likely to be considered a member of the Deaf Culture?

   a. Jan, who was born with a severe-to-profound hearing loss and learned to speak and listen. She does not use sign language, because her deaf friends also speak and listen.

   b. Tom, who attended a residential school for the deaf and married his high school sweetheart.

   c. Steve, who went completely deaf at the age of 21.

   d. Jean, who lost her hearing at the age of 35 and learned sign language so she could communicate with other members of the Deaf Culture.

6. Which statement is true of tinnitus?

   a. Fifty percent of persons with hearing loss suffer from tinnitus.

   b. Tinnitus is correlated with age.

   c. Tinnitus is caused by an aberration in the cochlea.

d. Etiology may relate to every level of the auditory system.

7. Tinnitus can best be treated with:
   a. Aspirin.
   b. There is no treatment that is always effective.
   c. Neurophysiological medications.
   d. Meditation.

8. Aural rehabilitation begins during which phase in the time course of acquired hearing loss?
   a. Prehearing loss onset
   b. Onset of hearing loss
   c. Diagnosis
   d. Adjustment

9. Mrs. Davidson has anxiety that she is getting old. For this reason, she is reluctant to visit an audiologist clinic and have her hearing loss confirmed by an audiologist. This fear is an example of:
   a. Communication handicap
   b. Psychological consequence of hearing loss
   c. Life factor influences
   d. Nonmonetary costs of seeking aural rehabilitation services

10. A common tendency for persons with acquired hearing loss is to:
   a. Quit or change jobs
   b. Feel as if hearing loss has destroyed their lives
   c. To spend more time at home because of their hearing loss
   d. To achieve an equilibrium state in which they have overcome their embarrassment about their hearing difficulties and their uncertainty about their social identity

11. One way in which a speech and hearing professional can better serve his or her patient case load is to:
   a. Attend cultural events in the community and develop a relationship with a person who can serve as a cultural informant
   b. Adopt a sales orientation
   c. Learn how to better serve those members of the Deaf Culture who receive cochlear implants
   d. Become a certified interpreter

CHAPTER 12

Aural Rehabilitation Plans for Adults

TOPICS

- A strategy for plan development
- Counseling
- Hearing aids for adults
- Assistive listening devices and other assistive devices
- Follow-up
- Other kinds of intervention
- Case study
- Final remarks
- Key chapter points
- Multiple choice questions
- Key resources

In the last chapter, we discussed demographics for the adult population, progression of hearing loss, and steps for evaluating the magnitude of hearing loss and communication difficulties. In previous chapters we have discussed services that might comprise an aural rehabilitation plan, such as provision of amplification, assistive devices, and communication-strategies training. In this chapter, we bring these topics together and consider a systematic process for designing a patient-oriented aural rehabilitation plan for hard-of-hearing adults. This process usually requires the orchestration of a number of interventions, and these services often can be integrated in such a way as to achieve maximum benefit for the individual.

■ A STRATEGY FOR PLAN DEVELOPMENT

Figure 12-1 outlines the three component stages of developing a plan. These include: evaluation, strategy, and implementation.

Evaluation

First, the individual will be assessed, and his or her current status, wants, problems, and needs will be evaluated. This evaluation will allow the topics posed in Table 12-1 to be addressed. These topics pertain to patient demographics (e.g., Where is this person in terms of stage of life?), audiological and conversational needs (e.g., Is this person a candidate for a hearing aid?), and ecological concerns (e.g., Does the person work? If so, what are the communication demands associated with the workplace?). Topics to be evaluated also will include economics and psychosocial adjustment. For example, can the individual afford hearing aids? Is the person motivated to use them? During the evaluation stage, you will likely administer some of the assessment instruments we reviewed in Chapter 3, where we considered assessment of conversational fluency and communication handicap. These instruments include patient questionnaires and interviews. You will likely utilize the assessment instruments reviewed in Chapter 6 too, where we considered the assessment of hearing and speech recognition. These instruments include the audiogram, tests of speech recognition, and tests of lipreading and speechreading enhancement. These same measures may also be administered in the third stage of the aural rehabilitation plan, *implementation*.

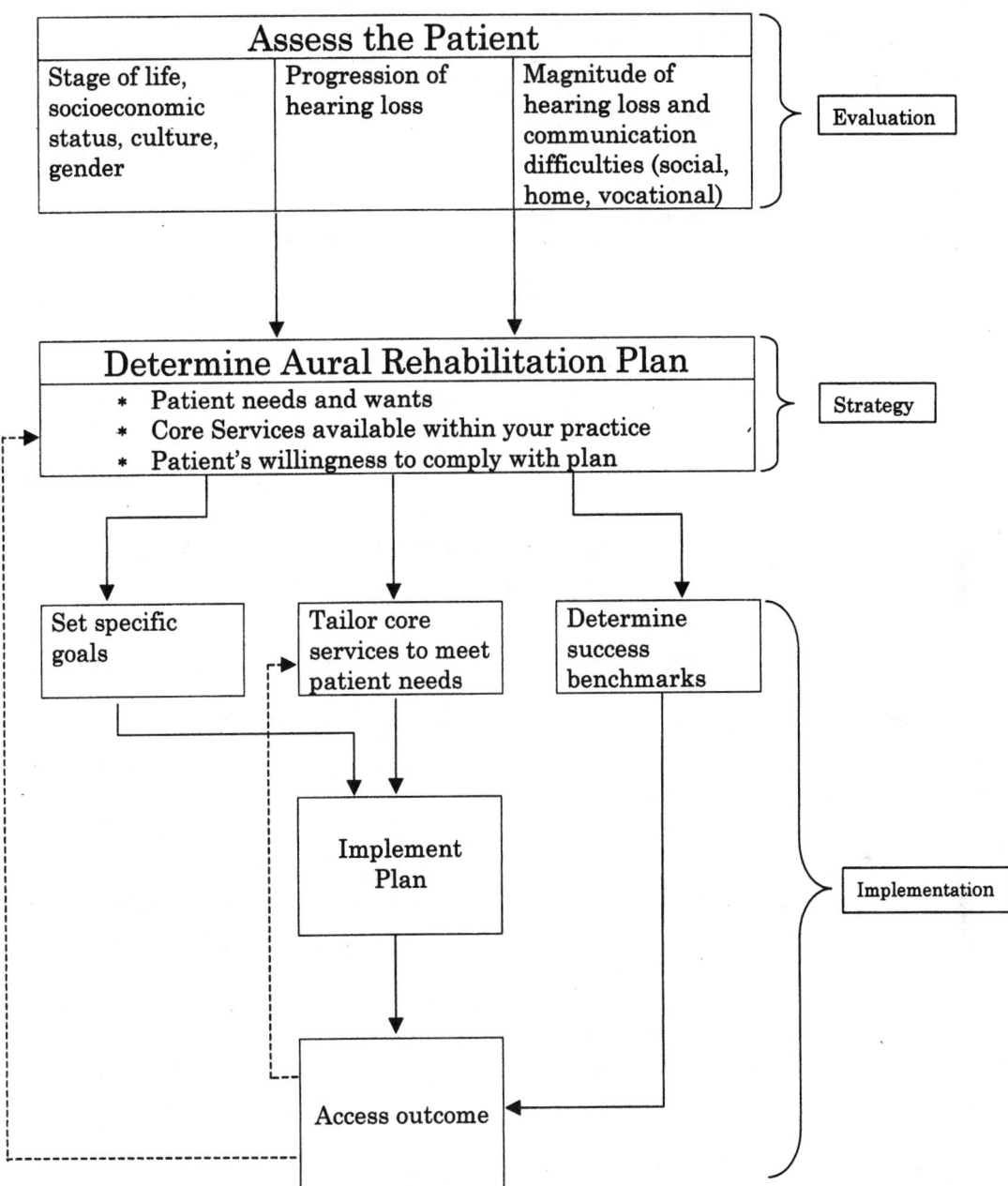

FIGURE 12-1. Stages in the design of an aural rehabilitation plan.

Table 12-1. Assessing the individual in the scheme of designing an aural rehabilitation plan.

A. Demographic

What is the individual's stage of life, socioeconomic status, culture, gender, and other relevant life factors?

B. Audiological and Conversational

What is the individual's hearing loss?

How well can the individual recognize speech using only audition? Using vision and audition?

What is the individual's communication handicap?

Does the individual use communication strategies effectively?

What listening devices does the individual currently use? Are they appropriate?

C. Ecological

What are the individual's communication demands in the home?

What are the individual's communication demands in the workplace?

What are the individual's communication demands in the social arena?

D. Economic

What are the financial resources available to support the individual's aural rehabilitation plan?

How does the individual make buying decisions?

How does the individual perceive aural rehabilitation services in terms of monetary costs and benefits?

E. Psychosocial

What are the psychosocial concerns related to the individual's hearing loss and communication difficulties, and how can they be addressed?

What are the nonmonetary costs related to seeking and receiving aural rehabilitation services for the individual, and how can they be minimized?

How motivated is the individual to receive services and to participate in aural rehabilitation interventions?

One way to conceptualize the evaluation stage is illustrated in Figure 12-2 (in the spirit of Hyde & Riko, 1994). This figure presents a decision tree, which outlines the decisions that might be made in the initial stages of an aural rehabilitation plan. The squares in this decision tree indicate that a decision must be made at this time. For instance, you might recommend that the patient receive an audiogram and take a test of speech recognition in an audition-only condition (moving from left to right, this

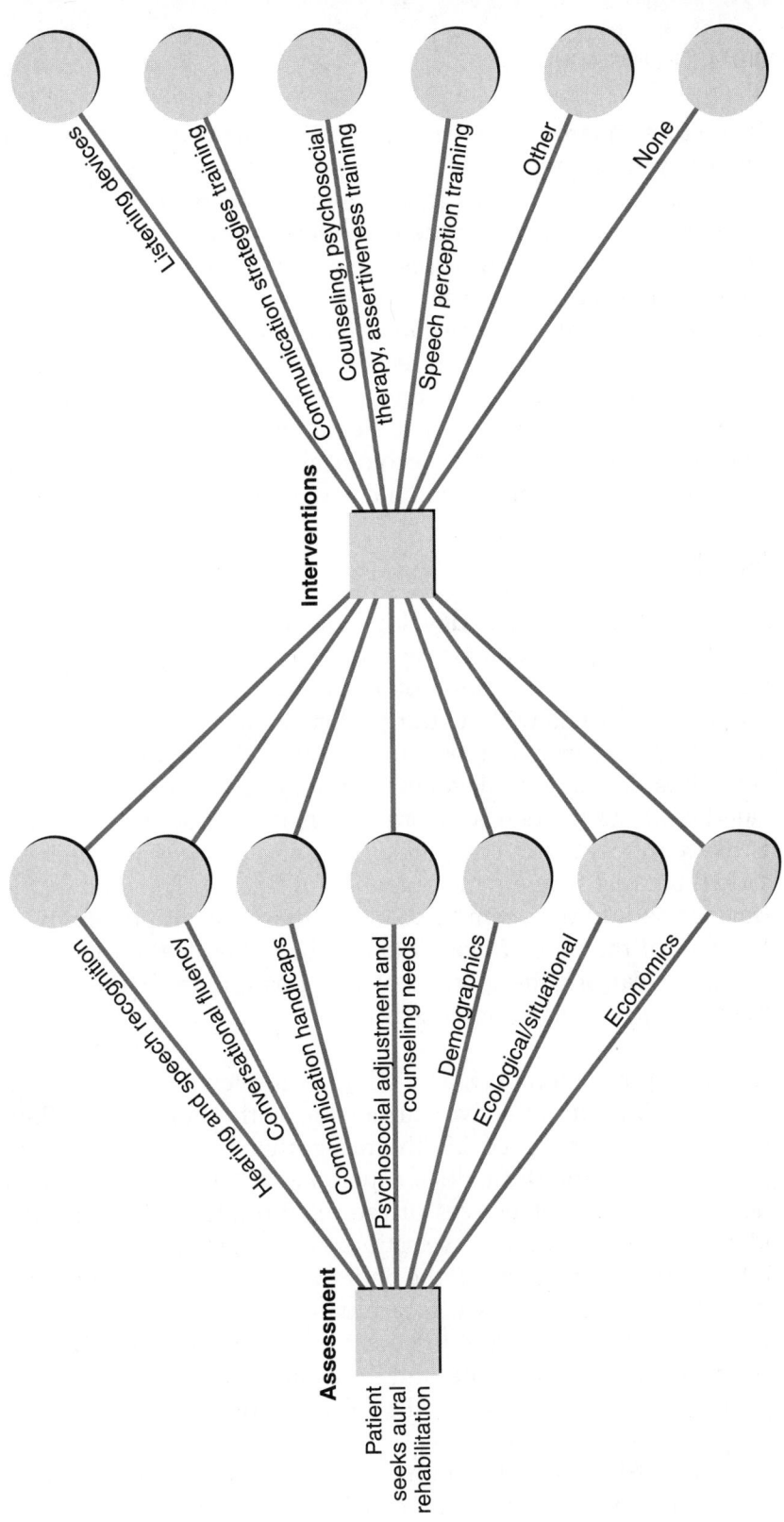

FIGURE 12-2. A decision tree for the initial stages of an aural rehabilitation plan. Squares denote a point in time where a decision is made. Circles indicate points in the temporal flow of the plan that may be beyond the control of the clinician or patient.

447

is the first square in the temporal flow of the decision tree). The circles in the decision tree indicate points that may not be under the clinician's or patient's control, such as the patient's performance on a hearing test or the outcome of a particular intervention. The outcome of the assessments will point the way to particular interventions (or no intervention) being selected. The interventions will be determined by the results of your assessment of hearing and speech recognition, conversational fluency, communication handicap, and psychosocial adjustment and counseling needs, and by what the patient tells you about his or her demographic variables, ecological/situational communication circumstances, and economic wherewithal.

Strategy

The next stage will be to develop a broad strategy to guide your aural rehabilitation efforts. An aural rehabilitation strategy will be based on a consideration of an individual's needs, the availability of offerings within your particular practice, and the individual's ability or willingness to comply with the specifics of the plan. It is desirable to develop a strategy that can be communicated easily to the hard-of-hearing person. It should be one that is likely to meet with compliance, and it should excite the individual because it offers the potential for benefit. The plan that is devised should not seem to be out'of the realm of possibility in the eyes of the patient. For instance, the patient's immediate reaction on learning the specifics of a proposed plan should not be, "I would *never* wear a hearing aid!"

In developing a strategy, as well as in implementing the plan, you will develop an active partnership with your patient. Both of you will be involved in "the recognition, identification, and description of the difficulties experienced; the negotiation and definition of the objectives of the rehabilitation program; the identification, evaluation, selection, and implementation of the intervention strategy itself; the definition of the desired outcome including the criteria used to evaluate the outcome of the program; the identification of the positive and negative factors that contributed to the outcome; and the evaluation of the effects, impacts, and consequences of the rehabilitation program on the person's activities outside the clinical setting" (Gagné, McDuff, & Getty, 1999, p. 48). Through the development of this partnership, and the implementation of what Gagné et al. (1999) call a solution-centered, problem-solving strategy, patients will allevi-ate those listening challenges that motivated them to seek pro-fessional help in the first place (see also Chapter 5, where we consider problem-solving techniques in the context of psychoso-cial therapy). Developing and implementing an aural rehabilita-tion plan will entail developing specific goals (objectives). Defin-ing the goal serves to identify strategies to solve the listening problem and also provides a standard by which you can evalu-ate the effectiveness of your intervention.

How Do You Develop an Objective for Your Aural Rehabilitation Plan?

Following McKenna (1987), Gagné et al. (1999) present the following guidelines for formulating aural rehabilitation objectives:

"The specific objective should be formulated in a way that identifies:

- all of the individuals involved in the pursuit of the objective;
- the role of and responsibilities of each person involved in the intervention program;
- the conditions under which the personalized and customized objective will be accomplished while taking into account the expressed needs, willingness, and capabilities of all of the partic-ipants;
- the criteria that will be used to evaluate whether or not the objective has been reached;
- a time frame within which the objective should be reached." (p. 49)

One instrument that has proved helpful in identifying problems and focusing objectives is the Client Oriented Scale of Improve-ment (COSI) (Dillon et al., 1997). This scale is presented in the Key Resources at the end of this chapter. Originally developed to as-sess hearing aid benefit, it can also be used to guide the overall au-ral rehabilitation plan and to assess outcome. At the onset of inter-vention, the patient nominates up to five situations in which the patient would like to communicate better or cope better. The patient is encouraged to be as specific as possible when writing down the situations. The five situations are listed in order of importance. At the end of the intervention, the patient reviews the original descriptions. For each one, the patient indicates (a) how much better or worse the situation is now relative to before aural rehabilitation began, and (b) what is the absolute ease of communication following intervention.

For example, Mr. Chou wrote in the first row of the COSI form, "My most common challenge is to understand and be understood in a noisy room." The clinician encouraged him to be more specific, so Mr. Chou added, "I want to hear at clubs, because I enjoy going to clubs. Especially I like going to Maxwell's on Friday nights after work." Specificity pinpoints the intervention and better permits the assessment of outcome. On the second row, Mr. Chou wrote, "I have trouble hearing people over the telephone, especially when I'm at work and there are people talking all around me." By completing this form, Mr. Chou established that there are specific situations in which he would like to communicate more effectively, that is, he acknowledged that a disability related to his hearing loss exists. Second, he conveyed to the clinician the order of importance of his communication needs. After intervention, and after an appropriate adjustment period (about 3 months), Mr. Chou revisited his original responses. He indicated that his ability to communicate in noise was "better," and that his final ability could be described as "occasionally." The use of two ratings, that of "improvement" and "final ability," indicates the effectiveness of the aural rehabilitation intervention and potential areas for continued attention. Importantly, the patient develops a sense of having received an individualized intervention program.

Implementation

The final stage in developing an aural rehabilitation plan is implementation. Specific goals (e.g., enhanced communication on the telephone) will be set, and existing services within the particular aural rehabilitation setting will be tailored to meet individual needs (e.g., the person may be invited to attend a communication-strategies training program that includes other adults of similar age and hearing loss).

The goals set will be in direct response to the patient's particular problems. For example, if a patient has difficulty listening at professional meetings that are conducted at a rectangular table, an FM system might be recommended. On the other hand, if the patient rarely attends meetings, and complains primarily of experiencing problems in conversing during one-on-one interactions, a hearing aid might serve to alleviate the listening difficulties.

The clinician will want to assess whether the plan is working. This will entail establishing success benchmarks and means for assessing them. In addition to assessing communication handicap, conversational fluency, or hearing and speech recognition (Chapters 3 and 6), you might also assess satisfaction with and benefits from using hearing aids and other listening devices (perhaps using some of the assessment instruments reviewed in Chapter 7). In addition, you might ask open-ended questions that are specific to the objectives that you and the patient have identified for the aural rehabilitation plan. For example, you might explicitly ask, *Is this situation still a problem for you? How often does it occur? Has the situation improved as a result of our aural rehabilitation efforts? How do you perceive that it affects your quality of life now? Compared to before you began aural rehabilitation, how is the problem now?* Figure 12-3 presents a continuation of the decision tree we began in Figure 12-2. For example, one intervention selected for a particular patient might have been provision of a behind-the-ear hearing aid. A variety of measures might indicate the success of this intervention, including a self-assessment questionnaire, sound-field testing in an

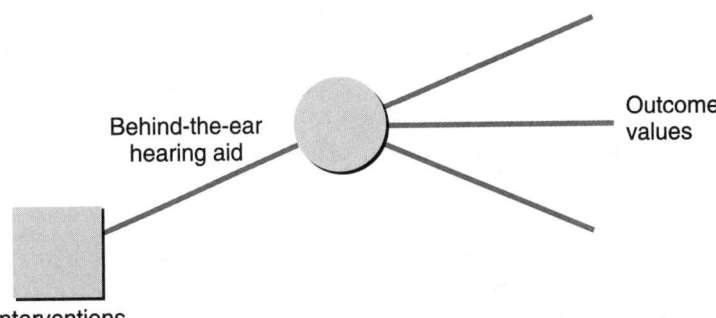

FIGURE 12-3. A continuation of the decision tree begun in Figure 12-2. The consequences of a particular intervention may be assessed with a variety of outcome measures.

audiological test suite, and a self-report of how many hours a day the patient wears the hearing aid. If conversing with her fellow volunteers at a community organization had been a primary impetus for the patient to seek aural rehabilitation, then you might ask, "Has the hearing aid helped you to hear your friends at the [community organization]? Tell me about how you're doing and what kind of successes and difficulties that you are experiencing."

The aural rehabilitation plan should be flexible. If new problems arise or the intervention proves unsuccessful, the plan should be adaptable. Always keep in mind that patients and their predicaments often change, so the aural rehabilitation plan may require fine-tuning and adjusting as it unfolds. By *predicament*, we mean the sum of the relevant variables affecting the patient, including the hearing loss, situation, attitudes, aptitudes, lifestyles, and communication behaviors. For example, Mrs. Crown originally sought aural rehabilitation because she could not understand speech in quiet situations. Her audiologist fitted her with a behind-the-ear hearing aid that was equipped with a telecoil. She is delighted with the hearing aid and now finds she wants to use the telephone, something she has avoided using for 3 years. Mrs. Crown would now like to incorporate telephone training and telephone-related conversational strategies into her aural rehabilitation plan. This situation is an example where the aural rehabilitation plan must be adapted to the changing needs of the patient.

Mrs. Crown's situation is illustrated graphically in Figure 12-4. Before aural rehabilitation, she desired to converse more effectively in quiet. After her aural rehabilitation intervention, in which she received a hearing aid and possibly communication strategies training, the intervention has had an impact on her lifestyle because she can now talk to friends and family with more success. This impact has given her the desire and confidence to begin using the telephone and the desire to solve her telephone-related communication problems.

Predicament: The "sum of all pertinent aspects of client state and situation, including disorders, impairments, disabilities, handicaps, environments, demands, resources, attitudes, behaviors, and so on."

—*Hyde & Riko, 1994, p. 351*

Most aural rehabilitation services include counseling, dispensing of hearing aids and assistive devices, and provision of formal communication training classes. Less often, the plan entails psychosocial therapy, assertiveness training, and speech perception training. More frequently of late, plans include other interventions, including therapy aimed at telephone training and the alleviation of tinnitus. As aural rehabilitation specialists plan their

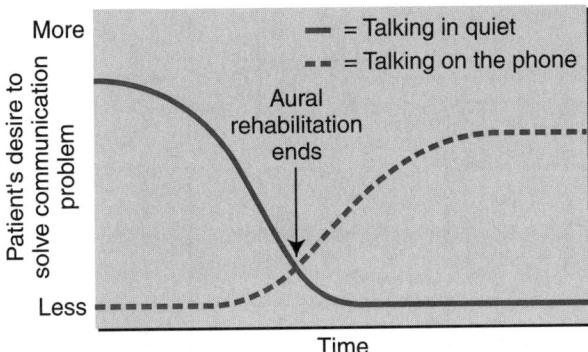

FIGURE 12-4. The aural rehabilitation plan may require fine tuning as patients' predicaments change.

strategy and implementation procedures, they consider how these services can be tailored to meet individual needs. For best results, patients should be involved in defining the plan and, together, clinician and patient should prioritize and update the key goals as circumstances change and evolve.

The typical progression of events involved in providing aural re-habilitation are represented in Figure 12-5. The hard-of-hearing person is evaluated and then receives counseling. Counseling can lead to discussions about psychological adjustment to hearing loss, receipt of hearing aid(s) and/or assistive listening device(s), and participation in communication strategies training classes. Counseling is ongoing during these activities. Follow-up is pro-vided regularly thereafter, often on an annual schedule.

■ COUNSELING

In Chapter 5, we considered three types of counseling: informa-tional counseling, rational acceptance and adjustment counsel-ing, and emotional acceptance and adjustment counseling. After the patient is evaluated, you will typically provide information-al counseling. Depending on the particular patient, other types of counseling might also be appropriate. As you progress in the aural rehabilitation plan, you might offer more counseling or other types of counseling. For instance, if the patient has some unresolved emotions related to accepting the hearing loss, emo-tional acceptance and adjustment counseling may focus in this

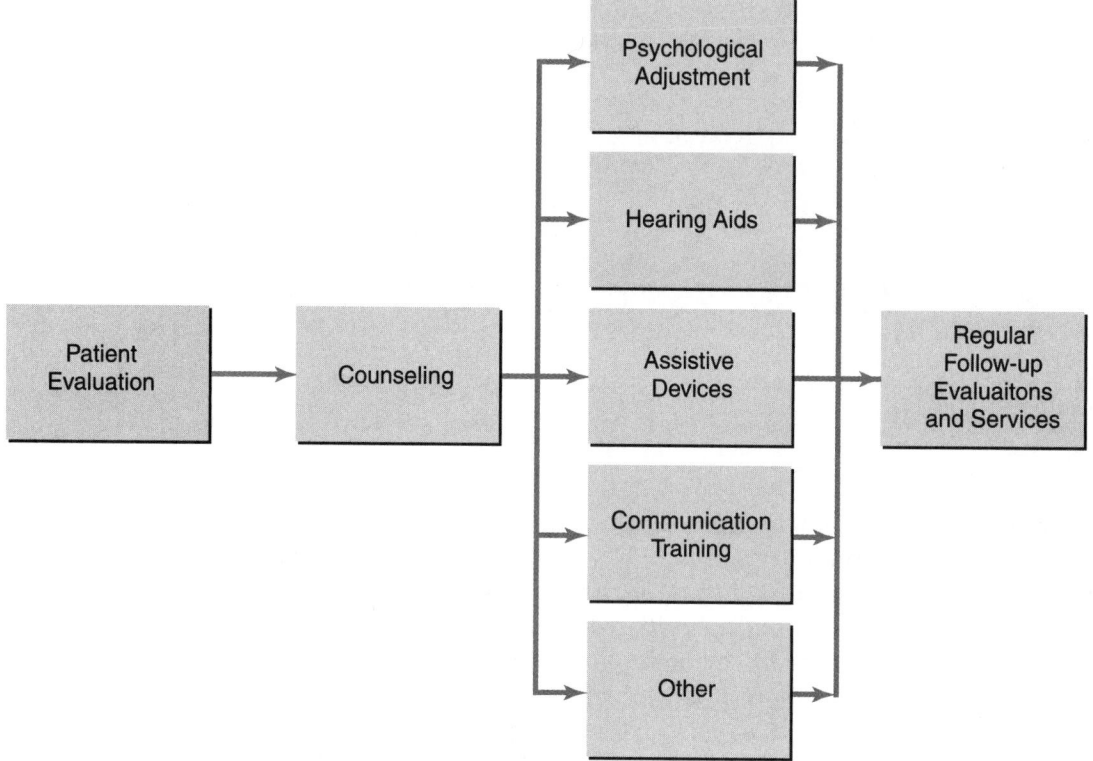

FIGURE 12-5. Components of an aural rehabilitation plan.

direction. Also, as some issues are resolved, it is not uncommon for other issues to surface.

During initial informational counseling, you will explain the results of the hearing and speech recognition tests and talk about the options available for solving specific communication problems. How you go about counseling will depend in part on what you have learned about the patient when you took the case history, what you learned from the COSI or another self-assessment instrument if you administered either one, and what you perceive about the patient's level of knowledge and the patient's personality. For example, if during the case history the patient has told you he or she suspects a hearing loss, then you might begin the counseling session by confirming this suspicion. The language you use in explaining an audiogram to an electrical engineer will differ from that which you will use if explaining it to a fiction writer. There are some patients who want closure as quickly as possible (e.g., "So, what do we do about it?" a patient might ask as soon as you finish describing the hearing loss.), and others who will want to mull over the information and who will need you to explain their situation in many different ways (e.g., "Gee, this is so much to think about. Let me come back later, after I've had a chance to read this pamphlet you gave me and after I talk to my daughter. What kind of loss did you say I have?")

Although there are no cookbook "right" ways to counsel at the onset of aural rehabilitation, there are definitely "wrong" ways. It is important that you not bombard the patient with professional jargon, nor provide him or her with more information than he or she can process or may want at that time. You will also want to be sensitive to the patient's situation. For example, in the case where a patient has been reluctant to come in, you will not turn to the spouse and say, "You're right Mr. Jones, your wife has a whopping hearing loss." Rather, you might begin, "I can understand Mrs. Jones why you think people mumble all the time. Your hearing test suggests that you can tell when someone is talking, but you may not hear many of the speech sounds being said." Then you can go on to explain the effects of a sloping high-frequency loss on speech recognition.

Always keep in mind the three central tenets that we considered in Chapter 5: (1) congruence with self (i.e., act as yourself and not as some idealized professional), (2) unconditional positive regard (assume the patient knows best and assume he or she has the inner resources to manage the communication difficulties), and (3) empathetic understanding (listen to the patient's concerns and feelings and be genuinely curious about what the patient has to tell you). And never forget the patient orientation discussed in Chapter 11. Your job is not to sell patients a fancy hearing aid or listening technology; your job is to figure out a patient's concerns and how you can best assist him or her in alleviating those hearing-related problems that are most troublesome.

▰ HEARING AIDS FOR ADULTS

When determining whether to include provision of hearing aid(s) in an aural rehabilitation plan, an audiologist first must determine whether an individual is an appropriate candidate. If he or she meets the audiological criteria, the audiologist will perform a hearing-aid evaluation and provide a hearing-aid fitting and orientation session. Establishing an appropriate use-pattern will be a prominent goal in the aural rehabilitation plan.

You Want How Much?

Some people will demonstrate *consumer anxiety* when acquiring a hearing aid for the first time. This is a fear that they are being taken advantage of because they do not know much about hearing loss or hearing aids. Their concerns may include the following (Reiter, 1995):

- How do I know I am being sold the proper hearing aid?
- Why is the person down the street cheaper?
- Why are hearing aids so expensive?
- Do I really need two hearing aids?
- How do I know this dispenser is really any good?
- How do I know I am not being ripped off?
- Why should I buy hearing aids when they really are not any good because my friend does not wear his any place but the chest of drawers? (p. 10)

Through good service, open communication, and mutual respect and goals, you can alleviate consumer anxiety. To this end, it is important that you provide adequate pre- and postfitting counseling and follow-up aural rehabilitation services. As you establish satisfied consumers, they will begin to recommend you to others.

Candidacy

Who is a candidate for a hearing aid? The answer depends on the degree and the nature of hearing loss and on patient motivation.

Hearing aids are available to alleviate a wide range of hearing losses. A traditional view is that individuals with an average sensorineural hearing loss between 40 and 90 dB HL are most likely to benefit from conventional amplification. Those at the extremes of hearing acuity, with mild or profound loss, are least likely to benefit. In recent times, this view has changed. Even adults with mild high-frequency loss may experience difficulty in recognizing speech, but nowadays may be fitted with a high-frequency emphasis hearing aid.

Whether a hearing loss is significant enough to warrant amplification relates at least in part to the individual's lifestyle and occupation. For example, a retired gardener and a school teacher may have similar hearing losses. The gardener may believe amplification is unnecessary for days spent weeding flower beds, whereas the teacher may find it critical for hearing children's voices emanating from the back of the classroom.

Motivation to use a hearing aid is an important but often overlooked issue when determining whether someone is an appropriate candidate. Many people who have hearing loss simply are not interested in obtaining a hearing aid. In fact, it has been suggested that only about 5.8 million of the 23.5 million persons (or 23%) in the United States who have hearing loss actually own hearing instruments (Kochkin, 1992). Factors that commonly influence persons to obtain a device include (Mueller & Bender, 1988):

- Communication problems at home, on the job, or in social situations
- Encouragement of family members
- Direction from a medical professional, usually their audiologist or otolaryngologist

Reasons why individuals may not be motivated include vanity, financial constraints, or fear of aging. Some persons fear a social stigmata associated with using a hearing aid and are concerned they will be devalued by others. Some harbor a fear of operating a mechanical device or are not willing to commit time and effort to using an aid on a regular basis. Finally, many people believe their hearing loss is not problematic enough to warrant use of an aid.

In a survey of 2,300 adults 50 years and older, The National Council on the Aging identified barriers to the wearing of hearing aids (The National Council on the Aging, 1999). The survey asked respondents to cite the reason or reasons why they do not wear hearing aids. Half of the respondents cited the expense of purchasing a hearing aid as a roadblock, and about 20% expressed concerns about vanity and the stigma attached to hearing aid use. Interestingly, the most common responses were, "My hearing is not bad enough," and "I can get along without one." A third of the respondents reported that, "[hearing aids] will not help with my specific problem."

These findings from the National Council on the Aging (1999) mesh well with those reported in a study that examined expectations and adjustment to hearing loss and the relationship between these two variables and hearing aid outcome (Jerram & Purdy, 2001). The results of this latter study showed that people who use their new hearing aids for more hours a day are more likely to have greater acceptance of their hearing losses, even before receiving their hearing aids, and are more likely to have higher prefitting expectations. Persons who have not accepted their hearing loss and who have lower expectations wear their hearing aids fewer hours. The predictive influence of acceptance of hearing loss and prefitting expectations on eventual hearing aid use implies that we should develop motivation in patients' prefitting and provide follow-up counseling.

In developing motivation in patients, you might implement the 10-step hierarchical model presented in Figure 12-6. These steps are based on a marketing model designed to change the behavior of a target audience (Kotler & Andreasen, 1996). The 10 steps are grouped into five sets of tasks for the clinician.

1. **Education:** To become successful hearing-aid users, individuals must have a clear understanding of the magnitude of their hearing loss and realize that the loss is not medically reversible. They also need to understand their options in managing their communication problems and understand the value and limitations of hearing aids.

2. **Value change:** Individuals must believe that hearing aids will not result in devaluation of them by others. Others will not see them as old or as damaged goods. Additionally, they must come to realize that hearing aids can reduce communication difficulties and that they are relevant to their own lives. This step may entail a discussion of current beliefs and values and

Audiologist's Task	Step	Patient Stage
Educate	1.	Understands nature of his/her hearing loss.
	2.	Understands what a hearing aid can and cannot do.
Change Values	3.	Realizes hearing aids are not necessarily a sign of aging.
	4.	Considers using a hearing aid.
Change Attitudes	5.	Learns about appropriate hearing aid styles.
	6.	Perceives that the benefits accrued from using a hearing aid exceed monetary and nonmonetary costs.
Motivate Patient To Act	7.	Understands steps for obtaining a hearing aid.
	8.	Acquires hearing aid.
Establish Use Pattern	9.	Completes trial period with hearing aid.
	10.	Continues appropriate usage.

FIGURE 12-6. A model for developing motivation in adults to use hearing aids for the first time.

an eventual disregard for the influences of family, friends, or co-workers who may have negative views about hearing-aid use.

3. **Attitude change:** The audiologist may discuss appropriate hearing aid styles and ask patients about preferred styles. They may discuss the monetary and nonmonetary costs associated with obtaining a hearing aid. Ideally, the patient will come to believe that the benefits received from using a hearing aid outweigh the costs.

4. **Action:** The audiologist must describe the steps involved in obtaining a hearing aid. The person then undergoes a hearing aid evaluation and fitting.

5. **Establishment of use pattern:** Once an individual has obtained a hearing aid, the aural rehabilitation process is not over. In particular, the individual should continue using the hearing aid in appropriate communication interactions.

Hearing Aid Evaluation for Adults

Once motivation is established and candidacy is determined, the individual receives a hearing aid evaluation. The audiologist selects the appropriate electroacoustic properties for the hearing aid, commonly by means of a prescriptive procedure. The amount of gain is prescribed, usually so that more gain is provided for the poorer frequencies and less for the better frequencies. The maximum sound pressure level output (SSPL-90) is also determined, after measuring loudness discomfort levels (LDLs) (see Chapter 7).

During the hearing-aid evaluation, the audiologist and patient determine the style of hearing aid. This decision is based on a combined consideration of the magnitude of the individual's hearing loss and his or her personal preference. For instance, an audiologist might conclude that a BTE device is most appropriate for a person who has a severe sensorineural hearing loss. However, after discovering he is adamantly opposed to wearing a visible device, the audiologist may prudently recommend an ITE hearing aid. By following the patient's lead, the audiologist averts certain non-use of the hearing aid by the patient.

Other decisions that will be made during the hearing-aid fitting include whether the person will use one hearing aid (monaural amplification) or two (binaural amplification), the type of hearing aid microphone (e.g., omnidirectional versus directional), and whether various features are desired, such as a telephone switch or a remote control switch for adjusting volume.

Hearing-Aid Fitting and Orientation

Once a hearing aid has been selected, ordered, and received, the patient returns to the audiological clinic for a hearing aid fitting and orientation. This is an important segment of the aural rehabilitation process. The person must become comfortable in handling the device and must feel confident that he or she can manage this new piece of technology.

Mail-In Daily Logs

A simple method to provide follow-up after the initial hearing-aid orientation is through the use of daily logs, similar to the procedure we considered in Chapter 3. The audiologist creates seven postcards, each addressed with the audiologist's business address and each with a stamp. On the other side of each card, a date is printed, with the seven cards having seven consecutive dates. Each day, the patient's task is to complete three items printed on the back of that day's card: The time the hearing aid was put on, the time the hearing aid was taken off, and any additional comments. The patient mails a card every day, so the audiologist is assured the cards were not completed on one occasion.

This daily log allows the audiologist to monitor the patient's progress during the initial period of adjustment. The audiologist can determine whether the patient is gradually increasing use time and whether the patient is experiencing any difficulties. For example, one patient commented that her hearing aid squealed, on three separate days. Any time a patient seems to be having difficulty in adjusting to the hearing aid (e.g., if the patient reports a problem on two or more days), the audiologist can call the patient and discuss the difficulties, and if necessary, schedule an appointment.

The hearing-aid is fitted to the patient's ear. Performance with the hearing aid is then evaluated, often first with real-ear measurements, in which a miniature microphone attached to a plastic tube is placed in the ear canal to measure loudness of sounds, both with and without the hearing aid. Speech recognition performance also is measured with and without the hearing aid. Finally, the new user is asked about sound quality. The clinician may ask such questions as the following:

- **Can you understand my voice? Does it sound natural? Am I too soft or too loud? Do I sound tinny?**
- **How does your own voice sound? Does it sound hollow? Do you feel like you are talking inside a cave or a barrel?**
- **How do environmental noises sound? Can you hear the telephone ring? How do your footsteps sound?**

Once the hearing aid is introduced, an overview of its operation and maintenance is presented. This overview includes a demonstration of how to clean it, how to troubleshoot problems, and how to turn it on and off. The new hearing-aid user might be given simple printed guidelines for maintaining the device, such as those presented in Table 12-2.

If the device has a telephone switch, the individual should practice turning on the switch, placing the telephone handset over the hearing aid, and then conversing on the clinic telephone. If the hearing aid does not have a telephone switch, the person might practice placing the telephone handset at a short distance from the hearing aid microphone. The patient should insert and remove the device several times and adjust the volume.

Individuals also practice putting the battery into the battery compartment and taking it out, and they are shown the battery's negative and positive sides. They should receive information about where to purchase batteries, how much they might cost, and how long they should last. They also should receive printed materials concerning the proper disposal of batteries, because dead batteries pose a danger to children and pets.

Table 12-3 describes appropriate expectations for hearing aid use. The patient and the audiologist will probably review the benefits and limitations of hearing aids, even if they have done so already during a previous appointment. Other topics will include feedback (what it is, why it occurs, and how it can be minimized), adjustment (one must become accustomed to listening to amplified speech), and how to know when the aid is not functioning normally (what to try at home to fix it and when to return to the audiologist).

Printed information about the trial period and warranty are provided during the hearing-aid orientation. Usually, patients receive a 1-month trial period with a new hearing aid and may return it for a full or partial refund if they are not satisfied. Patients should be encouraged to have a hearing evaluation and a hearing-aid check on an annual basis. Some may return to the clinic more often because they are experiencing difficulties. For instance, the earmold may not fit properly. During this period of early use, the patient probably will be administered speech recognition tests to assess benefit of amplification and to validate

Table 12-2. This handout can be provided to patients as a guide to maintaining their hearing aids.

Do's and Don'ts for Maintaining Your Hearing Aid

Do:

- Regularly remove earwax from the earmold or sound-outlet of the hearing aid, using a wax removal brush or a wax loop remover.
- Routinely wipe the hearing aid with a clean, dry tissue.
- Open the battery case every night.
- Store hearing aid in your carrying case with a dry-pack and place in a safe place.
- Ensure your hands are clean and dry and free of creams before handling the hearing aid.
- Keep the hearing aid away from moisture.
- Carry a spare fresh battery with you when you are out.
- Check your batteries and replace when necessary.
- Turn off the hearing aid before taking if out of your ear to prevent feedback.
- Keep hearing aid away from dogs and cats.
- Remove your hearing aid when you are perspiring, such as on a very hot day or during strenuous exercise.
- Clean the earmold and tubing on a weekly basis.

Don't:

- Leave a dead battery in the battery drawer.
- Apply hair spray or face powder when wearing a hearing aid.
- Bathe, shower, walk in the rain, or swim when wearing a hearing aid.
- Take your hearing aid out while standing on a hard surface such as a tile floor; hearing aids are fragile and may break if dropped.
- Wear your hearing aid when using a hair dryer.
- Discard batteries in a place that is accessible to children or pets.
- Force the battery compartment closed; if it won't close, recheck the battery position or try another battery.

Source: Adapted from *Hearing Aids: Who Needs Them?* by D. P. Pascoe, 1991. St. Louis, MO: Big Bend Books.

performance. In addition, self-assessment questionnaires about the benefit of hearing aid use may also be completed. Common instruments used for this purpose include the Hearing Aid Review (Brooks, 1990), Profile of Hearing Aid Performance (Cox &

Table 12-3. Appropriate expectations for hearing-aid use.

1. Many hearing aids may make speech somewhat clearer because they are adjusted to amplify the sounds you have the most difficulty hearing.

2. Hearing aids not only amplify speech, but also noises in the background, so you will probably have difficulty understanding speech in noisy environments.

3. Hearing aids make soft sounds loud enough for you to hear, but are designed to keep strong sounds from being uncomfortably loud.

4. Even when wearing a hearing aid, you will probably experience problems understanding people who are talking from a different room and locating where sound is coming from.

5. Hearing aids may not be helpful in reverberent listening conditions, such as rooms that have hard walls and floors and no draperies or carpet.

6. Your voice and the voices of others may sound different; you might feel that your voice is emanating from inside of a barrel.

7. Hearing aids will let you hear some sounds that you have not heard for a while, such as your own breathing or clothes rustling.

8. You will still have difficulty understanding speech, even though you are wearing a hearing aid.

9. Your hearing aid should be comfortable to wear; if it is not, then contact your audiologist.

Source: Adapted from *Hearing Aids: Who Needs Them?* by D. P. Pascoe, 1991. St. Louis, MO: Big Bend Books.

Alexander, 1991), and the Hearing Aid Performance Inventory (Kricos, Lesner, Sandridge, & Yanke, 1987).

Establishing a Use Pattern

Research suggests that 18% of adults who own hearing aids do not utilize them. Forty-seven percent are dissatisfied with their devices (Kochkin, 1997). There are several possible reasons why people may not use their hearing aids. Some individuals find hearing aids uncomfortable to wear or difficult to handle. Some experience overwhelming problems when listening in the presence of background noise. Others may have had unrealistic expectations about what a hearing aid can and cannot do, and they may receive less than expected benefit. For some, speech may sound "tinny" or loud. In some instances, patients may have wanted one kind of hearing aid (such as an in-the-ear aid) but the audiologist pre-scribed another, one that may be more appropriate for the hearing loss configuration (such as a behind-the-ear style). Research sug-gests that this state of affairs may lead to overall dissatisfaction (Mueller, Bryant, Brown, & Budinger, 1991). Prefitting counseling, allowing the patient to choose the hearing aid style, and ample postfitting follow-up can increase patient satisfaction and lead to greater hearing-aid use.

There are at least three identifiable ***hearing aid use patterns*** to describe the ways in which adults use hearing aids (Figure 12-7). Those who eventually become full-time users often increase the number of hours per day they use the new hearing aid, so that after several days or weeks, it is used during almost all waking hours. Commonly, persons who reject their hearing aids either return them to their audiologist or put them away in a drawer, trying them for only a brief trial period of a few days or weeks. Finally, some individuals never achieve fulltime use nor do they reject the hearing aid(s). They may try wearing the hearing aid in a variety of situations initially, and then decide they need it only for specific places. An intermittent use pattern is best established on the basis of experience, so the individual actually tries the device in a variety of situations before deciding when it is and is not helpful, rather than on assumptions made by either the pa-tient or the audiologist. Intermittent use patterns are most com-mon among those with a mild hearing loss.

Hearing aid use pattern: the times, situations, and locations in which a hearing aid user wears the hearing aids.

◼ ASSISTIVE LISTENING DEVICES AND OTHER ASSISTIVE DEVICES

Individuals may use assistive listening devices either in addition to or in lieu of a hearing aid. The need for various devices relates to a person's degree of hearing loss, his or her ability to recognize speech in quiet and noise, social and occupational demands, and motivation to use hearing aids or assistive devices. Probably the most common requests for assistive devices pertain to telephone amplification systems and then television viewing. Although there are many exceptions, it is a general rule of thumb that the greater the hearing loss the greater the interest in and need for as-sistive listening devices. This situation is especially true for alert-ing devices, when individuals with severe and profound losses

Full-time Use Pattern

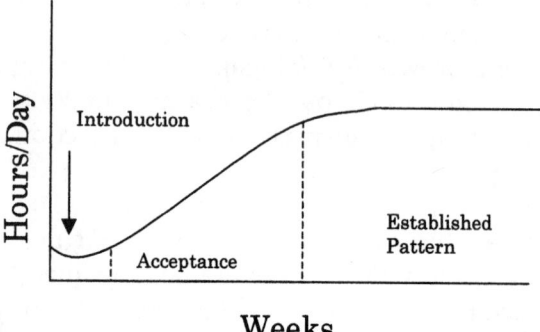

Rejection Pattern

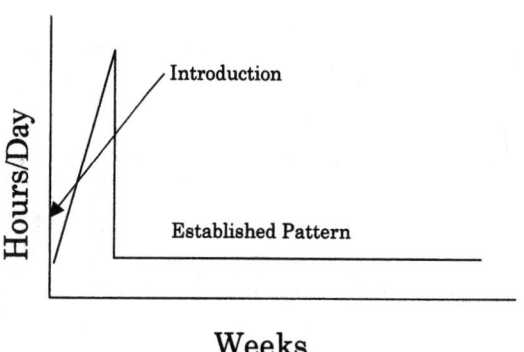

Intermittent Use Pattern

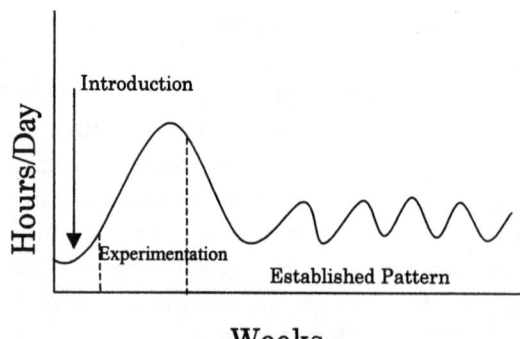

FIGURE 12-7. Patterns of use found in first-time hearing-aid users.

must rely on alerting stimuli to warn them of such conditions as fire or other emergencies, whether they are awake or asleep (and not wearing a hearing aid).

During the evaluation stage of designing a patient's aural rehabilitation plan, you will investigate the patient's capabilities, preferences, situational needs, and lifestyle as they pertain to his or her need for assistive devices. For instance, you may ask a person who has a severe hearing loss about interest in assisted listening for television viewing.

In assessing the need for assistive devices, the clinician might determine those communicative situations for which devices might be indicated. For example, Table 12-4 suggests those circumstances in which alerting, listening, and visual support systems might be appropriate for adults who have severe or profound hearing losses. In this framework, communicative interactions are classified as interactive or noninteractive, and warning needs are classified as basic or lifestyle-specific.

To obtain information about a person's need for and current use of assistive listening devices, some clinicians have employed written checklists like those presented in the Key Resources section at the end of this chapter. Preferably after a person has had an opportunity to gain experience with a hearing aid, the audiologist can review this checklist with him or her and ask about situations that still are problematic. As problems are identified, the clinician can refer the individual to the checklist and then demonstrate systems that currently are not used, but that are appropriate for alleviating communication difficulties.

Issues that might be considered as the aural rehabilitation strategy is put together and recommendations for assistive devices are being formulated include (Compton, 1995):

■ **Affordability:** How expensive is the device? Especially if an individual has recently purchased a hearing aid, affordability is an important issue to consider when recommending assistive devices. It may be desirable to have the patient prioritize listening needs, and then to select the most useful/versatile assistive device(s) accordingly.
■ **Reliability and Durability:** Will the device work as promised, and will it hold up over repeated usage? Many

Table 12-4. Circumstances in which patients with profound or severe hearing losses may desire assistive listening devices.

I. Basic Warning Signals
- **A.** Smoke alarms
- **B.** Doorbell/knock
- **C.** Telephone ring
- **D.** Intruders

II. Lifestyle-specific Warning Signals
- **A.** Vehicle, such as sirens or horns
- **B.** Alarm clock
- **C.** Children/infants
- **D.** Household appliances, such as microwave or washer/dryer signals

III. Interactive Communication
- **A.** Face-to-face
- **B.** Telephone conversation
- **C.** Group
  - **1.** home
  - **2.** workplace
  - **3.** social gatherings
  - **4.** meetings
  - **5.** classrooms

IV. Noninteractive Communication
- **A.** At home
  - **1.** television
  - **2.** radio
  - **3.** stereo
- **B.** At work
- **C.** At public sites
  - **1.** religious services
  - **2.** movies
  - **3.** concerts
  - **4.** dramatic arts presentations
  - **5.** lectures
  - **6.** professional conferences
  - **7.** sports events
  - **8.** airport terminal

Source: Adapted from "Alerting and assistive systems: Counseling implications for cochlear implant users," by L. K. Schum and N. Tye-Murray, 1995. In R. S. Tyler and D. J. Schum (Eds.), *Assistive Devices for Persons with Hearing Impairment* (pp. 86–102). Needham Heights, MA: Allyn & Bacon.

manufacturers are now producing assistive devices, some of which vary in reliability, quality, and durability. When recommending an assistive device, you will want to balance the features of a particular device against its cost. Reliability may be of paramount consideration when safety is an issue, as in emergency alerting systems like fire detectors.

■ **Operability:** How does it work? The person must be able to manage the device. For instance, he or she should be able to replace the batteries, if applicable, and be able to operate the device. Sometimes formal instruction is necessary; therefore, the patient must have the time and the cognitive (and possibly financial) wherewithal to participate in a training session.

■ **Portability:** Can the device easily be transported from one locale to another? In some instances, portability is an issue. If someone travels frequently, for example, then the person will want a telephone amplifier that can easily be transported in a purse or coat pocket. A replacement handset amplifier would be inappropriate in this instance.

■ **Compatibility:** Can the device be used with a hearing aid? In many cases, patients wear their hearing aids at all times and will opt to wear the aid with any assistive listening device.

■ **Cosmetics:** What does it look like when in use? Some people may be self-conscious about using an assistive listening device. For example, pulling out a wireless FM listening device at a restaurant may be difficult. Counseling and opportunity for practice under the supervision of an audiologist may minimize cosmetic concerns.

In dispensing an assistive listening device, the following steps usually are followed (Sutherland, 1995):

■ Demonstrate how to use the device(s).
■ Review the advantages and disadvantages of the device and its capabilities and limitations.
■ Describe how the devices work and how to install them.
■ Demonstrate how to troubleshoot the devices.
■ Demonstrate the device to family members.
■ Answer any questions.
■ Review the Americans with Disabilities Act and talk about patients' legal rights.

▰ FOLLOW-UP

Ideally, new hearing-aid users will participate in a group aural rehabilitation program following receipt of a hearing aid or other listening device. Information about the care and use of the device that was presented during the hearing-aid orientation may be reiterated and provision made for supervised practice in handling the device and in using the telephone. Other class topics likely will include communication strategies, listening, and speechreading. The Key Resources section presents an example of a course syllabus for a 6-week adult aural rehabilitation group class.

For individuals who cannot or will not participate in a formal aural rehabilitation program, the clinician might provide written materials via the mail and occasionally write short letters inquiring about the patient's satisfaction and progress with amplification. Communication through e-mail can be effective, as well as the use of Internet Chat rooms centered on hearing loss and aural rehabilitation.

Apart from learning about their listening devices and communication strategies, patients also may learn about legislation concerning the rights of persons with hearing impairment. Several laws that are relevant to adults are presented in Table 12-5, along with a brief description of each.

Individuals might be encouraged to join self-help organizations for hard-of-hearing adults. One such organization is Self Help for Hard of Hearing People, Inc. (SHHH), one of the largest in existence for hard-of-hearing adults. It is comprised of hundreds of local chapters and a national office that disseminates information about hearing loss and communication. The Key Resources section presents addresses for this group as well as other self-help organizations. In addition, it lists professional organizations that serve hard-of-hearing and Deaf adults.

You probably will want to follow up later on an individual's progress with using any assistive devices, and evaluate whether the device is working for the person and meeting the targeted needs. In addition, you will want to ensure the individual is using a device properly If the person is embarrassed to use a device in public when appropriate, you might include assertiveness training in your formal aural rehabilitation classes.

Table 12-5. Legislation that hard-of-hearing and Deaf adults should be familiar with.

LEGISLATION	EFFECT
Section 504 of the Rehabilitation Act of 1973	Prohibits discrimination against qualified disabled people in any federally supported program or activity
Hearing Aid Compatibility Act of 1988 (P.L. 394)	Mandates that all telephones manufactured for sale in the United States after August 16, 1989 (cordless phones by 1991) must be hearing-aid compatible
1988 Telecommunications Accessibility Enhancement Act (P.L. 100-542)	Requires that the General Services Administration make provision for telecommunications access to federal agencies, both for employees to be able to use the telephone and for deaf and speech-impaired individuals to have access to federal offices
Television Decoder Circuitry Act (Chip Bill) (P.L. 101-431)	As of July 1993, all television sets sold in the United States with screens 13 inches or larger must have built-in circuitry that can decode and display closed captions
The Americans With Disabilities Act (ADA) (P.L. 101-336)	Signed into law on July 17, 1990, this legislation extends civil rights protection for people with disabilities in private sector employment, public accommodations, state and local government services, transportation, and telecommunications relay services

Source: Adapted from "New perspectives in audiological rehabilitation, by C. A. Binnie, 1991. In G. A. Studebaker, F. H. Bess, and L. B. Beck (Eds.), *The Vanderbilt Hearing-aid Report II* (pp. 233–243). Parkton, MD: York Press.

Typically, individuals should return to their audiologists on an annual basis for a hearing test and a hearing-aid check. During these visits, the audiologist can access whether hearing has worsened and whether the hearing aid is still functioning properly. Assessment usually includes an aided and unaided audiogram and word recognition testing. Sometimes, self-report scales are administered to access subjective hearing-aid benefit. Example scales are presented in Table 12-6.

Table 12-6. Self-assessment scales for measuring hearing-aid benefit.

SCALE	AUTHOR(S)
Hearing Problem Inventory	Hutton (1980)
Hearing Aid Performance Inventory (HAPI)	Walden, Demorest, & Helper (1984)
Hearing Handicap Inventory for the Elderly (HHIE)	Newman & Weinstein (1988)

The Americans With Disabilities Act

You might provide your patients who are interested in The Americans With Disabilities Act (ADA) with this summary of their rights. The ADA guarantees persons with disabilities the following rights (Wood & Sandsone, 2000):

Employment

A person with a disability may not be denied employment or promotion solely because of their disability. If the person can perform the job duties without placing "undue hardship" on the employer, the person cannot not be denied the right to work or a promotion.

Government Programs

A person with a disability may not be denied the right to government programs or benefits.

Public Accommodations

The person with a disability must have full and equal access to hotels, restaurants, stores, schools, parks, museums, auditoriums, and other public buildings. Owners of existing buildings must alter them, and new buildings must include access to the disabled in their design.

(continues)

Public Transportation

All new buses, taxis, and trains have to be accessible to disabled persons, including those in wheelchairs.

Telephones

Telecommunications devices for hearing- and speech-impaired people must be available to the extent possible and in the most efficient manner. (p. 334)

OTHER KINDS OF INTERVENTION

Sometimes adult patients will seek aural rehabilitation because they suffer from tinnitus, or because they desire to be more effective communicators on the telephone, even though they have telephone-related technology. For these patients, you might provide tinnitus therapy or you might indicate what kinds of interventions are available for tinnitus and where patients might receive them. For those who desire it, you might provide telephone training.

Tinnitus Intervention

As noted in Chapter 11, tinnitus is a symptom associated with a variety of ear disorders. These disorders include ear infections, excessive cerumen or foreign objects in the ear canal, otosclerosis, Ménière's disease, acoustic neuroma, and acoustic trauma. It often co-occurs with hearing loss, especially noise-induced hearing loss. Tinnitus may also be symptomatic of cardiovascular disease, including anemia, vascular malformations, aneurysm, head tumors, and occlusion of the carotid arteries. Because tinnitus is often symptomatic of medical conditions other than hearing loss, a patient should see an otolaryngologist to rule out medical or surgically treatable ear pathology before entering into a tinnitus management program. A visit to an otolaryngologist is especially important if the tinnitus is unilateral, as that may be symptomatic of an acoustic neuroma (ear tumor).

In addition to answering questions about the tinnitus and possibly completing a questionnaire about its nature (e.g., What does it sound like? Where is it located? See Chapter 11), the patient may also undergo some of the following audiological and medical procedures prior to entering a tinnitus management regime:

- Comprehensive audiological testing, including site-of lesion testing (e.g., tone-decay testing and short increment sensitivity index)
- Impedance audiometry, to help establish the functional condition of the patient's middle ear, tympanic membrane, and Eustachian tube and to rule out blockage as a source of tinnitus
- Auditory brainstem response testing (ABR), which records the central auditory system's response to sound, to help distinguish between a cochlear and retrocochlear lesion (retrocochlear means the lesion lies between the cochlea and the brain)
- Vestibular and balance tests, such as eletronystagmography (ENG, where the eyeball is recorded in response to balance tests such as tracking, optokinetics, and positional testing), and rotary chair and pursuit tracking tests, to determine whether the vestibular system is involved in the patient's condition
- Head magnetic resonance imaging (MRI), to determine whether a tumor is present in the internal auditory canal
- Vascular studies, such as angiography, to explore the possibility of a cardiovascular cause

An audiologist might administer a tinnitus assessment battery. Using psychoacoustical measurement procedures, the battery typically consists of pitch and loudness matching tasks, perceptual location, minimum masking level, and postmasking effects. For example, when determining the minimum masking level, the audiologist might present white noise to the patient through headphones, gradually increasing the level of presentation. The patient's task is to indicate when the noise is just loud enough to mask the percept of head ringing.

Unfortunately, there is no known cure for tinnitus. However, there are a variety of options that provide relief or some control over the sensation of tinnitus. Some of the more common treatments are summarized in Table 12-7. Treatments include masking the tinnitus with an auditory signal, electrical stimulation, relaxation therapy and biofeedback, acupuncture, counseling, herbal extracts and vitamins, and other forms of pharmacological interventions (which include sleep aids and medications to reduce anxiety).

Table 12-7. Summary of a variety of methods available for managing and controlling tinnitus (Wilson & Henry, 2000; Vernon & Meikle, 2000).

METHOD OF TINNITUS TREATMENT	DESCRIPTION
Relaxation training	The patient is taught to decrease muscular tension through a series of exercises, sequentially tensing and relaxing targeted muscle groups. Discussion focuses on tinnitus as a source of stress, and the use of relaxation both at home and in real-life situations to relieve stress and associated tinnitus.
Biofeedback	This method is a form of relaxation training in which changes in a person's muscle tension or skin temperature are reinforced with a simple signal, such as a tone that changes in pitch or loudness. This signal helps the patient control arousal level.
Cognitive therapy and counseling	Patients learn to control where their attention is directed or change the content of their thoughts. For example, they learn to replace maladaptive thoughts with constructive thoughts and learn to direct their attention away from the tinnitus.
Masking devices	The patient wears a masking device (behind the ear) that delivers a sound to the ear that masks the tinnitus, or the patient sets a radio or CD player to make continual sound. The masking sound may be easier to tune out because it is a constant sound, and it also gives the patient a sense of control over the condition because the patient determines whether to hear the masking sound. Often, the pitch of the masking sound is adjusted to match the pitch of the patient's tinnitus.
Tinnitus retraining therapy (TRT)	TRT involves a combination of counseling and sound therapy. During counseling, three main points are considered: (1) tinnitus is a form of compensation by the auditory system due to damage or dysfunction within the auditory pathways; (2) tinnitus becomes a problem because of emotional and autonomic responses; and (3) the brain can learn to attenuate these abnormal activations (Jastreboff, 2000). During sound training, patients receive constant broadband low intensity noise, allowing the patient to still hear tinnitus. The noise generators facilitate habituation and reverse the distress experienced as a result of tinnitus.

One treatment that has received attention in recent years is tinnitus retraining therapy (TRT), which relies on the natural ability of the brain to "habituate" to a signal and filter it out on a subconscious level so it never reaches conscious awareness. Just as persons can habituate external auditory signals such as air conditioner fan noise and a refrigerator hum, they can learn to ignore the sound of their tinnitus. In this neurophysiological approach, patients receive counseling then listen to broadband white noise for approximately 6 hours a day for 12 to 18 months to habituate themselves to the phantom signal. Eventually, they do not attend to it, nor experience an emotional reaction, even though the tinnitus may still be present. There is some evidence this treatment works for some patients (Jastreboff et al., 1996; Berry, Gold, Frederick, Gray, & Staecker, 2002).

Persons who suffer severe tinnitus often benefit by enrolling in a self-help group. The American Tinnitus Association (ATA) is the umbrella organization for many such groups. ATA provides patients with information about the problem and current techniques for managing it. The organization sponsors workshops, regional meetings, and seminars, allowing patients to interact with each other and with professionals. They also sponsor self-help groups in the majority of the states in the United States. These self-help groups provide guidance to members and help them relieve distress and regain hope by allowing them to share their experiences and solutions with other individuals with tinnitus. Often an audiologist or other speech and hearing professional serves as the group facilitator who shares professional knowledge (and often personal experiences as they frequently experience tinnitus too). Persons interested in starting a self-help group can contact the ATA (the address is provided in the Key Resources section at the end of this chapter) to receive start-up materials (Reich, 2000).

What You Might Do as a Group Leader for a Tinnitus Support Group

Reich (2000) presents the following example of how a hearing professional who has both the professional knowledge about tinnitus treatments, and who has experienced tinnitus, might lead a group discussion:

"A person who is alone at night worries the tinnitus will become too loud to tolerate. The person may believe there is no escape from the internal

(continues)

noise and that it will drive them mad. Consequently, the person is anxious, panicky, and feels helpless. The group leader, hearing this, might ask others how they handle worrying about tinnitus when they are alone and it is quiet. That will surely elicit ideas from others such as, 'I turn on the radio and leave it on all night so that even if I wake up, I hear something other than my tinnitus.' They might also comment that listening to music not only takes their mind off of the tinnitus, it also is a pleasant and soothing pastime. Someone might suggest a soothing hot beverage before going to bed. There are a myriad of activities by which people encourage restful sleep. The important thing here is that by taking charge of the situation, the person no longer needs to feel anxious, panicky, or helpless." (pp. 432–433)

Dancer (2001) reported the top five tinnitus management methods used by audiologists who responded to a survey. In order of popularity, the treatments are counseling (64%), masking (51%), support groups (41%), drug therapy (22%), and herbal extracts and vitamins (21%).

Telephone Training

Patients sometimes express a desire to communicate more effectively on the telephone, even if they have received an assistive device that facilitates telephone conversations (e.g., a telephone amplifier) or if they have a listening device with a telephone adapter. Often, these people are new cochlear implant users who have not used the telephone for a long period prior to receiving their implant. After many years of not using the telephone, some people need assistance in overcoming apprehensions and fears. There are training programs available specifically designed to promote success using the telephone (e.g., Castle, 1988; Erber, 1985; Wayner & Abrahamson, 1998).

Telephone training may begin with a discussion of useful tips. For example, you might encourage the patient to practice some of these lines (Wayner & Abrahamson, 1998, p. 32):

- "I can't listen as fast as you can talk. Will you slow down for me?
- I'm not good at recognizing voices. Who is calling please?
- Let me repeat that back to you to make sure I heard you right.
- I think I could understand you better if you would talk a little softer.
- Did you just say that (for example) the meeting is next Sunday at 7:00?"

Initially, the patient will practice speaking to familiar persons, such as the clinician or a family member, about familiar topics. The communication partner might read from the newspaper or from a simple passage. With practice, the conversations can become more interactive and less structured. For instance, you may coach a patient as he or she calls the bank and checks the balance in an account or calls a restaurant to make a reservation.

CASE STUDY 1

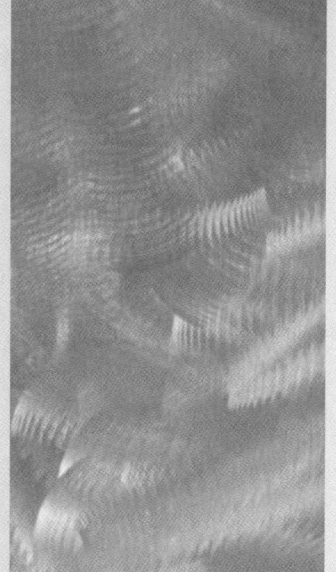

Now let us consider a case study, as an example how the goals of the aural rehabilitation plan might be tailored to meet the individual needs of a specific patient.

Mrs. Kerley is a mid-level manager in an investment brokerage house. She is 49 years old. She recently has experienced difficulty in talking on the telephone, which is why she is seeking aural rehabilitation. She does not report any other difficulties in her home or workplace. There is some evidence Mrs. Kerley is reluctant to admit a hearing loss and may be underplaying the magnitude of her communication difficulties. For instance, she mentions that her teenage boys tend to mumble, but dismisses it as a "stage they are going through."

(continues)

Mrs. Kerley and her clinician identified the following aural rehabilitation goals:

- **Assessment of hearing status.** Mrs. Kerley will receive a complete audiological evaluation, including speech recognition testing.
- **Provision of counseling.** Counseling will be aimed at helping Mrs. Kerley accept and cope with her hearing loss.
- **Consideration of a hearing aid with a telecoil.** In early discussions, she has indicated to her audiologist that she has mixed feelings about using a hearing aid, because she is afraid her employer may think her old. In turn, this may limit her career advancement. The audiologist will work with her to develop motivation to use a device.
- **Receipt of a telephone amplifier.** Mrs. Kerley's work telephone will be fitted with a telephone amplifier.
- **Practice in using communication strategies on the telephone.** Mrs. Kerley will receive one-on-one communication strategies training, with special emphasis placed on telephone use.

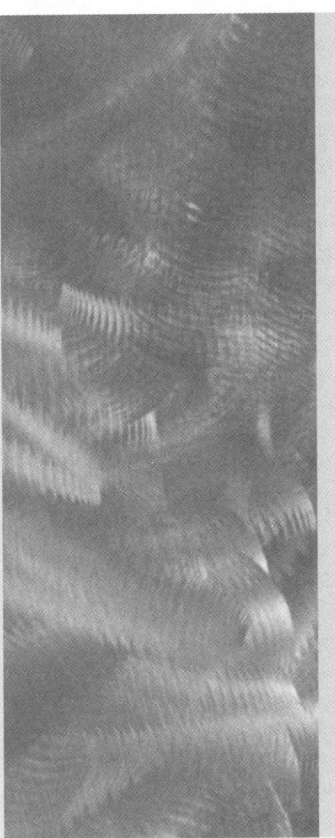

■ FINAL REMARKS

Technology has opened new vistas for the rehabilitation of individuals who have hearing loss. Sophisticated hearing aids, various assistive listening devices, and cochlear implants have made it much easier for clinicians to alleviate listening difficulties. Ironically, these very advances sometimes make us lose sight of the fact that many adults continue to have problems with communication even after receiving high-technology devices. They still need to receive aural rehabilitation follow-up services.

Many aspects of aural rehabilitation can be labor-intensive, expensive to provide, and time-consuming. Some services require much individualized attention for the patient, over the course of hours, weeks, and even months. As a professional, you may feel sometimes that you simply do not have enough time nor the financial resources to provide the high-quality aural rehabilitation you desire. However, many professionals are attempting to develop effective and efficient procedures that might alleviate these difficulties. VHS audiovideo tapes and home VHS players, personal computers with built-in audio stereo speakers, compact disc (CD)-ROM, and digital versatile disc (DVD) portend a broadened array of aural rehabilitation services for adults who have hearing loss. Moreover, the time spent in providing quality services will have a long-term payoff in patient satisfaction and in referrals to your practice.

KEY CHAPTER POINTS

- ✔ There are three stages involved in developing an aural rehabilitation plan: evaluation, strategy, and implementation. At each stage, the focus will be on customizing the plan for the individual.
- ✔ The evaluation state of the aural rehabilitation plan may be conceptualized as a decision tree, which outlines the decisions that might be made in the initial stages of a plan.
- ✔ In developing a strategy, and in implementing a plan, you will develop a partnership with your patient and develop a solution-centered, problem-solving strategy. You will focus on those listening challenges that motivated the patient to seek professional help.
- ✔ The COSI is a self-assessment instrument used to guide the overall aural rehabilitation plan and to assess outcome, and in particular, can be used to assess hearing aid benefit.
- ✔ Patients' predicaments change over time, so the aural rehabilitation plan must be fine-tuned and adjusted as it unfolds.
- ✔ You may need to develop motivation in a patient to use a hearing aid. This goal may entail an education process, a change in the patient's value system and attitude, and establishment of a hearing-aid use pattern.
- ✔ Hearing aids are available to alleviate a wide range of hearing loss. Candidacy depend on degree of loss and also on a person's lifestyle, occupation, and motivation to use a hearing aid.
- ✔ A significant number of adults who receive hearing aids do not use them. There are several reasons for non-use. For ex-

ample, some people find the sound unacceptable, and others are disappointed that their hearing aids do not provide greater benefit.

✔ Issues to consider when recommending an assistive device include affordability, durability, operability, portability, compatibility, and cosmetics.

✔ A patient who suffers from tinnitus may undergo a variety of medical and audiological tests.

✔ Although there are no cures for tinnitus, tinnitus retraining therapy (TRT) has been found to be successful in helping many patients manage their problem. Other management strategies include counseling, relaxation therapy, and self-help support groups.

✔ Some patients will desire telephone training, and you may serve as a "coach" for the patient, starting with easy, structured listening tasks to less familiar, more open conversations over the telephone.

MULTIPLE CHOICE QUESTIONS

1. Mr. Garcia has arrived for his first audiological procedure. An audiogram has confirmed what he has long suspected: a bilateral moderate sensorineural hearing loss. What would probably not happen on this first visit?

   a. The audiologist would take an impression of his ear for an all-in-the-ear hearing aid.

   b. The audiologist would provide him information about the irreversible nature of sensorineural hearing losses.

   c. Mr. Garcia would complete a self-assessment instrument.

   d. Mrs. Garcia would receive an explanation about her husband's audiogram.

2. In assessing the individual in designing an aural rehabilitation plan, you would most likely consider the following variables first:

   a. Ecological considerations, the patient's credit rating, and audiogram

    b. Demographics, ecological issues, and audiological variables

    c. The patient's workplace needs, medical history, and family support

    d. The patient's communication mode, educational history, and attitude towards hearing aids

3. In a solution-centered, problem-solving framework:

    a. Patients focus on those listening challenges that brought them to the professional to begin with.

    b. One solution may lead to another problem, which in turn may lead to another solution.

    c. The clinician asks the patient to develop a decision tree to address listening problems.

    d. A and B above.

4. The Client Oriented Scale of Improvement (COSI):

    a. Is a multiple choice inventory of communication handicap

    b. Is designed to assess conversational fluency in difficulty listening situations

    c. Was originally developed to assess hearing aid benefit, although can be used to guide the overall aural rehabilitation plan

    d. Is comprised of a checklist of listening difficulties and corresponding rating scales assessing both the importance of the listening task associated with the difficulty and the severity of the difficulty

5. In the context of an aural rehabilitation plan, a *predicament* is best defined as:

    a. An instance in which a patient has a listening difficulty in which the professional can offer little relief, as may happen with a patient who suffers severe tinnitus

    b. A summary of the patient's listening difficulties, and reasons why that person sought services from a speech and hearing professional in the first place

    c. The totality of a patient's state and situation, including disorders, impairments, disabilities, handicaps, environments, demands, resources, attitudes, and behaviors

    d. The truism that a solution to one problem often creates the onset of another problem

6. What is likely not a reason for consumer anxiety?
    a. Concern as to whether a patient really needs two hearing aids instead of one
    b. Concern that some other provider could provide aural rehabilitation services for less money
    c. Concern that the audiologist won't let a patient return the hearing aid if after a few days it proves unsatisfactory
    d. Concern about the competency of the clinician

7. What is a primary reason that many people decide not to obtain a hearing aid?
    a. They believe their hearing is too good to warrant use of an aid.
    b. They do not want to wear something behind their ear.
    c. They realize that hearing aids only make speech louder, not necessarily easier to understand.
    d. Their families are embarrassed about having a family member with a hearing impairment.

8. In developing motivation for hearing aid use, the first step is usually:
    a. Attitude change
    b. Education
    c. Value change
    d. Understanding steps for acquiring a hearing aid

9. During the hearing-aid fitting and orientation, a patient typically learns:
    a. How to change the frequency response of the hearing aid
    b. How to adjust the maximum level sound pressure level
    c. How to troubleshoot problems
    d. How to exchange the hearing aid for a more sophisticated model if the patient decides he or she wants more "bells and whistles"

10. You will probably begin to think about possible assistive devices for your patient during:

    a. The evaluation stage of designing the aural rehabilitation plan, as you investigate the individual's capabilities, preferences, and lifestyle

    b. During the follow-up, when you know how much benefit the person receives from a hearing aid

    c. After the patient requests information

    d. During the implementation stage of the aural rehabilitation plan, when you determine what works and what does not

11. Mrs. Menendez has severe arthritis. For this reason:

    a. You might recommend an assistive device with large user controls rather than a traditional hearing aid.

    b. You re-evaluate her lifestyle to determine just how much intervention is warranted.

    c. You do not recommend a telephone amplifier because it will make the receiver too heavy to hold.

    d. You recommend a behind-the-ear hearing aid.

12. Mr. Rampart comes to you complaining of unilateral tinnitus. You recommend:

    a. That he receive impedance testing.

    b. That he see an otolaryngologist because it might be symptomatic of an auditory neuroma.

    c. You send him to a vestibuologist for balance testing.

    d. You send him to a cardiologist for vascular studies because it might be symptomatic of cardiovascular disease.

13. During tinnitus retraining therapy, a patient:

    a. Receives biofeedback to minimize his anxiety relating to the tinnitus

    b. Receives cognitive therapy

    c. Wears a tinnitus masker designed to eliminate the perception of the head noise

    d. Receives counseling about how the brain learns to attenuate emotional and autonomic responses

14. One of the first steps in telephone training is:

    a. To ask the patient to call someone outside the clinic using a clinic phone

    b. To ask the patient to role-play with the clinician ways to instruct the telephone conversational partner

    c. To practice conversing with a familiar conversational partner

    d. To perform a task such as making a dinner reservation at a restaurant or making an appointment for a hair cut, while the clinician stands by as a "coach"

KEY RESOURCES

The NAL Client Orientated Scale of Improvement (COSI). (Used with permission from Oticon.)

COSI
The NAL Client Oriented Scale of Improvement

Name: _____
Audiologist: _____
Date: 1. Needs established _____
      2. Outcome assessed _____

SPECIFIC NEEDS

Indicate Order of Significance

☐	☐	☐	☐	☐

Degree of Change
"Because of the new hearing instrument, I now hear..."

					Worse
					No Difference
					Slightly Better
					Better
					Much Better

Final Ability (with hearing instrument)
"I can hear satisfactorily..."

					Hardly Ever 10%
					Occasionally 25%
					Half the Time 50%
					Most of Time 75%
					Almost Always 95%

486

Alerting, Assistive, Listening, and Visual Support Systems Checklist

Date: _____

Instructions to the clinician: Place an (X) in the column that best describes client's use of, interest in, or need for, each listed system.

SYSTEM	CURRENTLY USES	USED TO USE	IS INTERESTED IN	DOES NOT NEED
Assistive Listening Systems				
Closed-caption decoder for TV	☐	☐	☐	☐
Telecommunication for the Deaf (TDD)	☐	☐	☐	☐
Direct audio input (to speech processor from battery-operated radio, tape-player, or portable stereo)	☐	☐	☐	☐
Telephone adapter				
Telephone amplifier	☐	☐	☐	☐
Telephone answering machine				
TDD Relay Message Service	☐	☐	☐	☐
Group System (FM, loop, hardwire, infrared)	☐	☐	☐	☐
Fax machine	☐	☐	☐	☐
Oral interpreter	☐	☐	☐	☐
Alerting Systems				
Telephone signaler	☐	☐	☐	☐
Doorbell signaler	☐	☐	☐	☐
Door Knock signaler	☐	☐	☐	☐
Smoke alarm signaler	☐	☐	☐	☐
Alarm clock signaler/vibrater	☐	☐	☐	☐
Baby cry signaler	☐	☐	☐	☐
Pet cat or pet dog	☐	☐	☐	☐
Trained hearing ear dog	☐	☐	☐	☐
Other (specify):	☐	☐	☐	☐

Comments: _____

_____

_____

Source: Adapted from "Alerting and assistive systems: Counseling implications for cochlear implant users," by L. K. Schum and N. Tye-Murray, 1995. In R. S. Tyler and D. J. Schum (eds.), *Assistive Devices for Persons with Hearing Impairment* (pp. 86–122), Needham Heights, MA: Allyn and Bacon.

Overview of a 6-Week Communication-Based Aural Rehabilitation Class for Hard-of-Hearing Adults[1]

Week 1

1. Introduction of class members
2. Pretraining assessment (self-assessment questionnaires, audiovisual, and vision-only speech recognition assessment)
3. Hearing loss and communication handicap
4. Hearing aids: Care, maintenance, and benefits
5. Discussion: How to be a good listener
6. Homework assignment

   a. Review listening strategies

   b. Identify difficult listening situations encountered during the week

   c. Review handout materials about assertive, aggressive and passive communication behaviors

Week 2

1. Discuss homework
2. Discuss handouts: What does assertive behavior have to do with hearing loss?
3. Assertive, aggressive, and passive communication behaviors exercises
4. Speechreading practice
5. Discuss second set of handouts: Factors that influence communication success
6. Topicon exercises (see Chapter 3, this text)
7. Homework

   a. Identify difficult communication situations encountered during the week

   b. Identify one situation in which you had a successful conversation, and describe factors that contributed to success

[1]Modeled after a program offered at Central Institute for the Deaf (Mauźe & Frederick, 1995).

Week 3

1. Discuss homework

2. Group discussion: How to take control of the communication environment and optimize your residual hearing and speechreading skills

3. Environment exercises (with handouts)

4. Speechreading practice

5. Group discussion: Communication is more than just hearing

6. Continuous discourse tracking exercises (see Chapter 4, this text)

7. Homework

   a. Use repair strategies during the following week, and be prepared to describe use to class

   b. Describe an incident in which you optimized the communication environment

Week 4

1. Discuss homework

2. Group discussion: Communication breakdowns and repair strategies

3. Speechreading practice

4. Group discussion: Communication is more than just hearing (continued from last week)

5. Role playing: Using repair strategies effectively

6. Homework: Construct examples of message-tailoring remarks (see Chapter 2, this text)

Week 5

1. Discuss homework

2. Group discussion: When hearing aids aren't enough: Assistive listening devices for the hard-of-hearing adult

3. Speechreading practice

4. Quest-Ar practice (see Chapter 3, this text)

5. Homework: Review handout materials concerning the communication environment

Week 6

1. Posttraining assessment

2. Group discussion: Putting it all together

Self-Help and Professional Organizations That Serve Hard-of-Hearing and Deaf Adults

Alexander Graham Bell Association for the Deaf
3417 Volta Place, N.W.
Washington, DC 20007

American Deafness and Rehabilitation Association
P.O. Box 55369
Little Rock, AK 72225

American Athletic Association of the Deaf
2015 Wooded Way
Adelphi, MD 20783

American Hearing Research Foundation
55 E. Washington Street, Suite 2022
Chicago, IL 60602

American Tinnitus Association
P.O. Box 5
Portland, OR 97207-0005

Association of Late Deafened Adults (ALDA)
P.O. Box 641763
Chicago, IL, 60644-1763

Better Hearing Institute
P.O. Box 1840
Washington, DC 20013

Canadian Hard of Hearing Association (CHHA)
P.O. Box 3176, Station "D"
Ottawa, Ontario, Canada KlP 6H8

Canadian Association of the Deaf (CAD)
205-2435 Holly Lane
Ottawa, Ontario, Canada KIV 7P2

Hearing Society for the Bay Area, Inc.
20 10th St., Suite 200
San Francisco, CA 94103

Ménière's Network
The Ear Foundation
2000 Church Street
Box 11
Nashville, TN 37236

National Association of the Deaf (NAD)
814 Thayer Avenue
Silver Spring, MD 20910

National Captioning Institute (NCI)
5203 Leesburg Pike, Suite 1500
Falls Church, VA 22041

National Center for Law and the Deaf
800 Florida Avenue, NE
Washington, DC 20002

National Center on Employment of the Deaf National Technical Institute for the Deaf
Rochester Institute of Technology
1 Lomb Memorial Drive
Rochester, NY 14623

National Crisis Center for the Deaf
University of Virginia Medical Center
Box 484
Charlottesville, VA 22908

National Information Center on Deaf
Gallaudet University
800 Florida Avenue, NE
Washington, DC 20002-3625

Oidos, Inc. (Organizacion Internacional de Orientacion al Sordo)
APTDO. 41122 Minillas Station
Santurce, Puerto Rico 00940

Self-Help for Hard of Hearing People (SHHH)
7800 Wisconsin Avenue
Bethesda, MD 20814

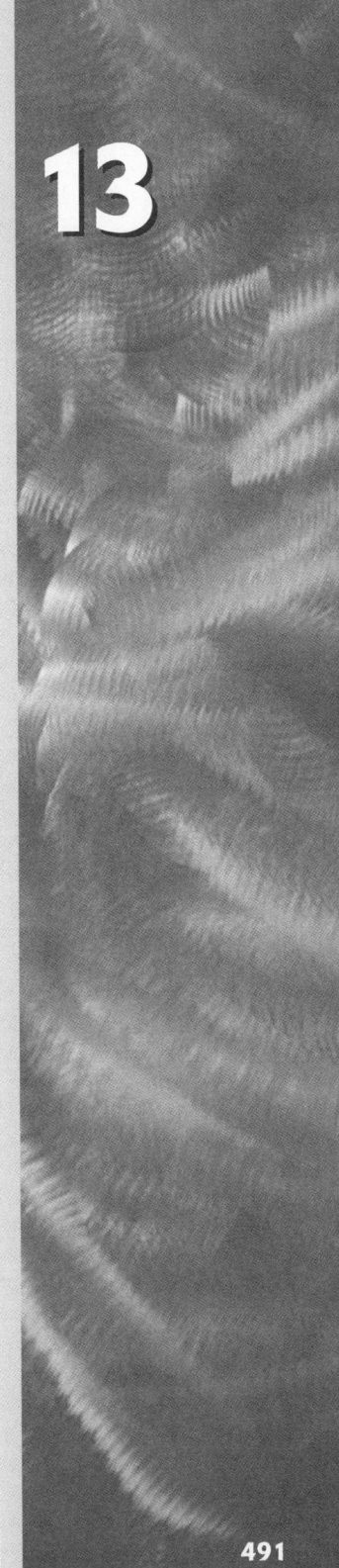

CHAPTER 13

Aural Rehabilitation Plans for Older Adults

TOPICS

- Presbycusis
- Speech recognition
- Factors that influence the impact of hearing loss
- Aural rehabilitation plans for older persons
- What happens if hearing loss goes untreated?
- Hearing aids, assistive listening devices, and follow-up aural rehabilitation
- Aural rehabilitation in the institutional setting
- Case study
- Final remarks
- Key chapter points
- Multiple choice questions

In many ways, the listening challenges faced by older persons mirror those faced by younger adults who have similar degrees of hearing loss. No matter how old you are, a hearing loss will render some parts of the speech signal inaudible, and hence, will reduce your ability to recognize words. However, there are some differences too. Older persons will have a harder time recognizing words, even though they may have the same degree of hearing loss, and they will be more adversely affected by the presence of background noise and other competing sounds, and by the presence of a reverberant listening environment. For example, an older person will have a harder time understanding a talker at a noisy cocktail reception than will a younger person, even if their audiograms are identical. The older person will experience more difficulty conversing in a reverberant convention hall that has tile floors and hard-surfaced walls and ceiling. Older persons may also tire more easily when listening and find their attention wanders. Many times, the older person will have other medical and social issues to deal with in addition to hearing loss, issues that are less commonly faced by younger persons. For instance, the older person may have declining health or may have less social support due to deaths of loved ones and contemporaries. In this chapter, we consider the older members of our society and focus on designing an aural rehabilitation plan to meet their communication needs.

For our purposes, older persons are individuals who are 60 years of age and older. However, this age is a somewhat arbitrary benchmark, and people, agencies, and other concerns vary in how they define the term "older." Theaters, shops, and national parks confer the status of "senior citizen" to any individual over the age of 55 years. On the other hand, Congress has extended the mandatory age for retirement from 65 years to 70 years. Certainly, one reason for these ambiguous definitions relates to the heterogeneity of the population. For instance, one 65-year-old woman may be vibrant and healthy and be a "youthful old," whereas another woman who is 60 years old may be sedentary and afflicted with illness.

It is likely that, as a speech and hearing professional, you will at some point in your career work with older people (Figure 13-1). The elderly represent the fastest growing segment in American society. More than 30 million people in the United States are over the age of 65 years. This number is projected to rise to 39 million by

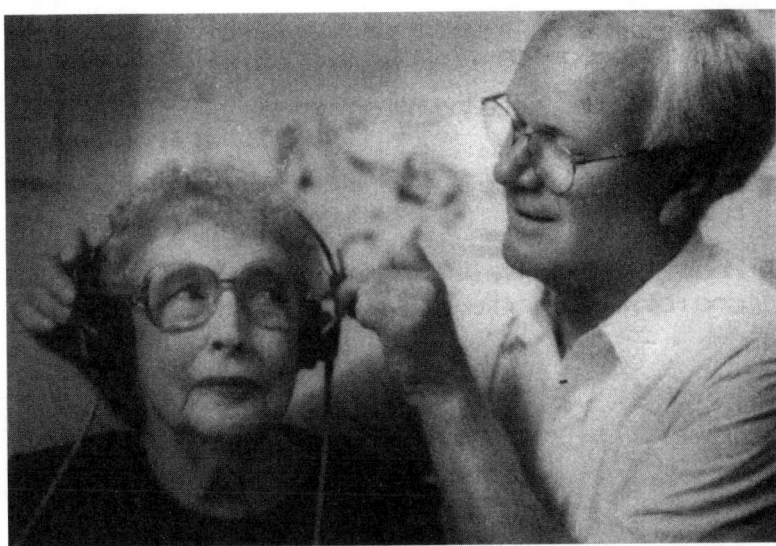

FIGURE 13-1. The number of elderly in the U.S. population is increasing. It is likely they will comprise a significant segment of a speech and hearing professional's case load. (Photograph by Marcus Kosa, courtesy of the Central Institute for the Deaf)

the year 2010 (U.S. Census Bureau, 1986). In 1988, individuals 65 years and older comprised approximately 12% of the United States population. By the year 2020, this figure may swell to 13–18% as the baby boom generation ages (Cunningham & Brookbank, 1988). This group has the highest demand for medical care and social services than any other population group.

Baby Boomers differ from traditional seniors who also comprise today's elderly population, both in terms of their values and their purchasing habits (Bloom, 1999; McGuire, 2002). Traditional seniors, sometimes known as the "Just Good Enough" generation, have experienced the deprivations of the Depression and World War II. They tend to save their money, and many dislike carrying debt and even using a credit card. Although they may enjoy perusing the Internet, many are unlikely to buy services or products from an Internet source. Traditional seniors value trust, service, and quality. They might be characterized by the following qualities and tendencies (McGuire, 2002, p. 4):

■ More homogenous
■ Team/family approach
■ Lately retired, less active

Baby Boomers comprise the generation born between the years 1945 and 1965. Every 7.5 seconds, a member of the Baby Boom turns 50 years old, although many are "in major age denial."

—Bloom, 1999

- More resistant to technology
- Save and bargain
- Avoid credit
- Follow advice
- Price oriented

By comparison, many Baby Boomers are working adults who value active, youthful lifestyles. They desire more to enhance their strengths than to shore up their weaknesses. Whereas the older generation may have accepted that bodies decline physically with age, this is the generation who knows that teeth can be whitened and hair revived with squirts of Rogaine. Convenience and cosmetics are likely to supercede price when they consider whether to use a hearing aid and whether to seek other aural rehabilitation services. This generation tended to marry at an older age, and to bare children later, so many of the Baby Boomer generation provide financial and other kinds of support to both their parents and their children. As a result, they have to juggle work and family commitments (Goodale, 2003). They are more highly educated, more savvy with technology, and more demanding in their expectations and less patient in waiting for results than were their parents. They might be characterized by the following qualities and traits (McGuire, 2002, p. 4):

- Very diverse [About three in ten describe themselves as African-American, Hispanic, or Asian-American. (Goodale, 2003)]
- Individual "me" approach [Boomer patients were born to parents raised during the Depression and World War II, and so they reaped the fruits of pent-up consumer demand in the flush years that followed these eras.]
- Still working, very active [For many, time is of the essence, whereas for the older patients, who might be retired, the visit to the audiologist is both a clinical and a social visit.]
- Technologically proficient [This is the generation that came of age during the personal computer revolution.]
- Bargain and spend [Choices abound, and Boomers have always lived in a consumer-oriented society.]
- Use credit or time-plans [This generation is comfortable with debt and used to instant gratification.]
- Want control of own decisions/care [This generation questions authority, be it as a result of Viet Nam or Watergate; they don't accept expert opinions at face value, and

they want to have input into what happens in their treatment plans.]

- Value oriented [This generation grew up in a time when the quality of life improved rapidly for the average citizen, when good quality could be had for low price.]

As we begin our consideration of the older population, we start from the same platform from which we dove off when considering aural rehabilitation plans for adults: Consider who the patient is, what the person's concerns are, and how to best tailor the intervention plan to meet the patient's needs. The traditional senior and the Baby Boomer may share many of the same needs, but they will also pose different challenges as you begin to design and implement an individualized aural rehabilitation plan.

Victor

An audiologist and her family visit her husband's parents once a year. One year, the audiologist noticed that her father-in-law, Victor, seemed depressed as compared to the year before. He spent most of the pretty summer days sitting on an easy chair with his dog wedged beside him. When the family gathered in the family room to talk, Victor said little and often even read the newspaper. Victor refused to attend social functions and had discontinued his daily walks with the dog. The audiologist noticed that Victor sometimes did not respond to his name being called from another room and often responded inappropriately to questions. For example, to the question, "Do you want peas or corn tonight?", he might grumble, "yes."

After several days of observing Victor, the audiologist began to suspect he might have a hearing loss and broached the possibility with Victor and her mother-in-law. With much coaxing, the audiologist convinced her father-in-law to have a hearing test while she was still in town. Victor was found to have a bilateral, moderate-to-severe sensorineural hearing loss. Driving home from the clinic that day, he turned to his daughter-in-law and confided, "Just between you and me, I was beginning to think I was losing my marbles. People were looking at me strange when I would try to join into a conversation, as if I said something peculiar, and I was thinking I

(continues)

was forgetting everything anyone told me. Maybe it is my hearing that's all that's wrong." Victor received a hearing aid shortly thereafter. The next summer, the audiologist found her father-in-law to be more his outgoing and gregarious self.

This narrative hints at several important points relevant to the older population:

- Hearing loss can be misinterpreted for other signs of aging, and might co-occur with depression. In fact Williamson and Fried (1996) demonstrated that it is not uncommon for older adults to attribute hearing difficulties to old age instead of to a specific condition that can be alleviated with treatment.
- Hearing loss can decrease social engagement and increase social isolation.
- Provision of aural rehabilitation services can have a positive effect on the quality of life for many older individuals.

PRESBYCUSIS

Many older persons experience hearing loss. In fact, hearing loss is the third most common chronic condition afflicting the noninstitutionalized elderly (Hazard, Andrews, Bierman, & Blass, 1990). Although estimates vary, about 30% of individuals over the age of 65 years who dwell in the community have some degree of hearing impairment. Fifty percent of those between the ages of 75 and 79 years have some degree of hearing loss (U.S. Bureau of the Census, 1997). Up to 90% of seniors living in institutions have hearing loss (Hull & Griffin, 1992). Similarly, incidence of hearing loss is also high in the European elderly. For instance, two and a half million people in the United Kingdom over the age of 70 years have enough hearing loss to benefit from using a hearing aid (although only one third of them own one, and 10% of these persons do not use them) (see Hanratty & Lawlor, 2000, for a review). Hearing impairment is more common among older men than women, and men are more likely to begin losing their hearing at a younger age (Gordon-Salant, 1987).

Presbycusis is age-related hearing loss.

Presbycusis is the global term used to refer to hearing loss associated with the aging process. The exact cause of presbycusis is not known. No doubt, age-related degeneration and one's genetic make-up are important factors. It appears that physiologically, two major causes of age-related hearing loss are (1) neural, meaning a loss of nerve fibers and neural tissue and (2) metabolic or strial, meaning a change in the blood supply to the cochlea. Neurologically, the cell bodies of the auditory nerve that comprise the *spiral ganglion* may degenerate. Metabolically, the membranes of the cochlear tissues begin to thicken, causing occlusion of the capillaries and a loss of blood supply. In addition to neural and metabolic causes, some evidence suggests that the central auditory system may also undergo age-related histopathology. For instance, the volume of the *cochlear nucleus* may shrink as the myelin surrounding the neural axons begins to thin (see Boettcher, 2002, for a review). A lifetime of noise exposure in a modem society, in both recreational and occupational settings, also takes its toll in the later years. Disease and exposure to ototoxic agents can be contributing factors in some individuals.

> The **spiral ganglion** is comprised of the nuclei of the nerve fibers that connect to the hair cells and meet in the central core (which is called the *modiolus*) of the cochlea.
>
> The **cochlear nucleus** is a cluster of cell bodies in the brain stem where the nerve fibers leading from the cochlea enter and synapse.

Pure-Tone Thresholds and Auditory Processing

Figure 13-2 presents median thresholds for males for each decade of life between the ages of 20 and 80 years. As can be seen, hearing loss increases with age, and the audiogram displays evolve from a fairly straight line in youth, from 500 to 6000 Hz, to a precipice in the mid-years, with the fall-off frequency at about 2000 Hz. By the eighth decade, the display presents a falling slope, with the greatest loss occurring in the high frequencies. The decline in hearing thresholds accelerates over time, with the rate becoming more pronounced after individuals pass into their forties. The hearing loss may become significant enough to seek audiological help only in the sixth or seventh decade, when the PTA might be 20 dB or greater than it was during young adulthood (Chessman, 1997).

In addition to sensorineural hearing loss, some older individuals experience changes in their auditory processing abilities. These changes are indexed by performance on psychophysical tests and on tests of altered speech or demanding listening tasks. For example, some older persons have a reduced ability to discriminate two sounds that differ in pitch, intensity, or duration (Schneider, 1997). If you present a 60 dB tone and a 65 dB tone to an older listener, he or she may say they are the same instead of different, whereas a younger person will clearly perceive them as different. Some persons have difficulty understanding time-compressed or

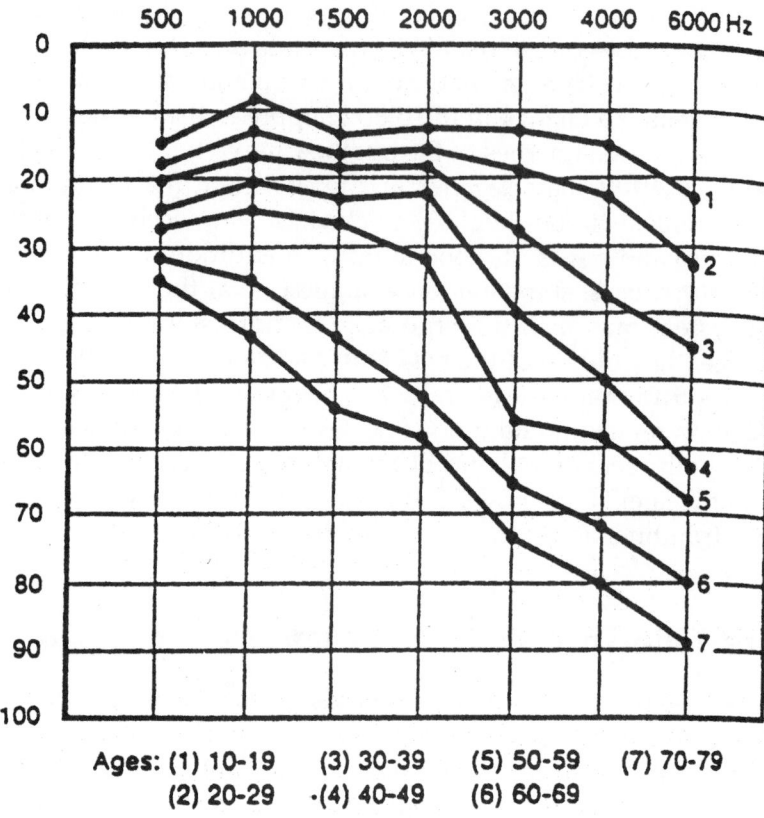

FIGURE 13-2. Audiograms as a function of decade of life. (From *Aural Rehabilitation: Serving Children and Adults* (4th ed.), by R. H. Hull, 2001, p. 321. Clifton Park, NY: Delmar Learning. Reproduced with permission.)

frequency-filtered speech. Moreover, when a competing signal is presented to one ear, and the target speech signal to the other, many elderly adults experience greater difficulty in understanding the target signal than do younger listeners.

■ SPEECH RECOGNITION

A concomitant decline in speech recognition accompanies presbycusis. Beyond the age of 60 years, monosyllabic word recognition scores decline by 13% per decade in males and 6% per decade in females (Chessman, 1997). Speech recognition difficulties are exacerbated when an older person attempts to listen in a noisy environment, more so than is the case for younger listeners (Pederson, Rosenthal, & Moller, 1991; Plath, 1991).

Much research has been conducted to determine the extent to which speech recognition difficulties are caused by peripheral cochlear pathology and the extent to which they result from changes in the central nervous system and central auditory processing. This is a complex issue. We know that the aging brain demonstrates a number of changes, including the following (Willott, 1996):

■ A loss of neurons
■ A reduction in the number of synaptic connections between neurons
■ Changes in the excitatory and inhibitory neurotransmitter systems
■ Changes in neural transmission along the auditory pathway
■ Possibly, changes in cognitive processing of the acoustic signal (e.g., information processing, labeling, retrieval, and storage)
■ A decrement in long-term memory

These global changes in brain functioning might have some effect on an older individual's ability to process rapid streams of speech information. They also may affect how well the individual comprehends the gist of a message.

Although these factors likely affect speech recognition, it appears that decreased word recognition is related primarily to changes in a person's hearing sensitivity at the cochlear level. Hearing sensitivity for the higher frequencies in particular relates to speech recognition performance. An older person's average hearing loss at the frequencies 1000, 2000, and 4000 Hz is the single best predictor of a variety of different speech recognition tests (Humes, 1996).

What Older Persons Have to Say About Hearing Loss

Sometimes you will hear comments that will clue you to the possibility of a hearing loss. Here are some remarks often made by older patients (Pichora-Fuller, 1997):

■ "I hear, but I have trouble understanding."
■ "Sounds seem all jumbled up."

(continues)

- "It is difficult to tell where sounds are coming from."
- "I understand when it is quiet, but I have trouble when it is noisy."
- "I understand when I'm talking to one person, but I have trouble in a group."
- "In a group, if I know who is talking then I can follow the conversation, but I have trouble when someone else starts talking,"
- "When someone else starts talking sometimes I have to look around to see who it is."
- "If I know the topic of conversation then I do pretty well, but I often get lost when the topic changes."
- "People seem to talk too fast; I need more time to make sense of what has been said."
- "It is not so much that I can't understand what is said but that it is tiring to listen."
- "I sometimes pretend to understand because it isn't worth it to ask the talker to repeat because I'm afraid that it would be an imposition and it could annoy or make the talker impatient."
- "I don't know for sure when I hear correctly and when I don't."
- "It's hard to get jokes; you have to get the punchline right away or it isn't funny."
- "When I'm with two or more people, they start talking to each other and leave me out."
- "I don't enjoy social events any more" (p. 125).

FACTORS THAT INFLUENCE THE IMPACT OF HEARING LOSS

Figure 13-3 indicates that a large number of factors influences the effect that hearing loss has on an older person's life. This figure provides a blueprint for compiling a profile of who the patient is and to develop an understanding of the impact of hearing loss. Impact will vary with an individual's economic circumstances, social circumstances, emotional status, and physical status, and cognitive status. You will want to take into account these factors as you develop an aural rehabilitation plan for a particular patient and seek to minimize or eliminate specific communication problems.

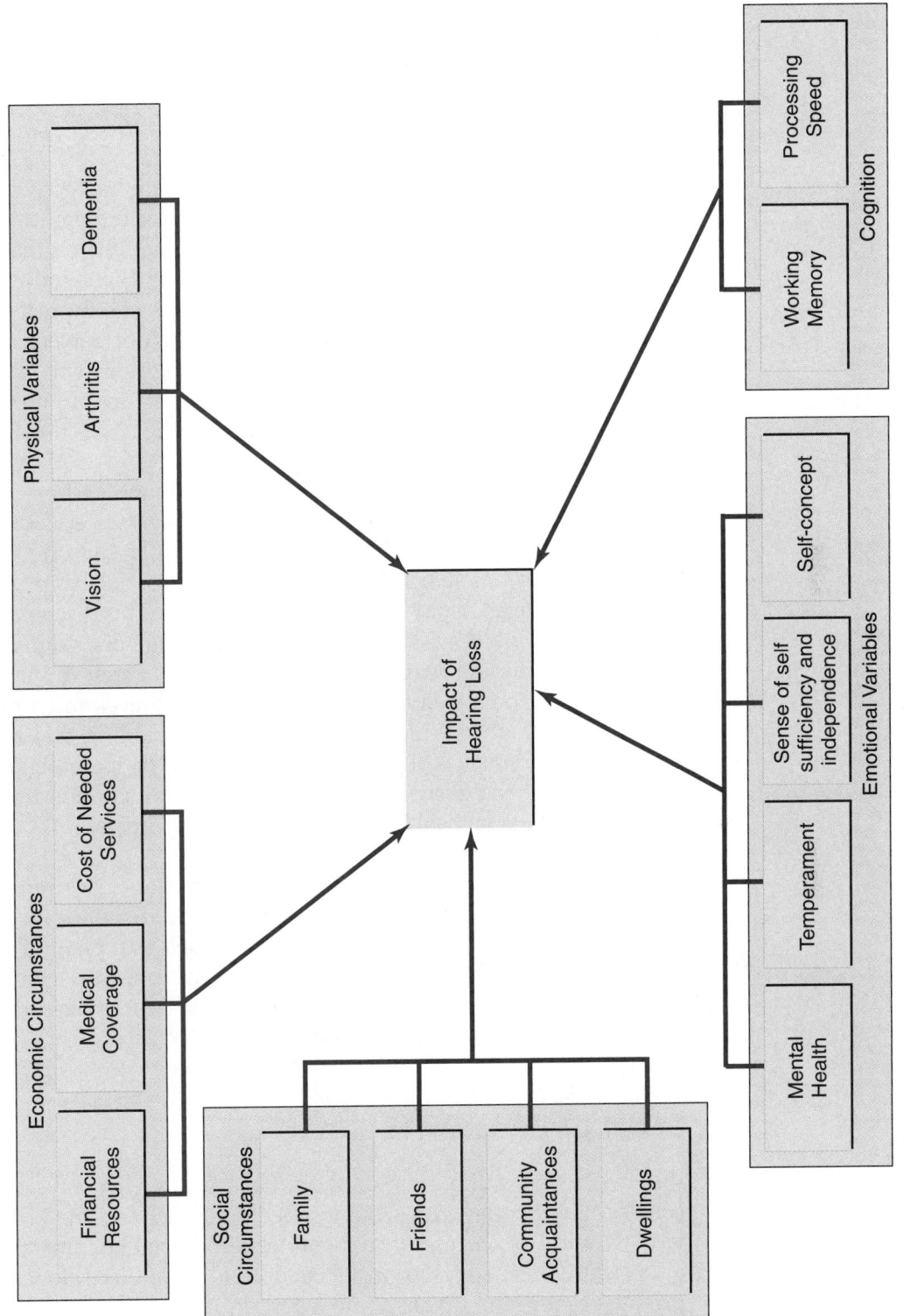

FIGURE 13–3. Factors that influence the effects of hearing loss for an older person.

Economic Circumstances

Longer lifespans and forced retirements have resulted in greater numbers of older persons living in poverty. Schulz (1992) suggested that the majority of elderly persons have only a modest income, and a significant minority live below the poverty level. However, the elderly as a group are not necessarily bereft financially as many stereotypes would suggest. In fact, their situation has actually improved since the 1960s and 1970s. Some individuals have prepared for retirement, and rely on Social Security incomes and/or work pensions. There are some older persons who do not have many expenses except those associated with health care, because their house is paid for, their children are grown, and other life expenses have been paid (Traynor, 1995).

Older women tend to be economically disadvantaged as compared to their male counterparts. For example, twice as many women over the age of 85 years live in poverty than do men (United States Census, 1984). Many women do not have independent resources to pay for hearing health care. This discrepancy in financial worth arises from such factors as wage discrimination and years of unpaid work in the home (Zones, Estes, & Binney, 1987). Largely because of social forces, many older women have not received higher education and technical training and have lived a life of financial dependence on a mate. The increase in divorce rate and the existence of no-fault divorce has undermined further the financial health of the nation's older females.

A patient's economic status may affect the impact of hearing loss and the aural rehabilitation plan, particularly if the individual does not have medical coverage. Decisions such as monaural versus binaural amplification or the selection of assistive listening devices may be influenced by a patient's financial resources, medical coverage, and cost of the devices and related services.

Social Circumstances

When examining the issue of social circumstances, we typically consider the people with whom patients interact and those individuals with whom they feel a connection. Social circumstances also include residency. For instance, does a patient live alone in a private home? In a private home with family members? In a nursing facility? Knowing the identities of a patient's communication partners and where the individual resides are important when designing an aural rehabilitation program.

A Family Affair

Sociologists and demographers tell us that most older persons have living children, and many older persons live within a 30-minute driving distance of at least one of their offspring. The majority of older persons see their children at least once a week, and three quarters of them talk to their children on the telephone on a weekly basis. As these data indicate, there typically is great potential to involve children in their parents' aural rehabilitation plan.

SOCIAL CONTACTS

The number of people a patient interacts with and the frequency of interaction influence the person's morbidity, mortality, and physical functioning (Strawbridge, Cohen, Shema, & Kaplan, 1996). Older people who have five or more contacts are less likely to suffer from loneliness and depression and more likely to have a higher quality of life than persons who have fewer social contacts. For example, a person who lives within a 30-mile radius of children and grandchildren and who works as a volunteer at the local zoo is more likely to have good mental health and be more interested in participating in an aural rehabilitation program than someone who has no family nearby and few interests outside of the home (Figure 13-4).

The extent to which an older individual maintains frequent and significant contacts with family, friends, and community acquaintances can ameliorate or exacerbate the impact of hearing loss. Social contacts allow an individual to feel more a part of life and more involved in the community and provide motivation to address a hearing loss. Individuals who do not have communication partners available often do not seek aural rehabilitation services (Figure 13-5).

Just as social relationships influence the impact of hearing loss, hearing loss can affect social relationships. It is not uncommon for a hearing loss to trigger a negative feedback loop like that illustrated

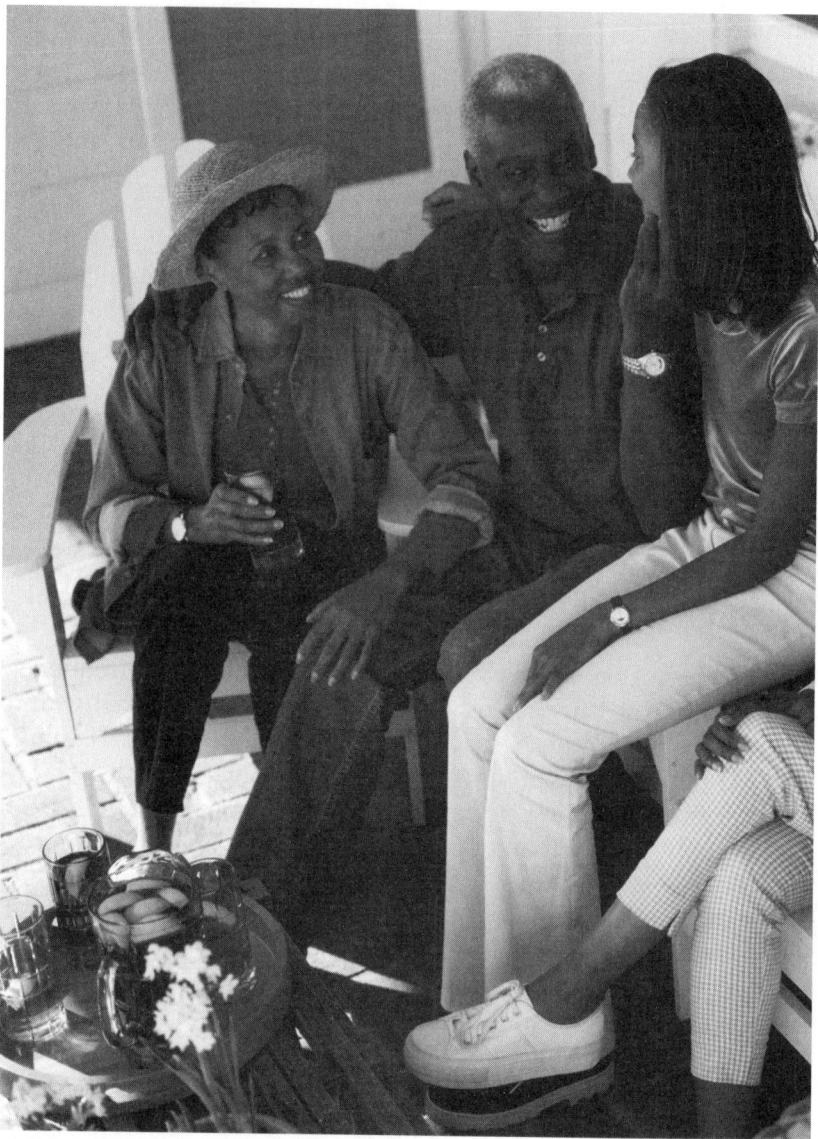

FIGURE 13-4. The number of social contacts and the frequency of contact can affect an older person's desire for aural rehabilitation. Persons who live near family members often are motivated to improve their communication effectiveness. (Copyright Photodisc/Getty Images)

in Figure 13-6. Lindblade and McDonald (1995) suggested that older persons may withdraw from social interactions because conversation becomes too effortful. In turn, family and friends may begin to perceive them as unsociable, preoccupied with health

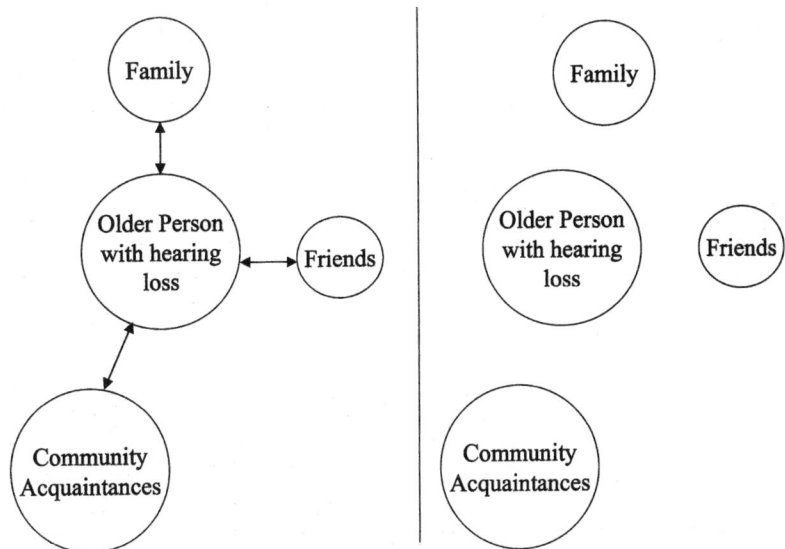

FIGURE 13-5. The number and frequency of social contacts influence a patients motivation to seek aural rehabilitation services.

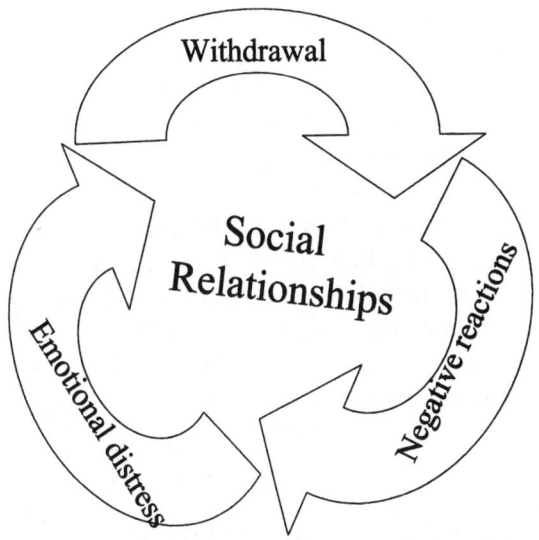

FIGURE 13-6. Hearing loss can trigger a negative feedback loop.

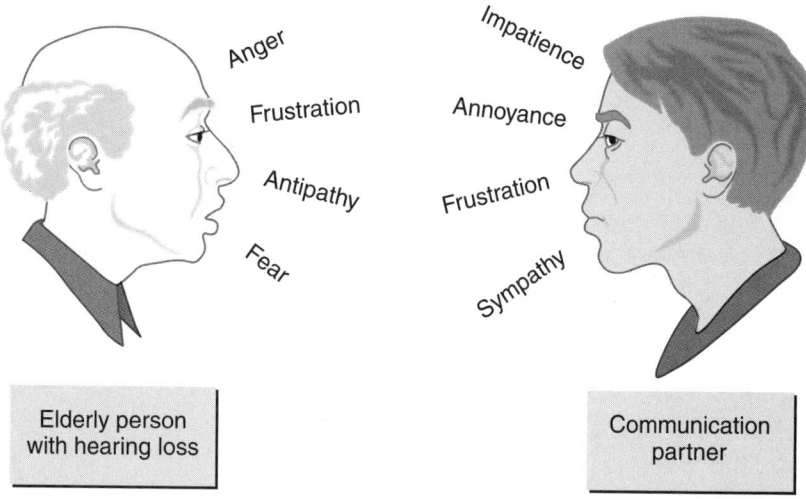

Anger
Frustration
Antipathy
Fear

Impatience
Annoyance
Frustration
Sympathy

Elderly person
with hearing loss

Communication
partner

FIGURE 13-7. Hearing loss can create miscommunications between an older person and a frequent communication partner and sometimes results in the older person withdrawing from social interactions.

matters, forgetful, or paranoid (Figure 13-7). These perceptions may lead to an older individual mistakenly being labeled as demented, confused, hostile, or senile. For example, a son might find that his father frequently responds inappropriately to questions and suspect that he is experiencing cognitive decline. It may only be that the father has hearing loss, or has both hearing loss and mild confusion. As an older person withdraws, and appears to be less cooperative or less effective as a conversational partner, family and friends may begin to drift away and decrease contact. The older person may increasingly experience anger, frustration, apathy, and anxiety. This situation may lead to more withdrawal and more negative reactions from communication partners.

To the extent possible, professionals working with an older individual should do all in their power to prevent this serial cascade of events. You may include in your aural rehabilitation plan ways to encourage the patient to join small social activity groups that are not too demanding on his or her communication skills. For instance, if the patient enjoys playing cards, then you might encourage a bridge group. If the patient enjoys reading, then a book club might seem inviting.

Provision of counseling for family and friends about the ramifications of hearing loss in general and characteristics of the patient's particular loss is crucial if this negative feedback loop depicted in Figure 13-6 is to be broken. Family, friends, and caretakers can learn how to counteract an older person's tendency to withdraw and avoid conversational interactions and encourage the individual to obtain aural rehabilitation services. In addition, they can actively participate in the aural rehabilitation program. They can learn how to use communication strategies effectively or learn how to help the older person handle a hearing aid or assistive listening device, or to handle the device for the person if necessary.

RESIDENCY

Most older persons live in private residencies, with only about 5% residing in nursing homes (Nussbaum, Thompson, & Robinson, 1989). The majority of nursing home residents have hearing loss, and half of these have severe losses (Schow & Nerbonne, 1980; Voeks, Gallagher, Langer, & Drinka, 1990).

The residential-care population require special attention, as they are likely to have a multitude of impairments and health conditions, and their environments are likely to be more noisy than private home environments (Figure 13-8). Noisy environments can magnify communication handicap, and may result in individuals withdrawing from communication interactions and social activities.

Emotional Variables

Now let's consider emotional variables and how one's emotional state can influence the impact of hearing loss. It is not unusual for older people who have hearing loss to experience depression, isolation, anger, insecurity, and loneliness. Sometimes individuals feel shame, either from a sense of inadequacy or from a sense of being a burden on family, friends, and co-workers. They may be ashamed that they must ask for message clarifications and that their ears may not be "what they used to be." They may hesitate to ask their communication partners to exert the extra effort needed to communicate with them. Some older persons feel an overwhelming sense of wanting to "save face" and "save pride" to hide from people that they need help in facilitating communication. These kinds of emotions and mindsets may lead older adults to undergo lifestyle changes and to experience a diminished quality of life.

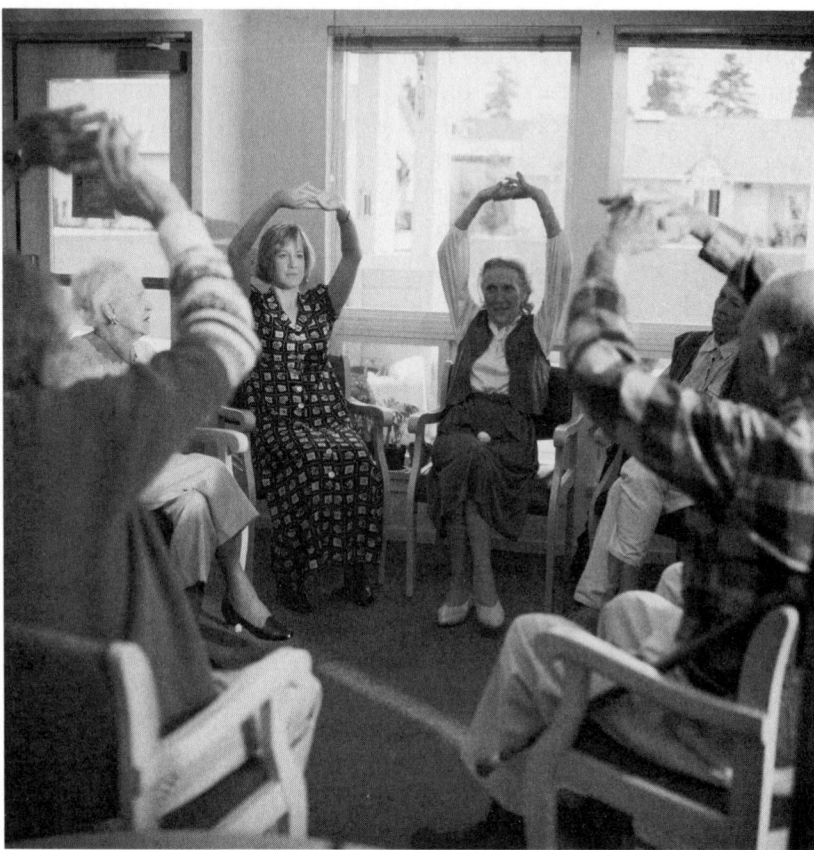

FIGURE 13-8. A patient's residence can have an impact on an aural rehabilitation plan. A person in a health-care facility or nursing home may have a particular need for assistive listening devices. In addition, health-care workers may need special instruction about how to communicate with an older person who has hearing loss; for example, making sure their mouth is clearly visible to the patient.

The emotional state of an individual will not only be influenced by the onset of hearing loss, but in turn, how the individual reacts to hearing loss will be influenced by the individual's psychoemotional profile. A profile of a person's emotional state can be constructed by considering the following variables:

■ Mental health
■ Temperament
■ Sense of self-sufficiency and independence
■ Self-concept

MENTAL HEALTH

A person is said to have a *mental health problem* if he or she has psychopathology or clusters of other acute or chronic symptoms. As with any age group, older individuals vary widely in their mental health. However, it is not uncommon for an older person to suffer from depression. The following situations may trigger depression:

- Loss of or separation from friends and loved ones
- Decreased ability to perform physical activities
- Retirement
- Empty-nest syndrome
- A decline in general health

A hearing loss can magnify feelings of hopelessness, loneliness, and helplessness, and depression may decrease desire to seek hearing health care. Other mental conditions, such as anxiety, obsessive-compulsiveness, and neuroticism, also may increase the communication difficulties associated with a particular degree of hearing loss.

A **mental health problem** is defined as psychopathology or clusters of other acute or chronic symptoms.

TEMPERAMENT

Some people are, by temperament, more or less able to cope with hearing loss. *Temperament* refers to stable personality traits. Such traits as introversion versus extroversion, assertiveness versus passiveness, and optimism versus pessimism will relate to the impact of hearing loss (e.g., Knutson & Lansing, 1990). For instance, an older person might routinely be frustrated by minor irritations, such as getting stuck in traffic, breaking a pencil lead, or forgetting to set an alarm clock. This person may be more affected by hearing loss than someone who has a more easy-going temperament. He or she may be intolerant of talkers who are difficult to understand and may over-react when a remark is missed or not recognized.

Temperament refers to stable personality traits.

SENSE OF SELF-SUFFICIENCY AND INDEPENDENCE

Self-sufficiency and independence relate to whether an individual can conduct day-to-day activities without undue reliance on others. There appears to be a relationship between perceived control and adherence to an aural rehabilitation plan (Garstecki & Erler, 1998). In particular, older women who feel a sense of internal

Self-sufficiency and independence relate to whether a person can conduct day-to-day activities without undue reliance on others.

control over what happens in their lives tend to experience a heightened sense of control over their hearing loss than women who do not experience this feeling.

Many older people feel increasingly dependent on others for daily activities. Some can no longer drive, some cannot do their own shopping, and some must have intermediaries accompany them to medical appointments. Hearing loss can be yet another signal of increased dependence, as an older person with hearing loss may have to rely on others to manage communication difficulties. One man complained, "My wife has to make all my telephone calls for me, and I hate it. It makes me feel like I'm 3 instead of 83!" One goal of the aural rehabilitation plan is to increase the older patient's sense of self-sufficiency and independence.

SELF-CONCEPT

Self-concept refers to how people view themselves.

Self-concept relates to how people view themselves; for example, does someone think of him- or herself as having a hearing impairment? Does the person think that he or she is capable of coping with a disability? Often one's self-concept does not match other person's perceptions, or an audiological report. One patient commented to her audiologist, "I don't feel old, and I certainly don't think of myself as a senior citizen. But the way people treat me reminds me I'm not young anymore. Someone will take my arm to help me up the stairs, or I go to buy a movie ticket, and they give me the senior citizen rate without even asking me if I'm eligible. It's weird." This woman was dismayed when her audiologist proceeded to describe the results of her hearing tests, and she learned she had a bilateral moderate hearing loss.

Persons' self-concepts interact with hearing loss. Some may experience difficulty in accepting aging altogether, and may refuse to wear a hearing aid. Conversely, another may accept hearing loss and have no problem maintaining a healthy self-concept.

Physical Variables

Physical variables as well as emotional variables influence the impact of hearing loss. Several physical changes occur as people age. Their skin wrinkles, age spots appear, hair may turn gray, joints stiffen, and muscles become weaker. Manual dexterity begins to decrease. The rate at which these changes occur varies among individuals, and some people are physically fit well into their eighties and even nineties. Physical fitness interacts with hearing loss to the extent that it may determine the kinds of communication interactions the individual engages in (e.g., Does the person attend parties? Still work?) and the kinds of listening devices that can be used (e.g., Is manual dexterity a problem if the patient desires an in-the-canal hearing aid?).

In addition to changes in physical fitness, many older persons experience chronic ailments, and these may influence the impact of hearing loss. The most common chronic ailments include (in order of frequency of occurrence, National Center for Health Statistics, 1987):

■ Arthritis
■ Cardiac disease
■ Hearing loss
■ Hypertension
■ Orthopedic problems
■ Cataracts

Three common physical conditions are especially relevant when we consider the impact of hearing loss for an older person. These are reduced vision, arthritis, and dementia.

REDUCED VISION

Between about 30 and 40% of individuals over the age of 70 years have impaired vision (Vinding, 1989), and this percentage increases as a function of age. Visual impairment is defined as a vision loss that cannot be corrected through the use of eyeglasses or contact lenses alone. Almost all persons over the age of 70 years use prescription lenses. Of these, 18% must use a magnifying glass for reading and close work. The frequency of blindness rises with age and peaks at 85 years of age and older. The prevalence of blindness in both eyes is about 1% for individuals 74 years old and almost 3% for individuals 85 years and older (Centers for Disease Control and Prevention, 2001). Unfortunately, the majority of individuals who have severe vision impairments also have significant hearing loss (Kirchner & Peterson, 1980). It is a sad twist of fate that, in the face of hearing loss, when someone could utilize the visual signal probably more so than at any

Cataract: progressive retinal disorder that entails a clouding of the lens; causes blurred vision and impairs contrast sensitivity.

Glaucoma: caused by the malfunction of the eye's drainage system that results in irreversible damage to the optic nerve.

Diabetic retinopathy: results from longstanding diabetes, causing blurred and distorted vision in the central visual field and sometimes a detached retina.

Macular degeneration: a progressive loss of both reading vision and distance vision.

other time in life for the purpose of speech recognition, this sense also begins to decline. Visual difficulties may relate to *cataracts, glaucoma, diabetic retinopathy,* or *macular degeneration,* as well as other conditions.

Trends in Vision and Hearing

Older persons are more like to seek intervention for impaired vision than impaired hearing. The Centers for Disease Control and Prevention (2001) report the following statistics:

■ Percentage of people age 70 years and older with a visual problem who:
Have seen a doctor: 99%
Wear glasses: 93%
■ Percentage of people 70 yrs older with a hearing problem who:
Have seen a doctor: 76%
Use a hearing aid: 34%

In some cases, visual skills cannot be enhanced through the use of corrective lenses or ophthalmologic intervention. Reduced visual acuity has the following implications for the impact of hearing loss and the design of an aural rehabilitation plan:

■ Speechreading: The individual will not be able to utilize the visual signal maximally so likely will experience more difficulty in day-to-day speech communication than a person who has similar hearing loss but normal vision.
■ Speech recognition training: Speechreading training may not be appropriate when vision is reduced, because the patient may not be able to adequately see lip movements and other facial gestures. Speech perception training might be aimed at helping the patient be alert to auditory stimuli and to utilize residual hearing to the fullest extent possible.
■ Communication environment: A patient who is less visually able will need optimal lighting in his or her communication environment to maximize what clues are available from speechreading. Sometimes, the environment cannot

be lit optimally for communication because bright lights cause the patient ocular discomfort.

- **Hearing aids and assistive listening devices:** Reduced vision may mean an individual is unable to manipulate the controls of a hearing aid. This consideration may influence the kind of listening devices you recommend, and you will want to be sure to instruct a family member or caregiver on how to check the batteries and handle the hearing aid. Any written materials should be reiterated with a different format. If a hearing aid is recommended, it is important to spend time with the patient so he or she learns to feel the parts of the hearing aid and learns to adjust it by touch (Lindblade & McDonald, 1995).

ARTHRITIS

Arthritis is a painful inflammation of the joints that decreases an individual's ability to perform fine motor activities. For this reason, arthritis can decrease a patient's ability to use listening devices. For example, arthritis may pose the following difficulties for tasks related to using a hearing aid:

- Putting the hearing aid on and taking it off
- Opening the battery compartment and inserting batteries
- Removing ear wax and performing other cleaning tasks
- Operating the controls

Recommendations for listening devices will hinge on a patient's ability to handle them. In some cases, it might be more appropriate to recommend an assistive listening device that has large controls and is easy to manipulate than to recommend a hearing aid. It also may be appropriate to instruct family members or caregivers how to handle the listening devices.

DEMENTIA

Another common physical problem among older persons is dementia. The symptoms of dementia include gradual memory loss, disorientation, decline in the ability to perform everyday tasks, and loss of language skills. ***Alzheimer's disease*** is a form of dementia. Approximately 10% of individuals over the age of 65 years has Alzheimer's disease. This percentage increases almost

Alzheimer's disease is a form of dementia that affects approximately 10% of people over the age of 65.

fivefold for persons over the age of 85 years. Seven out of 10 afflicted people live at home and receive care from family or friends.

Hearing loss often co-occurs with dementia; in fact, older people with dementia are significantly more likely to have hearing loss than older people without dementia. If a hearing loss is present, it is more likely to be greater if the patient has dementia than if he or she does not.

Aural rehabilitation may be especially important for these people. Mulrow, Aguilar, and Endicott (1990) demonstrated that use of hearing aids may improve cognitive functioning. Instruction for family caregivers also may improve communication functioning.

Cognitive Variables

Even if an older person does not manifest symptoms of dementia, which we included in the preceding section as a physical variable, the person may display changes in cognitive functioning that occur as a natural process of aging. In particular, the person may have slowed processing speed and reduced working memory. The extent to which these cognitive declines are present may affect how well the individual can comprehend speech. For example, if someone has a deficit in processing speed, that person may not understand connected discourse very well, especially if the talker speaks quickly. If the person has decreased working memory, the individual may forget the beginning of an utterance by the time the talker has reached the end of what he or she has to say, or the individual may not be able to process the meaning of the message because full attention has to be focused simply on remembering the words.

Processing speed: the rate at which information is conducted and manipulated throughout the nervous system.

PROCESSING SPEED

Older adults, on average, are slower than younger adults when performing speeded cognitive tasks. Evidence suggests they are slower in processing both visuospatial and verbal information (e.g., Hale & Myerson, 1996). For example, older persons have a harder time comprehending sentences that are spoken quickly than do younger persons, and they have poorer recall for speeded speech. If you asked an older person to decide, *as quickly as possible,* whether two words rhyme, that person will probably take longer to reach a decision than if you ask a younger person to perform the same task.

WORKING MEMORY

Older adults also do not perform as well as younger adults on tasks that require them to held material in memory for a short period and then to recall it (Salthouse, 1994). Moreover, older adults have greater difficulty in simultaneously holding onto and manipulating information over and above problems with simply holding on to spoken words in their short-term memory (Wingfield, Stine, Lahar, & Aberdden, 1988). For example, when asked to recall information verbatim, older adults will not perform as well as younger adults. After watching a newscast, they may find the question, "What type of election did the reporter refer to at the beginning of the news brief?" difficult to answer. This kind of age-related deficit will be exacerbated if they are required to answer questions that require an inference or an integration to be made. For instance, they might show less skill in answering the question, "Did the reporter of the three local elections seem biased when she assessed the possible influence of the president's support of the candidates in each election?" than will a younger adult.

> **Working memory:** the ability to store simultaneously and manipulate items in memory.

■ WHAT HAPPENS IF HEARING LOSS GOES UNTREATED?

The National Council on Aging (1999) asked the question, *What happens to the quality of life if hearing loss goes untreated in an elderly person?* To answer it, they surveyed 2,304 seniors who have hearing loss. The survey centered on the use of hearing aids and did not focus on the larger domain of aural rehabilitation. None the less, the findings illustrate what might happen if an older person fails to receive adequate aural rehabilitation intervention. A summary of the survey responses appear in Tables 13-1 and 13-2.

As can be seen in Table 13-1, respondents who do not use hearing aids were more likely to report feeling sad or depressed for a period of 2 weeks or more during the previous year than respondents who used hearing aids, and they were more likely to report feeling worried, tense, or anxious for a month or more during the past year. They were also more likely to experience paranoia

Table 13-1. Responses to a nation-wide survey indicating the emotional status of older persons who have hearing loss. Those who responded affirmatively to the item pertaining to sadness and or depression had felt either emotion for 2 more weeks for the previous year. Those who responded affirmatively to the item pertaining to worry, tension, and anxiety had felt these states for a month or more during the past year.

EMOTION	MILDER HEARING LOSS, USES HEARING AID %	MILDER HEARING LOSS, DOES NOT USE HEARING AID %	MORE SEVERE HEARING LOSS, USES HEARING AID %	MORE SEVERE HEARING LOSS, DOES NOT USE HEARING AID %
Sadness/Depression	14	23	22	30
Worry/Tension/Anxiety	7	12	12	17
Paranoia	13	24	14	36
Insecure/Irritable, Fearful/Tense	8	10	11	17

Source: Adapted from The National Council on the Aging. (1999). *The consequences of untreated hearing loss in older persons.* Washington, DC.

("Other people get angry at me for no reason," when they misunderstand or ask people to repeat themselves). In fact, non-hearing-aid users were almost twice as likely to report that "people get angry with me for no reason" than were hearing-aid users. Finally, non-hearing-aid users were more likely to describe themselves as feeling insecure, irritable, fearful, or tense than were hearing-aid users. These differences between users and non-users were robust, even when other variables such as income level and age were taken into account. The percentage of persons reporting negative emotions increased with the severity of the hearing loss.

Older persons who have hearing loss and who do not use hearing aids often suffer social consequences in addition to emotional consequences. As implied by Table 13-2, isolation becomes a real possibility. The survey showed that older persons who do not use hearing aids were more likely to avoid social activities, such as interacting with neighbors and participating in structured events and were less likely to engage in activities sponsored by senior centers.

The results of this study demonstrate that older patients who have hearing loss, be it more mild or severe, experience both emotional

Table 13-2. Responses to a nation-wide survey indicating the emotional status of older persons who have hearing loss.

ACTIVITY	MILDER HEARING LOSS, USES HEARING AID %	MILDER HEARING LOSS, DOES NOT USE HEARING AID %	MORE SEVERE HEARING LOSS, USES HEARING AID %	MORE SEVERE HEARING LOSS, DOES NOT USE HEARING AID %
Participates Regularly in Social Activities	47	37	42	32
Participates in Senior Center Activities	24	15	21	16

Source: Adapted from The National Council on the Aging. (1999). *The consequences of untreated hearing loss in older persons.* Washington, DC.

and social consequences if the hearing loss goes untreated. Untreated individuals are more likely to experience depression, anxiety, worry, tension, paranoia, and emotional inner turmoil than are hearing-aid users. In contrast, hearing-aid users remain more active in their neighborhoods, in organized social activities, and in senior citizen centers.

In light of these negative consequences that go hand in hand with untreated hearing loss, it is imperative that older persons receive adequate diagnosis, treatment, and follow-up. Now we consider aural rehabilitation plans for older persons.

■ AURAL REHABILITATION PLANS FOR OLDER PERSONS

An aural rehabilitation plan for older patients will include assessment of hearing, communication handicap, and conversational fluency. It then may be appropriate to provide a hearing aid, a hearing aid orientation, assistive devices, speech perception training, or communication strategies training. To consider the special needs of a patient, and develop a good understanding of the relevant factors that have an impact on the patient's hearing status and communication, a hearing professional often begins with a case study and, sometimes, questionnaires.

Learning About the Patient

During the first interactions with an older person, you likely will take a case history and conduct an interview. As with younger adults, you will want to learn about the patient's current communication needs and conversational settings. You also might gather information from other sources, such as members of the family, or administer a questionnaire. Audiological testing will be performed to determine the presence of hearing loss and problems in speech recognition.

THE CASE HISTORY

The case history will provide information about the patient's subjective impression of communication difficulties and a description of listening problems. It also will furnish information about the patient's living arrangements, social interactions, vocational status, and hobbies. The case history also may include conversation with a family member or caregiver, during which you might ask about the patient's memory emotional state, motivation to participate in an aural rehabilitation program, and the feasibility of doing so. It is important also to gather medical data about the following topics (Groher, 1989):

- **Strokes, memory loss, vision problems, dizziness, and medications taken,** because they may have an effect on the patient's ability to participate in testing and subsequent aural rehabilitation.
- **Arthritis and muscle weakness,** because, as we noted earlier, these conditions may interact with a patient's ability to handle a listening device.
- **Ambulation, behavioral changes, and other pertinent conditions,** because they may affect the kinds of communication activities in which the patient may engage.
- **Dementia and Alzheimer's disease,** as patients will require assistance from caregivers or family members to use hearing aids. There is some evidence that hearing loss can magnify cognitive dysfunction and accelerate dementia (Garahan, Waller, Houghton, Tisdale, & Runge, 1992), so it is important that hearing-aid use be encouraged, when appropriate.

During the case history, it is wise to be alert for symptoms of dementia. For example, if someone cannot remember his or her birth date or seems confused by simple tasks, such as completing a questionnaire, the audiologist may want to alter the test procedures. Otherwise, performance may not reflect true hearing ability.

COMMUNICATION HANDICAP AND CONVERSATIONAL FLUENCY

As we have noted in previous chapters, communication handicap relates to the psychosocial effects of hearing loss. You might ask your patient to complete a questionnaire about perceived handicap, such as the Hearing Handicap Inventory for the Elderly (Ventry & Weinstein, 1982). Such instruments provide information about how the respondent perceives social and emotional consequences of hearing loss.

Conversational fluency, or the ease and effectiveness with which a patient can carry on a conversation with a communication partner, often is assessed informally when the patient is older. You might engage in conversation and note the frequency of communication breakdowns and the ways in which the patient attempts to repair them. You might question family members about how well the individual can engage in conversation.

Audiological Testing

In addition to learning about the patient and his or her communication handicap, it is important to quantify degree of hearing loss. Audiological testing for an older person typically includes collection of air- and bone-conduction thresholds for pure tones, speech reception thresholds, and speech recognition scores.

Traditional testing procedures may need to be adapted for the elderly. The audiologist will want to have ample time for patient instructions and may need to double-check to ensure that instructions are understood. If a patient is in the early stages of Alzheimer's disease, reinstruction. may be necessary if the patient takes a short break because the person may forget the task. For someone in the later stages of dementia, testing may not be possible.

Other accommodations for the older patient that may be necessary include the following:

- During air- or bone-conduction testing, tone stimuli may need to be presented for a longer duration of time than for younger persons. Some older persons have difficulty in grasping the concept of listening for a soft, brief tone.
- Stimuli for speech recognition testing may need to be presented live-voice rather than recorded voice, outside of the test booth, so that the patient and clinician can sit face-to-face (Hull, 1995). Some older persons are disconcerted by listening to a disembodied, impersonal voice over headphones.
- Time for rest periods may need to be allocated, or testing spread over more than one day, as some individuals may suffer from fatigue.
- Before testing begins, a visual examination should be made to ensure that there is not impacted cerumen in the outer ear. In some older persons, cerumen removal may be necessary.
- The use of insert earphones may be required to ensure that a correct audiogram is obtained. Softening of the cartilaginous tissue of the ear canal and pinnae occurs with aging.

■ HEARING AIDS, ASSISTIVE LISTENING DEVICES, AND FOLLOW-UP AURAL REHABILITATION

If audiological testing reveals a hearing loss, it may be appropriate to schedule the patient for a hearing-aid evaluation. However, many patients who receive an evaluation either opt not to purchase a hearing aid or do not use the device once it is acquired. In fact, only about 10–30% of older persons who have hearing impairment actually own a hearing aid (Weinstein, 1991) and, of these, only a fraction use them on a regular basis.

The audiologist will want to assess carefully motivation to use amplification before the fitting and then ensure that support systems for hearing-aid use are in place following fitting. Table 13-3 presents factors that affect a patient's motivation to use a hearing aid.

Table 13-3. Factors that may affect an older person's motivation to use a hearing aid.

- Degree of hearing loss
- Communication difficulties
- Self-concept
- Opinion of hearing-aid users (e.g., "Only really old people use hearing aids, and I'm not there yet.")
- Number and quality of conversational interactions in which a patient engages
- The availability of communication partners
- Physical health (such as manual dexterity and visual acuity)

Many of the procedures we have reviewed for selecting hearing aids for adults (Chapter 11) are applicable for the elderly population. When selecting the hearing aid, the audiologist might select one that has oversized touch-type volume controls or one that has easily manipulated battery compartments, especially if manual dexterity is problematic for the patient. Other factors that will influence the recommendation include finances (Can the patient afford the device?), monaural versus binaural hearing aids, and whether assistive listening devices might be appropriate instead of, or as a supplement to, the hearing aid.

Another section of the survey conducted by the National Council on Aging (1999, which we reviewed earlier in this chapter when we considered the effects of no aural rehabilitation), focused on the benefits of hearing aid use. In addition to including responses from older persons who use hearing aids, this section also included responses from family members. Overall, both users and family members reported that following receipt of a hearing aid, improvements occurred in the patient's confidence, independence, relationships with family, and overall outlook on life. Interestingly, the families on average perceived greater improvements than even the users, suggesting that the patients' new ability to hear enhanced the family dynamics of communication. The findings are summarized in Table 13-4. Bess (2000) summarizes a series of other studies that present complimentary findings. Hearing aid use by older persons improves their conversational fluency, helps maintain their psychosocial well-being, reduces communication handicap, and improves overall quality of life.

Table 13-4. Percentage of hearing aid users who reported improvements as a result of hearing aid use.

IMPROVEMENT	% HEARING AID USERS	% FAMILY MEMBERS
Relationships at home	56	66
Feelings about myself	50	60
Life overall	48	62
Mental health	36	39
Self-confidence	39	46
Relationships with children and grandchildren	40	52
Willing to participate in group activities	34	44
Sense of independence	34	39
Sense of safety	34	37
Ability to play card/board games	31	47
Social life	34	41
Physical health	21	24
Dependence on others	22	31
Relationships at work	26	43
Ability to play sports	7	10

Source: Adapted from The National Council on Aging. (1999). *The consequences of untreated hearing loss in older persons.* Washington, DC.

Sometimes the older patient will desire an assistive listening device in addition to or in lieu of a hearing aid. For instance, sometimes an elderly person is unable to handle a hearing aid or earmold because of arthritis and may need a simple FM system instead. Kaplan (1996) suggested that, when arthritis or reduced tactile sensation is present, a simple hardwired system with earphones may be most appropriate. During conversation, a communication partner can talk into a microphone while the older person can wear earphones.

The same microphone-headphone system also can be used for viewing television or listening to the radio. The patient can simply place the microphone by the system's speaker. Alternatively, an older person may be interested in obtaining a listening system that plugs directly into the earphone jack of the television set or radio. For watching television, there is also the option of closed captioning.

When an elderly person lives alone, security is often an issue. It may be important to consider alerting devices to signal the door-bell and telephone ringing and the smoke alarm going off.

One Versus Two?

Jerger et al. (1995) suggested that for some older adults, one hearing aid might be better than two:

"Conventional wisdom suggests that, because humans are normally two-eared listeners, two hearing aids (binaural amplification) ought to provide more benefit than only one (monaural amplification). This is indeed the case in most young people and in many older persons with hearing loss. It is not, however, a universal finding. Some older persons actually seem to do better with a monaural than with a binaural fitting. They report too much confusion of sounds when they wear two aids and that they do better when listening through only one. It is as if the second hearing aid interferes with the first to produce a confusion of sounds in which speech understanding suffers." (p. 934)

The importance of the hearing-aid orientation cannot be overemphasized, and whether the older person becomes a successful hearing-aid user may well hinge on the audiologist's willingness to take the time necessary to give a thorough orientation. There can be no shortcuts here. Ample time must be devoted to instructing the patient on how to insert and remove the earmold and how to handle the hearing aid. One patient, who stopped using his hearing aid shortly after purchasing it, was asked why he never developed a consistent use-pattern. He responded that he did not know how to work the wax removal device, that the battery door was too difficult to operate, and that it hurt his ear to remove the aid at night. This man's audiologist may or may not have provided information about these topics during the hearing-aid orientation. However, the audiologist obviously did not take enough time to ensure that the patient had an adequate understanding of how to handle the hearing aid and did not provide enough follow-up support to ensure successful use.

In addition to receiving a traditional hearing aid orientation after receiving a hearing aid, the audiologist might address specific difficulties that older persons often encounter with their hearing aids. These include changing batteries, inserting the aid into the ear (Figure 13-9), and adjusting the volume control. (Some hearing aid manufacturers accommodate the older patient by constructing aids that have a raised volume control and extraction handles.)

A component of a hearing-aid orientation may be instruction for family members, caregivers, and others involved in the patient's health care. They may learn about caring for the hearing aid, and also develop realistic expectations about what the hearing aid can and cannot do for the patient.

Many older people participate in group aural rehabilitation programs following receipt of a hearing aid, or even without obtain-

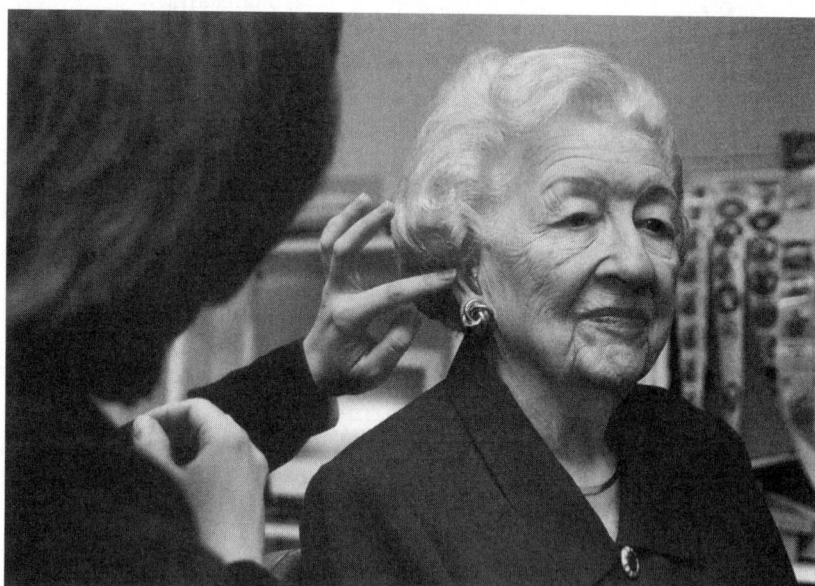

FIGURE 13-9. The older patient might require extra time to learn how to insert the aid into the ear and to extract it. (Photograph by Kim Readmond, courtesy of the Central Institute for the Deaf)

ing one. The program may include such topics as the following (Kricos and Lesner, 1995):

■ Hearing aids and their functions
■ Counseling about issues that are important to the participants
■ Hearing and hearing loss
■ Assistive listening device technology
■ Auditory and visual nature of speech
■ Communication strategies

Often, family members will participate in the aural rehabilitation program with their older relatives (Figure 13-10).

Research suggests that some older patients benefit from participating in formal aural rehabilitation programs. Information counseling and communication strategies may be especially helpful.

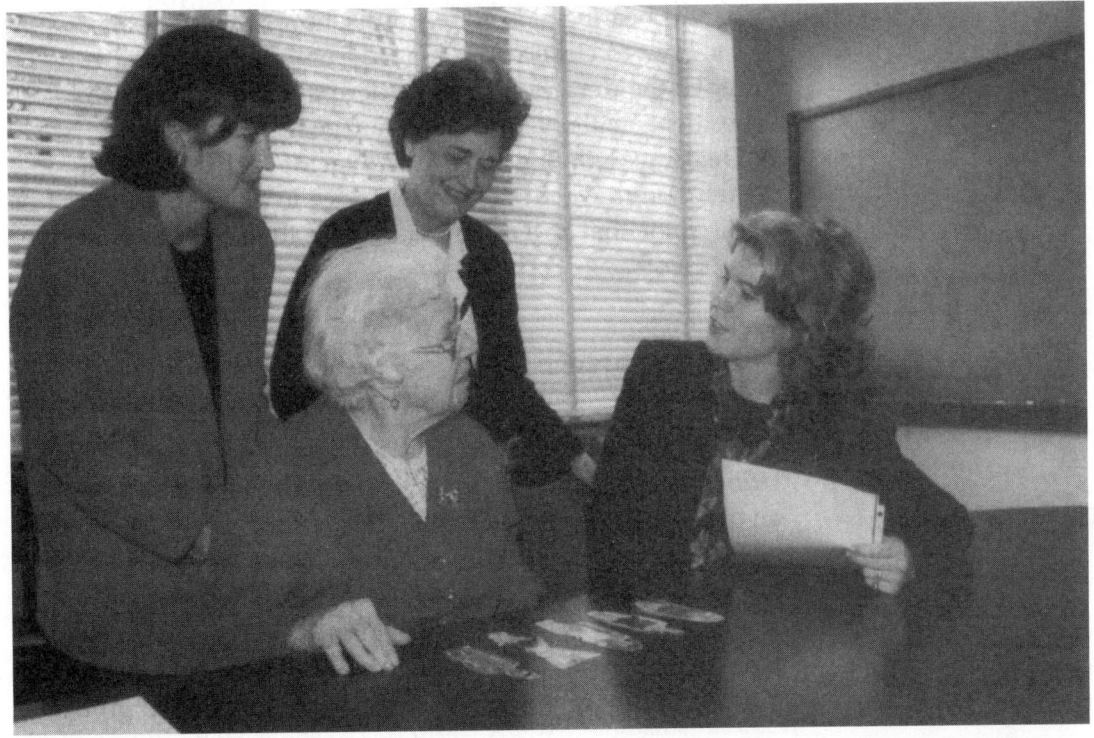

FIGURE 13-10. Family members and other close acquaintances might be encouraged to participate in the aural rehabilitation program for and older adult. (Photograph by Kim Readmond, courtesy of the Central Institute for the Deaf)

For instance, research experiments suggest that many people may experience less perceived communication handicap following a counseling-based aural rehabilitation program (Ventry & Weinstein, 1983). Some benefit from participating in a program that provides analytic auditory training coupled with communication strategies training, but not a program that provides only analytic auditory training (Kricos & Holmes, 1996). Perhaps the individuals who are most likely to benefit are those who have the greatest communication difficulties prior to the onset of training (Kricos & Holmes, 1996).

There are less tangible benefits for older persons who participate in group aural rehabilitation programs in addition to these just listed (see Taylor & Jurma, 1999). First, elderly patients benefit from affiliating with peers who are similar to themselves in a variety of ways, and the group experience permits them to expand the network of social contacts. The social contacts not only alleviate age- and hearing-related loneliness, but they may also elevate their involvement and motivation for seeking help in managing their hearing difficulties. In the aural rehabilitation program, seniors can exchange stories and solutions, share frustrations, and talk about their hearing aids. Finally, the opportunity to interact with an audiologist or other speech and hearing professional can bolster their store of information and increase their number of opportunities to receive counseling.

■ AURAL REHABILITATION IN THE INSTITUTIONAL SETTING

If you are designing an aural rehabilitation program for a patient in a nursing home setting, you may need to adjust the program for the institutionalized setting. Shultz and Mowry (1995) noted some of the problems associated with providing hearing health care to patients in a nursing home. These include:

- Managing the hearing loss when the patient may also have dementia or Alzheimer disease. Often patients with dementia also have depression, which can decrease motivation to participate in an aural rehabilitation plan.
- Preventing hearing aids from being lost. For instance, a patient may place the hearing aid in a bathrobe pocket,

and the robe may end up in the laundry before the aid is removed.

■ **Involving the staff in the aural rehabilitation plan and providing inservice training.** Personnel should be aware of the communication difficulties associated with hearing loss. They should be familiarized with communication strategies and learn how to optimize the listening environment. Finally, they need to know how to handle hearing aids; for example, how to change batteries, how to clean earmolds, and how to insert and remove the devices from an older person's ear, as many residents will not be able to manage them alone.

■ **Dealing with the high turnover of facility personnel.** You may provide an inservice in August, only to discover that in December, half of the staff has been replaced.

An administrator of a nursing home may approach you to perform an inservice for the staff who work with the patients, or you may approach the nursing home personnel. An inservice may be scheduled for a length of time ranging anywhere from a couple of hours (more common) to several half-day sessions (less common). Scheduling is often difficult because staff changes occur about three times during a 24-hour shift, so all workers may not be available at any given time. In addition, staff may not be financially compensated for the time they devote to receiving training, and some attendees may have just finished working an 8-hour shift and may be anxious to end their workday. Often the staff will have little knowledge about hearing loss, and some may not have received higher education so may lack appropriate background knowledge to understand some of the material you would like to present.

The way in which you present material must be at level of difficulty that is appropriate for the audience and done in a way that maintains their interest and attention. The use of visual materials and hands-on teaching aids help achieve these guidelines. In addition, the presentation of case studies, demonstrations (e.g., "Please try on the ear plugs in the package I gave you at the beginning of the class. Once you have them in place, I'll ask you to try to understand the sentences that I will read."), and group discussion ("Please help me generate a list of conditions that might make speechreading difficult.") serve to engage the staff in the learning process. The goal of an inservice is to provide basic information about hearing loss and hearing aids, to develop empathy for the person who has hearing loss, and to teach strategies for enhancing communication with patients. The program designed at Central Institute for the Deaf includes three units: hearing loss and hearing aids, speechreading, and communication strategies. Sample objectives for the speechreading unit include:

- Participants will identify characteristics of a good speechreader.
- Participants will identify factors that influence the speechreading task.

CASE STUDY 1

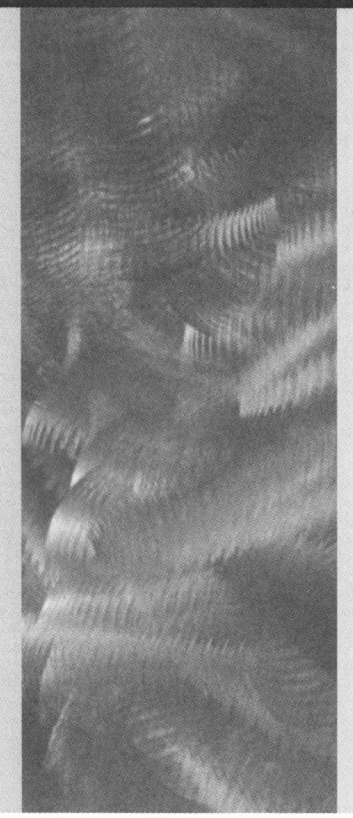

The following example illustrates appropriate aural rehabilitation objectives that might be incorporated into a program for an older adult.

Mr. Gifford is a 70-year-old man who recently retired from his position at the post office. He is married, and his daughter and her family live nearby. Mr. Gifford is concerned that his severe hearing loss may prevent him from giving tours to groups at the zoo. Although he is reluctant to admit this, he also feels that he is sometimes left out of the conversation at family gatherings, because he misses so much of what is said. Mr. Gifford tried using a hearing aid about 5 years ago, when he first noticed a hearing problem, but was dissatisfied with the sound quality. Besides, while delivering mail he found he rarely engaged in conversation with many persons. Mr. Gifford's aural rehabilitation goals are to improve his ability to hear while working outside at the zoo and to improve his ability to participate in family conversations. Mr. Gifford is in fairly good health, although he does have arthritis in his hands.

(continues)

Mr. Gifford and his clinician agreed they were to establish goals for both his volunteer work and for his home setting. Aural rehabilitation goals included:

- Assessment and fitting of an appropriate hearing aid. Mr. Gifford's ability to handle a hearing aid and work the controls also would be assessed. An instrument that he can handle, given his dexterity limitations, would be recommended.
- Provision of extensive follow-up-fitting support. This goal would include establishing a use-schedule for the first few weeks of use, and a brief program of speechreading and listening training, to acclimate him to the amplified signal.
- Development of effective use of constructive facilitative communication strategies (i.e., strategies aimed at structuring the environment for optimal communication by minimizing background noise and ensuring a favorable view of the talker, as discussed in Chapter 2). Instruction would be provided to maximize Mr. Gifford's listening potential in both indoor and outdoor environments.
- Development of effective use of other facilitative communication strategies and repair strategies to facilitate communication with family members and visitors to the zoo.
- Involvement of family members in the aural rehabilitation plan. Mrs. Gifford and her daughter would be encouraged to participate in a communication-strategies training program with Mr. Gifford, and to develop their use of communication strategies. Mrs. Gifford would also be invited to attend the hearing-aid fitting, and develop realistic expectations about what a hearing aid can do.
- Enrollment in a support group for hard-of-hearing individuals, such as Self-Help for Hard-of-Hearing People (SHHH). An attempt would be made to identify a group that has at least some other senior citizen members.

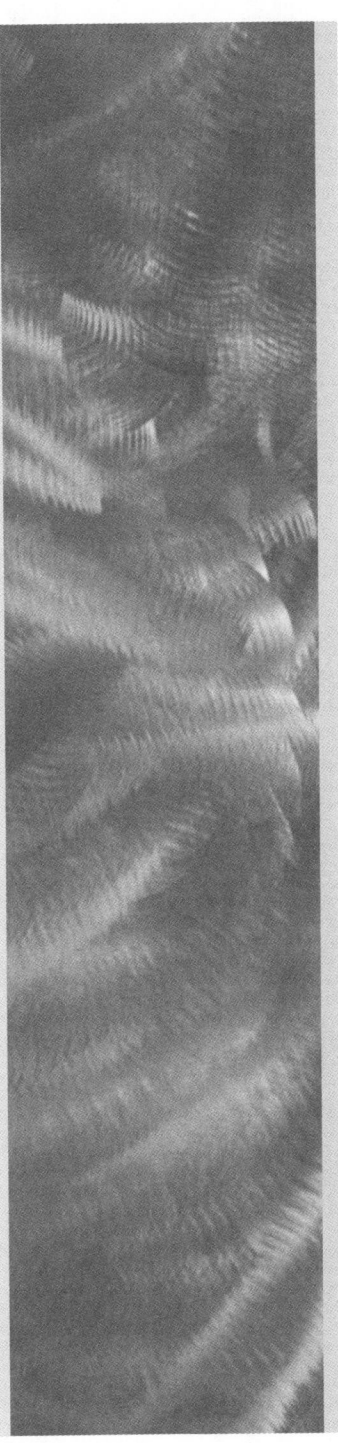

■ FINAL REMARKS

You may discover that working with older people provides some of your most rewarding professional experiences. One audiologist described how she tested an elderly woman who had terminal cancer. "Mrs. Kramer had a moderate, bilateral hearing loss," the audiologist related. "I knew by talking with her, and reviewing her medical records, that she only had a few months to live. I suggested that she might not be interested in purchasing a hearing aid." Much to the audiologist's surprise, Mrs. Kramer not only wanted to buy a hearing aid, she wanted to buy two. She also wanted to borrow a VHF videotape that provides speechreading training. Mrs. Kramer's rationale was simple: "There is so much going on in my body that I can't control. It feels good to be able to actually do something positive about my hearing problem."

■ KEY CHAPTER POINTS

✔ The elderly represent the fastest growing segment of the U.S. population. Approximately 30% of the elderly population has hearing loss.

✔ Degree of hearing loss increases with age. Age-related hearing loss is called presbycusis.

✔ The impact of hearing loss on the older individuals may vary as a result of the person's economic status, social circumstances, social contacts, and emotional and physical health. Two persons may be of the same chronological age, yet vary greatly on these variables.

✔ Three physical conditions that may influence dramatically the design and success of an aural rehabilitation plan include reduced vision, arthritis, and dementia.

✔ Some changes may need to be made in the procedures for assessing hearing status, and for providing a hearing-aid orientation. In particular, more time usually must be scheduled to provide aural rehabilitation services for an older adult than for a younger adult.

▪ MULTIPLE CHOICE QUESTIONS

1. Although the aural rehabilitation needs of older persons resemble those of younger adults, there may be some differences, due to the fact that older persons:
    a. Are often less likely to want to have money to spend on a hearing aid because they grew up during the Depression
    b. Are less likely to want to wear a hearing aid because they are part of the Baby-Boom generation
    c. May have more difficulty recognizing speech in noise, and may tire more easily when listening
    d. May be hypersensitive to high-frequency tone pips

2. The differences between older adults who were born before 1945 and those who were born between 1945 and 1965 include the following:
    a. The former group tends to be more resistant to technology and more likely to follow advice.
    b. The former group likes to use credit or time-plans.
    c. The latter group will want to avoid credit.
    d. The latter group often endorses a family or team approach.

3. Hearing loss in the elderly is:
    a. Often best characterized as a flat audiogram configuration
    b. The number one chronic condition in this population
    c. Most commonly the result of a lifetime of noise exposure
    d. More common among men than women

4. Physiologically, the most common cause of presbycusis is:
    a. A loss of hair cells
    b. Cochlear conductive
    c. A combination of neural and metabolic factors
    d. A deterioration of the tectorial membrane

5. Which of the following is not typically thought to be a classic manifestation of presbycusis?

   a. Reduced speech discrimination

   b. Poor temporal resolution, where the patient cannot distinguish two tones that differ in duration

   c. Poor ability to recognize speech in larger convention rooms

   d. A sensation of fullness in the ear

6. You are about to administer the NU-6 Test to a person who is 80 years old. What is the best predictor of the patient's performance?

   a. The patient's PTA

   b. The patient's thresholds at 1000, 2000, and 4000 Hz

   c. The patient's central auditory processing capabilities

   d. The patient's processing speech and working memory

7. Which of the following statements is false?

   a. Older women are less able financially to implement a comprehensive aural rehabilitation plan.

   b. Most older persons live in private residencies.

   c. Older women who do not sense an internal locus of control are more complacent and are more likely to adhere to an aural rehabilitation plan.

   d. Temperament might affect adherence with the aural rehabilitation plan.

8. What is macular degeneration?

   a. Progressive retinal disorder that results in a clouding of the lens.

   b. Due to low blood sugar, it causes distorted vision in the central visual field.

   c. A progressive loss of both reading vision and distance vision.

   d. A decline in an older person's macula in both the utricle and saccule.

9. An older person may have reduced processing speed. For example, this person might:
    a. Take longer than a younger person in deciding that the words *bat* and *book* do not rhyme
    b. May become disoriented when taking a long walk away in his or her neighborhood
    c. May have difficulty in making inferences after listening to a lecture
    d. May have poor word discrimination as a result

10. An older person who opts not to use a hearing aid, even if needed, is more likely than someone who does use a hearing aid to:
    a. Seek social support from a senior center
    b. Seek support from a network of family and friends
    c. More likely to be fearful and tense
    d. Is more likely to feel an internal locus of control

11. Mr. Thomson has arrived at your clinic for a hearing test. Mr. Thomson is 79 years old. During pure-tone testing, you might make the following adjustment in your test procedures:
    a. Forego word recognition testing because Mr. Thomson likely will have poor speech discrimination
    b. Forego bone conduction testing because Mr. Thomson will likely tire before you are able to complete the procedure
    c. Use insert earphones to eliminate the possibility of collapsing ear canals
    d. Perform the testing as quickly as possibly to prevent fatigue

12. There are many difficulties inherent in preventing an inservice to personnel in a nursing home facility. One of the prime difficulties is that:

    a. Most nursing homes do not cater to the needs of persons who have hearing loss.

    b. Inservices are difficult to schedule, because of work shifts.

    c. Most nursing home directors do not know about the importance of audiology and aural rehabilitation.

    d. There are no instructional designs available that maintain staff attention.

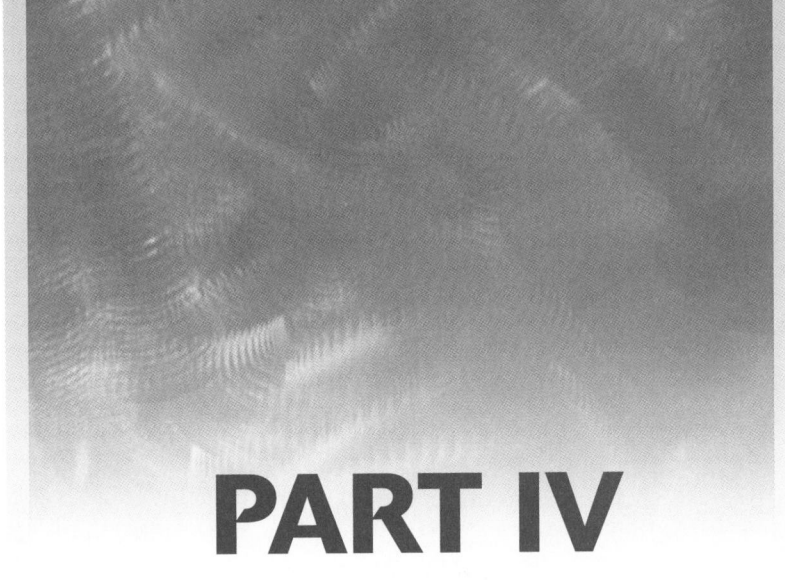

PART IV

Aural Rehabilitation
for Children

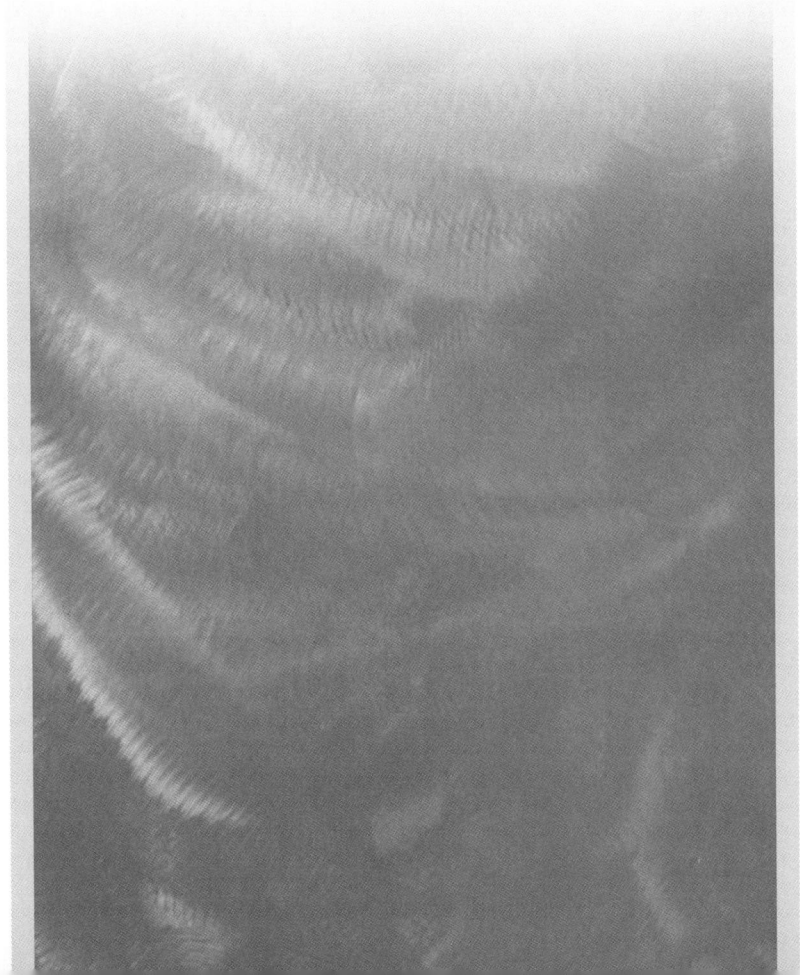

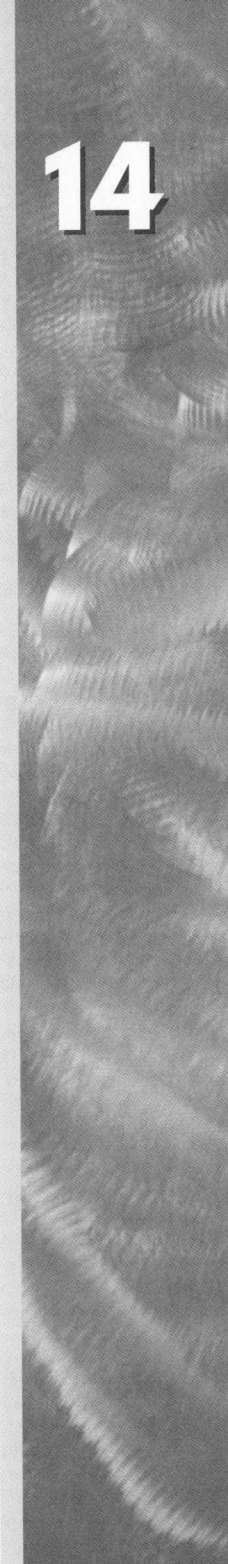

CHAPTER **14**

Children Who Have Hearing Loss

TOPICS

- Demographics
- Causes of hearing loss
- Hearing and speech recognition skills
- Screening
- Identification and quantification of hearing loss
- Other hearing-related conditions
- Coping with a child's diagnosis
- Amplification
- Case study
- Final remarks
- Key chapter points
- Multiple choice questions
- Key resources

Parents react in many different ways when a hearing professional tells them that their baby has a severe or profound hearing impairment. One common reaction is for parents to say, "O.K. We'll get hearing aids for her, and she can learn to lipread us." They assume hearing aids and lipreading lessons can make the hearing loss inconsequential. Unless the parents know someone who has had a significant hearing impairment from birth, they may not realize initially that their child's speech development, language acquisition, conversational skills, and literacy likely will differ from what is common for children with normal hearing. Parents may become aware of these consequences only gradually, as they receive counseling from speech and hearing professionals and as they acquire many months and even years of firsthand experience in watching their child grow. They also will learn to appreciate the long-term commitments that will be required of them, the child, other members of their family, and the child's school system in order for the child to realize his or her full potential.

With this chapter, we begin our consideration of children who have hearing losses. First we focus on demographic issues and then hearing measurement. In subsequent chapters, we focus on intervention plans and speech, language, literacy and conversational skills.

Prelingual: hearing loss incurred before the acquisition of spoken language.

In this chapter, we are concerned primarily with children who have prelingual hearing loss. As noted in Chapter 1, children who are *prelingually* hearing-impaired had their hearing losses when they were learning language and speech. They may have been born with hearing loss (in which case they have congenital hearing impairment) or they may have lost their hearing early in life, perhaps as a result of meningitis, high fever, or head trauma. An

An **intervention program** for children includes family counseling, hearing-aid fitting, selection of appropriate assistive listening devices, speech perception training, and other aspects of a child's educational and rehabilitation program.

intervention program includes family counseling, hearing-aid fitting (or cochlear-implant fitting), selection of appropriate assistive listening devices and follow-up support, and speech perception training. It also encompasses other aspects of a child's educational and rehabilitation program, such as speech and language therapy, educational and classroom placement, and communication mode. The intervention program also may include instruction for the child's parents about how to nurture their child's language, listening, and conversational skills.

■ DEMOGRAPHICS

Over 1 million children in the United States have a hearing loss (Figure 14-1). For every 1,000 children in this country, 83 have what is termed an *educationally significant hearing loss* (U.S. Public Health Service, 1990). Severe and profound losses in infants have an incidence of 1 to 2 per 1,000 (Feinmesser, Tell, & Levi, 1982; Parving, 1985). Among school-age children, severe to profound hearing loss occurs in about 9 children of every 1,000. If we consider children who have any degree of hearing loss, even a mild loss, then the incidence rises to as high as 1 in 25 (Teele, Klein, & Rosner, 1989).

Two important statistics to consider when reviewing the demographics of children who have significant hearing loss pertain to the occurrence of other disabilities and the hearing status of their parents.

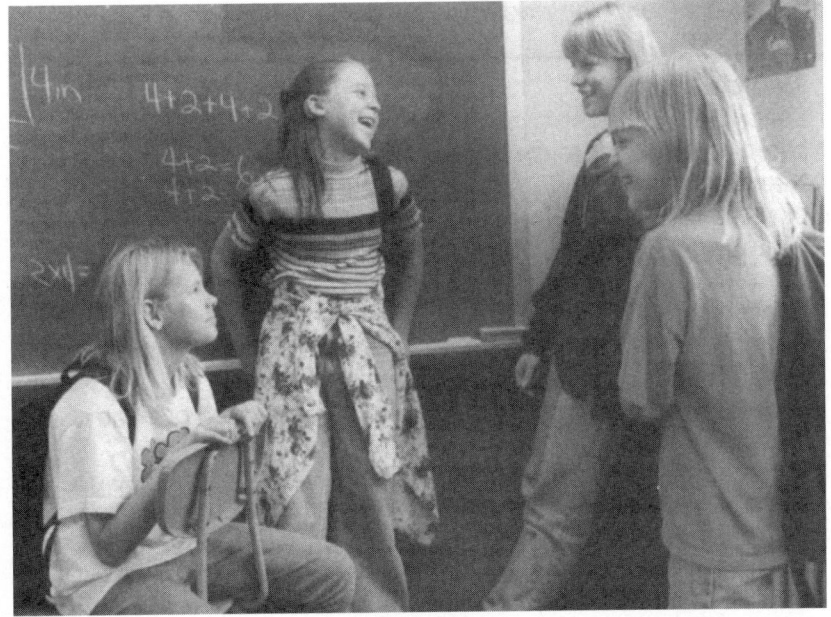

FIGURE 14-1. Over 1 million children in the United States have a profound hearing loss. (By Patti Gabriel, courtesy of the Central Institute for the Deaf)

Other Disabilities

Approximately 30% of hearing-impaired children have a disability in addition to hearing loss (Wolff & Harkins, 1986). Co-occurring conditions include mental retardation, significant visual impairment, learning disabilities, and attention deficit disorder. Emotional or behavioral problems, cerebral palsy, and orthopedic problems also may co-occur with hearing loss. Sometimes, the multiple disabilities stem from similar causes, such as trauma at birth or prematurity. Causes may also relate to ethnic background and heredity. Table 14-1 presents conditions that commonly co-occur with hearing loss. The relatively high frequency of co-occurring conditions suggests that the speech and hearing professional will need to take these into account when developing a child's intervention plan and aural rehabilitation strategy and when working as a member of the child's multidisciplinary team.

Table 14-1. Conditions that may co-occur with hearing loss.

- Mental retardation
- Behavior or psychiatric disorders
- Learning disability, related to reading and/or writing
- Nervous system ailments, such as seizures, vestibular disturbances, or spina bifida
- Eye disease, including optic degeneration, ocular lens abnormalities, and retinitis pigmentosa
- Renal disease
- Musculoskeletal abnormalities in the skull, oral cavity, face, outer and/or middle ear, limbs, or joints
- Musculoskeletal disease, such as growth retardation or bone disease
- Growth retardation
- Skin disease, such as pigmentary disorder (e.g., albinism, white forelock, iris bicolor or heterochromia), keratosis, sun sensitivity, thick, coarse hair, and malformed fingernails and toenails
- Metabolic disease such as diabetes, goiter, liver and spleen enlargement, or impaired metabolism or carbohydrates
- Cardiac and vascular disease

Parent's Hearing Status

Ninety to 95% of children who have a severe or profound sensorineural hearing loss have parents who are normally hearing (Northern & Downs, 1991). This means that, prior to their child's birth, they may have been unfamiliar with the many ramifications of hearing loss. They probably will not know sign language. They also are unlikely to be members of the Deaf Culture (Chapter 11). Thus, they will have much to learn about hearing loss and aural rehabilitation, and they will need to make a decision as to whether to try to learn how to sign. They may also need to consider issues concerning the Deaf Culture. They may not (or may) be in agreement with the goal of enculturating their child into a culture that is different from their own.

■■■ CAUSES OF HEARING LOSS

Hearing loss that is severe or profound usually is sensorineural or mixed. Sensorineural hearing loss, in which the hearing loss is centered in the inner ear or auditory nerve, may stem from either environmental or genetic causes.

Environmental Causes of Sensorineural Hearing Loss

Environmental causes may be *prenatal* (occurring before birth), *perinatal* (occurring at birth), or *postnatal* (occurring shortly after birth). Prenatal factors that may affect a child's hearing status include the following:

Prenatal: before birth.
Perinatal: during birth.
Postnatal: after birth.

■ Intrauterine infections, including rubella, cytomegalovirus, and herpes simplex virus
■ Complications associated with the Rh factor (wherein maternal antibodies affect the Rh-positive blood cells of the baby)
■ Prematurity
■ Maternal diabetes
■ Parental radiation
■ Toxemia during pregnancy
■ *Anoxia* (lack of oxygen)
■ Syphilis

Anoxia: deficiency or absence of oxygen in the body tissues.

Hearing loss may be incurred during birth, in which case it stems from a perinatal cause. Perinatal causes of hearing loss include anoxia, which may be caused by a prolapse of the umbilical cord and a subsequent blockage of blood to the infant's brain. Although rare, the use of forceps during birth may cause damage to the cochlea, as might severe uterine contractions.

A postnatal loss often occurs because of meningitis or use of ototoxic drugs. A listing of ototoxic drugs appears in Table 14-2. Other postnatal environmental factors include measles, encephalitis, chicken pox, influenza, and mumps.

Table 14-2. Medications that may be ototoxic.

■ Aminoglycoside antibiotics, which are often used against gramnegative bacteria. Hearing loss is often bilateral and sensorineural. Some of the drugs may be more vestibulotoxic than cochleotoxic.
Amikacin
Dihydrostreptomycin
Garamycin
Gentamicin
Kanamycin
Neomycin
Netilmicin
Streptomycin
Tobramycin
Viomycin

■ Salicylates, used in large quantities for the treatment of arthritis and other connective tissue disorders. Their use may result in sensorineural hearing loss and tinnitus.
Acetylsalicylic acid
Aspirin

■ Loop diuretics, used to promote urine excretion. Their use may result in sensorineural hearing loss.
Ethacrynic acid
Furosemide
Lasix

■ Other drugs that may be ototoxic and that are used in chemotherapy regimens.
Cisplatin
Carboplatin
Nitrogen mustard

Source: Adapted from *Comprehensive Dictionary of Audiology* (2nd ed.) by B. A. Stach, (2003). Clifton Park, NY: Delmar Learning.

Genetic Causes of Sensorineural Hearing Loss

Genetic factors are thought to cause more than 50% of all incidents of congenital hearing loss in children. More than 400 kinds of genetic-based hearing losses have been described, and with increased activity in genetics research and the Human Genome Project, new types continually are being identified.

Important vocabulary for talking about genetics and hearing loss is defined in the Key Resources section at the end of the chapter. *Genes* provide the blueprints for development and function and are arranged on the 23 pairs of *chromosome pairs,* 22 of which are *autosomes* and one of which is a pair of sex chromosomes. The human genome contains between 30,000 and 40,000 genes, which are segments located on the double helical DNA. A child inherits one set of chromosomes from each parent. The sex chromosome may be either X or Y. If both parents transmit an X chromosome, then the baby will be female. If the father transmits a Y chromosome, then the baby will be male. The nucleus of a cell contains the 46 chromosomes, with each chromosome consisting of a single molecule of deoxyribonucleic acid (DNA). DNA has a double helical structure and is composed of four bases called adenine (A), guanine (G), thymine (T), and cytosine (C). The double helix forms with a pairing with A and T, and C and G. Knowing the sequences of bases in a DNA strand automatically reveals the sequence on the adjoining strand. The constrained pairing means that DNA can replicate by separating the two strands of the helix, followed by each strand dictating a new complementary strand. A child inherits pairs of chromosomes, and hence pairs of genes, from the parents. Occasionally, one of the pairs may contain a mutation. This mutation may prevent the formation of a protein encoded by the gene. As a result, the child may manifest a clinically abnormal phenotype (which is the visible effect of the genotype), such as hearing loss (see Keats, 2002, for a review).

The different possible codes of a gene are called *alleles.* For example, an allele may specify blonde hair or red hair. If the same allele is inherited from both parents, then the resulting trait is *homozygous*. If the two are different, then the trait is *heterozygous*. Genetic hearing losses may be described as follows:

■ Autosomal dominant trait: One parent has a dominant allele for hearing loss which is passed on to the child, and

Chromosome pair: the basic units of genes; structures carrying the genes of a cell and made up of a single strand of DNA.

Autosomes: any of the 22 chromosome pairs that are not related to gender.

Alleles: the different possible codes of a gene.

Homozygous: having two identical alleles of the same gene; the same allele is inherited from both parents.

Heterozygous: having two different alleles of the same gene.

Autosomal dominant: one parent passes a dominant allele to the child; the probability of the trait being expressed in the child is 50%.

Autosomal recessive: both of a child's parents carry a recessive gene; the probability of the gene being expressed in the child is 25%.

X-linked: refers to the mother carrying a recessive allele for a trait on the sex chromosome, which is not expressed in female progeny but is passed to males.

Delayed-onset hereditary hearing loss: Hearing is normal at birth, then declines later in life as a result of a hereditary disorder.

typically, that parent has a hearing loss. The hearing loss is called ***autosomal dominant*** because a gene from only one parent is required for its manifestation. A child born to a parent with a dominant-trait hearing loss has a 50% probability of also having a hearing loss. If you examine the family history, you likely will find the reoccurrence of hearing loss in successive generations on one side of the family tree.

■ Autosomal recessive trait: A child may have parents who both carry a recessive gene for hearing loss, and yet both parents usually have normal hearing. The hearing loss is then related to an ***autosomal recessive*** trait. Approximately 80% of inherited hearing loss is of this type. The probability of a normally hearing couple's having a hearing-impaired baby, when both parents carry a recessive gene, is 25%. There may be no other family members who have hearing loss, and only a thorough examination of the family tree on either side of the family will reveal the rare occurrence of hearing loss. This is true only if both parents have normal hearing. If two deaf persons with the same recessive genes for deafness marry, all of their children also will be deaf.

■ X-linked trait: This rare kind of inherited hearing loss accounts for about 2% of genetic-based hearing losses. For a hearing loss to be related to an **X-*linked trait*,** the mother may have a recessive allele for hearing loss that is on the sex chromosome (labeled X on females and Y on males). When daughters inherit it, the trait is not shown, although they have a 50% chance of passing a hearing loss on to their sons. When males inherit the X-linked allele, they usually develop hearing loss.

Hereditary hearing losses are often classified according to (a) the mode of inheritance (e.g., *autosomal dominant*), (b) whether they are syndromic or nonsyndromic, (c) the audiological configuration, (d) whether they are bilateral or unilateral, (e) the progression (e.g., sudden or gradual) and age of onset of the loss, and (f) whether or not the vestibular system is affected. Many people who have a hereditary hearing loss experience a delayed onset that is nonsyndromic (Tomaski & Grundfast, 1999). Patients who have a ***delayed-onset hereditary*** disorder may have normal hearing at birth and then begin to lose hearing later (often not until they are in their twenties or thirties). A *nonsyndromic hearing loss* is one that has no other associated findings.

Many hearing losses based in genetics are part of a *syndrome,* which in medicine means a number of conditions that occur together and characterize a common disease. For example, Treacher-Collins is a syndrome that involves an autosomal dominant trait. In addition to hearing loss, which may range from mild to profound, the child with Treacher-Collins may manifest deficits in the oral cavity, nervous system, and pulmonary and renal systems. Another example of a syndrome that usually includes hearing loss is Goldenhar. In this syndrome, the afflicted child may have malformations in the mandible and outer ear, as well as a hearing loss that may range from mild to profound. Other systematic abnormalities associated with Goldenhar may manifest in the nervous system, eye, kidneys, and pulmonary and cardiovascular systems. This syndrome also involves an autosomal dominant trait. Other examples of autosomal dominant syndromes include Bjornstad syndrome, Harboyan sydrome, Stickler syndrome, and Waardenburg syndrome. Examples of autosomal recessive syndromes include Richards-Rundle syndrome, Alstrom syndrome, Usher syndrome, Pendred syndrome, and Brancio-Otorenal syndrome. Alport syndrome and Hunter syndrome are examples of X-linked recessive syndromes. These syndromes and examples of other syndromes that may involve the auditory system appear in Table 14-3.

Nonsyndromic hearing loss: a hearing loss that has no other associated findings.

A **syndrome** is a collection of conditions that co-occur as a result of a single cause and constitute a distinct clinical entity.

Table 14-3. Examples of syndromes that may include hearing loss.

SYNDROME	CO-OCCURRING CONDITIONS
Alport	Nephritis and sensorineural hearing loss
Alstrom	Pigmentary retinopathy, diabetes mellitus, obesity, malformation of the brain, and progressive sensorineural hearing loss
Bjornstad syndrome	Congenital sensorineural hearing loss and pili torti
Branchio-otorenal syndrome	Branchial anomalies, including branchial clefts, fistulas and cysts; otologic anomalies including malformed pinna or preauricular pits; renal abnormalities. Three fourths of patients have hearing loss, either conductive, sensorineural, or mixed
Crouzon	Premature closure of sutures, hypertension, downward displacement of eyeballs due to shallow orbits, mild to moderate conductive hearing loss, may entail mixed loss; closure of external auditory canal

(continues)

Table 14-3. (continued)

SYNDROME	CO-OCCURRING CONDITIONS
Down	Mental retardation, characteristic facial features, often accompanied by chronic otitis media, and associated conductive, mixed, and sensorineural hearing loss
Edward	Microcephaly, agenesis of bones, congenital heart disease, craniofacial abnormalities, mental retardation, and outer, middle, and inner ear anomalies
Epstein	Macrothrombocytopathia, nephritis, and sensorineural hearing loss
Fetal alcohol syndrome	Low birth weight, failure to thrive, mental retardation, wide-set eyes, recurrent otitis media, sensorineural hearing loss
Formey	Joint fusion, mitral insufficiency, and conductive hearing loss
Harboyan	Characterized by progressive sensorineural hearing loss of delayed onset
Hunter	Sensorineural, conductive, or mixed hearing loss, growth deficiency, mental and neurological deterioration, coarse facial features
Jervell and Lange-Nielsen	Electrocardiographic abnormalities, fainting spells, and accompanied by congenital bilateral profound sensorineural hearing loss
Latham-Munro	Myoclonus epilepsy, ataxia, and sensorineural hearing loss
Lemieux-Neemeh	Nephritis, motor and neuropathy with sensorineural hearing loss
Mondini dysplasia	Congenital anomaly of the osseous and membranous labyrinths, severe loss of hearing and vestibular function
Pendred	Goiter and moderate-to-profound congenital sensorineural hearing loss
Pfeiffer	Premature closure of sutures, broad thumbs, broad great toes, short fingers and toes, hypertelorism, high arched palate, downward sloping eyes, absent external auditory canals, conductive hearing loss
Richards-Rundle	Ataxia, muscle wasting, hypogonadism, mental retardation, and progressive sensorineural hearing loss
Robinson	Dominant onychodystrophy, coniform teeth, and sensorineural hearing loss
Stickler	Severe myopia, retinal detachment, flat facial profile, cleft palate, ocular anomalies, arthritis, sensorineural, conductive, or mixed hearing loss
Treacher Collins	Pinnae malformations, downslanting eyes, small chin, depressed cheek bones, large mouth, eyelid colobomar, conductive hearing loss related to atresia and ossicular malformation
Usher	Congenital sensorineural hearing loss and progressive loss of vision
Waardenburg	Widely spaced eyes, joined eyebrows, a broad nasal root, and a minimal to severe unilateral or bilateral hearing loss (about 30% of patients have a white forelock)

The gene that causes a hearing loss may be different from one person to the next. For instance, Usher's syndrome (see Table 14-3) may be related to at least 10 different genes. Moreover, the phenotypic expression of a gene mutation may vary from one patient to the next. Sometimes a gene mutation will result in hearing loss for one person, but not another (Keats, 2002).

A Pediatrician's Guide to Diagnose and Treat Hereditary Hearing Loss

The eponym *ALOUD* can guide a pediatrician in diagnosing and treating a baby who has a hereditary hearing loss (Tomaski & Grundfast, 1999):

"A: *Ask* about family history. [The family history might be a prime clue as to the presence of hearing loss. For example, if a family member incurred a hearing loss before the age of 30 years, or if a family member has a white forelock, one eye colored differently than the other, or kidney difficulties, the odds of the baby having a hereditary hearing loss increases.]

L: *Look.* Do a careful physical examination to look for physical findings known to be present in some types of [hereditary hearing impairment] [The physician will examine the face and head, eyes, ears, skin, hair, extremities, neck, and balance looking for such syndromic manifestations as skin tags, unsteady gait, and abnormal pigmentation.]

O: *Obtain* appropriate studies to include audiogram, urinalysis, temporal bone CT scan, possibly electrocardiogram, and other studies that may be indicated. [For example, if a physician suspects Jervell and Lange-Nielsen Syndrome, then an electrocardiogram might be ordered.]

U: *Use* consultants to include otolaryngologists experienced in dealing with [hereditary hearing impairment], pediatric ophthalmologists, clinical geneticists, and counselors. [For instance, an ophthalmologist might be consulted if an ocular symptom is noted. A clinical geneticist might confirm the presence of a hereditary syndrome, and might provide counseling regarding future pregnancies.]

D: *Determine* an appropriate plan of action for children newly diagnosed with [hereditary hearing impairment]. Depending on the severity of the child's hearing impairment, the family may need advice regarding the choice of educational setting and mode of communication. If the child is deaf, consideration is given to communication using American Sign Language and placement in a school for the deaf or aural-oral communication and mainstreaming the child in a regular public school." (p. 42) [See Chapter 15 for consideration of communication modes and classroom placement.]

Mixed and Conductive Hearing Loss

Some children have mixed hearing loss, which is a combination of both conductive and sensorineural components. The most common cause of the conductive component of a mixed hearing loss is otitis media, which is the second most common childhood ailment, second only to the common cold. Otitis media is an inflammation of the middle ear, often associated with the build up of fluid. The fluid may or may not be contaminated with infection.

Otitis media can result in a mild or moderate conductive hearing loss, particularly in the low frequencies, and can accentuate the amount of hearing loss in the presence of an existing sensorineural loss. The other symptoms of otitis media, besides hearing loss, and the severity, duration, and frequency of the inflammation vary between children. Some children will experience the condition one time and then never again and only experience slight pain and fever. Others will experience repeated bouts, with "glue-like" fluid, excruciating ear pain, and permanent hearing loss (due to damage to the ossicles and/or tympanic membrane).

In the absence of pain and fever, the condition may go unnoticed by the child, and hence, untreated. This is an undesirable state of affairs because the child may miss out on hearing important speech, language, and academic material. As a result, language and speech may be delayed, and academic performance may fall below the child's potential. Some of the symptoms that might alert parents to the presence of otitis media in their child include inattentiveness, reduced ability to discriminate speech, wanting the television turned up more loudly than usual, and undue fatigue.

Facts About Otitis Media

Here are some data about children in the United States and otitis media (Janota, 1999, p. 48):

- About 50% of children have a bout of otitis media by their first birthday and 80% by their third.
- Otitis media is two to four times less prevalent in African American children than in white children.

(continues)

- Otitis media is the most common reason a child under 15 years of age visits a physician.
- Thirty million doctor visits a year are caused by otitis media.
- Otitis media is the most frequent reason why doctors prescribe antibiotic therapy for children.
- The surgical treatment of middle ear effusion is the most frequent reason for administering general anesthesia to children.

■ HEARING AND SPEECH RECOGNITION SKILLS

Now let us turn our attention to the issue of listening skills in the child who has a severe or profound hearing loss. As Figure 14-2 illustrates, many different audiometric configurations fall under the rubric of severe and profound hearing impairments. For instance, the child denoted by the letter A in Figure 14-2 has a severe hearing loss. He has some hearing across a wide range of frequencies (250 Hz to 8000 Hz). With appropriate amplification, Child A may recognize some speech with audition only and may speechread very well. This child also may hear many of his own speech sounds while talking, such as the vowel segments (which tend to be louder than consonants) and consonants that have high amplitude, such as the nasals /m/ and /n/. This child likely will hear the rhythm and prosody of his own speech.

Child B, also represented in Figure 14-2, has a profound hearing loss. Like many people with profound hearing loss, she is not completely deaf. She has some measurable hearing in the low frequencies (250 and 500 Hz). This child probably will not recognize any speech in an audition-only condition, nor recognize her own speech (although she may hear the rhythm of her intonation). She may or may not be a good speechreader.

Many children have a combined severe and profound hearing impairment. Their hearing typically is better in the low frequencies than the high frequencies. For example, Child C in Figure 14-2 has a sloping hearing loss. This child will hear some words using only

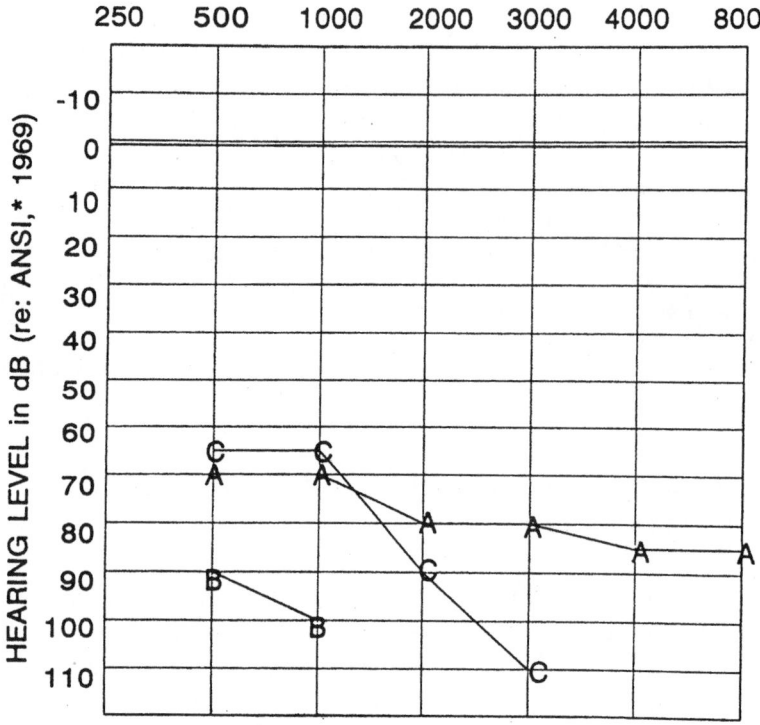

FIGURE 14-2. Audiometric configurations for three different types of hearing losses. Letters indicate the level at which a threshold was obtained. Child A has a severe hearing loss, Child B has a profound hearing loss, and Child C has a severe-to-profound impairment.

audition. His listening skills will appear to be more inconsistent than those of Child A or B. Because he has some hearing in the low frequencies, he will often detect the presence of speech and recognize some words. However, because much of the acoustic information that distinguishes one word from another is contained in the mid and high frequencies, he often will not discriminate the words even though he seems to hear them. Thus, his family and teachers may sometimes accuse him of "not listening" or "not paying attention." Child C may have reasonably good speechreading skills and probably will hear the rhythm and prosody of his voice while speaking. He will not hear many of his own consonant productions, particularly sounds that have high-frequency information, such as /s/ and /t/. He may hear his own vowel productions but they may all sound similar to him.

SCREENING

At least two events may trigger a parent or caregiver to bring a child to an audiologist for a hearing test. The first is that the child may have failed a screening test. The second is that a parent may have noticed the child is not responding to sound in the same way as normally hearing children.

It is critical that hearing loss be detected as soon as possible, and that an intervention plan of appropriate services be developed. Hearing is essential during the first 3 years of life if a baby is to develop normal speech and language. In this section, we consider screening.

Universal newborn hearing screening (often referred to in the literature with the acronym, UNHS), where every baby born is tested for hearing loss in the newborn nursery, has increasingly become the standard of care in the United States and in many places in Europe (the Key Resources section of this chapter presents terminology you might encounter if you work in a UNHS program). Prior to the proliferation of UNHS, children who had hearing loss were often not identified until the age of 2 years or older. This reality was in contrast to goals established by national health organizations for persons with hearing loss. These organizations called for identification to occur in the first few months of life (Hergils & Hergils, 2000); for example:

- National Institutes of Health, United States (1993) 3 months
- Socialstyrelsen (The National Board of Health and Welfare), Sweden (1994) before 1 year
- National Deaf Children's Society, United Kingdom (1994) 80% by 12 months

The U.S. initiative grows increasingly successful. As of November, 2002, 42 states and the District of Columbia had implemented UNHS. More than 85% of babies in the United States are screened before going home from the newborn nursery (Kirkwood, 2002). The advent of UNHS has changed the complexion of aural rehabilitation for children in many ways. Today, children in an aural rehabilitation program are more likely to be younger than in previous decades, and because they have received services early, they are more likely to develop better communication skills and develop them more quickly.

Screening is a "pass/refer" procedure, meaning that either the baby is found to have normal hearing or that there is reason to suspect a hearing loss exists. If hearing loss is suspected (i.e., a "refer" result is obtained), the baby is referred for a complete audiological workup that will assess the child's hearing bilaterally and at all of the audiometric frequencies. Babies who fail the screening test but who turn out to have normal hearing are examples of *false-positive* results. In a typical newborn screening program, the false-positive rate may range from 2% of babies tested to 7%. Many programs retest babies who fail the screening the first time before they leave the newborn nursery. This practice pushes the false-positive rate toward the lower end of 2%.

Methods used for screening include otoacoustic emissions (OAE) and automated auditory brainstem response testing (ABR), two procedures that will be described in the next section of this chapter. Screening is designed to detect hearing loss of 30 to 40 dB in the frequency region of 500–4000 Hz.

The impetus for UNHS stems from research showing that if hearing loss is identified before a child reaches the age of 6 months of age, and intervention is received, then that child will achieve language scores that compare favorably to children who have normal hearing, by the age of 3 years (Yoshinaga-Itano, Sedey, Coulter, & Mehl, 1998). This is not true of children who are not identified early and who do not receive concomitant intervention. Yoshinaga-Itano and Gravel (2001) summarize the importance of UNHS with the following checklist (pp. 63–64):

- Children with early-identified hearing loss who receive appropriate intervention services demonstrate significantly better language, speech, and social-emotional development than later identified children.
- Early-identified children with intervention have language development similar to their nonverbal cognitive development.
- Early-identified children with intervention and normal cognitive development maintain language development in the low average range throughout the first five years of life.

- The better the language development, the less parental stress there is, and the better personal-social development of children.
- Four out of every five children born in hospitals with newborn hearing screening programs have language development in the low-average range between 1 and 5 years of age when they have hearing loss only and no secondary disabilities. These statistics compare to outcomes of later-identified children in which only one in every five children have language development commensurate with that of children who hear normally.

Some babies are particular at risk for hearing loss. Risk factors associated with hearing loss include the following (Joint Committee on Infant Hearing, 1994):

- Low birth weight (less than 3.3 lbs)
- Family history for hearing loss
- In utero infections such as cytomegalovirus, rubella, or herpes
- Ototoxic medications
- Low *Apgar scores* (which reflect the normalcy of A = appearance, P = pulse, G = grimace, A = activity, and R = respiration at the time of birth)
- Need for use of a ventilator for 5 days or longer
- Cranial anomalies
- Physical manifestations consistent with a syndrome
- Bacterial meningitis
- Hyperbilirubinemia at levels that require an exchange transfusion

Apgar score: a numeric value between 1 and 10 assigned to newborns to describe their physical status at birth.

However, although these risk factors often trigger a suspicion of hearing loss, it is important to remember that almost 50% of children who have hearing loss do not have risk factors at birth.

Once a baby has been identified in a screening program as potentially having a hearing loss, then a follow-up evaluation must be scheduled as soon as possible. A baby who fails a newborn screening test should receive an appropriate audiologic and medical evaluation to confirm the presence of hearing loss by the age of 3 months. The baby with a confirmed hearing loss should begin to receive services before the age of 6 months (Joint Committee On Infant Hearing, 2000).

Even if a baby passes the newborn screening test, you might want to alert parents to watch for the tell-tale signs of hearing loss. A handout like that presented in the Key Resources section might be provided to parents when they leave the hospital with their new baby.

Childhood hearing loss can occur after birth, so it is essential that children undergo screening after leaving the hospital. At 6 months of age, babies with a risk factor for hearing loss should be retested, and then retested every 6 months thereafter until the age of 3 years.

For babies who are not at risk, parents might suspect a hearing loss, and bring the baby to their family physician or pediatrician for a screening. The physician may perform an informal gross test, using some type of noise-maker. If the baby does not respond to sound, a referral may be made for more extensive testing.

If the child is of school age (and hence, more likely to have a mild or moderate hearing loss), the loss might be identified during a school screening session. If a screening procedure indicates the possibility of hearing loss, the child is referred promptly for additional diagnostic audiologic testing.

■ IDENTIFICATION AND QUANTIFICATION OF HEARING LOSS

A child's hearing may be tested in a variety of ways. The selection of a measurement technique is dependent on a number of variables, including the age of the child, and his or her ability to participate in the test procedures. Once a hearing loss has been identified, hearing should be tested twice each year for young children, and four times or more annually if other problems are present or if there is concern about the accuracy of the test results. Older children usually need to be evaluated only once a year.

Objective Tests

Two objective tests are used to determine the presence of hearing loss: auditory brainstem response (ABR) and otoacoustic emissions (OAE).

AUDITORY BRAINSTEM RESPONSE TEST

Auditory brainstem response (ABR) testing often is used with babies between the ages of birth and 5 months. Electrodes are placed on the child's head, and brain wave activity elicited by the presentation of tone bursts or sound clicks is recorded. Usually, the child must be sedated for testing, as the patient must be very still in order to obtain accurate test results. ABR usually is used with individuals who cannot give behavioral responses or with individuals who provide inconsistent responses to sound stimuli. ABRs can be used to determine the severity of hearing in a baby and the degree of hearing loss at the different audiometric frequencies. ABRs yield thresholds within 10 dB of behavioral thresholds (Stapells, 2002). For this reason, ABRs provide the most comprehensive and accurate information for prescribing hearing aids for an infant or for justifying cochlear implantation.

Auditory brainstem response (ABR): an auditory evoked potential that originates from the eighth cranial nerve and is generated by electrical stimulation of the cochlea via an electrode.

For screening purposes, a variation of ABR might be used: ALGO. *ALGO* is an automated ABR screening device, which compares the baby's ABR response to a stored template of expected brain waveforms. The response is scored as either a pass or a failure.

ALGO: an automated ABR screening device used for screening newborns.

OTOACOUSTIC EMISSIONS TESTING

Otoacoustic emissions (OAE) are inaudible sounds that are the by-products of the mechanical actions of the outer hair cells in the cochlea. When sound stimulates the cochlea, the hair cells vibrate and initiate a signal in the eighth cranial nerve. Simultaneously, the vibration produces a sound that echoes back into the middle ear. The sound can be measured with a small probe inserted into the ear canal. Sound is presented, and the OAE is detected and traced. Persons who have normal hearing produce OAEs, whereas those who have hearing loss of 25–30 dB or greater do not. The procedure is widely used as a screening procedure. It is quick to administer and does not require the cooperation of the patient, other than to remain relatively still.

Otoacoustic emissions (OAE): low-level sound emitted spontaneously by the cochlea on presentation of an auditory stimulus.

When used for newborn screening, OAEs are often collected by a nurse, technician, or volunteer (although an audiologist may be on the hospital staff and will supervise the overall screening efforts). Only about 34% of the personnel who perform newborn screenings in the hospital are audiologists (Arehart,

Yoshingaga-Itano, Thomson, Gabbard, & Brown, 1998). The screener often uses a hand-held transient otoacoustic emissions screener, like the Echocheck (Otodynamics LTD, 1998). It flashes a green light when an OAE is present, a red light when it is not, and an orange light for an invalid test result.

OAEs are also often used to assess hearing status of babies during more comprehensive diagnostic evaluations. OAEs can be measured for frequency-select regions, which can help predict a baby's audiogram. Typically, an otoacoustic emission for a given frequency region may be recorded if the baby's hearing threshold for that region is better than 30 or 40 dB. It will likely be absent if the threshold is higher (Sininger, 2002).

Behavioral Tests

Behavioral tests include the audiogram (Chapter 5). However, when a child is very young, it may not be possible to obtain one. Thus, to obtain information about the child's ability to detect a range of frequencies, the audiologist may utilize behavioral/observational audiometry (often referred to with the acronym BOA), visual reinforcement audiometry (VRA), or conditioned play audiometry.

BEHAVIORAL/OBSERVATIONAL AUDIOMETRY

Behavioral/observational audiometry (BOA): method of testing a child's hearing in which the tester presents a sound stimulus and observes the child's behavior for change.

In *behavioral/observational audiometry (BOA),* the audiologist presents a sound stimulus and observes the child's behavior. Response to sound may be manifested by a change in sucking pattern, eye widening, cessation of activity, or a head turn.

One shortcoming of BOA is that babies vary in their responsiveness to sound stimulation. Some 3-month-old babies will react to sound presented at 20 dB HL, whereas others will not until the sound reaches 80 dB HL. For this reason, the procedure can reliably only eliminate the possibility of profound hearing loss. In addition, babies respond differently to sound, depending on their level of arousal, on how many times they have heard the sound (i.e., habituation occurs), and whether the sound is of interest to them (e.g., speech as opposed to tone pips). Finally, the observer's expectations can color the results: When you want to see a response from a baby, you may see it, whether it really occurred or not (Widen & O'Grady, 2002).

VISUAL REINFORCEMENT AUDIOMETRY

Visual reinforcement audiometry (VRA) is used with children between the ages of 6 months and 2½ years. VRA takes advantage of a baby's natural inclination to turn toward sound. It is an example of an operant-conditioned response. The child is tested in a sound-treated room. Sound is presented through an audiometer. When sound is presented initially, a box in the room lights up. Inside of the box is a toy that moves. For example, a box may light up to reveal a toy monkey clashing cymbals. The child is trained to look at the box when the sound is presented, and then testing is begun to determine the threshold for the frequencies of the audiogram.

Visual reinforcement audiometry (VRA): method of testing young children in which presentation of the sound is coupled to lighting of a toy for reinforcement of the child's response.

CONDITIONED PLAY AUDIOMETRY

Conditioned play audiometry is used to assess children, starting at about the age of 2 to 2½ years. Children may place a peg into a pegboard each time a sound is presented through the audiometer (Figure 14-3). He or she may drop a block into a jar. The child is trained to wait and listen for a sound and then perform the response task when the sound is presented. Often, the child's parent may sit in the sound-treated room with the child during testing, while the audiologist may be in the adjacent room with the audiometer, watching through the window. The parent must be coached to sit quietly and not provide cues about the presence or absence of sound to the child.

Conditioned play audiometry: method of testing children 2.5 years and older in which child is trained to perform a task in response to presentation of a sound.

▬ OTHER HEARING-RELATED CONDITIONS

Children may suffer from other hearing-related conditions besides sensorineural, conductive, and mixed hearing loss. Three such conditions are central auditory processing disorder (CAPD), auditory neuropathy, and tinnitus.

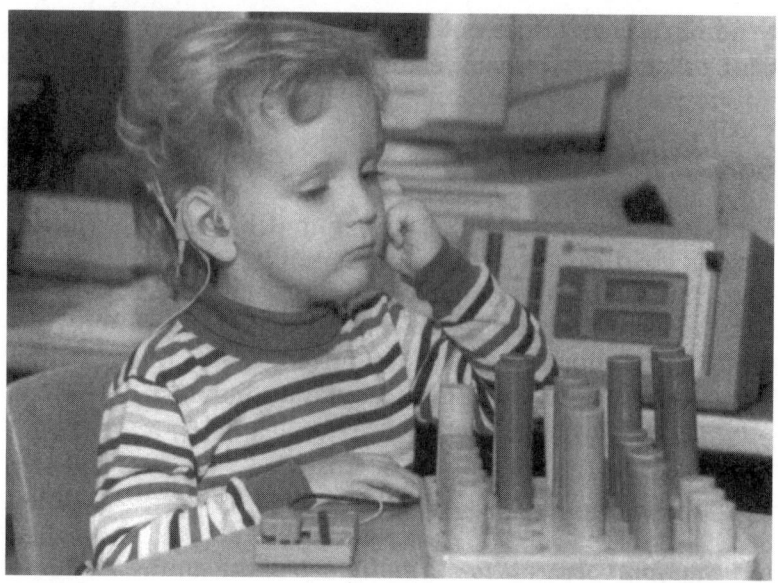

FIGURE 14-3. A young child is tested with conditioned play audiometry. He listens for a sound and places a peg into the pegboard every time he hears one. (Photograph by Patti Gabriel, courtesy of the Central Institute for the Deaf)

Central Auditory Processing Disorders (CAPD)

Some hearing losses are due to *central* causes, which means that sound transmission between the brain stem and the cerebrum is disrupted, either as a result of damage or a malformation. Thus, the temporal cortex of the brain may receive incorrect information, or the information may not be processed correctly. These deficiencies in auditory processing skills sometimes are referred to as a ***central auditory processing disorder (CAPD).***

Central auditory processing disorder (CAPD): functional auditory disorder that is centered in the brainstem or cortex, and not the peripheral hearing system (outer, middle, or inner ear).

CAPD may result from head trauma, brain tumors, autism, or neurologic vascular changes. Sometimes, a cause cannot be found. This is a difficult diagnosis to make. Many times, the problem is not implicit in the audiogram. A parent might comment, "He hears me, but many times I have to repeat myself several times before he gets what I'm saying." A teacher might note, "Whenever I talk to Mary, I find myself slowing down how fast I talk and accentuating my articulation. Otherwise, she gets this blank look on her face, as if her mind is somewhere else."

Children who have central hearing loss usually experience difficulty in one or more of the following:

- Localizing and lateralizing sound
- Auditory discrimination
- Auditory pattern recognition
- Associating meaning to sound
- Listening in noise
- Understanding degraded speech signals, fast speech, or speech with an unfamiliar accent
- Following rhythmic and melodic aspects of music
- Reduced auditory memory

Auditory Neuropathy

Auditory neuropathy is thought to be related to CAPD, albeit different because it involves the peripheral auditory system. Children who receive a diagnosis of *auditory neuropathy* typically have a mild to moderate sensorineural hearing loss, and they exhibit OAEs. They either have absent or abnormal ABRs and poor word recognition, poorer than that which would be predicted by their audiological thresholds. Because OAEs are present, while ABRs are not, the disorder is believed to stem from problems with the auditory nerve or spiral ganglion, although the exact cause is unknown. Unfortunately, for many children who have auditory neuropathy, hearing aids are not very helpful.

Auditory neuropathy: a condition where the patient has a pure-tone audiogram that shows any degree of hearing loss, from mild to profound, and shows normal OAEs. ABRs are either absent or degraded.

Tinnitus

Not only adults suffer from tinnitus (Chapter 11). Children too may experience sound in their heads that has no external cause. In fact, tinnitus may be experienced by 25–55% of children who have hearing loss. Just like adults, tinnitus may inflict deleterious effects, including insomnia, emotional trauma (e.g., fear and worry), physical symptoms, attention difficulties, and listening challenges (Kentish, Crocker, & McKenna, 2000). Tinnitus may be hard to detect in children because they may have always had it (so it seems like the normal state of affairs) or they may lack the words to describe the phenomenon.

▰ COPING WITH A CHILD'S DIAGNOSIS

Grief Reactions in Parents

The family must make many adjustments when they learn that one of their young members has a hearing loss. Carney and Moeller (1998) summarized some of the research that has examined the consequences of learning about the presence of hearing loss:

> It is common for parents to experience grief reactions and feelings of loss of control when a child is diagnosed with a hearing impairment. There is considerable evidence in the literature of negative consequences of such variables as high parental stress on child development. Quittner and Steck (1989) completed interviews with over 1000 mothers of hearing-impaired children in Canada. They documented a high prevalence of maternal stress, with impact on family satisfaction and child development. Dunst (1985) reported that poorer feelings of well-being on the part of parents contributed to their lack of responsiveness to infant attention bids. Several researchers have found that parental language input can be seriously affected by the psychological state of the parents, which in turn can have far-reaching consequences for the child (Greenstein, 1975; Schlesinger & Acree, 1984; White, 1984). (pp. S64–S65)

This typically is a difficult period for families, and it is wise to be sensitive to the emotional turmoil that may be occurring.

After an audiologic appointment, the audiologist provides a written report to the child's parents as soon as possible. This provides a written documentation of what the audiologist has informed and counseled them about and also recaps the audiologist's recommendations.

When you talk with many parents of children who have significant hearing loss, you may find a recurring theme: Many parents harbor hostility toward the medical profession. This hostility may derive from at least one of two sources. The first can be labeled as *anger because their concerns were dismissed.* Parents may tell you how they suspected a hearing loss in their baby, and took the baby to their family doctor or pediatrician. The doctor may have dismissed the parents' concerns, and thereby may have delayed diagnosis for several months or even years. As a result, the child was delayed in receiving amplification and intervention services. Often parents feel not only anger but also guilt, because they did not follow their instincts and pursue second and third opinions more promptly.

Another source of hostility may be labeled as *anger because the hearing loss may have been prevented.* These feelings often arise after a child has lost hearing because of meningitis. Kravitz and Selekman (1992) noted:

> Many parents can identify the episode that resulted in their child's hearing loss; they blame it on improper medical care. In case after case, parents tell of their children being taken to hospitals because they had fever and appeared listless. The children were sent home with diagnoses of viral infection but within hours their conditions had worsened. The children spiked higher fevers, had seizures, and even arrested. The diagnosis was usually meningitis. While the children ultimately survived, they were left deaf and had other serious disabilities. Although years may have passed, these parents can vividly recall the harrowing details of their child's medical trauma. (p. 593)

In Chapter 11, it was noted that adults often pass through a series of emotional stages, just as most people who experience grief. These stages of emotional adjustment may include shock, denial, guilt, anger, and acceptance. Parents and family members may also pass through these stages when they learn of their child's hearing loss.

SHOCK, DENIAL, AND GRIEF

Shock and denial are ways of protecting oneself from a crisis and often result in parents focusing on minor details. An individual may deny that the hearing loss exists or may deny the enormity of its consequences. Grief then may occur, as parents realize that their ideal child has been lost.

ANGER AND GUILT

Anger and guilt may follow the denial stage, and often parents will become convinced that something they have done in the past may be responsible for the hearing loss. For example, one mother took anti-sea-sickness pills while on a cruise in the early weeks of her pregnancy. She experienced enormous guilt when her baby was diagnosed with profound hearing loss, because she was convinced the medication had resulted in abnormal fetal development.

ACCEPTANCE

Finally, acceptance may set in, as parents begin to accept that their child's hearing loss is a reality. Ideally, the parents and family are willing to take constructive steps to deal with their child's hearing condition.

Many parents feel confused and overwhelmed during the early stages following diagnosis, and these feelings may be magnified as they interact with a variety of different professionals who may provide abundant, and perhaps conflicting, advice about how to handle the child's loss. They may feel inadequate when they realize how much time and effort will be required on their part to maximize their child's potential. An important role of the speech and hearing professional during this time is to provide support and reassurance that the parents can handle the new demands and to empower them to interact effectively with their child.

The stages just described are not necessarily like the rungs of a ladder, which parents climb up one step at a time, and never climb back down. Rather, parents may pass from one stage to another, return to an earlier stage, and then advance again. For example, when a child enters kindergarten, the child's parents may look at his classmates who have normal hearing and realize more fully what a significant hearing loss may mean in terms of their child's academic achievement. This may trigger new feelings of grief, even if they have come to terms with the permanency of the hearing loss.

Dealing With Feelings and Moving Forward

Kozak and Brooks (2001) suggested ways for parents to deal with their feelings. These practical nuts-and-bolts recommendations are as follows.

- **Accept your feelings:** The situation is difficult and it is understandable and appropriate to be upset. Accept that it hurts and try to find something you can do to help your child. This will allow you to feel something more positive too.
- **Talk to others:** Find a spouse, parent, friend or parent of another child with a challenge. Tell them what you are feeling and listen to them [talk about] their feelings. Get some support and see if you can give any . . .
- **Write in a journal:** If thinking and feeling are not enough to help but talking is too much for you right now or if you can't find the right listener, try writing some notes about your feelings in a journal, notebook or even a letter . . .
- **Find a group to support you:** You can find good listeners, help, support and encouragement in a group of parents whose children have any special challenges . . . Your local children's hospital, clinics and schools may be resources for finding such a group . . . Most parents of children with challenges say that other parents of these children provided the most important help they received in the early years. This type of support can help you learn and move forward while you cope with all your feelings.
- **Other ways:** Some parents will look toward their ethical views or their religious values and comrades to help them find the way to feel better. Some people will delve into learning all they can about [hearing loss. Some may seek counseling] from a professional counselor or physician.
- **Give yourself a break:** Don't demand too much of yourself. Pat yourself on the back for doing what you've already done to help your child. Ask someone who cares about you for some words of encouragement. Get a hug from your child . . . Cry if it feels better to do so. Do something good for you, even if it's only taking time to watch the quiet beauty of a sunrise or sunset. Be thankful for your child. Don't expect yourself to do every job perfectly. No one is perfect in our imperfect world.

Infants

Much of what was just reviewed for coping with a child's diagnosis also applies to parents who have infants with hearing loss. Infancy is a time of great excitement and parent-baby bonding. When parents learn in the newborn nursery that their baby may not be who they had anticipated, the stages of grief that often accompany a child's diagnosis of hearing loss can be amplified. This occurs because parents of older babies and children have lived with their child and may have gradually grown to suspect a problem. They have observed their child not responding to sound, or have observed the child not developing vocal and listening behaviors that resemble those of his or her peers. Thus, they may not be totally caught off-guard at the diagnosis of hearing loss. In contrast, parents who learn that their baby might have a hearing loss while the baby is still in the hospital, and before they have had any chance to get to know and bond with the child, might be handed the news "cold turkey." *They had no clue!* Add to the natural emotions of grief the emotions associated with postpartum depression, the physical exhaustion of childbirth, and the stress of being a new parent, and the end result may be parents who feel flattened by what life has delivered them. It is critical that new parents receive counseling and support and that they have reason to believe there are mechanisms and support services that will steer them through this initial stage of considering and dealing with their baby's hearing loss.

Not every baby who fails a hearing screening test has a hearing loss. If a baby fails a screening test, then every attempt must be made to ensure that a comprehensive diagnostic evaluation is scheduled as soon as possible. Fast scheduling will minimize that period where parents worry, not knowing one way or the other whether their baby has a hearing loss.

Luterman and Kurtzer-White (1999) surveyed a group of parents of babies who had been identified as having hearing loss as a result of neonatal hearing screening. They found (p. 16):

- The majority of parents supported early identification of hearing loss and would have wanted to know the diagnosis at birth.
- A minority of parents (17% of the respondents) would have preferred to wait to learn of their child's hearing loss.

- Parents would prefer to be informed of their child's hearing loss by an audiologist who is not only a skillful clinician but also an empathetic counselor.
- Parents wanted unbiased information, particularly concerning the issues of communication and education methodology.
- The parents' predominant need was to meet other parents of children with hearing loss.
- Parents wanted and needed time to process what they experience and the amount of information they receive at the time of diagnosis.

Learning That Your New Baby May Have a Hearing Loss

Luterman (2001) describes eloquently the ordeal parents may undergo when they learn that their baby may have hearing loss:

"In data . . . gather[ed] from parents of children with hearing impairments who have failed the screening, we found that not one parent was told of the failure by an audiologist. Instead, they were informed by hospital personnel, none of whom could supply the parents with any information other than the test results. Instead of going home to enjoy their babies, these parents went home to worry and to test their infant's hearing. In many cases, it was several months before they could get an appointment to confirm the loss. In the words of one mother, "It was just Hell." Horror stories abound: parents finding out by seeing a note on their child's bassinet or being told as they are leaving the hospital by a nurse that "Your baby failed the screening test but don't worry about it." "And of course," said the mother, "That's all I worried about." (p. 87)

AMPLIFICATION

Children usually receive amplification as soon as a hearing loss is identified, even if the child is only an infant. The earlier a child receives amplification, the more he or she is likely to develop auditory speech recognition skills. Support for this assertion comes from research about both animals and humans, and about vision and audition.

Support for Early Amplification

Research with vision suggests that young mammals have a more plastic nervous system than adult mammals. For example, kittens raised with goggles that expose one eye to vertical stripes and the other eye to horizontal stripes go on to develop abnormal binocular feature detectors (Hirsch & Spinelli, 1970). Children who have strabismus (crossed eyes) for several years may not develop stereopsis, even after corrective surgery (Kaufman, 1979).

Research with audition has shown that birds who do not hear their species' song patterns during a critical period of maturation never develop those patterns (Marler, 1989). Similarly, adults who have prelingual hearing loss receive minimal, if any, benefit from receiving a cochlear implant (Tong, Busby, & Clark, 1988). Children who are younger at age of implantation are more likely to develop better speech recognition skills than children who are older (Fryauf-Bertschy, Tyler, Kelsay, Gantz, & Woodworth, 1997).

These kinds of research findings underscore the importance of early identification of hearing loss and the provision of amplification as soon as possible.

Selection of Hearing Aids

In Chapter 6, we considered the available styles of hearing aids. In this section, the selection of styles for children is considered in more detail. Children who may benefit more from receiving a cochlear implant are considered in Chapter 18.

Fitting hearing aids to children and infants differs in some ways to fitting hearing aids in adults (see Hoover, 2001, for a review). First, there are physical differences. Children, especially infants, have smaller ears and ear canals, so hearing aid style options may be limited. Ear canal size might increase the occurrence of feedback and squeal, and the tiny pinna might not hold a hearing aid behind the ear. Second, because sound is funneled into a small space before the tympanic membrane, the sound pressure delivered to a child's ear might be greater than when the exact acoustic signal is delivered to an adult ear. Thus, it becomes important to ensure that sound is not too loud to cause damage. Finally, babies and young children often cannot participate in the fitting process. They cannot tell you when sound is too loud, and they may not be able to take a word recognition test.

Traditionally, hearing aids for children included body aids, especially for children under age 3 years, because they are durable. More recently, body aids have become less popular, and most children receive behind-the-ear aids, no matter how young they are. Most behind-the-ear aids provide sufficient gain, even for profound hearing losses. Baby's ears typically are too tiny to accommodate an ITE, CID, or ITC style of hearing aid. Moreover, these styles are impractical because the baby is growing quickly, and thus, a new aid would be required to accommodate the ongoing physical changes that occur. Even with a BTE style, parents have to monitor changes in the baby's ear size. New earmolds may have to be made every 6 to 8 weeks.

In-the-ear aids usually are not provided to young children, for a variety of reasons. These include the following:

- The aid may not stay put in the ear.
- The child's ear canal is still growing, so the aid must be re-cast frequently.
- In-the-ear aids are difficult for parents to monitor. For example, parents may have a difficult time checking the position of the volume control.
- These aids permit no direct auditory input.

An advantage offered by behind-the-ear aids is that they can be connected to many FM assistive listening devices. These systems include a wireless microphone worn by a talker and a receiver the child uses, connected to the hearing aid.

Once a hearing aid is fitted on a child, the audiologist provides instruction to the parents or caregivers about how to care for the device and how to perform a listening check (Figure 14-4). Instruction may include how to wash an earmold, how to monitor the child's ability to hear with the device, and how to

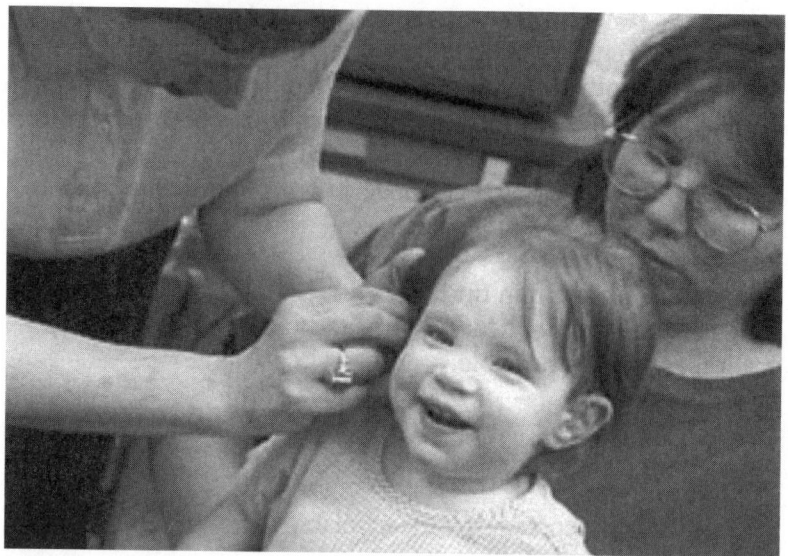

FIGURE 14-4. During the hearing-aid fitting, parents receive instructions about how to handle, maintain, and trouble-shoot the device. (From video footage by Rick Bernstein, courtesy of the Central Institute for the Deaf)

troubleshoot the hearing aid (e.g., what to do if the hearing aid will not turn on, if the sound is weak or distorted, or if the hearing aid squeals).

Special Considerations for Children and Amplification

Special considerations for providing amplification to children include ensuring appropriate fit of earmolds. Ill-fitting earmolds can lead to irritation of the ear canal, as well as feedback. Because the ear canal is growing, infants and preschool children may need to receive a new earmold every 4–6 months. When children are between 4 and 9 years of age, new molds may be necessary only on an annual basis.

Another issue relevant to children is the adjustment period for establishing use of the device. Some children reject their devices or want to control when they do and do not use it. Some children react negatively to amplified sound, and some may view the listening device as a means of asserting independence or gaining control over parents. A speech and hearing professional can encourage parents to take responsibility and foster full-time use of the listening device at home and school. With a younger child, parents may provide reassurance and support to the child. Initially, the device can be worn for short periods and then gradually increased over time. Routines of use should be established. Putting the listening device on in the morning should be part of getting dressed, and removing it should be part of getting undressed in the evening. For the older child, it is sometimes helpful to set a reinforcement system, in which some reward is received if the child wears the device for a specified amount of time every day.

CASE STUDY

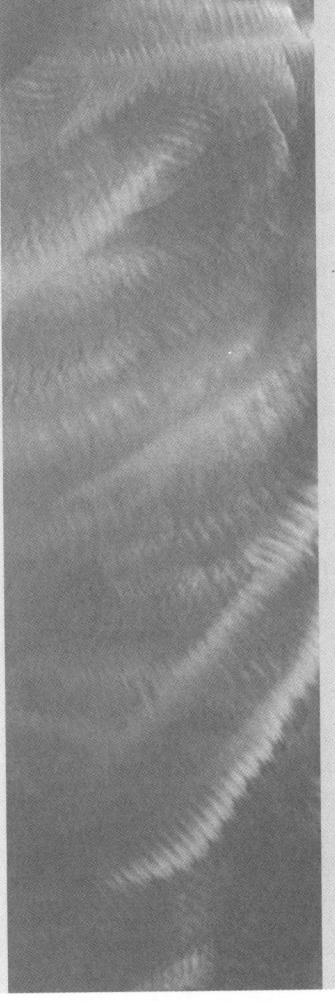

The following summary stems from one of the first universal newborn hearing screening programs in the United States. It tells about new parents who learned that their son, Matthew, had hearing loss and how they responded to the news. Luckily for little Matthew, his parents galvanized into action and provided a wonderful environment for developing speech and language (Cherow & Boswell, 1999, Page 24):

"[Gilbert Herer] and Eugene Sussman, chair of pediatrics at the Holy Cross Hospital in Silver Spring, Maryland—one of the largest birthing hospitals in the United States—joined forces to establish a universal newborn hearing screening program in 1996, while controversy over the cost-benefit of such programs was still raging.

Herer set out to institute a program that would establish a protocol to demonstrate that newborn hearing screening can be universal, that screening all babies before discharge can be done efficiently, and that parents had to return for a rescreen in the event that their child did not pass hearing screening before discharge.

'Matthew Reilly was the very first child we identified,' Herer said. Matthew's diagnostic ABR showed a 40 dB–70 dB hearing loss in his left ear and a profound hearing loss in his

(continues)

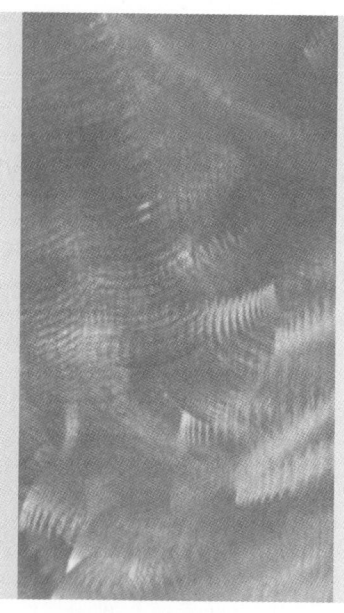

right. 'The minute his parents found out about his hearing loss, they swung into action,' Herer said. Matthew was fitted with a hearing aid with an FM boot so that he could get the clearest signal possible and remain in auditory contact with his mother who wore a wireless microphone. The FM system allows constant auditory stimulation, which enables the child's auditory/neurological system to pattern itself and helps support speech-language development.

Matthew is now 10 months old, and his parents have been keeping a diary of the words he is speaking. Herer says that, 'With appropriate amplification, babies who are identified early become immersed in a world of sound and take in auditory information and integrate it like hearing babies.'

"When my baby failed the hearing test at the hospital, I thought my world had come to an end. I looked at this beautiful baby and couldn't believe that she could be anything but perfect. I wish someone would have spent more time with me, telling me more about hearing loss and the meaning of a screening test."

—Mother of a child who failed the hospital screening test but who later was found to have normal hearing

FINAL REMARKS

In this chapter, we have focused on children who have severe and profound hearing losses. Children with lesser degrees of hearing loss also may experience listening difficulties. For instance, a child with a mild, high-frequency hearing loss may appear to have no problem in recognizing speech or responding to environmental sounds. However, the child may not be performing optimally in the classroom setting, because he or she may have degraded listening performance in the presence of background noise. A child with a mild-to-moderate hearing loss may have decreased speech recognition and may be delayed in both speech and language development if appropriate amplification is not provided.

Children who have a lesser degree of hearing loss represent a fairly significant segment of school children in the United States. Ross (1990) suggested that 16 of every 1,000 school-age children have pure-tone-averages (PTAs, Chapter 6) between 26 and 70 dB HL. These children may need special accommodations in the classroom, as we will discuss at the end of Chapter 15, and may benefit from the use of special assistive listening devices, such as FM trainers (Chapter 6).

■ KEY CHAPTER POINTS

✔ About 30% of children who have significant hearing loss also have another disability.

✔ Hearing loss may arise from a variety of causes that may be prenatal, perinatal, or postnatal. The hearing loss may be due to environmental factors or genetic factors.

✔ Some hereditary hearing losses have a delayed onset, and some are nonsyndromic.

✔ Otitis media overlaid on a sensorineural hearing loss results in a mixed hearing loss. If untreated, the child may suffer related speech and language delays.

✔ Children with severe and profound hearing loss present a range of listening skills.

✔ Universal newborn hearing screening has proliferated in this country and in Europe. As a result, children in aural rehabilitation programs tend to be younger at the onset.

✔ A variety of audiologic procedures are available for identifying hearing loss and determining the magnitude of loss. Whereas most of the procedures rely on behavioral responses from the children, two procedures (ABR and OAE) are objective.

✔ Parents often have difficulty in accepting their children's hearing loss and may pass through a series of psychological stages before acceptance occurs. A primary role of the speech and hearing professional is to empower parents to interact effectively with their child and to make important decisions about their child's aural rehabilitation plan.

✔ Early and appropriate amplification is critical for normal speech and language development. Children often receive behind-the-ear hearing aids. In-the-ear aids usually are not prescribed, for a variety of reasons, including the fact that children's ears may still be growing, so aids must be frequently recast.

■ MULTIPLE CHOICE QUESTIONS

1. The percentage of children who have hearing loss and who also have another disability is:
   a. Fifty percent
   b. Eighty percent
   c. Fifteen percent
   d. Thirty percent

2. The percentage of children who have hearing and who are born to parents who have normal hearing is:
   a. Fifty five percent
   b. Seventy-five to 80 percent
   c. Ninety to 95 percent
   d. Forty percent

3. Parental radiation that results in hearing loss is an example of what kind of cause for hearing loss?
   a. Nonsyndromic
   b. Environmental
   c. Genetic
   d. Autosomal dominant

4. A child may experience a delayed onset hearing loss most likely as a result of:
   a. Complications associated with the Rh factor
   b. Toxemia during pregnancy
   c. Meningitis
   d. Perinatal anoxia

5. Otitis media can result in what kind of hearing loss?
   a. Mild to moderate conductive
   b. Moderate to severe conductive
   c. Moderate sensorineural
   d. A high-frequency loss audiometric configuration

6. Alstrom is an example of:
   a. A syndrome
   b. A screening device
   c. A measuring unit for indexing a newborn baby's hearing thresholds
   d. A kind of inherited hearing loss that is related to an X-linked trait

7. The goal of the National Institutes of Health in the United States is that all children who have hearing loss are identified by:
   a. The first week of life
   b. The third month of life
   c. The first birthday
   d. The age of 2 years

8. Which of the following statements is false?
   a. Children who have hearing loss and who are identified early may have language development similar to their nonverbal cognitive development.
   b. Children who have hearing loss and who are identified early and who receive intervention maintain language development in the low average range throughout the first 5 years of life.
   c. The better the language development a child who has hearing loss has, the less stressed are the parents, and the better is the child's personal-social development.
   d. Children who fail a screening test in the newborn nursery have a hearing loss.

9. OAEs occur because:
   a. Of electrical activity generated by synapses in the auditory nerve
   b. Of the elasticity of the tympanic membrane
   c. The outer hair cells vibrate
   d. Of movement by the inner hair cells

10. ABRs can yield thresholds:
    a. Within 30 dB of behavioral thresholds
    b. Within 10 dB of behavioral thresholds
    c. Within 30 dB of behavioral thresholds, for the high frequencies only
    d. Within 10 dB of behavioral thresholds, for the low frequencies only

11. In audiology, the acronym BOA stands for:
    a. Benign OAE-ABR results
    b. Baby Otologic Awareness Campaign
    c. Brainstem Overview Assessment
    d. Behavioral Observational Audiometry

12. Auditory neuropathy is characterized by:
    a. Normal ABRs and absent OAEs
    b. Present OAEs and abnormal ABRs
    c. Normal bone conduction thresholds and normal ABRs
    d. Hearing loss that is centered at the level of the brainstem or cortex

13. Mary Jones has pure-tone averages of 10 dB in each ear. She has a hard time in distinguishing between a series of three tone pips and a series of four tone pips. Mary most likely has:
    a. CAPD
    b. Auditory neuropathy
    c. Severe tinnitus
    d. Syndromic hearing loss

14. Which statement is true?
    a. Parents often go through a stage of grieving when they learn their child has hearing loss. Once this stage passes, these emotions related to the hearing loss will likely not resurface.
    b. Guilt often precedes denial during parents' adjustment period to their child's hearing loss.
    c. Shock and grief often co-occur and are usually not thought to be separate stages of the adjustment period to a child's hearing loss.
    d. Good support from professionals typically allows parents to bypass the anger and guilt stages of adjustment to a child's hearing loss.

15. Most parents who have babies identified as having hearing loss as a result of neonatal hearing screening:
    a. Need time to process what they experience and the information they receive at the time of diagnosis
    b. Are referred to an educational consultant
    c. Are referred to a genetic counselor
    d. Would have preferred to wait to learn of their child's hearing loss until they have had a chance to bond with the baby

16. Babies who have hearing loss:
    a. Typically are fitted with body aids because they can be strapped to the body, so the baby won't lose it
    b. Typically are fitted with BTE
    c. Typically are fitted with ITE, because the pinna will not support a BTE
    d. Typically are fitted with CIC, so they will appear like any other infant

KEY RESOURCES

Important Terms to Know When Discussing Genetics[1]

Allele: one particular version of a gene.

Chromosome: structures bearing the genes of a cell and made of a single strand of DNA.

DNA: (deoxyribonucleic acid) nucleic acid polymer of which the genes are made.

Dominant allele: the allele whose properties are expressed as the phenotype.

Gene: a unit of genetic information contained within the chromosome that can be inherited.

Genotype: the total genetic make-up of an organism.

Heterozygous: having two different alleles of the same gene.

Homozygous: having two identical alleles of the same gene.

Mutation: an alteration in the genetic information carried by a gene.

Phenotype: the visible effect of the genotype.

Recessive allele: the allele for which properties are not observed because they are masked by the dominant allele.

Sex-linked: a gene is sex-linked when it is carried on one of the sex chromosomes.

Abbreviations and Acronyms

You might encounter these abbreviations and acronyms when reading the medical or audiological records for an infant or very young child (Mize & Wigley, 2002).

- BMT (bilateral myringotomy and tubes)
- Chemotx (chemotherapy)
- CHL (conductive hearing loss)
- CNT (could not test)
- DNT (did not test)
- F/u (follow-up)

[1] Definitions are from Clark and Russell, 1997, pp. 13–26.

- H/o (history of)
- M/o (month old)
- NBHS (newborn hearing screening)
- Pt (patient)
- R/o (rule-out)
- SF (soundfield)
- SLP (speech-language pathologist)
- SNHL (sensorineural hearing loss)
- S/p (status post)
- TM (tympanic membrane)
- Tymps (tympanogram)
- WNL (within normal limits)
- Y/o (year old)

A Parent's Guide to Hearing and Language Milestones[2]

Your baby will reach a series of milestones as he or she grows. If you suspect that your baby is not reaching these milestones, talk to your doctor or speech and hearing professional, because your baby may have a hearing loss or some other condition that is delaying development.

Newborn
- Cries
- Startles to loud and/or sudden sound

2 to 3 Months
- Laughs
- Forms sounds in the back of the mouth ("gah")
- Responds to your (parent's) voice
- Distinguishes changes in the tone of voice (happy versus sad)

4 to 6 Months
- Turns head toward sound
- Begins to put sounds together, typically a consonant and a vowel ("bah")
- Makes nonspeech sounds playfully (squeals, yells, makes "raspberries")

[2] Adapted from Hansen and Howard, 1992.

6 to 12 Months

- Babbles strings of syllables ("bah-bah-bah")
- Attempts nonverbal communication through facial expression, eye gaze, vocalization, and gestures such as pointing, reaching, and head shaking
- By 12 months, responds to name; understands the word "no" and simple instructions; gives a toy in response to a request

12 to 18 Months

- Strings sounds together that have an adult-like speech rhythm
- Speaks first words
- By 18 months, understands about 50 words and speaks up to 20 words, usually in isolation and not sentences or phrases.

18 to 36 Months

- Demonstrates rapid speech development: learns new words rapidly and puts them together in strings of two or more
- By 36 months, can understand up to 3,600 words; constructs sentences with an average of three to four words; can tell a simple story; can sing songs; can provide simple information verbally, such as the name of the family's street or his or her age

CHAPTER 15

Aural (Re)Habilitation Plans for Children

TOPICS

After the diagnosis of hearing loss is made and the child receives appropriate amplification, other rehabilitation services must be provided, including auditory training, language stimulation, and educational management. In this chapter, we consider the multidisciplinary team and the intervention plan. The bulk of the chapter is concerned primarily with children who have severe and profound hearing losses. At the end of the chapter, we consider children with mild and moderate hearing losses.

The Beginnings of Deaf Education in the United States

The beginnings of deaf education in the New World follow two threads, manual communication and aural/oral communication (or oralism). Although there were sporadic attempts to educate deaf children in the United States before Alice Cogswell, many historians date the dawn of deaf education in this country to her birth in 1805. Alice was born into a well-to-do family in New England. At the age of 2 years, she contracted "spotted fever" and lost her hearing. Treatments of salt water poured into her ears, leeches, and special creams could not return what was lost. An ear trumpet bought by her distraught parents allowed her to hear a church bell, but not much more.

Alice's father, Dr. Mason Fitch Cogswell, a physician who performed some of the first cataract surgeries in the United States, commissioned his young neighbor, Thomas Hopkins Gallaudet, to travel to Europe and learn instructional methods for the deaf. Gallaudet originally planned to visit the Braidwood family in England and Abbé Sicard in France, to gather instructional techniques in aural/oral communication and manual communication in the two countries, respectively.

(continues)

The Braidwood family proved to be secretive and unwilling to share their oral teaching methods. Thus, in 1816 Gallaudet left London for Paris, where he learned a manual communication system from Abbe Roch, Ambroise Sicard, and Laurent Clerc (himself deaf). Gallaudet returned to the United States, along with Clerc, and provided instruction to Alice. The two men went on to establish the American Asylum for the Education of the Deaf and Dumb (now the American School for the Deaf) in 1817, a school with a manual orientation. During the next 40 years, Clerc became one of the most influential educators of the deaf and the first (and one of the few) deaf teachers in the nineteenth century. Gallaudet's son, Edward Miner Gallaudet (1837–1917), became the president of the first college for the deaf in the new world, now named Gallaudet University.

The thread of oralism in the United States can be picked up several years later. This moment in time, too, was triggered when a young girl of a prominent family lost her hearing. Mabel Hubbard suffered scarlet fever in 1863 and, as a result, incurred an irreversible hearing loss. Her father, Gardiner Greene Hubbard, a lawyer in Massachusetts, helped to establish the Clarke School in Northampton, MA, in 1867, with the assistance of Samuel Howe, who also was the principal of the first school for the blind in the United States.

When Mabel Hubbard grew up, she married Alexander Graham Bell (Figure 15-1). In the latter half of the 19th century, Bell became an articulate and passionate advocate for oralism in the United States. In fact, an impetus for developing the telephone was a desire to develop an amplification device for his wife-to-be and for his mother, who also had a hearing loss. His counterpart who advocated an orientation that incorporated manual communication was Edward Gallaudet. In the late 1800s, these two men often were engaged in debate as to the merits of one method versus the other.

Throughout the 20th century, debates and controversies flared on and off as to which of the two basic educational approaches, manual or aural/oral, is most appropriate for educating deaf children. The debate continues into the 21st century.

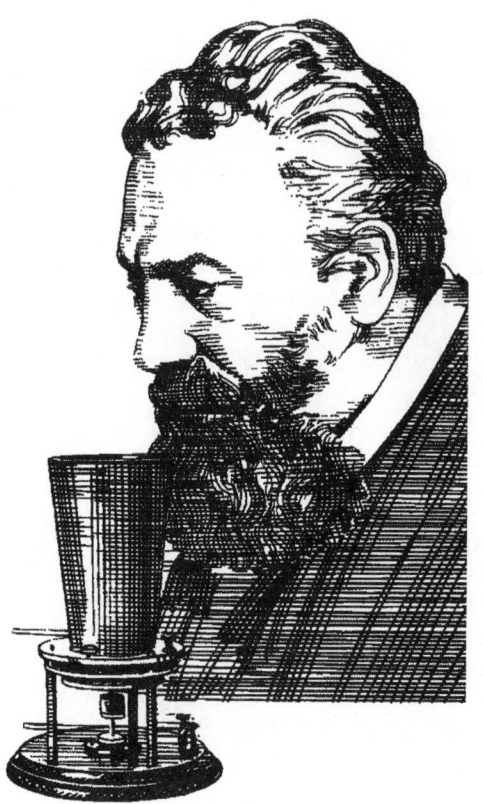

FIGURE 15-1. Alexander Graham Bell, advocate for oralism.

▰ EDUCATION LAW

Public Law 94-142 (Nov. 29, 1975): It is the purpose of this Act to assure that all handicapped children have available to them, within the time periods specified in section 612(2) (B) a free appropriate public education which emphasizes special education and related services designed to meet their unique needs, to assure that the rights of handicapped children and their parents or guardians are protected, to assist States and localities to provide for the education of all handicapped children and to assess and assure the effectiveness of efforts to educate children.

Major legislation for children who have disabilities dates back to 1975, when Congress passed the Education for All Handicapped Children Act of 1975, known as PL 94-172 or the EHA law. This law guaranteed a free and appropriate education for all children with disabilities between the ages of 3 and 18 years of age, in the least restrictive environment possible. The disabilities covered included hearing loss, as well as specific learning disabilities, speech and language impairments, emotional disturbances, cognitive deficiencies, orthopedic impairments, visual impairments, and others. The term *free and appropriate public education* meant that children would receive special education and supporting services at public expensive and under public supervision. These services were to comply with the standards of the state educational agency. A *least restrictive environment* was described as one in which a child who has a disability could be placed with the least limitations and still thrive when compared to peers who did not have a disability. The environment had to meet the child's unique needs and allow the child to be educated to the maximum extent appropriate with peers who have typical development.

Making Sense of the Numbers

Federal laws usually are designated with a tag number like PL 94-142. The *PL* is an acronym for *Public Law*. The first two numbers, *94*, correspond to the number of the Congress that passed the law. The remaining three numbers indicate the piece of legislation. For instance, PL 94-142 was the one hundred-and-forty second piece of legislation passed by the ninety-fourth Congress of the United States. The Congressional number advances once every 2 years (in even years).

In 1990, PL 94-142 was amended and reauthorized as PL 101-476, and became known as the Individuals with Disabilities Education Act (IDEA). IDEA also encompasses earlier amendments made to the original act, including PL 99-457 and PL 101-476, which mandate services for infants and toddlers and their families. IDEA changed the term *handicapped children* to *children with disabilities*. It expanded the age range of children covered by PL 94-142 to individuals from birth to the age of 21 (up to the 22nd birthday). The key additions afforded by IDEA are the (a) provision of public services for infants and toddlers and their families, (b) assistance to individuals making a transition from secondary school to postschool settings, and (c) the inclusion of assistive technology services in educational planning. The services for infants might include any or all of the following:

■ Family training, counseling, and home visits
■ Special instruction

- Speech pathology and audiology
- Occupational therapy
- Psychological services
- Case management
- Medical services for diagnosis or evaluation
- Screening and assessment

Under the amended law, rehabilitation counseling and social work were also included as related services. The definition of disability was expanded to include children with autism and traumatic brain injury.

IDEA was amended in 1997 by PL-105-17. The reauthorization underscored parent participation in decision making, made provisions for addressing the general education curriculum in education planning, and promoted high expectations for achievement. Key provisions of the IDEA include the following (Messina & Messina, 2004):

"1. *Identification*—the state and local education agencies must actively seek out and identify children who have special education needs (Child Find).

2. *Evaluation*—A child must be evaluated appropriately prior to placement. All methods used for testing and evaluation must be in the primary language or "mode of communication" of the child. No one test may be the determining factor for placement. [The Evaluation procedures cannot be racially or ethnically biased. Before a child is placed in an intervention program, a full and individualized evaluation will be conducted to determine the child's educational needs.]

3. *Individualized Education Plan (IEP)*—An IEP must be prepared for each child based on their individual educational needs.

4. *Parents* are equal participants in the decision-making process and students may be participants in their IEP development.

5. *Related Services*—Shall be provided on an individualized basis to assist the child to benefit from special education.

6. *Least Restrictive Environment (LRE)*—Each child shall be educated to the maximum extent appropriate with children who are nonhandicapped and children should be educated in more

restrictive (different) settings only when less restrictive alternatives are not appropriate.

7. *Private School*—When children are placed in private schools by state or local education agencies in order to receive an appropriate education, this must be done at no cost to parents; private school programs must meet standards set by law.

8. *Early Intervention and Preschools*—The IDEA now makes early intervention services available to children ages 0–5.

9. *Due Process*—Rights of parents and children must be guaranteed by states and localities; including notice, right to hearing, and appeal procedures. [If parents have a complaint, they will have an opportunity for a due process hearing that is conducted by the state educational agency, the local educational agency, or intermediate educational unit. They have the right to be accompanied by counsel and other individuals with special knowledge with respect to their child's disability.]

10. *Advisory Board*—Each state must set up an advisory board, including individuals who have disabilities, teachers, and parents of children who have disabilities.

11. *Funds*—IDEA/PL 94-142 provides flow through funds per child per year to supplement state and local program efforts. Funds may be withheld for noncompliance. Payments by the state to local school districts may also be suspended for noncompliance.

12. *Records*—Parents have access to their child's educational records and can request that they be amended."

Individualized Education Program (IEP)

An IEP is a written statement developed for children who have a disability. The plan includes a description of the child's current levels of performance, a statement of annual goals (e.g., a listing of language structures that will be mastered), a recommendation for special education support with an indication of how support will be provided and to what extent, and objective criteria for evaluating progress. The IEP also indicates the extent to which a child will be able to participate in regular educational programs. An example segment of an IEP appears in Table 15-1.

Individualized Education Plan (IEP): a federally mandated plan for providing education to children with disabilities, which is updated annually.

Table 15-1. Example segment of an Individual Education Program.

DOMAIN	STATUS	ANNUAL GOAL	SHORT-TERM OBJECTIVE
Audiologic	Can discriminate two utterances that differ in syllable length and intonation, such as *hello* from *how are you?*	To achieve closed-set identification of monosyllabic everyday words	Will correctly identify a spoken word when presented in the context of four then six alternatives with 80% accuracy
Language	Does not use bound morphemes, such as *-ed* or *-ing*	To establish consistent use of word endings in expressive and written communication	Will demonstrate use of past tense endings in 80% of written samples 70% of spontaneous and spoken language samples
Speech	Neutralizes vowels and omits final word consonants	To improve speech intelligibility	Will distinguish between /I/, /a/, and /u/ in imitated speech tasks with 80% accuracy, and produce final consonants in at least 50% of words spoken during a spontaneous speech task
Psychosocial	Does not follow classroom rules	To demonstrate grade-appropriate classroom behavior	Will receive positive reinforcements for adhering to classroom regulations, and accumulate 100 points during a 3-month period
Educational	Reading is delayed by one grade level; can read aloud but has reduced comprehension	To improve reading comprehension	Will demonstrate comprehension on 85% of grade-appropriate reading samples

The IEP is developed in a meeting attended by representative(s) of the local educational agency, the teacher, the parents or guardians, and sometimes, the child and/or other individuals at the discretion of the parents. These meetings are held at least annually.

Individualized Family Service Plans (IFSP)

Whereas IEPs are formulated for children over the age of 3 years, an IFSP is formulated for a child under that age. These services, called *early intervention services,* may be extended for a child through the age of 5 years. IDEA requires that states that receive funding for early intervention provide services to a child who experiences developmental delays, as measured by appropriate test instruments. Unlike an IEP, the IFSP concerns both the needs of the child and the child's family.

Once a child has been deemed eligible, a service coordinator is assigned to the family and child. The service coordinator coordinates the child's evaluations and assessments, facilitates and helps develop the IFSP, assists the family in receiving appropriate services, then helps develop a transition plan to preschool services if appropriate. Appropriate services might be provided by audiologists, family therapists, physical therapists, psychologists, social workers, speech and language pathologists, special educators, pediatricians and other medical specialists, and nutritionists.

The IFSP is a written document developed by a team, including the family. It describes the programs and services for a child, lists goals and objectives and procedures to be undertaken to ensure they are met, and identifies equipment that the public agency will provide the child and/or the child's family. Included in the IFSP are the following:

- A description of the child's present levels of physical, cognitive, emotional, social, and communication development, based on objective testing
- An overview of the family's resources and priorities, and their concerns about the child's status
- The goals and objectives targeted for the child and the family
- The services and procedures that will be implemented to achieve the targeted outcomes, including how often and when they will be provided, and when they will begin and end
- A statement of the criteria that will be used to establish whether the goals and objectives have been achieved

Individualized Family Service Plan: a federally mandated plan for the education of preschool children, which emphasizes family involvement and is updated annually.

> **Acronyms You Might Encounter in the Educational System**
>
> Some of the acronyms used when talking about children and their educational needs include the following:
>
> - FAPE: Free appropriate public education
> - IAT: Intervention assistance team, a multidisciplinary group of professionals who work together to provide intervention for a child
> - IDEA: Individuals with Disabilities Education Act
> - IEP: Individualized Education Program
> - IFSP: Individualized Family Service Plan
> - LRE: Least restrictive environment
> - SST: Supplemental services teacher, who interacts with a child's regular teacher to help the child

THE MULTIDISCIPLINARY TEAM

A **multidisciplinary team** is a group of professionals with different expertise who contribute to the assessment, intervention, and management of a particular individual.

An aural rehabilitation specialist usually works as a member of a *multidisciplinary team.* This team may include an audiologist, a speech-language pathologist, an educator, an otolaryngologist, and a psychologist. (In fact, the child's aural rehabilitation specialist may also be the child's audiologist or speech-language pathologist.) Depending on the situation, the team also may include a social worker or special education teacher. Each professional provides a different perspective of the child's abilities and needs. For instance, an audiologist collects information about the magnitude of hearing loss, a speech-language pathologist provides information about speech and language skills, and a psychologist and educator assess cognitive skills, learning patterns, psychosocial adjustment, and academic performance. A multidimensional portrait of the child emerges and provides a foundation for making recommendations about the best course for intervention.

Team members share their information with one another, perhaps in the form of written reports, or as a group in a formal staff meeting. One person serves as a case manager and coordinates and integrates the various recommendations and services.

The team interacts with parents so they can make wise decisions about a child's intervention plan. For babies and toddlers, IDEA requires that a team of professionals focus on the family system and address issues specific to the particular family. As noted in the preceding section, an IFSP must be formulated and include procedures for the identification of children with hearing loss (by means of at-risk criteria and audiologic screening methods), determination of extent of hearing loss, appropriate referral for medical and other services, provision of aural rehabilitation services such as auditory training, and determination of need for amplification and other listening devices. It includes a description of a child's current status and a report of the family and the expected outcomes of intervention. Specific details are included, such as the location and plan for service delivery, how long services will last, and how and when the child will be promoted into the public school systems.

The importance of early family-focused intervention cannot be overstated. Numerous studies suggest that families who receive counseling early, on a regular basis (such as weekly), who receive regular input from a teacher of the deaf, and who have an opportunity to interact with other families who have deaf children tend to have children who have better overall communication skills than families who do not receive this kind of support (Greenberg, Calderson, & Kusche, 1984; see also T. Clark, 1994; Greenberg, 1983; Greenstein, 1975; but also Musselman, Wilson, & Lindsay, 1988, for less definitive results).

Team management of children also occurs in the school setting. The multidisciplinary team formulates an IEP, which, as was noted in the preceding section, includes a description of the child's current levels of performance, a statement of annual goals (e.g., a listing of language structures that will be mastered), a recommendation for special education support with an indication of how support will be provided and to what extent, and finally, objective criteria for evaluating progress.

ROLES OF THE AUDIOLOGIST AND THE SPEECH-LANGUAGE PATHOLOGIST

Because an audiologist or speech-language pathologist may serve as the aural rehabilitation specialist on a multidisciplinary team as well as a child's case manager, we briefly consider their roles as team members. Exactly who does what is a gray area, as the roles of an audiologist and speech-language pathologist in the management of a child who is hard-of-hearing or deaf often overlap. What may be one person's responsibilities in one setting may belong to someone else in another location. In this section, we consider what are often the responsibilities of each professional.

The Audiologist

An audiologist may perform any of the following duties:

- Evaluate hearing and speech recognition skills
- Select, fit, and help maintain appropriate listening devices, including hearing aids and FM trainers
- Provide speech perception training
- Provide consultation to parents and other professionals on the multidisciplinary team

Audiologists identify and evaluate children's hearing capabilities and speech recognition skills. Although very young children may not be able to participate in word recognition testing, assessment of hearing thresholds can be performed with almost all age groups. Following identification, the audiologist may make any necessary referrals, such as to a physician or other health-care professional. The audiologist also may initiate the formation of the multidisciplinary team and the case-management process.

Audiologists also select and ensure proper use of listening devices. They will select and fit a hearing aid or make a recommendation for the child to receive a cochlear implant. They likely will explore the child's home and school environments, either through parent and teacher questionnaires or through site visits to the home and school. For instance, the audiologist may see that the child is in a noisy classroom and often misses much of the teacher's speech. The audiologist then may recommend that the child and teacher use an FM auditory trainer to reduce the effects of background noise. Follow-up maintenance and repair also will be provided.

Sometimes audiologists provide formal speech perception training rather than, or in addition to, the speech-language pathologist or classroom teacher. In some cases, they may make recommendations to the person who provides training.

Finally, audiologists consult with parents and teachers about the child's listening potential and difficulties and ways to encourage the development of listening skills.

The Speech-Language Pathologist

A speech-language pathologist may perform any of the following functions:

- Evaluate speech and language performance
- Provide speech and language therapy
- Consult with parents, and classroom teachers
- Provide instruction in sign language to child, classroom teacher, and parents, if appropriate
- Maintain bridges of communication between clinical setting, classroom and home, and ensure that therapy objectives are reinforced informally throughout a child's day
- Advise audiologists about appropriate language levels for audiological tests
- Provide speech perception training

A speech-language pathologist evaluates speech and language performance. If the child is 2 years old or younger, a speech and language evaluation may not be possible, simply because the child has so little speech and language to evaluate.

The speech-language pathologist also provides speech and language therapy. Test results are used to identify initial therapy objectives, and a hierarchy of steps to be followed over time is developed. Often, the objectives coincide with a curriculum that has been developed specifically for hard-of-hearing and deaf children.

A third role assumed by speech-language pathologists in the intervention plan is to provide consultation to parents, teachers, audiologists, and other members of the multidisciplinary team. Speech-language pathologists often provide general information. For instance, they may familiarize parents and teachers with their child's speech and language skills and how the child's skills compare to those of other children. They also can describe how speech and language skills progress in normally hearing children and children with hearing loss and factors that may accelerate or impede progress. Such information helps those who know the child to develop appropriate expectations. It also may provide them with ideas about how best to nurture their child's development.

For families who use simultaneous communication or ASL, speech-language pathologists can help parents and teachers learn sign language. They may recommend printed or video resources that include sign dictionaries and even provide direct instruction and practice.

Speech-language pathologists also can suggest ways for helping children generalize what they learned in therapy to more real-world settings by informing parents and teachers about their child's current therapy objectives and by suggesting practice materials. For example, a speech-language pathologist might observe a child in the classroom and then suggest ways the classroom teacher can integrate speech and language practice into the daily routine.

Speech-language pathologists may provide information about the child's language skills to audiologists and help them select appropriate audiological tests. For instance, if the speech-language evaluation reveals that a child has an extremely limited vocabulary, the audiologist may opt not to evaluate the child's speech recognition skills with recorded sentence lists.

In some cases, the speech-language pathologist provides formal speech perception training. The child's audiologist typically provides information about the child's listening performance, and this information is used to design training objectives. Again, the speech-language pathologist interacts with teachers and parents so they can reinforce auditory and speechreading training in everyday communication situations.

■ DECISIONS ABOUT THE INTERVENTION PROGRAM

Before an audiologist, speech-language pathologist, or educator begins to think about the specifics of an aural rehabilitation plan, such as auditory training objectives, four key decisions must be made about a child's intervention program. Typically, a child's parents or primary caregiver make them, although they receive information and recommendations from the multidisciplinary team before doing so. The decisions are summarized in Figure 15-2. All four decisions have an impact on how well a child develops listening, speech, and language skills, and affect academic and psychosocial development. It is important to understand that no single route is appropriate for all children, and hence, each child must be considered on an individual basis.

One decision often affects or determines another. For instance, if a family opts for an aural/oral program, they also may opt for a private day school if an aural/oral program is not readily available in their local public school system. Decisions also may be revised many times during the course of the intervention program.

School Placement

One of the first decisions parents must make about their child's intervention plan relates to school placement. They must decide whether their child will receive services from a public or private institution and whether the child will attend a day or residential program. Since the passage of U.S. Public Law (PL) 94-142 (the

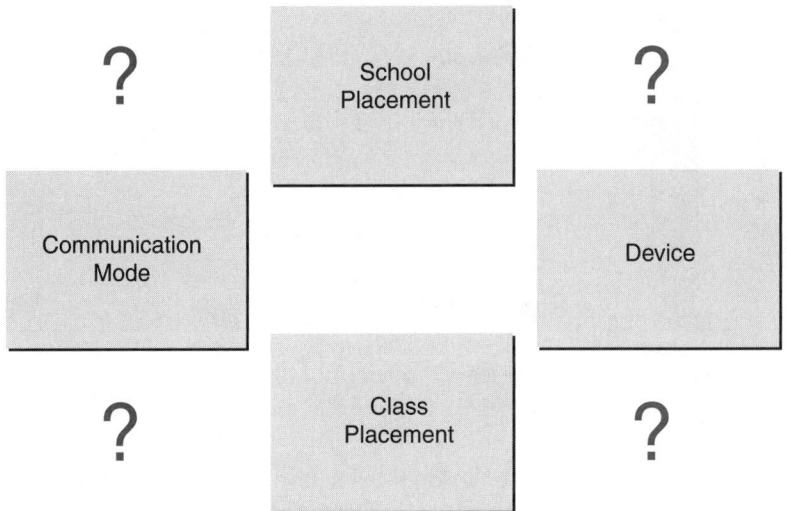

FIGURE 15-2. Decisions that must be made about a child's intervention program.

Education for All Handicapped Children Act) in 1975, there has been a substantial increase in the number of children who remain in their home communities and receive a public education. Concomitantly, there has been a decrease in the number of children who attend residential schools.

School placement enrollments are illustrated in Figure 15-3. Public school placements increased in the decade between the 1985–1986 school year and the 1994–1995 school year. Overall, the majority of children who have hearing loss attend public schools with children who have normal hearing. As we will learn in the next section, many of these children attend a resource room or self-contained classroom within the confines of the public school.

Classroom Placement

A second decision relates to program placement. This decision is influenced by the age of a child at the time of diagnosis. For instance, if a child is a baby, than parents might consider either a center-based program or a home-based program, or a combination of the two. In a *center-based program,* children attend

In a **center-based program,** children attend therapy for a designated number of hours per week.

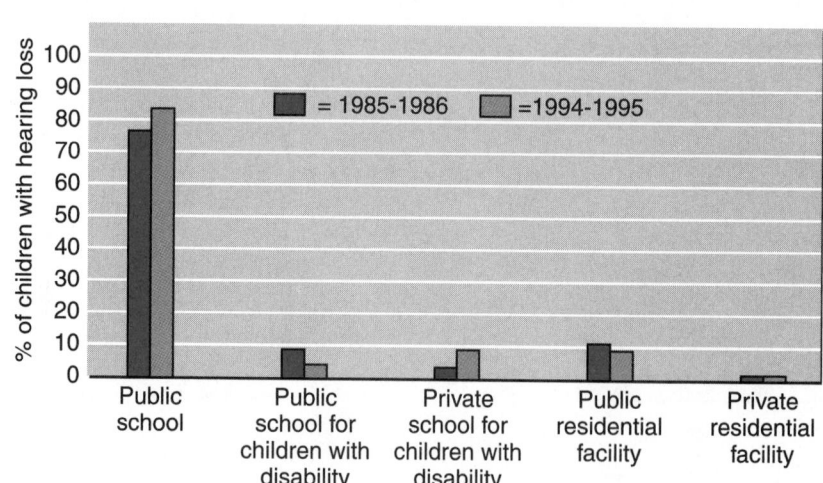

FIGURE 15-3. Percentage of children who have hearing loss in different school placements. (Data come from U.S. Department of Education, 19th Annual Report to Congress on the Implementation of the IDEA, Appendix A, 1998)

therapy for a designated number of hours each week. Their parents may participate too. In *home-based programs,* an early-intervention specialist visits the infant's home and provides instruction to the parents and child (Figure 15-4). Home-based programs occur in the home and emphasize one-on-one rather than group training (Scheetz, 1993).

In a **home-based program,** an early interventionist visits the infant's home and provides instruction for the child and parents.

Beyond infancy and early preschool, two distinct classroom placement options, self-contained and mainstream, are available in many school districts and a third (a combination of the two), resource rooms, may also be available. *Self-contained class-rooms* are contained within neighborhood or community schools and include only deaf and hard-of-hearing students (Figure 15-5) or may include children who have other disabilities, in which case it is classified as a *multicategorical self-contained* classroom. In *mainstream classrooms,* deaf and hard-of-hearing children attend classes together with children who have normal hearing. Often children attend a self-contained classroom for part of the school day and a mainstream classroom for some

Self-contained classrooms include only deaf or hard-of-hearing children.

In **mainstream classrooms,** deaf or hard-of-hearing children attend classes with their normally hearing peers.

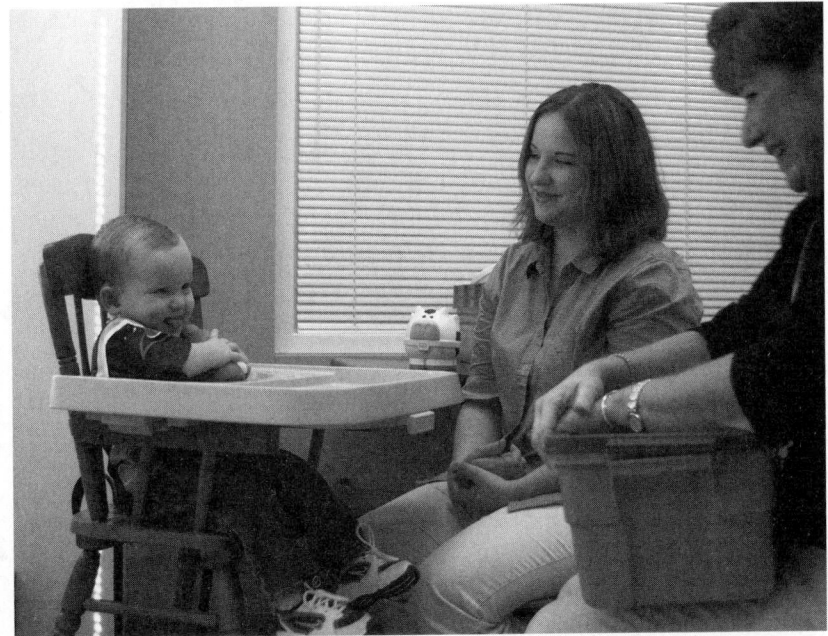

FIGURE 15-4. Home-based programs occur in the home. A professional provides one-on-one services for the baby, and works with the baby's family. (Photograph by Kim Readmond, courtesy of the Central Institute for the Deaf)

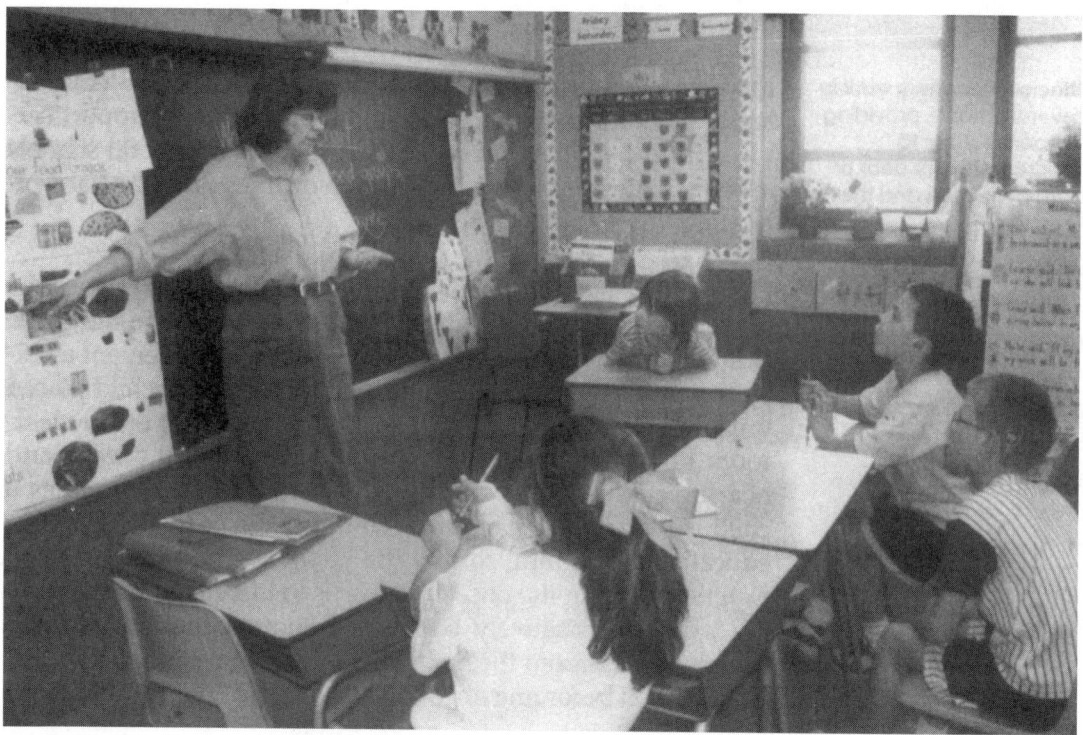

FIGURE 15-5. Self-contained classroom placement. Class sizes are usually small, and children sit in a circle around the teacher. (Photograph by Kim Readmond, courtesy of the Central Institute for the Deaf)

Resource rooms provide instruction in particular areas for children who spend part of their day in regular classrooms.

Itinerant teachers work in several schools, providing support services to children who are deaf or hard-of-hearing and their teachers.

subjects, such as art and physical education (Figure 15-6). When in a mainstream classroom, children often utilize support services, such as the use of a sign or oral interpreter and/or an FM trainer. Some children attend a mainstream classroom and also receive individualized instruction in a resource room. Children who attend *resource rooms* spend some part of their school day in a regular classroom, and receive instruction from an early intervention specialist for certain topics, such as language. An alternative or a supplement to a resource room is an *itinerant teacher.* The child attends school in a regular classroom, but receives support services from an itinerant teacher, who works in several schools and has expertise in issues related to deafness and the hard-of-hearing.

Figure 15-7 illustrates the classroom placement of children who have hearing loss. Data are shown for that segment of the population who attend public day schools. Most children attend either regular classrooms or separate classrooms, with about an equal percentage in either.

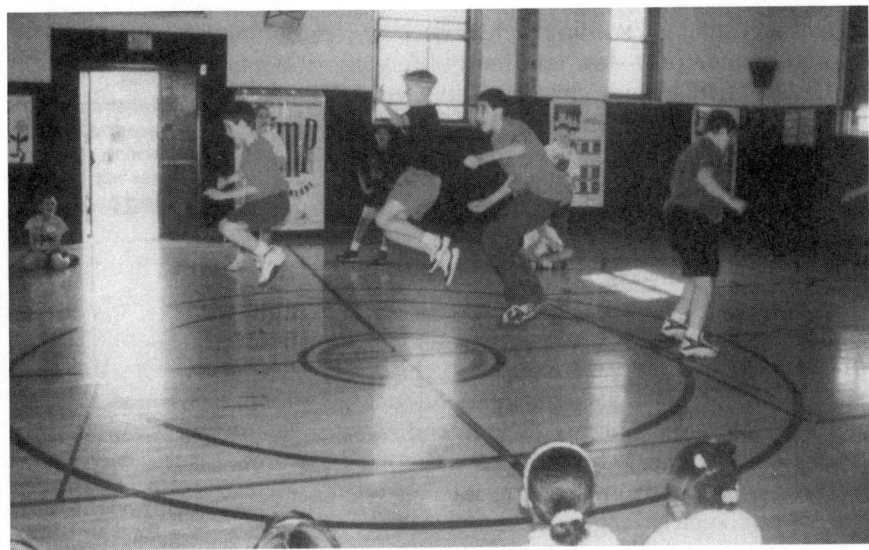

FIGURE 15-6. Partial mainstream classroom plassment. Children may be mainstreamed for nonacademic subjects during the school day, such as physical education class. (Photograph by Kim Readmond, courtesy of the Central Institute for the Deaf)

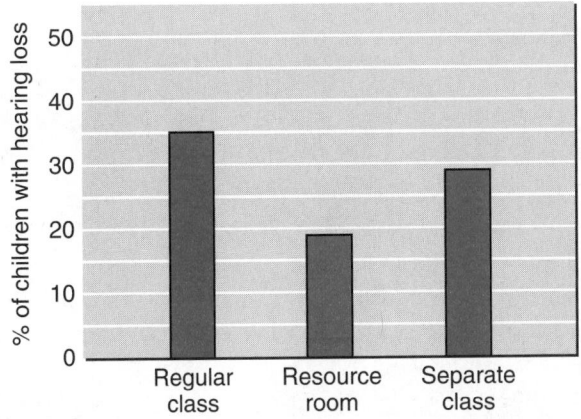

FIGURE 15-7. For those children who attend public school, percentages displayed as a function of classroom placement. (Data from U. S. Department of Education, 19th Annual Report to Congress on the Implementation of the IDEA, Appendix A, 1998)

Two derivatives of mainstreaming are classroom options of *inclusion* and *co-enrollment*. Like mainstreaming, inclusion entails placing children who have hearing loss in classrooms with children who have normal hearing. The difference is that in a

Inclusion: inclusion integrates all students and activities into the daily routine of the general education classroom.

mainstream placement, a child will often attend the resource room and attend special classes. In some scenarios, children are treated more like "visitors" to the regular classroom than active members (Anita, Stinson, & Gaustad, 2002). Because of academic or behavioral considerations, the classroom teacher might believe a child is best served in the special classrooms. The upside of this model is that in some ways the child might get the best of both worlds. He or she receives needed support and still has an opportunity to interact with a peer group. The downside of this model is that a student's "visits" to the classroom might be disruptive to the classroom routine, and the child may not be able to slip into the flow of what is happening at the moment (e.g., the child might not have performed an assignment that is under current discussion).

In contrast, a child in an inclusion classroom is included in all aspects of the class life and the school (Figure 15-8) (Anita et al., 2002; Marschark, Young, & Lukomski, 2002). The classroom teacher has the primary job of educating every child in the class-

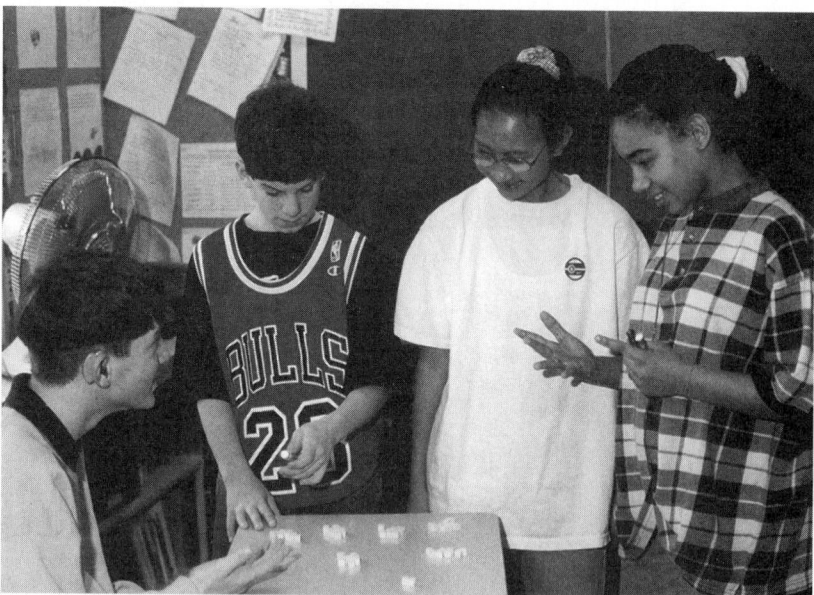

FIGURE 15-8. In an inclusion classroom, the child who has hearing loss is an active member of the classroom, participating in all academic and social interactions. (Photograph by Marcus Kosa, courtesy of the Central Institute for the Deaf)

room. The classroom teacher may have a partnership with a special education teacher in making adjustments to the curriculum and structuring the classroom environment to meet the learning needs of the child with hearing loss. The philosophical difference between mainstreaming and inclusion is that, in the former, the child must adapt to the classroom, whereas in the latter, the classroom must adapt to the child (Stinson & Anita, 1999). Inclusion is not without its challenges. Many classroom teachers feel unprepared to handle the multifaceted needs of both children who have normal hearing and children who have hearing loss, and sometimes the child with hearing loss has problems integrating socially with his or her peers who have normal hearing (e.g., Israelite, Ower, & Goldstein, 2002) and feels "different" than classmates (Leigh, 1999).

In a *co-enrollment model,* the classroom is conducted by two teachers, a regular classroom teacher and a teacher for children who have hearing loss (Jimenez-Sanchez & Anita, 1999). This model aspires to put children who have hearing loss on the same playing field as children who have normal hearing. This kind of team-teaching gives all students exposure to their own culture, and that of others and languages, and helps students establish a self-identity and self-esteem.

Co-enrollment: a model of educating children who have hearing loss that entails a team of teachers, one a regular classroom teacher and the other, a trained teacher for children who have hearing loss.

School Days

High school students who had hearing losses ranging from moderate to profound were queried about their school experiences and interactions with their peers. These students live in Toronto, Canada. They attended special classes for hard-of-hearing students for their elementary schooling and now attend a regular public high school with children who have normal hearing. Here are some of their comments about fitting into the mainstream (Israelite et al., 2002, pp. 141–142):

About fitting in, a student named Sam said: "My biggest challenge was grade 9. Trying to fit in a school where I had never been, where people from my neighborhood attended too. . . . When I was there, people would put me down because I was

(continues)

different from them. But my challenge was to fit with them, to tell them that I could do the same thing as [them] or possibly better."

About revealing her hearing loss to peers, a student named Kate said: "I realized when I first entered my mainstream English class they don't know I'm hard-of-hearing so they treat me like everyone else. If I say I'm hard-of-hearing, then they will treat me differently. . . . So I don't say anything so they treat me the same as everyone else."

About interactions with the classroom teacher, a student named Jade said: "One thing I hate is when I was in grade 9, one of my English teachers told a teacher I was going into her grade 10 class, and my teacher told her that I was hard-of-hearing. My teacher was making sure [my grade 10 teacher knew] I was hard-of-hearing. Every need of mine would be granted. I hated that [grade 10] class so much. The teacher was so nervous around me. I don't need special treatment. I don't like it when I come to a classroom and the teacher knows me because I'm hard-of-hearing."

Figure 15-9, adapted from Deno (1970), illustrates one model for determining classroom placement. The goal is to move the child toward a regular mainstream classroom placement as expediently as appropriate. Only when necessary is a child placed outside of the mainstream classroom or taken out of the classroom to receive special support services. Not all speech and hearing professionals adhere to such a model. Sometimes a child is placed in a regular classroom at the onset of his or her educational program, so that the youth has normal classroom experiences from the onset and learns to identify with the hearing world. Alternatively, some children are educated in a self-contained classroom throughout their school years, with special emphasis on becoming enculturated into the Deaf community.

There is not a great deal of research data available to help parents make choices about classroom placement. Some evidence suggests children who attend mainstream and inclusion classrooms have better speech and language skills than those who attend self-contained classrooms. However, the selection process deter-

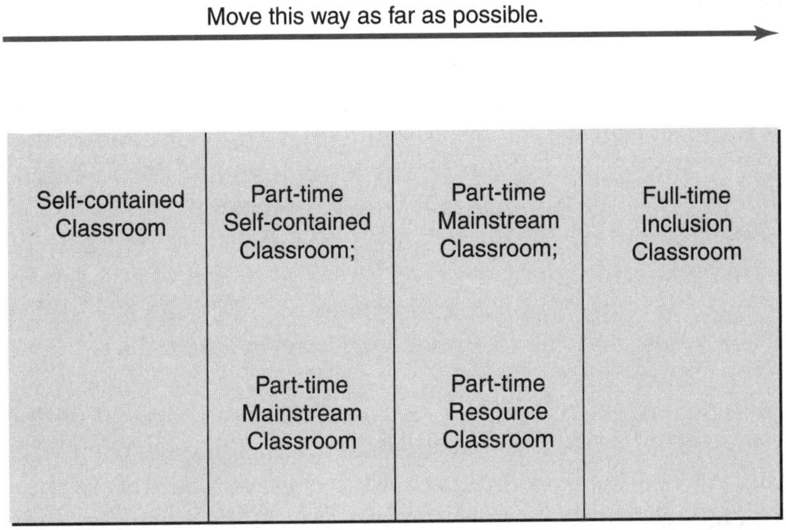

Move this way as far as possible. →

Self-contained Classroom	Part-time Self-contained Classroom;	Part-time Mainstream Classroom;	Full-time Inclusion Classroom
	Part-time Mainstream Classroom	Part-time Resource Classroom	

FIGURE 15-9. One model for determining classroom placement.

mining classroom placement is often designed to place children with better skills in programs that provide fewer specialized services. As such, mainstreaming per se may not necessarily result in better communication skills. Northcott (1990) noted that children who are placed in mainstream classrooms usually have the following characteristics: "early fitting of hearing aids, early family oriented infant/preschool programming, auditory-oral approach to language learning and . . . speech as the primary mode of communication." (p. 15)

Communication Mode

A third decision to be made about the intervention program relates to communication mode. Will the child use primarily speech to communicate? Manually coded English and speech? ASL? If a sign system is selected, the family also must learn the system, as well as the child. Before we consider the decision process, let us first review the various communication modes.

The majority of persons with profound hearing impairments use one of three modes to communicate: *American Sign Language* (ASL), manually coded English, and spoken language. A relatively small minority use a system called Cued Speech.

American Sign Language (ASL) is a manual system of communication used by members of the Deaf Culture in the United States.

AMERICAN SIGN LANGUAGE

ASL is a manual system of communication. A person does not use ASL and speak at the same time. ASL has a different grammar than spoken English. One ASL sign might represent a concept that would require many English words to express. Facial expressions and body language can impart a variety of meanings to the signs. In both ASL and manually coded English, fingerspelling may be used if there is no sign for a particular word or concept. In fingerspelling, one handshape corresponds to each letter of the alphabet. The American manual alphabet appears in Figure 15-10.

Bilingual/bicultural model: teaching children with significant hearing loss ASL as their first language and then later English in school as they develop reading and writing skills.

A great deal of attention in recent years has been focused on the use of a ***bilingual/bicultural model*** for educating children with significant hearing loss. In this model, children use ASL as their first language for communication and then, later, learn English in school as they develop reading and writing skills. The premise is that, if children develop a language system for thought and expression first, basic skills will transfer to learning similar skills in a second language. The fact that deaf children of deaf parents (who use ASL) often have better language and literacy achievement than deaf children of hearing parents provides a primary rationale for this approach. A number of educational programs in the United States, Sweden, and Denmark have implemented this model.

MANUALLY CODED ENGLISH

Manually coded English is a form of communication in which manual signs correspond to English words.

As the name implies, ***manually coded English*** is comprised of manual signs corresponding to the words of English. It also has the same syntactic structures. Typically, a person who uses manually coded English speaks simultaneously while signing. For instance, as a boy says, "The cat is inside," he will sign the article *the,* and then one sign each for *cat, is,* and *inside.* The combined use of sign and speech as an educational philosophy is referred to as ***simultaneous communication.*** The child uses every available means to receive a message, including sign, residual hearing and lipreading. The majority of very young deaf and hard-of-hearing children use simultaneous communication. However, this could change in the future. The increased use of cochlear implants may mean that more children use an aural/oral mode. Conversely, the resurgence of Deaf pride and the Deaf Culture movement (which we considered in Chapter 11) may lead to more children using ASL.

Simultaneous communication: combined use of sign and speech.

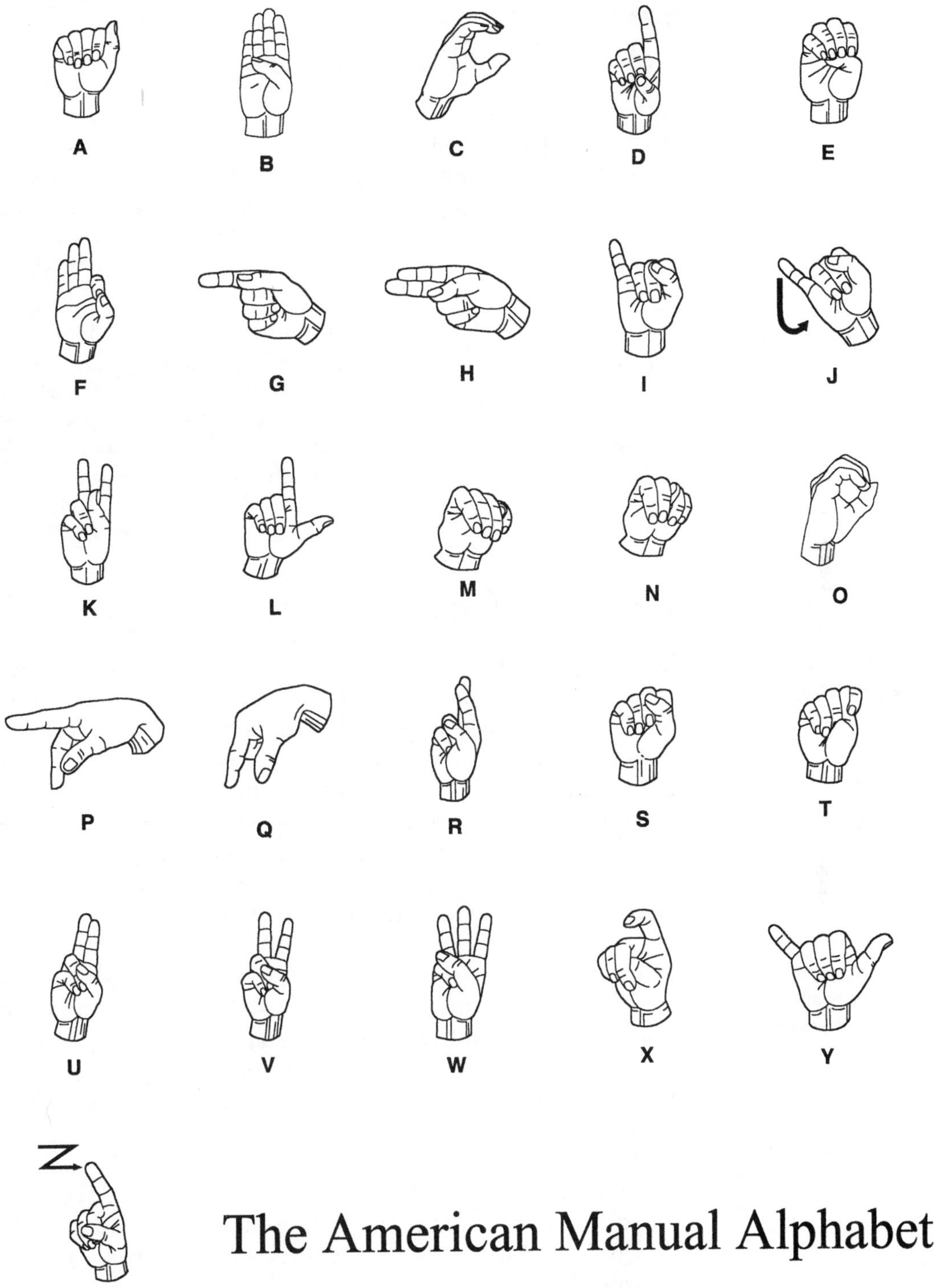

A B C D E

F G H I J

K L M N O

P Q R S T

U V W X Y

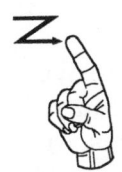

The American Manual Alphabet

FIGURE 15-10. The American manual alphabet.

More on Manually Coded English

There is no universally accepted English-based sign system. For example, under the rubric of manually coded English fall the systems of Signed English, Seeing Essential English (SEE 1), Signing Exact English (SEE 11), Linguistics of Visual English (L.O.V.E.), and the Rochester Method. People in one region of the country may sign a word one way, whereas those in another region sign it in a different way.

Many teachers and children who use manually coded English actually sign a Contact form of English, omitting function words such as *the* and morphemes, including those that mark past tense and plurality (Marmor & Pettito, 1979; Nix, 1983). Children who receive a Contact model of English may be at relatively high risk for developing deficits in language syntax.

AURAL/ORAL LANGUAGE

Aural/oral language is the language used by persons with normal hearing.

Aural/oral language is the same language used by persons with normal hearing. The child with a hearing impairment who uses aural/oral language will speak messages and use speechreading to receive messages. Most children who use aural/oral language are educated with a multisensory approach, but a small number are educated with a unisensory approach. Children in a *multisensory approach* utilize both vision and hearing to recognize speech. In learning to talk, children rely on residual hearing, speechreading, and in some instances, touch.

Multisensory approach: use of both vision and hearing, and sometimes touch, to recognize speech.

Unisensory approach: use of only residual hearing to receive spoken messages.

Children in a *unisensory approach* rely only on residual hearing to receive spoken messages. The classroom teacher may sometimes expect a child to recognize the signal auditorilly, even if the youngster has minimal residual hearing. This approach is sometimes referred to as an *acoupedic approach,* and is defined by Pollack (1970) as follows:

The acoupedic approach is a comprehensive habilitation program for infants and their families that emphasizes auditory training without formal lipreading instruction.

The term acoupedics refers to a comprehensive habilitation program for the hearing impaired infant and his family, which includes an emphasis upon auditory training without formal lipreading instruction. (p. 13)

CUED SPEECH

Cued Speech is a communication mode that is used by a handful of children with profound hearing loss. This communication system uses phonemically based hand gestures to supplement speechreading (Comett, 1967). Thus, the talker speaks while simultaneously cueing the message. By themselves, the hand signals are uninterpretable. When coupled with the audiovisual signal, speech recognition increases because viseme members are distinguished from one another.

Cued Speech, a system for enhancing speechreading, uses phonemically based gestures to distinguish between similar visual speech patterns.

In the Cued Speech system, eight different handshapes are used to distinguish consonants, and six locations on the face and neck are used to distinguish vowels. For instance, the consonants /p/ and /b/ resemble one another on the mouth. The consonant /p/ is distinguished by a 1 handshape and the consonant /b/ is shown by a 4 handshape. Thus, if a talker said the word *pea*, he or she would hold a 1 handshape to the corner of the mouth, because a 1 handshape indicates the phoneme /p/, and a placement at the mouth comer indicates an /i/ vowel. If the talker instead said *bee*, he would hold a 4 handshape at the mouth corner. The word *boo* would be signaled by a 4 handshape at the throat. Figure 15-11 presents the Cued Speech system.

SELECTION OF A COMMUNICATION MODE

Much debate and controversy surround the issue of communication mode, and many speech and hearing professionals take firm stands in favor of one mode versus another. Of all the decisions parents must make about their child's intervention plan, this decision can be the one they revisit most often.

Selection of communication mode is an area where there are no clear answers to the best way to go, and it is likely the best route is different for different children. With this said, there is some evidence that children educated with an aural/oral emphasis program achieve better speech and language performance and literacy development than children educated in a program that uses sign language. For instance, Markides (1988) found that children from an aural/oral emphasis program were more likely to achieve better speech intelligibility than children from simultaneous communication programs, and their speech intelligibility was less likely to deteriorate over time.

Vowel Positions

Consonant Handshapes

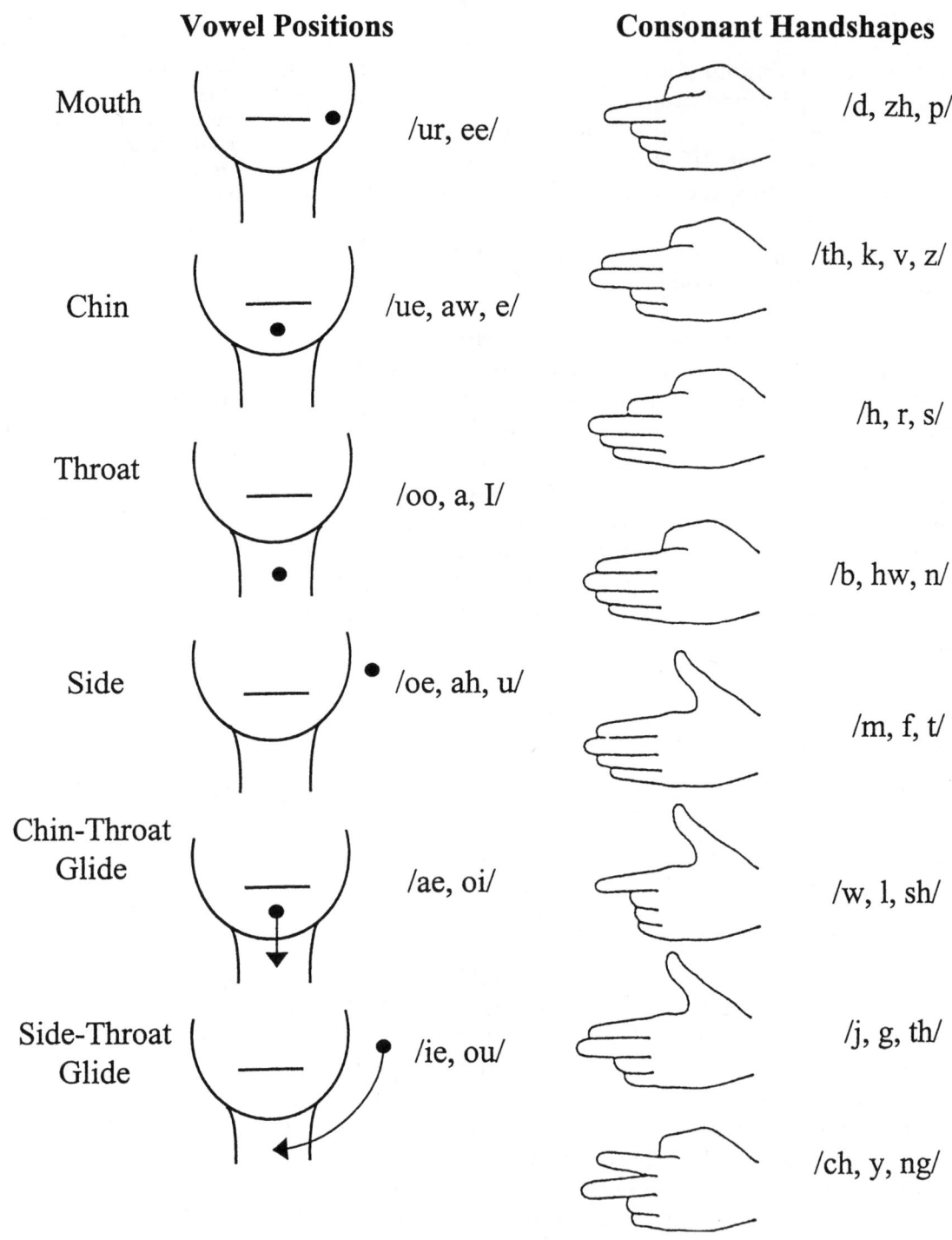

Mouth — /ur, ee/

Chin — /ue, aw, e/

Throat — /oo, a, I/

Side — /oe, ah, u/

Chin-Throat Glide — /ae, oi/

Side-Throat Glide — /ie, ou/

/d, zh, p/

/th, k, v, z/

/h, r, s/

/b, hw, n/

/m, f, t/

/w, l, sh/

/j, g, th/

/ch, y, ng/

FIGURE 15-11. Hand configurations and hand placement positions for Cued Speech.

Although such studies suggest differences may exist between programs that implement different communication modes, most research investigations have provided relatively little control over other factors such as socioeconomic status or intellectual abilities. This is because there are many difficulties inherent in relating communication mode to outcome measures such as literacy or speech intelligibility. Complex interrelationships exist among demographic variables and the use of speech and sign. For example, children who use an aural/oral mode are more likely to have more hearing, to attend preschool, to come from higher-income families, and to use a hearing aid more often (Jensema & Trybus, 1978).

Perhaps where the issue of communication mode advantage is best resolved is in the population of cochlear implant users. Numerous studies have shown that children who use a cochlear implant and an oral method of communication develop better speech and language skills than do children who use simultaneous communication (e.g., Kirk, Miyamoto, Ying, Perdew, & Zuganelis, Osberger & Fischer, 2000). For instance, a group of researchers at Central Institute for the Deaf studied one hundred eighty-one 8- and 9-year-old children from across North America. They found that children who were in an oral education program developed better speech (Tobey, et al., 2003), language (Geers, Nicholas, & Sedey, 2003), conversational fluency (Tye-Murray, 2003), and reading (Geers, 2003) than did children who were enrolled in a simultaneous communication environment. The oral communication advantage proved robust, even after they factored out child, family, and educational variables. The researchers also found that following cochlear implantation, more children switched from using a simultaneous communication mode to an oral mode than the converse. Cochlear implantation was also associated with a shift from private school and special education settings to public school and mainstream programs.

Some metrics have been developed for helping families choose communication modality. For example, Northern and Downs (1984) developed the Deafness Management Quotient (DMQ), a formula that factors in residual hearing, central intactness, intellectual factors, family constellation, and socioeconomic situation. Similarly, Geers and Moog (1987) developed the Spoken Language Predictor (SLP), which is a sum of five weighted predictor factors that include hearing capacity (which is determined by speech recognition performance), language competence, nonverbal intelligence, and family support. If a child achieves a certain score or better with one of these metrics, an aural/oral mode is recommended. If not, a modality that includes sign language is advised. More recently, a system has been devised that bases this decision both on family- and child-centered measures, as well as the progress a child makes during a 6-month period in a program conducted by speech and hearing professionals. This program, called Diagnostic Early Intervention Project (DEIP) (Moeller, Coufal, & Hixson, 1990), appears to be highly effective in determining optimal placement in an education program, and relatedly, optimal communication mode (Moeller et al., 1990).

Listening Device

In addition to deciding about school and classroom placement, and selecting a communication mode, a decision must be made about a listening device. The decision usually is made fairly soon after diagnosis of hearing impairment as to whether a child will be fitted with a hearing aid or a cochlear implant. Before receiving a cochlear implant, the child must have a trial period with a hearing aid (Chapter 18).

Parents have a plethora of information available to help them make a decision about a listening device. For instance, research suggests that children who use cochlear implants surpass hearing-aid users who have similar degrees of hearing impairment in their speech recognition, speech production performance, and language and reading (see Chapter 16). Moreover, children who are younger when they receive a cochlear implant are more likely to perform better than children who are older.

In light of such experimental findings, it is likely that cochlear implant use will become more prevalent in the future. Indeed, there is potential for the cochlear implant to become the most commonly used listening device by young deaf children.

■ FACTORS THAT INFLUENCE INTERVENTION DECISIONS

Now that we have reviewed some of the decisions that must be made about a child's intervention program, let us consider the factors that often influence how these decisions are made. Figure 15-12 lists some factors that might influence a family's decisions. In many ways, the factors overlap.

Location		A.	Urban
		B.	Rural
Professional Counseling		A.	Pediatrician
		B.	Otolarynogologist
		C.	Speech and Hearing Professional
		D.	Educator
		E.	Psychologist
		F.	Other
Family Variables		A.	Income
		B.	Acceptance
		C.	Education
		D.	Expectations
		E.	Participation
		F.	Structure
		G.	Familiarity with Deafness
		H.	Other
Child Variables		A.	Age
		B.	Residual Hearing
		C.	Age at hearing loss onset
		D.	Vocalizations
		E.	Behavior
		F.	Language

FIGURE 15-12. Factors that influence the decision-making process.

Locale

Because urban and rural areas of the United States afford different educational opportunities, decisions about the intervention plan are to some extent dependent on geographic location. In large cities, parents often have a choice between intervention approaches. In rural areas, familial choice may be minimal. Because of limited resources, many rural school districts historically have endorsed only one intervention option and offered few publicly supported education services. Thus, for children who do not live in urban areas, many decisions about intervention may be made at the district and state level, by persons other than the family.

Locale

Brackett (1990) describes how school factors can affect the design of an intervention program:

> Some school districts, especially those in rural communities, do not have staff specifically trained or with appropriate credentials for working with hearing-impaired students. With no teacher of the hearing impaired to provide academic support, and with only one itinerant speech-language pathologist to cover a 150-mile area and visit schools twice weekly for the most severe cases, the question arises, "Is it possible to provide a quality program with the personnel who are available?" The answer may be "no" if caseloads are heavy and coordination time is difficult to arrange. Or the answer may be a resounding "yes." Many highly individualized programs have been implemented by support personnel who, with some inservice consultation, provide exactly what a child needs even though they do not possess the "correct" professional credentials.
>
> The school district's attitude . . . can affect the service delivery model selected. A district may not want the bother of generating a local program, preferring instead to send the student to an already existing out-of-district program. Conversely, a small district may be able to hire that special teacher who can effectively design a suitable program for a specific child. Economics also affect the choice of a model for a particular child. It may be less expensive to initiate a program locally, rather than pay a large tuition to centralized special education services. However, it is difficult to effectively implement a quality program without sufficient resources. (p. 92)

Professional Counseling

Most families of recently diagnosed children who are deaf or hard-of-hearing receive advice and counseling from a fleet of professionals. In addition to members of the multidisciplinary team, they also may receive advice from their family doctor and other professionals in their communities. The intent of professional counseling is to provide families with information, support, and opportunities for participation. Such counseling can be invaluable to families who are wrestling with issues that were unfamiliar to them before they had a hard-of-hearing or deaf child. Perhaps one of the most important roles you will play in a family's life will be to provide informational and emotional adjustment and acceptance counseling to families.

What Parents Say They Want From Professionals

Jackson Roush invited a group of parents to write about their experiences with speech and hearing professionals and to describe what was helpful in their interactions. Roush (1994) summarized the responses in the passage below:

1. The early stages of identification are among the most stressful some parents will experience in their entire lives. Families want professionals to provide facts and information, but also to consider the affective domain. A sincere, caring attitude from professionals, even if they don't know all the answers, is noticed and appreciated. This is particularly important during the early stages of identification and intervention. Consideration of the parents' emotional state apart from the specific needs of the child, is especially appreciated.
2. Early on, many parents want the "right choices" presented to them; but eventually, most want to make their own decisions. They must depend on professionals, however, to provide honest, unbiased information, delivered at a level appropriate to their knowledge and experience. Most families seek professionals who will support and encourage them along the path of their own choosing.

(continues)

3. Families want flexibility in methodology and placement decisions. What may be the "right decision" at a given point in time may change later on. Families want to be supported in the options they choose, and not made to feel "locked in" to these important decisions.

4. Families need to be praised and supported for what they are able to do, and not 'judged' for what they are unable to do.

5. Parents want and need the support of other parents. Many families report an emotional 'turning point' when they connected with a supportive group of other parents.

6. Professionals should consider the impact of hearing loss on the entire family. Parents are particularly appreciative when professionals seek creative ways to encourage the participation of all family members rather than designating a given individual, usually the mother, as the family expert and decision maker. (pp. 349–350)

Family Variables

In addition to locale and professional counseling, a third factor that influences decisions about the intervention plan is the family. Certainly home reinforcement and support is desirable no matter what program options are chosen.

Many family variables potentially affect the design of the intervention program. How these family variables interact and affect the decision making process are no doubt complex. These variables include at least these, the family's:

- Socioeconomic status, and availability of medical insurance
- Acceptance of the hearing loss
- Level of education and professional interests
- Expectations about who the child will become, and what he or she will achieve
- Willingness to participate in an intervention program
- Structure, including the number of siblings and whether both parents live in the household
- Familiarity with deafness

The impact of these kinds of variables may be great. Let us consider four of them in more detail to demonstrate this point:

- **Socioeconomic status:** A wealthy family may have the resources to afford extensive private speech language therapy and hence opt to use an aural/oral mode of communication with their deaf child. They are more likely to have medical insurance and their insurance policies may provide coverage for cochlear implants. A family with little income and no insurance will not have these resources.
- **Acceptance of hearing loss:** A family that has not accepted a child's deafness may not seek intervention services for several months or even years following diagnosis.
- **Family structure:** A family headed by a young, single mother with several children may participate less in decisions made about her child's intervention program, or participate less in the implementation of the program. For example, one mother enrolled her 1-year-old daughter in a center-based program. She had two other young children and also worked the evening shift in a factory. She soon dropped out of the intervention program, unable to follow the program routine while coping with other life demands.
- **Familiarity with deafness:** Families who are familiar with deafness, perhaps because of another relative's hearing loss, may be influenced by choices familiar to them. They also may be more accepting of the child's deafness and seek assistance quickly.

Child Variables

Not only general family-related variables influence intervention choices, so do characteristics of the individual child. These characteristics might include the presence of other disabilities, the child's intelligence, or degree of residual hearing. For example, if a child has mental retardation as well as significant hearing loss, an aural/oral communication mode likely will not be selected. On the other hand, if the child has residual hearing and receives good benefit from amplification, this option may be chosen. Less tangible child variables, such as whether the child is an introvert or an extrovert and whether the youngster is willing to accept challenges and competition, also will affect intervention decisions.

A child's progress and success also influence choices about intervention. For example, parents may enroll a child in one kind of program, but a lack of progress may lead them to enroll the child in a different program. A child's progress in developing receptive and expressive language, intelligible speech, and a positive self-concept impinge on whether and when a plan of intervention is modified.

A psychoeducational assessment usually is performed to obtain information about the child. The *psychoeducational assessment* usually includes an evaluation of the following child variables (Heller, 1990, p. 62):

- Intelligence, both *verbal* (cognitive abilities demonstrated via language-based performance) and *nonverbal* (cognitive abilities demonstrated by performance that is not language-based)
- Verbal function, written language, and reading
- Arithmetic skills
- Visual-motor skills
- Visual and auditory memory and multimodal in tegration
- Social and emotional function and problem solving
- Attention

The results of this assessment may be used to design a child's intervention plan, and also, to assess whether the child is progressing within his or her current program.

■ FACILITATING LISTENING IN THE CLASSROOM

Classrooms are noisy environments. Shoes scuffling, children whispering, papers crackling, books slamming, chairs scraping, a student laughing, footsteps falling in the hallway, doors closing, air handling systems humming these are just some of the sources blasting sound into the classroom. Usually these sounds are bouncing from wall to wall, and from floor to ceiling, reverberating from one hard surface to another. Even for children with normal hearing, listening in today's classroom can be challenging because of background noise, especially as this noise may average 50 to 60 dBA in a regular classroom (Crandell & Smaldino, 1995). Children who have hearing loss will be at a double disadvantage in trying to attend to the teacher's speech and to hear other children in the class (Crandell & Smaldino, 2000). They experience difficulty even in quiet, and background noise and reverberation exacerbate already degraded word recognition and speech comprehension abilities.

Controlling Background Noise and Reverberation

Some simple steps can be taken to minimize the level of noise in a classroom and the amount of reverberation. These include any or all of the following (Johnson, 2000, p. 269):

■ Installing carpeting or cork on the floor
■ Applying rubber tips on chair and desk legs
■ Placing bookshelves or wall dividers to create quiet areas within the classroom
■ Angling mobile chalkboards to reduce the amount of reverberation
■ Applying window treatments such as draperies or shades to reduce the amount of reverberation
■ Covering ceiling with suspended acoustic tile
■ Using cushions in place of chairs

Other strategies include encouraging children to wear soft-sole shoes, such as tennis shoes, and keeping the door and windows closed during academic instruction.

More invasive and global initiatives can be taken to minimize noise and reverberation. The air handling system can be adjusted to minimize noise generation. Siebein, Gold, Siebin, and Ermann (2000) found that the primary noise source in classrooms came from heating, ventilating, and air-conditioning (HVAC) systems. The following air-conditioning systems were found to be especially noisy: (a) self-contained, wall-mounted units; (b) decentralized fan coil units; (c) central rooftop units that serve multiple

Background noise: any undesirable auditory stimuli that interferes with someone's ability to attend to a target signal or to concentrate.

Reverberation: the persistence of sound within a space because sound waves reflect off of hard surfaces.

rooms; and (d) central systems with variable air volume systems (p. 380). They suggested possible solutions to HVAC-related noise include the use of silencers, adequate duct length, and vibration isolators.

Selection of a classroom might be an option. Classrooms that are smaller, with lower ceilings and classrooms that are not perfect squares or rectangles will minimize reverberation. If the school administration has not selected a classroom for a self-contained or inclusion class, you might encourage them to allocate this kind of room. Moreover, you might select a room away from special purpose rooms (such as the gym or the band room) and away from environmental noise (e.g., a classroom facing a back alley would be preferable to a classroom facing a busy urban street).

Assistive Technology

In Chapter 7, FM systems were described. One of the more widely used options is an FM sound-field amplification system, which provides an optimal signal-to-noise ratio for both children who have hearing loss and children who have normal hearing. A signal-to-noise ratio is the relative difference in dB between the sound source of interest (e.g., the teacher's voice) and the background noise. The FM sound-field amplification system is like a public address system, comprised of an FM receiver and an FM microphone for the teacher. Rosenberg (1998) showed that these systems greatly improve classroom signal-to-noise ratios. For children who have severe and profound hearing losses, a personal FM system may be more appropriate. In this alternative, a child receives the teacher's voice. The teacher talks into a microphone placed near her mouth and the signal passes through to a FM personal receiver, which either stands alone or is incorporated into the child's hearing aid or cochlear implant.

■ CHILDREN WHO HAVE MILD OR MODERATE HEARING LOSSES

Heretofore, we have focused on children who have severe and profound hearing loss. However, there is a huge population of children who have mild and moderate hearing losses who may require services from a speech and hearing professional at some point. It has been estimated that about 15% of children in the United States (more than 7 million) have a low-frequency or high-frequency hearing loss in at least one ear (Niskar et al., 1998). Two factors thought to contribute to the high prevalence of hearing loss in children are otitis media and noise exposure.

Many of these children experience particular difficulty while listening in noisy and reverberant classrooms. As a result, they experience deficits in speech recognition, academic learning, social skills, and self-image. They may have difficulty recognizing speech that is spoken quietly or at a distance. For these reasons, children who have mild and moderate hearing losses also may need aural rehabilitation, although usually not to the same extent as children who have severe and profound hearing losses. Children with a mild hearing loss (hearing thresholds between 20 and 40 dB HL) are often diagnosed later in childhood, perhaps during an elementary school screening program, because they rarely seem to have significant problems in hearing or in developing speech and language.

Children with a moderate loss (thresholds between 40 and 70 dB HL) have difficulty understanding speech presented at a conversational level and may have difficulty comprehending speech in a group setting. However, children with either a mild or moderate loss tend to receive a great deal of benefit from the use of hearing aids.

Children with mild or moderate hearing losses usually have an IEP developed. In particular, they should receive a speech-language evaluation to determine whether their speech and language acquisition is progressing according to age-level normally hearing peers. Sometimes, children will have mild misarticulation errors, such as errors in the production of fricatives and affricatives. Children with moderate hearing losses may also have some delays in vocabulary development. Children with mild or moderate hearing losses may or may not need speech-language therapy, and they may need to use a free-field FM assistive listening device system (Chapter 7). Often a child's classroom teacher will consult with a speech and hearing professional about how to adjust the classroom environment to accommodate the child with hearing loss. Information such as that summarized in Table 15-2 might be provided to the classroom teacher.

Table 15-2. Guidelines for the classroom teacher.

The following suggestions should help _____ 's teacher understand although he/she receives benefits from his/her hearing aid, it does not make speech clearer, only louder. What he hears might be called indistinct speech since there are individual sounds that are distorted or that she may not hear at all. Therefore anything that can be done to improve the listening conditions would be helpful.

1. **Let _____ sit as close to the teacher as possible. In this way he/she will be able to benefit from both the auditory and visual cues.** This seat should be far away from noisy distractions of hallways, radiators, or windows. Expect _____ to have more trouble listening and paying attention when the room is noisy than when it is quiet.

2. **Speak naturally to _____ in a good clear voice. The hearing aid is an amplifier therefore it is unnecessary to shout.**

3. **If _____ does not understand something that was said, the teacher can:**

    a. repeat-perhaps a little slower.

    b. rephrase.

    c. write the word or sentence on the board.

4. **In order to follow a group discussion, it would be helpful if _____ could sit where she could see most of the faces, and if the teacher or children could try to let her know who is talking and let her look before the speaker begins to talk.** It is also ideal if the teacher can repeat the most important things said.

5. **In order to understand what is said, it is usually helpful for _____ to see the speaker's face and lips.** This is called speechreading. For speechreading it is helpful if

    a. _____ 's back is to the major light source.

    b. The speaker does not move around too much.

    c. The speaker speaks clearly and distinctly and faces _____ when talking.

6. **Sometimes the hearing-impaired child may miss the small words and misunderstand a sentence, especially if it is a long sentence and the room is noisy.** If _____ seems confused or gives a silly answer, repeat what was said and if he/she said something inappropriate let her in on the joke. _____ may not always tell the teacher if he/she has not understood, but she should be encouraged to do so. Hearing-impaired children are sometimes embarrassed to keep asking for repetitions.

7. **New vocabulary words may be difficult for _____ , and he/she may require a little extra help in vocabulary development.**

8. **In some cases a notetaker can be a help to the hearing-impaired student. Sometimes a "buddy" in the class can be assigned to repeat directions to the hearing-impaired child without disrupting the classroom routine.**

Source: A handout from Central Institute for the Deaf Hearing, Language, and Speech Clinics. Reprinted with permission.

In this section, we consider two different children, Marian Weiss and Kevin Tobias.

Marian Weiss

Marian was born with normal hearing, in Midland, Texas. The youngest of four daughters, Marian's sisters ranged in age from 17 years old to 3 years old. Her father is in the oil business and travels frequently; her mother is a full-time housewife. At the age of 11 months, Marian was struck with meningitis. Within a month, behavioral audiometry and an ABR test revealed a profound bilateral hearing loss. At the time of her illness, Marian already had a vocabulary of seven or eight words. Later cognitive testing revealed an IQ in the gifted range.

Within 1 month of identification of hearing loss, Marian was fitted with bilateral hearing aids. Marian's audiologist in Midland encouraged Mrs. Weiss to take sign language and to begin communicating with her daughter with simultaneous communication. The available preschool programs in the city were based on a simultaneous communication philosophy.

Mrs. Weiss balked at the idea of using a manual system of communication. As she told the audiologist, "I'm determined that someday Marian will go to college with normal hearing children, and that she won't be held back by this loss." For the Weiss family, money was no object. They were able to afford any available option.

Marian's mother combed the Internet for information about hearing loss. She learned about the cochlear implant, which was still fairly new for very young children, she learned about oral/aural communication, and she learned about private schools geared toward the needs of children who have

(continues)

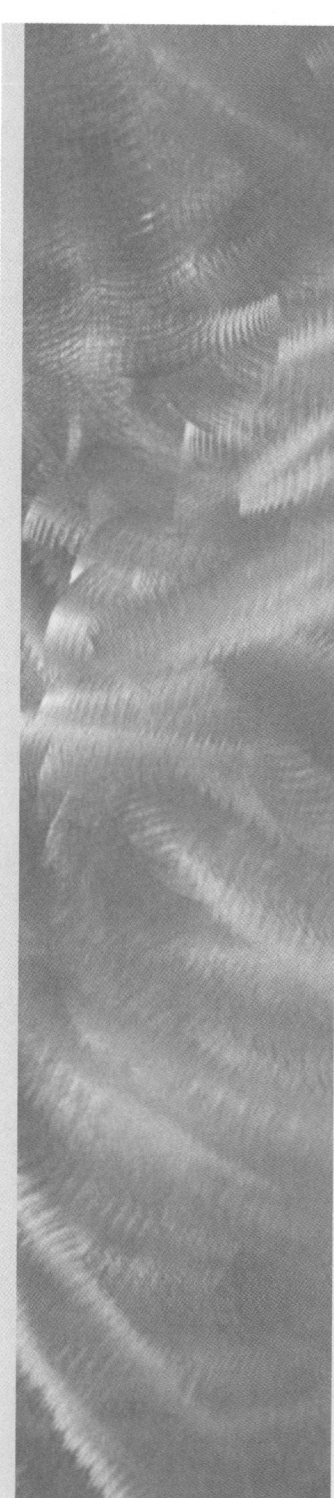

hearing loss. After conferring with her husband, they decided on cochlear implantation. The day after she turned 2 years old (at this time, the minimal age for cochlear implantation was 2 years), Marian traveled to Houston with her parents and received a cochlear implant.

For the next 3 years, Marian received weekly speech and language therapy from a private therapist. Mrs. Weiss enrolled in a distance learning program with the John Tracy Clinic in Los Angeles and received materials for promoting Marian's speech and language in the home environment on a regular basis. Mrs. Weiss became an active member in the Alexander Graham Bell Association, an organization that promotes aural/oral communication, and attended both regional and national conventions.

When Marian turned 4, the Weiss family made a momentous decision. They decided they would relocate the family to St. Louis, so Marian could attend a world-renowned oral school for the deaf. They sold their house and bought an apartment for Mr. Weiss in Midland. The older sisters relocated to public junior high and high schools in the St. Louis region.

For the next 5 years, the family resided in St. Louis, and Mrs. Weiss drove Marian to the private school. The second oldest child graduated from high school and went to college. Mr. Weiss continued his business travel and his work in Midland, spending about two weekends per month and holidays with the family in St. Louis. Marian attended the private school for 4 years then transitioned into a mainstream classroom for third grade. In the final year in St. Louis, the private school's mainstream support team provided support to her classroom teacher, and Marian continued to receive speech and language therapy.

At the age of 9, Marian relocated to Midland with her mother and the third sister, who is now in high school. The family bought a new house and now are reunited. Today, Marian is a confident and assertive child, who on occasion is even described as "bossy" by her classmates. She has excellent

(continues)

speech and language and performs at above grade level. Her friends in Midland all have normal hearing, and she considers herself to be part of the hearing world, although she is beginning to learn a few signs out of curiosity. She still calls her hearing friends in St. Louis and speaks to them on the telephone without difficulty.

This case is an example of a family who had definite ideas about what they wanted for Marian and who were willing to change their lifestyle so she could achieve it. The child's personality and her cognitive strengths, and her ability to benefit from the use of a cochlear implant, helped her to rise to the family's expectations. There is every likelihood that Mrs. Weiss's original vision will come true: Someday Marian will graduate from college and live the life of a person who has normal (or near-normal) hearing.

Kevin Tobias

Kevin Tobias was born with a profound hearing loss in Omaha, Nebraska. His mother, a single mother with one other son 2 years older than Kevin, suspected the loss early, although her primary care physician assured her that Kevin was fine.

It was Kevin's grandmother who convinced Ms. Tobias that Kevin's hearing problem was real. The grandmother took care of the boys while Ms. Tobias worked as a custodian in an office building. When he turned 14 months, Ms. Tobais and her mother took Kevin to a research hospital for an ABR. At that time, Kevin had no words. He communicated by screaming and throwing things. He should have had about 20 words by this time, and he should have been displaying vocal play, such as babbling syllables. When he was not angry or when he did not want something, Kevin was quiet.

An ABR test revealed a severe bilateral sensorineural hearing loss. A hospital audiologist became Kevin's service coordinator. Kevin's grandmother attended the sessions to develop Kevin's IFSP, as Ms. Tobias could not take time off work.

(continues)

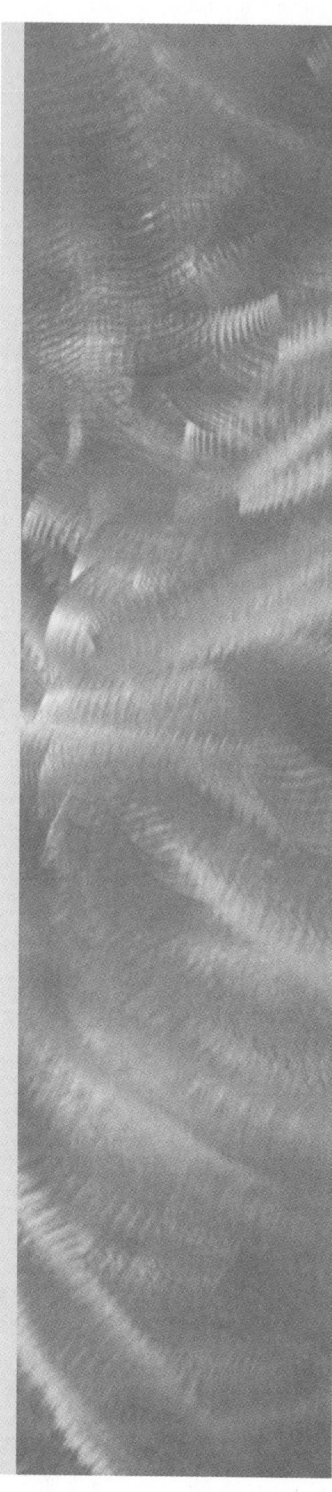

During meetings, one of the hospital nurses agreed to entertain Kevin and Kevin's brother, because the grandmother could not afford child care.

The audiologist applied to Nebraska's Medically Handicapped Children's Program to allow Kevin to obtain bilateral hearing BTE hearing aids. Kevin and his grandmother enrolled in a parent/toddler group at the research hospital's school. There, he received socialization and intensive language stimulation. The grandmother received sign language lessons and a series of signing videotapes.

Today, Kevin is 7 years old and is in first grade. He attends a self-contained classroom in the Omaha Public School system. He has speech that is about 40% intelligible, and the receptive and expressive language of a 5-year-old. His friends are comprised of his classmates in the self-contained classroom and his brother, who learned sign language through incidental learning at his grandmother's house. Kevin's teacher describes him as "all boy," someone who loves to tumble and roughhouse and play soccer.

His grandmother remains the person most active in his educational program, and Kevin now lives at least 5 out of 7 days at her house, including nights. Kevin's older brother has been diagnosed with several learning disabilities, so the grandmother has also taken responsibility for managing many of his needs. Ms. Tobias continues to remain in the boys' lives, although her long working hours and personal problems related to emotional health and relationship difficulties, serve as major distractions from her parenting.

Kevin's case is an example of a family that had to contend with many other pressures besides that of a child's hearing loss, including a single-parent household, low income, other instances of learning difficulties in a family member, and a parent's emotional and relationship difficulties. Because of the support of extended family and community services, Kevin appears to be on track to develop into an emotionally healthy and contributing member of his community.

◼️ FINAL REMARKS

This chapter presented an overview of children's intervention programs. We considered the decisions that must be made and factors that influence them. A variety of organizations exists that provide information about hearing loss in children and information about intervention plans. Many of these organizations are state speech-language-hearing associations. In addition to providing information, many of these organizations are comprised of professionals who provide speech, language, and hearing-related services to children and their families. The Key Resources section provides a list of many organizations and their addresses.

In the next two chapters, we consider the specifics of an aural rehabilitation plan. Unlike the situation with adults who have postlingual hearing loss (i.e., a hearing loss that was incurred after the acquisition of speech and language), the aural rehabilitation plan typically includes speech and language therapy as well as more traditional aural rehabilitation interventions.

◼️ KEY CHAPTER POINTS

✔ Public Law 94-142, passed in 1975, was a landmark event in the history of children who have disabilities. It guaranteed a free and appropriate education for all children between the ages of 3 and 18 years, in the least restrictive environment.

✔ The acronym IDEA stands for the Individuals with Disabilities Education Act and was passed by Congress in 1990. Stemming from Public Law 94-142, it expanded the range of children covered to individuals from birth to the age of 21. It was amended in 1997.

✔ An Individualized Education Program (IEP) is a written statement that describes the child's current levels of performance, a statement of annual goals, a recommendation for special education support with an indication of how support will be provided, and objective criteria for evaluating progress.

✔ An Individualized Family Service Plan (IFSP) specifies services to be provided to the child and the child's family. It is formulated for children aged 3 years or younger.

✔ A multidisciplinary team is assembled to evaluate a child and to provide support and services to the child and his or her family. The team may include an audiologist, a speech-language pathologist, an otolaryngologist, an educator, and a psychologist. The audiologist or speech-language pathologist often serves as the aural rehabilitation specialist and the case manager. The team interacts with a child's family to formulate an IEP or an IFSP.

✔ Some of the decisions parents must make about their child's intervention program relate to school and classroom placement, communication mode, and listening device.

✔ Classroom placement may be self-contained or mainstream. Variations of the latter placement include partial mainstreaming, inclusion, and co-enrollment.

✔ Communication modes include ASL, simultaneous communication, Cued Speech, and aural/oral language.

✔ Parents' decisions may be affected by several factors, such as their locale or their familiarity with deafness. You may play an important role in providing information and in making recommendations.

✔ Most children in the United States who have severe and profound hearing loss live at home and attend school in their home community. The majority of children use simultaneous communication.

✔ Most children with mild and moderate hearing losses can attend classrooms for normally hearing children. Usually, they will receive an IEP, although they may or may not require specialized speech and hearing services.

▬ MULTIPLE CHOICE QUESTIONS

1. Which of the following best describes PL 94-142:
    a. Ensures a free education for children birth to 21 years of age
    b. Ensures a free education for children in their home communities
    c. Ensures a free and appropriate education for children between the ages of 3 and 18 years
    d. Ensures support services for infants and their families

2. What is meant by the term, *least restrictive environment?*

   a. A child is placed in the home community.

   b. A child is placed in an environment that does not impede his or her academic development.

   c. A child is placed in an environment that imposes the least limitations while still allowing the child to thrive when compared to peers who do not have a disability.

   d. A child is placed in an environment that allows him or her to be included in all aspects of the general classroom's daily routines and activities.

3. What is IDEA-1997?

   a. One of the amended versions of the Education for All Handicapped Children Act, which underscores parent participation in decision making and the intervention plan and emphasizes high expectations for achievement

   b. The law that expanded the services provided to children who have handicap to include children below the age of 3 years

   c. The law that changed the terminology of "handicap" to "disability"

   d. The law that first made provision for family training, counseling, and home visits

4. What is due process with respect to an IEP?

   a. All children will receive a comprehensive evaluation of hearing, speech, language, cognition, and academic performance before goals and objectives are formulated for the IEP.

   b. Parents will have an opportunity to question the IEP, and if necessary, have a due process hearing. They have the option to be accompanied by counsel and other individuals with specialize knowledge about their child.

   c. Each state must set up an advisory board, including individuals with disabilities, teachers, and parents of children who have disabilities. This Board will ensure that due process is followed in providing education to children who have disabilities.

    d. For parents who opt to send their children to private schools, the state government will provide them the same funds toward tuition that would have been expended had their children received due process services in the home community via public education mechanisms.

5. What best describes the IFSP?

    a. A federally mandated plan for providing education to children with disabilities, which is updated annually

    b. Individualized Federal Service Plan

    c. An amendment made to IDEA in 1997

    d. A federally mandated plan for the education of preschool children, which emphasizes family involvement

6. Four decisions that must be made when planning a child's intervention program are:

    a. Communication mode, school placement, device, and class placement

    b. Locale, professional counseling, child variables, and family variables

    c. The use of spoken language, the selection of classroom placement, use of a coordinator, and device

    d. Device, educational plan, family plan, and school setting

7. A co-enrollment classroom is an example of:

    a. An educational placement where the child receives services from a resource room for part of the school day

    b. Mainstreaming

    c. Self-containment

    d. Educational models that entail a team of teachers, one a regular classroom teacher and the other, a teacher with specialized training

8. Which of the following statements is true?

    a. Proponents of bilingual/bicultural models of education often dissuade parents from teaching their children ASL.

    b. ASL has English syntax.

    c. Some ASL signs express meanings that would require several English words to convey.

    d. ASL is a form of simultaneous communication.

9. Which of the following statements is false?

    a. Cued Speech supplements lipreading.

    b. Cued Speech is equivalent to the manual alphabet.

    c. Cued Speech is used by a minority of children who are deaf.

    d. In Cued Speech, the position of the hand on the face and neck conveys vowel information.

10. For cochlear implant users, which mode of communication results in the development of optimal speech and language skills?

    a. Cued Speech

    b. Aural/oral

    c. Simultaneous communication

    d. ASL

11. Listening in a classroom may be facilitated by which of the following:

    a. Reducing reverberation by eliminating HVAC noise sources

    b. Reducing reverberation by placing the classroom away from special purpose rooms, such as the music room

    c. Keeping the window shades closed

    d. Reducing reverberation by placing carpet on the floor

12. What percentage of children in the United States have some degree of hearing loss in at least one ear?

    a. 5%

    b. 15%

    c. 25%

    d. 35%

KEY RESOURCES

Resources for Children Who Are Deaf and Hard-of-Hearing and Their Families

Alexander Graham Bell Association for the Deaf
3417 Volta Place NW
Washington, D.C. 20007-2778

American Academy of Audiology
8201 Greensboro Drive, Suite 300
McLlean, VA 22102

American Speech-Language-Hearing Association
10801 Rockville Pike
Rockville, MD 20852

American Society for Deaf Children
2848 Arden Way, Suite 210
Sacramento, CA 95825-1373

Auditory-Verbal International
2121 Eisenhower Avenue, Suite 402
Alexandria, VA 22314

Beginnings for Parents of Hearing-Impaired Children, Inc.
3900 Barrett Drive, Suite 100
Raleigh, NC 27609

Better Hearing Institute
P.O. Box 1840
Washington, DC 20013

Central Institute for the Deaf
4560 Clayton Road
St. Louis, MO 63110

Children with Attention Deficit Disorder
499 NW 70th Avenue, Suite 101
Plantation, FL 33317

Cochlear Implant Club International (CICI)
P.O. Box 464
Buffalo, NY 14223-0464

HEAR NOW
9745 E. Hampton Avenue, Suite 300
Denver, CO 80231-4923

John Tracy Clinic
806 West Adams Boulevard
Los Angeles, CA 90007

League for the Hard-of-Hearing
71 W. 23rd Street
New York, NY 10010

Learning Disabilities Association of America
4156 Library Road
Pittsburgh, PA 15234

National Association for the Deaf
814 Thayer Avenue
Silver Spring, MD 20910

National Captioning Institute
5203 Leesburg Pike, Suite 1500
Falls Church, VA 22041

National Cued Speech Association
Speech-Language Pathology Department
Nazareth College of Rochester
4245 East Avenue
Rochester, NY 14618

CHAPTER **16**

Speech, Language, and Literacy Development

TOPICS

In many ways, hearing loss has more far-reaching consequences for children than for adults. Not only may children not hear or understand the speech of others, but their own speech and language acquisition likely will be delayed as a result of their hearing loss. In this chapter, we consider their speech, language, and literacy development.

Data about children who have used cochlear implants for a prolonged period is also presented so that we may contrast their speech, language and reading skills with children who have similar hearing losses but use hearing aids. In this chapter, you learn that the advent of cochlear implants has had a dramatic effect on the outlook of speech, language, and literacy development in children who have significant hearing loss.

▰ SPEECH CHARACTERISTICS

Segmental errors: errors in speech sounds.

Suprasegmental errors: errors in speech rhythm and prosody, the pitch, rate, intensity, and duration imposed on phonemes and words.

Overall intelligibility *segmental errors* (errors in the sounds of speech), and *suprasegmental errors* (errors in speech rhythm and prosody) are often considered when compiling a description of children's speech (Figure 16-1). As a general rule, children with more residual hearing speak better and produce fewer segmental and suprasegmental errors than children with less residual hearing. However, how well a child speaks also depends on numerous other factors, including the speech therapy received, motivation to speak, the consistency of appropriate amplification use, the age of first receiving hearing aids, and the child's speech environment.

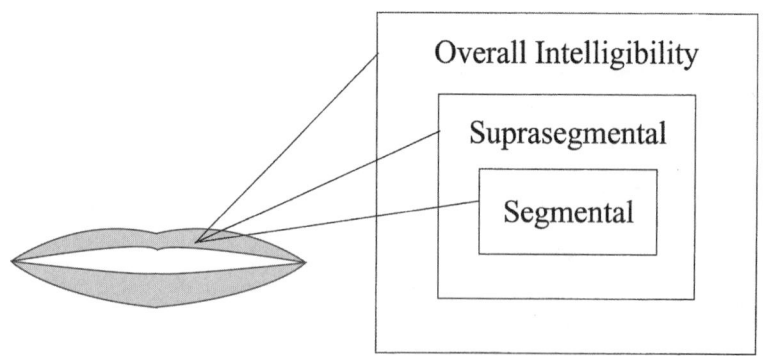

FIGURE 16-1 Speech proficiency is determined with a consideration of overall intelligibility, segmental errors, and suprasegmental errors.

For example, does the child hear speech often? Do those around the youngster provide good speech models? Is reinforcement provided when the child tries to speak?

Children who have mild to moderate hearing losses tend to have only mild speech and language difficulties, particularly if they use appropriate amplification. For this reason, in this chapter we focus on children who have more significant hearing losses.

Overall Intelligibility

Most children with profound and prelingual hearing impairments who use hearing aids are difficult to understand. On average, you will rarely identify more than 20% of the words they say (John & Howarth, 1976; Markides, 1970; Monsen, 1978).

Research suggests that children with significant hearing loss demonstrate different developmental patterns than normally hearing children and that they reach a plateau in their speech skills relatively early in their development. For example, the phonetic repertoires of deaf infants have been found to be restricted when compared to their normally hearing peers (Lach, Ling, Ling, & Ship, 1970; Stoel-Gammon, 1988). Children who have been studied longitudinally between the ages of 11 and 14 years demonstrate little change in the average number and types of vowel and diphthong errors they make over time (McGarr, 1987). Although children may be idiosyncratic in many aspects of speech production, many demonstrate similar error patterns when speaking.

Segmental Errors

Children with hearing impairments produce many segmental errors, both when speaking vowels and diphthongs and when speaking consonants. Markides (1970) attempted to quantify the articulatory errors. In a group of hearing-aid users who had a mean hearing level of 95 dB HL, 56% of all vowels and diphthongs and 72% of all consonants were rated by a group of listeners as deviant. Not surprisingly, there exists an inverse relationship between the number of vowel and consonant errors and overall intelligibility: As the number of errors in a child's speech increases, intelligibility decreases (Smith, 1975).

VOWEL PRODUCTION

Children who have significant hearing losses and who use hearing aids most commonly neutralize vowels, so a child might intend to say "Me too!" but instead produce, "Mah tah!" Some physiological studies have focused on how the tongue moves during vowel production. These studies suggest that talkers with profound hearing loss may not move their tongue bodies in the anterior-posterior (front-back) dimension as much as normally hearing talkers and may rely primarily on jaw displacement for distinguishing vowel height (e.g., the low vowel /a/ versus the high vowel /ɪ/) (Dagenais & Critz-Crosby, 1992; Tye-Murray, 1987, 1991). This restricted tongue movement is no doubt a primary component underlying the perceptual phenomenon of neutralized vowels.

A list of vowel error types includes the following:

- Neutralizations
- Substitutions
- Dipthongizations
- Prolongations
- Nasalizations

CONSONANT PRODUCTION

Children who have severe and profound hearing losses and who use hearing aids tend to produce characteristic consonantal errors. These errors include voiced/voiceless confusions, substitutions, omissions, distortions, and errors in consonant clusters. For example, a child might intend to speak the word *boat*, but actually say "poe." In this production, the youngster substituted the voiceless /p/ for the voiced /b/ and omitted the final /t/ sound. Many children produce consonants that are visible on the face more accurately than consonants that are not visible. For instance, a child is more likely to produce the word *pat* correctly than the word *cat*. The /p/ entails visible lip closure, whereas the tongue dorsum closing gesture for /k/ cannot be seen. Apparently, a child with a significant hearing impairment relies heavily on visual information for acquiring speech.

Manner of production errors are also common. Affricatives, fricatives, glides, and laterals are especially difficult for many children to produce.

The Roles of Auditory Information in Speech Acquisition

To understand the difficulties children with minimal hearing capability have in developing intelligible speech, it is helpful to think about the ways in which auditory information helps us learn to talk. Auditory information plays at least five important roles during a child's acquisition of speech:

1. *Auditory information potentiates the development of specific principles of articulatory organization.* By listening to the speech of others in their community, children learn how to regulate their speech breathing, learn how to flex and extend their tongue bodies, and learn how to alternate rhythmically between vowels and consonants. Children who cannot hear often do not learn to (a) manage their breath streams for speech, (b) rotate their tongue forward and backward in the mouth to establish vowel postures, and (c) move the articulators smoothly and continuously from one articulatory posture to the next.

2. *By listening to others, children learn how to produce specific speech events.* For instance, they learn to distinguish /p/ with a relatively rapid velocity opening gesture and /w/ with a slow velocity gesture.

3. *Children develop a system of phonological performance* (i.e., they learn the phonemes of their language community) through listening. Often children who cannot hear do not acquire some sounds in their language, especially those associated with high-frequency auditory information, such as /s/ and /ʃ/.

4. *Auditory feedback informs children about the consequences of their articulatory gestures and how these consequences compare to sounds produced by other talkers.* For example, if a talker explodes air through his lips, he learns that this will produce a plosive sound. If he does it with too much vigor, he will hear a sound that may be inappropriately loud, when compared to other talkers of his language. It is not uncommon for a deaf talker to produce a slight popping sound when producing plosives.

5. *Auditory feedback may provide information for monitoring ongoing speech production and for detecting errors.* For instance, you might hear yourself say "See went," and then quickly

(continues)

correct yourself and say "She went." Deaf talkers are unable to monitor themselves in this way.

When a child does not have a sensory mechanism that fulfills these five roles, acquiring speech and maintaining appropriate articulatory patterns is a formidable task (Tye-Murray, Spencer, & Woodworth, 1995).

Suprasegmental Errors

Children with significant hearing loss and who use hearing aids tend to have a distinctive speech quality. Their speech often sounds breathy, labored, staccato, and arrhythmic. Errors in suprasegmental patterns contribute to this aberrant speech quality. These include errors in stress, speaking rate, coarticulation, breath control, pitch, and intensity.

STRESS

Many children place equal stress on all syllables or stress words inappropriately. For instance, the word *baby* may be produced with the stress on the second syllable instead of the first, as in "bah-BEE." Research suggests that talkers with significant hearing loss may be able to produce the articulatory maneuvers necessary for producing appropriate stress, for example, greater jaw and lip displacement for stressed syllables and less displacement for unstressed syllables. As such, the absence of auditory feedback may not limit children's potential to produce stress appropriately, but other factors such as unfamiliarity with stress patterns may come into play (Robb & Pang-Ching, 1992; Tye-Murray & Folkins, 1990).

SPEAKING RATE

Typically, children with severe and profound losses speak very slowly, pausing often, both within words and between words. They may insert extraneous sounds and prolong words. Voelker (1938) found that children with profound hearing loss spoke 70 words per minute as compared to 164 words per minute spoken by children with normal hearing.

COARTICULATION

Many children do not coarticulate sounds in the same way as normally hearing talkers. For instance, a child might say the word *basket* as "ba-a-sa-ka-a-ta." In this production, the child has articulated each sound as if it were an isolated unit.

Normally hearing talkers tend to begin preparing for an upcoming vowel position during a preceding consonant position, such that the jaw is in a higher position during the /p/ that precedes the /i/ in the word *peep,* and is in a lower position during the /p/ that precedes the /a/ in the word *pop.* Talkers with profound hearing loss tend not to demonstrate this coarticulatory effect (Tye-Murray, Zimmermann, & Folkins, 1987). Acoustic studies also support the lack of coarticulation (Monsen, 1976; Rothman, 1976). For example, the acoustic characteristics associated with consonant-vowel transition segments of monosyllables tend to be similar, regardless of phonetic context.

BREATH CONTROL

Most hard-of-hearing and deaf children produce relatively few syllables per breath, as they often manage their airflow inefficiently. In fact, often the first objective in a speech therapy curriculum is to establish better breath control in the young deaf talker.

Adult talkers who have profound and prelingual hearing loss demonstrate normal respiratory and aerodynamic behaviors for nonspeech tasks and aberrant behaviors for speech (Forner & Hixon, 1977; Itoh, Horii, Daniloff, & Binnie, 1982). Poor breathing behavior correlates highly with poor speech intelligibility.

Deaf talkers often inefficiently manage the speech airstream, as characterized by higher air volume expenditure during connected speech (Forner & Hixon, 1977; Metz, Whitehead, & Whitehead, 1984). For example, they demonstrate higher air consumption and shorter durations for sustained vowels and higher airflow rates than normally hearing talkers. This practice means they let out more breath when speaking a syllable than do normally hearing talkers. Unstable airflow also occurs. McGarr and Lofqvist (1982) suggested that air wastage may occur because deaf talkers fail to establish biomechanical resistance either with the larynx or other supralaryngeal articulators.

VOICE QUALITY

Children's voice quality may be unpleasant. Their pitch may sound excessively high or variable. Some children speak with a monotone. Pitch breaks, with pitch abruptly changing from high to low, are common.

INTENSITY

Children may speak too softly or too loudly, and often their intensity may fluctuate inappropriately. It is not surprising that children often cannot adjust their speaking intensity as a function of context. That is, they may not raise intensity when talking in a noisy gymnasium nor lower it when speaking in a quiet library.

▄▄▄ LANGUAGE

In light of the many segmental and suprasegmental errors, it is not surprising that many children with severe hearing impairments have poor intelligibility When these speech problems coexist with language problems, communication becomes difficult indeed. In this section, we focus specifically on the kinds of language problems many children with significant loss manifest.

Regardless of which communication mode they use most frequently, be it simultaneous communication, aural/oral, ASL, or Cued Speech, most children who are profoundly deaf and who use hearing aids do not learn the English language well. One way to appreciate how hearing impairment affects language development is to compare normally hearing and hard-of-hearing groups. Eight-year-old normally hearing children have a better knowledge of grammar than do adults with profound hearing loss. Moreover, most adults with significant hearing loss never acquire a vocabulary better than that of a normally hearing fourth grader (Bamford & Saunders, 1985).

We often categorize language difficulties as either problems of form (syntax and morphology), content (semantics and vocabulary), or pragmatics (use).

Form

The list comprising problems of *form* is extensive (see Seyfried & Kricos, 1996). Children with hearing loss may overuse nouns and verbs and rarely use adverbs, prepositions, or pronouns. They may omit function words. Most of their sentences have a simple subject-verb-object structure, and their sentences have few words compared to those produced by normally hearing children. Compound or complex sentences are rare, as are morphemes that mark plurality or past tense. In telling a story about her cat, one child said, "Socks jump. Cup fall over. Mess big. Mom mad about Socks." In this narrative, the child omitted functions words such as *was* and tense markers such as *ed*. Her syntactic structures were simple. Although you might follow her story, you probably will think that her sentences sound telegraphic.

Form: proper use of the elements of language, such as nouns and verbs, prepositions, and so on.

Sometimes children order their words incorrectly. A child may say, "Saw cat big," meaning she saw a big cat.

Not only do they rarely speak compound or complex sentences, children with significant hearing loss usually cannot interpret them when they speechread or read. For example, you might say to a child, "The cat was chased by the dog." The child may interpret this sentence as though it were in the active tense. Thus the meaning becomes: *The cat chased the dog.*

You might speak a nominal sentence to a child, such as, "The ending of the school year saddened the teacher." The child might interpret it in an objective sense and derive this meaning: *The school year saddened the teacher.*

Children with significant hearing loss sometimes show similar developmental trends as normally hearing children, albeit delayed. Deaf children between the ages of 5 and 7 years often acquire syntactic structures in the same order as normally hearing children, but at a much slower rate. However, children who show a great degree of language delay are at higher risk of following deviant patterns of development (Levitt, McGarr, & Geffner, 1987). That is, they are likely to follow developmental patterns that are different than those of normally hearing children.

Content: extent of vocabulary and use of words.

Content

Perhaps one of the most pervasive language problems among children with significant hearing loss is a restricted vocabulary. These children often learn only common everyday words. They may have gaps in their vocabularies, wherein they do not know words relating to an entire concept, such as outer space. Hence, words such as *planet, Martian, star, spacemen,* and *rocket* may be unfamiliar. They often use words in limited ways. For instance, a child may use a word such as *happy* as a predicate (e.g., *The boy is happy*) but not as a modifier (e.g., *The happy boy is here*). Many children cannot identify synonyms and antonyms or understand idioms such as *She was mad as a hornet.* Similarly, they frequently have difficulty handling words with multiple meanings. For example, children may understand the word *stand,* when you say, "Please *stand* by the piano." But when you ask them to, "Please move the music *stand,*" they may shrug their shoulders and say, "Huh?" In this example, the meaning of the verb form of *stand* is clear, but not the noun form.

In general, children who have significant hearing loss will learn words that are concrete more readily than they will learn words that are abstract. They will quickly associate meanings to words like, *bird, chair, sit, telephone,* and *ball.* But words that you cannot pair up with a physical object or an overtly observable behavior will be more difficult to learn. Words such as *rephrase, sentimental, admirable,* and *wise* will be much harder to absorb.

Longitudinal studies of the vocabulary of young children who are deaf reveal delays when compared to those of normally hearing children. For instance, White and White (1987) studied 46 prelingually deafened infants over a 3-year period. The infants ranged in age between 8 and 30 months at the time of entry into the study. By the third year, children had attained a receptive and expressive vocabulary that matched those of normally hearing children only 1 year of age.

Pragmatics: the study of how language is used.

Pragmatics

Children with a hearing impairment sometimes use questions inappropriately. For instance, one child's first question to a new acquaintance was, "How much money does your father make?"

A child may not know how to initiate or maintain a conversation or know how to repair breakdowns in communication. In some circumstances, the child may nod and bluff, pretending to understand.

A child also may not know many of the social graces of conversation. For example, he or she may not know how to take turns while conversing, how to acknowledge that the message has been heard, and how to change the topic of conversation. Overall, the child probably will not use language functionally as well as his normally hearing peers. In the following conversation, a child with hearing loss introduced a topic abruptly and did not respond to the adult's request for clarification:

Adult:	"Do you want to come with me?"
Child:	"Car fell off table, boom!"
Adult:	"What did you say?"
Child:	"Mine."

These inappropriate responses may relate both to the child's hearing loss (he may not have recognized the adult's utterances) and his unfamiliarity with conversational rules.

In general, there at least three reasons why some children do not learn conversational pragmatics well. These are:

- **First, they do not receive extensive practice in using language.** Their unfamiliarity with many language structures and reduced vocabulary limit their ability to converse. Moreover, if they do not use an aural/oral communication mode, they have fewer conversational partners to interact with because few normally hearing persons know manually coded English or ASL.
- **Second, they cannot overhear their parents or other people talking.** Thus, they do not receive the everyday, incidental models of how to use language.
- **Third, they do not receive the same formal instruction as normally hearing children.** For instance, a parent may carefully explain the rules of politeness to a child with normal hearing (do not interrupt, say "thank you"; let someone else say something). The parent may not explain the rules to her child with a hearing loss, either because of

A child using **manually coded English** or ASL may not receive the same language experiences as a normally hearing child, as few people in the child's environment will be familiar with these means of communication.

the child's limited language or because of the parent's limited skill in using *manually coded English* or ASL.

LITERACY

Literacy is an issue closely related to language development. Literacy is indexed by performance on reading and writing measures. Given many children's difficulties using English language, it is not surprising that many also have difficulty learning to read and comprehend and to compose written text.

Reading

Children who are deaf and hard of hearing and who use hearing aids often show delays or differences when compared to children who have normal hearing. The average reading and writing levels of deaf high school students are at a third or fourth grade level (Allen, 1986). This level is barely adequate to allow them to read a newspaper. Rarely does a deaf or hard-of-hearing student exceed a 7.5 grade reading level (Trybus & Krachmer, 1977). Reading difficulties are a resilient problem: There has been little improvement in the average reading performance of hard-of-hearing children relative to their normally hearing peers over the past 80 years.

There are at least two major reasons for reading deficits and several other contributing factors. First, reading problems no doubt stem largely from an inadequate language system. Deficits in vocabulary and unfamiliarity with groups of related words (as in the planets and space-related terms) and unfamiliarity with complex syntactic structures interfere with deaf children's ability to understand printed text.

In addition to having inadequate language, which precludes them from mapping language they already know to the printed word, children who have profound hearing loss do not develop an auditory basis for mapping sound to print (Golding-Meadow & Mayberry, 2001). This situation is a second major reason why these children experience reading difficulties. Typically, when children crack the code of deciphering the written word, they grasp the principles of associating sound to words. Access to a phonological code allows them to "sound out words" for sound-print mapping. Many children who have never heard sound, or who have had access to degraded speech signals, do not develop the phonological awareness of their normal-hearing counterparts.

Other factors that compound the reading task include deficits in experience and world knowledge and, perhaps, deficits in children's abilities to take on another's (i.e., the author's) point of view. For example, if a child has never overheard a news report on television, he or she may have difficulty reading articles related to current events. If a child has difficulty viewing the world from another's perspective, he or she may not be able to digest fictional stories and narratives.

In addition, their restricted ability to engage in conversation may affect their reading performance. For example, skills related to the conversational-based form of language may include a child's ability to carry on a meaningful dialog with an adult or another child. These skills may facilitate the comprehension of printed dialog and narratives.

Finally, additional factors that may affect reading performance include the type of instruction a child has received. For instance, children who have been educated with a whole-word (or look-say) type of instruction may have different reading skills than children who have been educated with a phonetic-based system (letter analysis). The design of the curriculum, the expertise of the teacher(s), and the involvement of the family may also interact with reading performance.

Writing

Deaf children often lag behind their normally hearing peers in writing skills. Their writing samples often contain syntactic errors, such as omission of articles, inappropriate use of pronouns, and omission of bound morphemes (e.g., 's and -ed). Deaf writers tend to use a preponderance of subject-verb-object sentences, and rarely construct complex syntactic structures. Rarely do deaf writers use synonyms, antonyms, metaphors, or cohesive forms of substitution or ellipsis. They may introduce a variety of topics without elaborating on them (Yoshinaga-Itano, Snyder, & Mayberry, 1996).

Some children have difficulty writing narratives, in which there is a clear beginning, middle, and end to their story. Sometimes, they have difficulty focusing on the important parameters of a story. For example, a third-grade boy, when asked to write a story about a girl holding a scorched dress and an iron, wrote the following sample:

Girl have red sweater. Hair yellow. Girl work hard!

In this example, the child appears to have focused on surface details of the picture rather than the underlying story. The child also used inappropriate verb tense (e.g., *have* instead of *has*) and omitted function words. Most children progress beyond this level of expression and often demonstrate gains in their narrative skills (including semantic linkages by use of surface structure and topic and event, connectors, logical sequence, temporal sequencing, physical causality, and psychological causality) between the ages of 7 and 18 years of age, although they rarely achieve the competency of normally hearing age-matched peers (Yoshinaga-Itano & Downey, 1996).

■ CHILDREN WHO USE COCHLEAR IMPLANTS

In the foregoing discussion, we were concerned with children who use hearing aids. Children who have a significant hearing loss but who use cochlear implants represent a relatively new group of children, a group that performs more similarly to children who have better hearing than to children who have a profound hearing loss. In this section, we consider the speech, language, and literacy of young cochlear-implant users.

Implantation of children with multichannel cochlear implants was approved by the FDA in 1990. We are now in a time period when longitudinal information about their performance is available, and we can make statements about their long-term performance.

Speech

Children who use cochlear implants typically tend to speak better than children who use hearing aids, and you may recognize considerably more than 20% of their words. For example, in a study of one hundred eighty-one 8- and 9-year-old children who had used cochlear implants since before the age of 5 years, Tobey et al. (2003) found that listeners understood on average more than 60% of the children's words. More than half of the children produced words that were 80% intelligible or better.

VOWEL PRODUCTION

There is evidence that children with prolonged cochlear-implant experience achieve better vowel production than children who use hearing aids and who have similar hearing losses. Figure 16-2 shows the vowel production of 36 children who have prelingual deafness and use cochlear implants (Tye-Murray, Tomblin & Spencer, 1997). These data were collected between 1990 and 1997 as part of the University of Iowa Hospitals' Cochlear Implant Program. The children were 5 years, 6 months of age on average at the time of implantation, with a range of 2 years to 11 years. The children used simultaneous communication and attended public school in their local communities. To have been included in the study, they had to have worn their cochlear implants for at

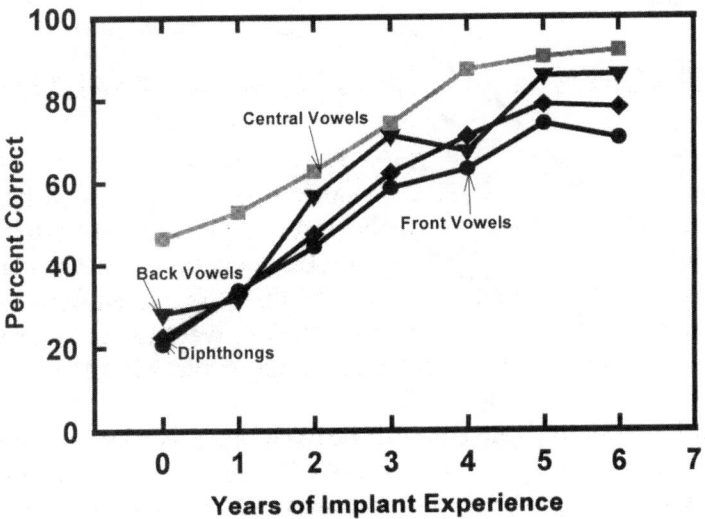

FIGURE 16-2. Vowel production over time for 36 young cochlear-implant users.

least 5 years. They were tested one time before implantation and then every year thereafter. Data were obtained during a story-retell task, a task described in more detail later in the chapter.

Percent correct results are plotted as a function of place of articulation and averaged across children. Figure 16-2 suggests that, after 5 or 6 years of implant use, children produce vowels with about 80% accuracy, on average. This is considerably better than the 44% accuracy levels reported by Markides (1970) for young hearing-aid users.

CONSONANT PRODUCTION

Receipt of a cochlear implant also enhances a child's ability to produce consonants. Figures 16-3 and 16-4 portray a description of the 36 children's consonant production, as a function of both place and manner of production.

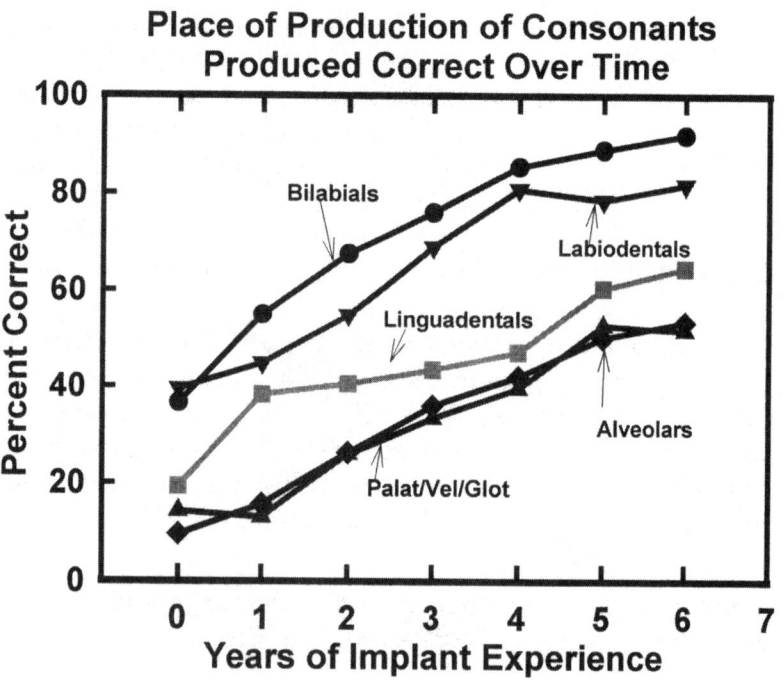

FIGURE 16-3. Consonant production over time as a function of place of articulation from 36 young cochlear-implant users (Palat = palatals, Vel = velars, Glot = glottals).

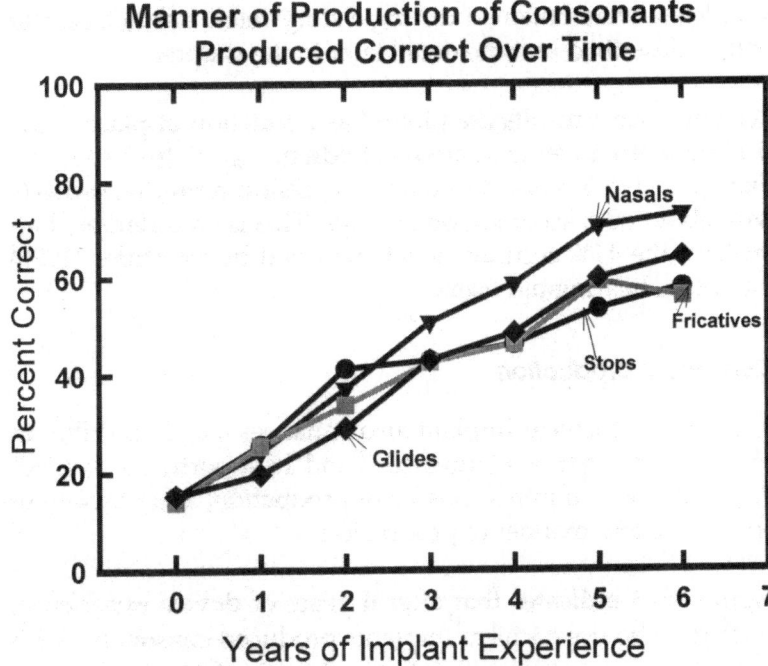

FIGURE 16-4. Consonant production over time as a function of manner of articulation from 36 young cochlear-implant users.

Figure 16-3 indicates that after 6 years of device experience, children who use cochlear implants produced consonants with about 70% accuracy, which is better than the 28% accuracy level reported by Markides (1970) for hearing-aid users. Interestingly, just like children who have similar hearing losses but who use hearing aids, the young cochlear-implant users tended to produce the more visible bilabial consonants correctly more often than the less visible palatals, velars, and glottals. The relatively good overall performance and the exceptionally good production of more visible sounds suggest young cochlear-implant users rely both on auditory and visual signals for acquiring consonant sounds.

Figure 16-4 presents manner of consonant production over time. The young cochlear-implant users showed about the same amount of improvement for all manner classes. Perhaps the most interesting finding shown in this figure relates to the production of fricatives. By the sixth year of cochlear-implant use, children produced such sounds as /s/ and /z/ with almost 60% accuracy.

Many children with similar losses who use hearing aids never acquire these sounds (Smith, 1975).

RELATIONSHIP BETWEEN HEARING ABILITIES AND SEGMENTAL SPEECH PRODUCTION IN COCHLEAR-IMPLANT USERS

In addition to completing a speech test, the children in the cochlear-implant study described here also completed the Word Intelligibility Picture Index (WIPI) (Ross & Lerman, 1971), which is a 6-choice monosyllabic word recognition task. This test was scored by percent phonemes correct.

Figure 16-5 illustrates the relationship between speech production (in a sentence-imitation task rather than a story-retell task) and performance on the WIPI. The data were collected after each child had accumulated 5 years of experience with their cochlear implants. There is a strong relationship between children's abilities to produce phonemes and their abilities to recognize them. A Pearson correlation, which tests how well one set of data predicts another, was $r = .88$, which is a remarkably strong correlation. No doubt many factors affect children's speech acquisition with a cochlear implant, including family commitment to the cochlear implant process and a child's intervention plan. However, the findings in Figure 16-5 suggest a direct correspondence exists between a child's ability to speak and a child's ability to recognize speech sounds.

SUPRASEGMENTAL SPEECH PRODUCTION

Children who use cochlear implants tend to produce fewer suprasegmental errors than children who have similar hearing losses but who use hearing aids (Tye-Murray, Spencer, & Woodworth, 1995). In fact, clinicians sometimes notice changes in the voice quality of children within the first year after they receive a cochlear implant, and these changes often precede changes in segmental speech production.

Language: Content and Form

Children who receive cochlear implants may have accelerated and enhanced language acquisition. Tomblin, Spencer, Flock,

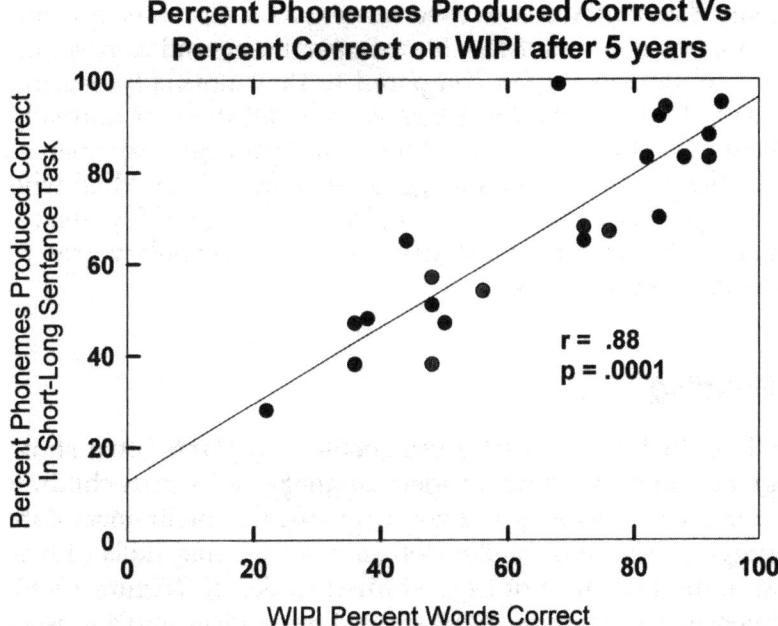

FIGURE 16-5. The relationship between children's speech production and speech recognition skills after 5 years of cochlear-implant experience.

Tyler, and Gantz (1999) looked at the syntax of a group of 29 young cochlear-implant users and a comparable group of 29 young hearing-aid users with a measure called the Index of Productive Syntax (IPSyn) (Scarborough, 1990). They determined the cochlear-implant users demonstrated greater rates of growth in English grammar over time than did the hearing-aid users. Other studies confirm the robust development of syntax. For instance, Geers, Nicholas, and Sedey (2003), in a study of one hundred eighty-one 8- and 9-year-old implant users, found that about half of the children demonstrated English syntax at a level comparable to their peers who have normal hearing. It also appears that postimplant language acquisition rate parallels that of normal development (Svirsky, Chute, Green, Bollard, & Miyamoto, 2002).

Vocabulary acquisition is also enhanced by the use of a cochlear implant. Waltzman et al. (1997), who obtained language data from 38 children who received their cochlear implants before the age of 5 years, reported they demonstrated 4 years of vocabulary growth during a 3-year period.

Reading

Given that children who use cochlear implants often show greater improvements in their language skills than children who use hearing aids, it is not surprising that data suggest they go on to develop superior reading skills (this issue has not been studied in depth) (Figure 16-6). Spencer, Tomblin & Gantz (1997) studied 34 cochlear-implant users who have prelingual deafness. At the time they were tested, they had 62 months of implant experience, with a range of 24 to 108 months. They ranged in grade level from kindergarten to senior high school. On average, they were at the fourth grade level. The investigators also tested a comparable group of hearing-aid users. Children completed the Woodcock Reading Mastery Test, which assesses children's ability to comprehend short two- to three-sentence paragraphs. The investigators found that 50% of the children who used cochlear implants were reading at grade level. They achieved higher reading levels than the hearing-aid users and exhibited faster performance growth rates over time.

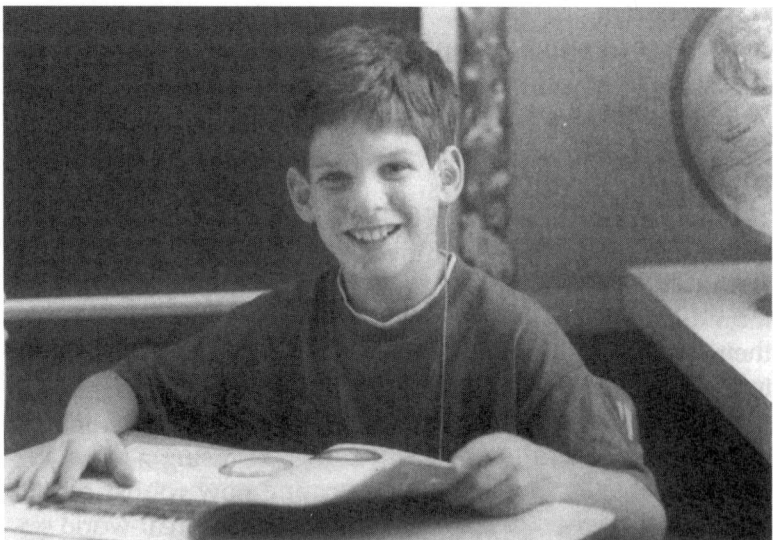

FIGURE 16-6. Use of a cochlear implant appears to lead to better reading skills than use of conventional amplification. This result is probably because enhanced hearing capacity allows children to acquire English language more readily, which in turn has a salutary effect on literacy. (Photograph by Patti Gabriel, courtesy of the Central Institute for the Deaf)

■ SPEECH AND LANGUAGE EVALUATION: GENERAL PRINCIPLES

Now that we have described speech, language, and literacy development, let us turn our attention to the assessment of speech and language performance. First we consider general principles, then more specific issues.

There are several general principles to remember when testing the speech and language of children who have hearing loss. The principles pertain to the following topics:

- Task type
- Mode of communication
- Rapport
- Test procedures
- Test norms

Task Type

The first principle is that children often use speech and language differently in one setting than in another, and they perform differently on varying tasks. For example, children are more likely to produce a sound correctly when they imitate their speech-language pathologist than when they tell a story to their classmates. For this reason, it is wise to construct a profile of the child's speech and language proficiency from numerous formal and informal measures. By using a variety of speech tasks, a clinician can determine how robust certain skills are and whether they have generalized to real-world settings. This information can guide the development of therapy objectives and can be used to evaluate progress.

Mode of Communication

The second principle to remember when evaluating speech and language is that the evaluation should be performed with a child's preferred mode of communication (Figure 16-7). For example, the child may use *simultaneous communication.* If the speech-language pathologist does not know the child's sign system, then a sign language interpreter should be secured. The child must understand the tasks and the test items to provide a true reflection of speech and language skills.

Simultaneous communication: an educational approach used with children with severe and profound hearing loss that integrates aural/oral communication and manual communication.

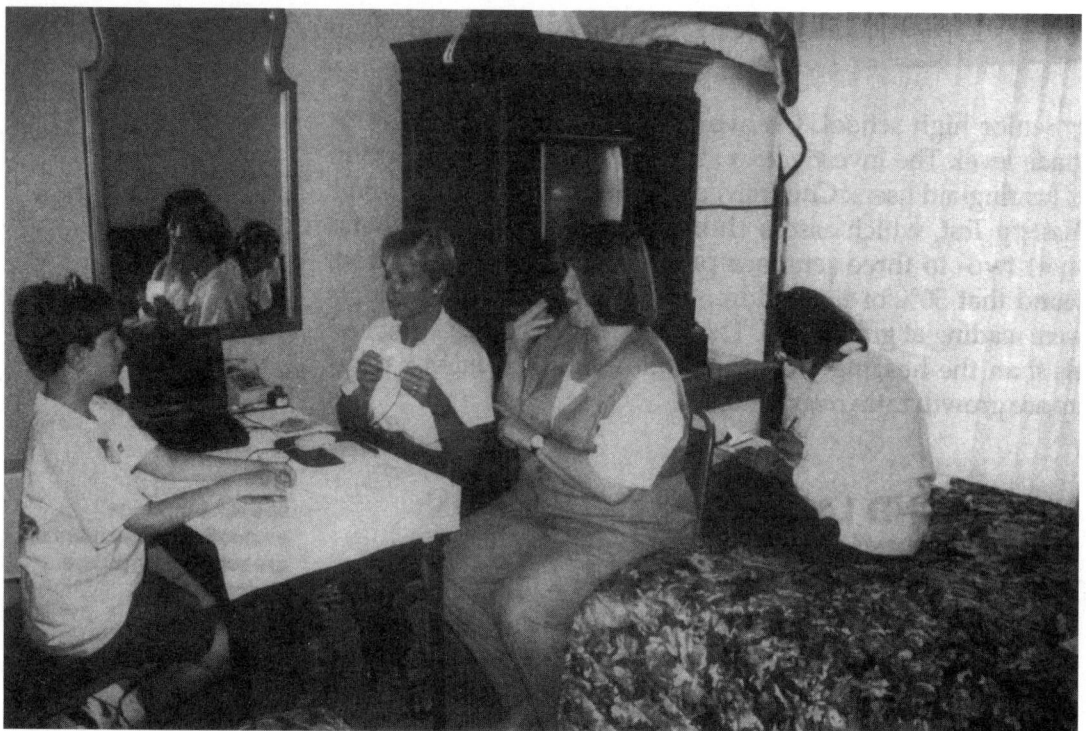

FIGURE 16-7. A speech and language evaluation usually is performed with a child's preferred mode of communication (in this picture, simultaneous communication). Here, an interpreter cues the messages of a speech-language pathologist, who does not know Cued Speech. (Photograph by Kim Readmond, courtesy of the Central Institute for the Deaf)

Rapport

The third principle is that, before formally evaluating a child, a rapport must be established between tester and child. You may find that many children with hearing losses are shy about using their voices, especially among strangers. If children do not feel comfortable in the tester's presence, they will not provide speech or language samples that represent their true skills. In fact, they may not provide samples at all.

Test Procedures

Fourth, it is important to select specific test procedures appropriate for the child's age and language. For example, if an articulation test has picture cards, the child must have the vocabulary necessary to name the pictures.

Test Norms

Finally, the speech-language pathologist should try to use at least some tests that have been developed for children with hearing loss (although this may not always be possible, because few tests are available). For children who use simultaneous communication, you will find that many tests have not been designed to be administered with sign. Moreover, norms of many tests reflect the performance of normally hearing children and not children with hearing loss.

ASSESSING SPEECH SKILLS: INTELLIGIBILITY, SEGMENTALS, AND SUPRASEGMENTALS

Now that we have considered general principles for a speech-language evaluation, let us review procedures for assessing speech. The evaluation may include an overall assessment of intelligibility. It also may include assessment of segmentals and suprasegmentals.

Speech Intelligibility

To assess speech intelligibility, a speech sample first must be collected and then evaluated. To obtain a speech sample, the speech-language pathologist might ask a child to perform any or all of the following tasks:

- **Imitate a series of isolated words or sentences.** For example, a speech-language pathologist might say, "The boy saw the cat," and the child then repeats the sentence. This procedure typically elicits a child's best performance (Figure 16-8).
- **Create a citation speech sample.** A speech-language pathologist might instruct a child, "Tell me the name of the picture," or, "Tell me what is happening here." The child then speaks the name or describes what is occurring in the picture. This task is highly structured like an imitated-sentence task, but the child does not receive a speech or vocabulary model to imitate.

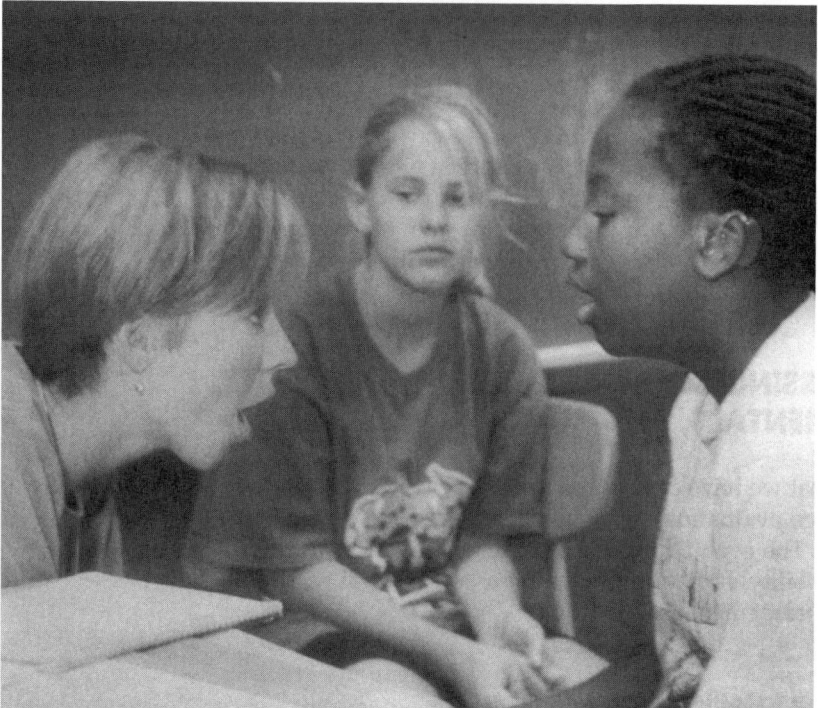

FIGURE 16-8. One way to collect a speech sample from a child is to use an imitation task. The clinician speaks an utterance and the child imitates it. (Photograph by Marcus Kosa, courtesy of the Central Institute for the Deaf)

- **Retell a story.** A speech-language pathologist may show the pictures in Figure 16-9 to a child one at a time and tell a corresponding story, picture by picture. The child then retells the story. This procedure constrains the language that children use in the sample, but still allows for the evaluation of spontaneous speech and language production.
- **Speak spontaneously, using continuous speech.** A speech-language pathologist might observe informally a child in therapy, in the classroom, or on the playground while he or she speaks to other children. In the therapy session, they may engage in casual conversation, and the speech-language pathologist pays close attention to the child's articulation proficiency and language structures.

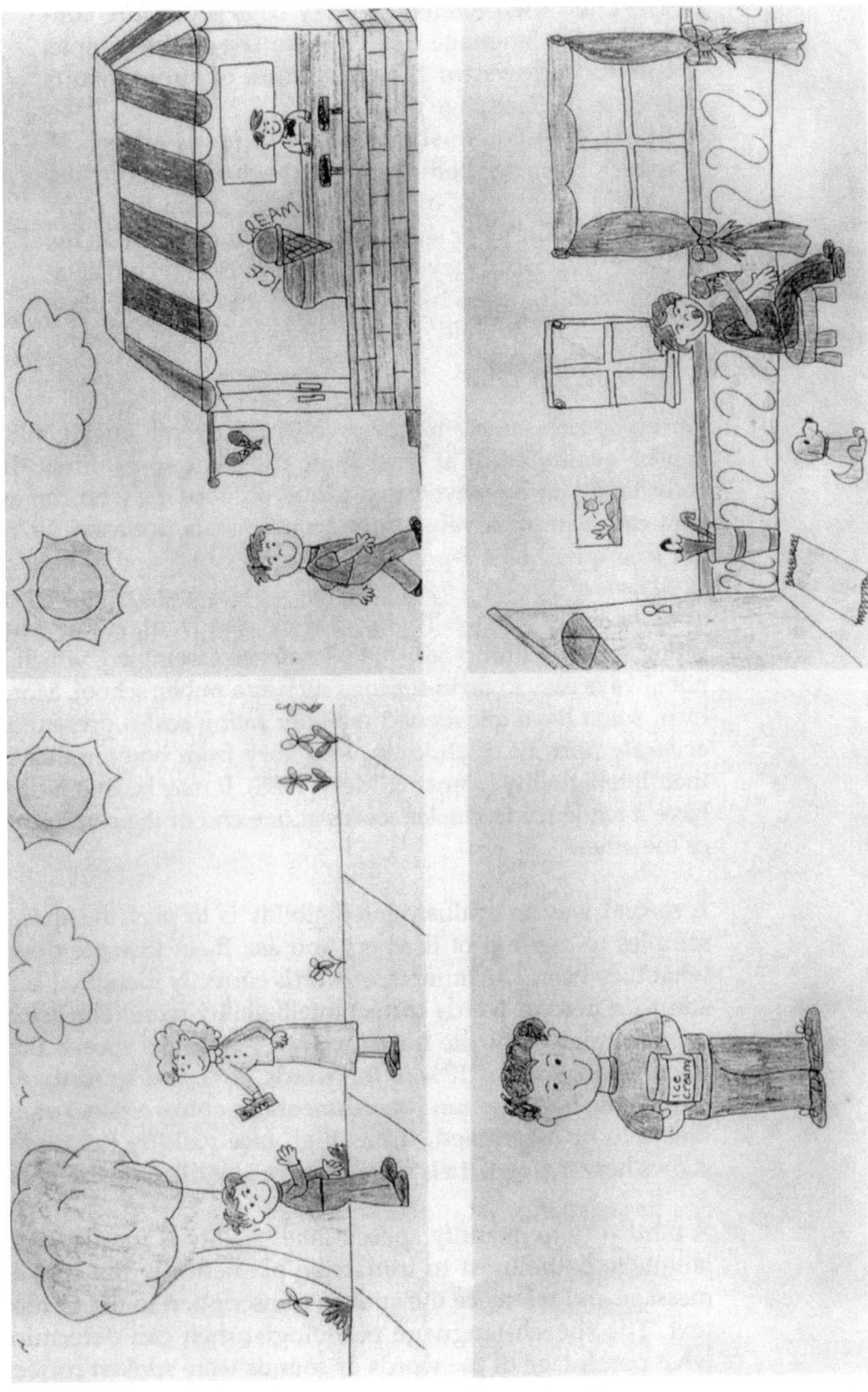

FIGURE 16-9. Picture cards that might be used to elicit a story-retell speech and language sample. A clinician first tells a story, using a prepared text that corresponds to each picture in the picture series (here, organized clockwise, beginning with the top left-hand corner). Then the child tells the story back.

Once a speech sample has been collected, overall intelligibility can be evaluated in at least three different ways. First, the recordings can be played to a group of listeners who can assign each sample a value from a rating scale (Johnson, 1975). For example, 1 on a 5-point scale might correspond to *I understood none of the child's message,* and 5 correspond to *I understood all of the child's message.* There are some disadvantages to using rating scales. A group of listeners must be assembled, which is not always easy to do in settings such as a public school. Moreover, some have questioned whether rating scales present an accurate portrait of children who vary from one another in their intelligibility (Samar & Metz, 1988). It may be that judges have a tendency to cluster scores at one end of the continuum or the other.

A second way to evaluate intelligibility is to play the speech samples to a group of listeners, and ask them to write down what they hear. The number of words correctly identified constitutes a percent words correct intelligibility score. The listeners also might estimate how much of the child's speech they understood, such as 10% of the words, 20%, and so forth. Although the transcription procedure also requires a panel of listeners to be assembled, it has high face validity because it shows how many of their words can be identified by listeners.

A third way to quantify speech intelligibility is for a speech-language pathologist to transcribe phonetically the spoken message and reference the spoken transcription to the printed text. The speech-language pathologist then can determine what percentage of the words or sounds were spoken correctly. This way is probably the most commonly used procedure for assessing intelligibility in clinical and educational settings.

Measures of speech intelligibility vary as a function of several different variables (Figure 16-10). For instance:

- A child will be more intelligible when reading a paragraph than speaking a list of unrelated sentences.
- Listeners will understand more of a child's speech if they have heard the speech of other children with hearing loss before, than if they are naive listeners.
- Listeners will recognize more speech if they can hear and see children rather than only hear them.

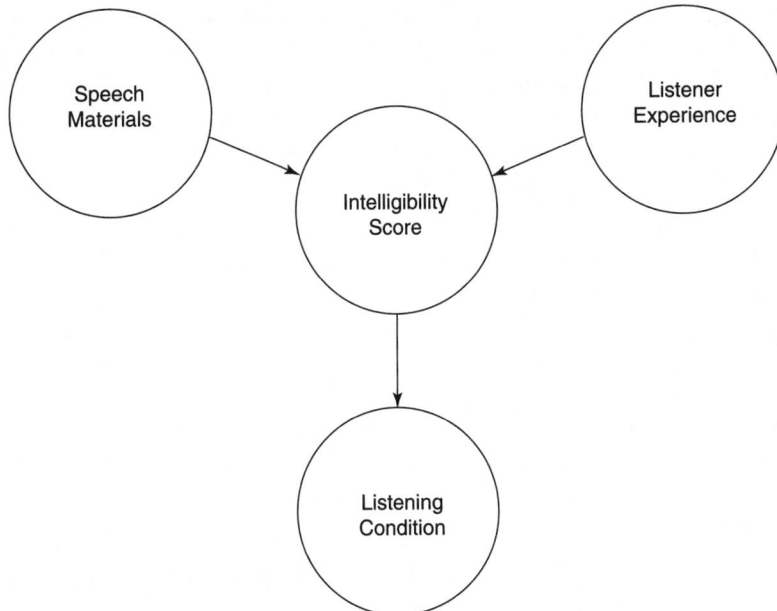

FIGURE 16-10. Factors that may affect a speech intelligibility score.

When recording intelligibility scores it is wise to comment on these variables, especially if the child's progress is to be monitored over time. If this is not done, the child's intelligibility score might improve because of a change in an extraneous variable. This may be misinterpreted as an improvement in the child's speaking proficiency.

Segmentals

Segmental speech testing determines which sounds children can articulate and which sounds they cannot. Variables to consider when selecting test procedures include context, methodology, and whether to use conventional tests of articulation.

Segmental speech production can be evaluated with a variety of contexts, including nonsense syllables, isolated words, sentences, and spontaneous speech. It is common to evaluate how well children produce various features of articulation, such as place and manner.

Methodologically, a child may imitate the speech-language pathologist or might produce the sounds by naming picture cards or reading printed words aloud. The child also may speak spontaneously, and then the speech-language pathologist can determine what sounds were produced in a set number of words (say, the first 200 words spoken by the child).

Often, conventional articulation tests are used to assess segmental speech skills, such as the Goldman-Fristoe Test of Articulation (Goldman & Fristoe, 1969) and the Test of Minimal Articulation Competence (T-MAC) (Secord, 1981). Some speech-language pathologists modify the tests by eliminating test words that are not in the child's vocabulary. If modifications are made, they should be recorded alongside the child's scores. Tests designed specifically for children with hearing loss include the Phonologic Level Speech Evaluation (Ling, 1976), the CID Phonetic Inventory (Moog, 1988), and the Speech Intelligibility Evaluation (SPINE) (Monsen, 1981).

Suprasegmentals

Suprasegmental speech skills can be evaluated by rating children's spontaneous speech as described by Subtelny, Orlando, and Whitehead (1981) or by asking them to perform specific speech tasks. For instance, a speech-language pathologist might determine whether a child can sustain the vowel /a/ for 5 seconds (to assess breath management) or whether the child can speak two-syllable phrases with correct stress and pitch variation (to assess his or her ability to imitate stress patterns) (Levitt, 1987).

■ ASSESSING LANGUAGE SKILLS

Table 16-1 presents examples of language tests sometimes used with children who are hearing impaired. They are organized according to whether they primarily assess form, content, or pragmatics.

Assessment procedures generally can be classified as checklists (e.g., Moog & Geers, 1975), tests (e.g., Quigley, Monranelli, & Wilbur, 1976) or language sample analyses (e.g., Kretschmer & Kretschmer, 1978). In compiling a checklist, a speech-language

Table 16-1. Language tests that are sometimes used to test children who have hearing loss. Assessment instruments designed specifically for hard-of-hearing children and teenagers are denoted with an asterisk (*).

Form

Rhode Island Test of Language Structure (RITLS) (Engen & Engen, 1983)*

Grammatical Analysis of Elicited Language (GAEL) (Moog & Geers, 1979)*

Grammatical Analysis of Elicited Language, pre-sentence level (GAEL-p) (Moog, Kozak, & Geers, 1983)*

Test of Syntactic Ability (TSA) (Quigley, Monranelli, & Wilbur, 1976)*

Written Language Syntax Test (WLST) (Berry, 1981)

Berko Morphology Test (Berko, 1984)

Test for Auditory Comprehension of Language (TACL) (Carrow, 1973)

Developmental Sentence Analysis (DSA) (Lee, 1974)

Index of Productive Syntax (IPSyn) (Scarborough, 1990)

Content

Semantic Content Analysis (Kretschmer & Kretschmer, 1978)

Peabody Picture Vocabulary Test-Revised (PPVT-R) (Dunn & Dunn, 1981)

Reynell Developmental Language Scales (Reynell, 1977)

Function

Pragmatic Content Analysis (Kretschmer & Kretschmer, 1978)

Performative Content Analysis (Hasenstab & Tobey, 1991)

---

pathologist checks whether a particular behavior is present. For example, the speech-language pathologist might check *yes* or *no* for the statement, *The child recognizes the meaning of subject-verb-object sentences.*

Many tests contain items that assess formally a child's ability to use language structures. For example, if negation is assessed, the child might be asked to change the sentence, *He will go* to *He will not go.*

Language sample analyses usually are performed on samples of both the child's receptive and expressive language. A clinician might describe the semantic classes children use and recognize, their complex sentence productions, and their communication proficiency.

ASSESSING READING SKILLS

Although few assessment tools have been designed specifically for children who have hearing loss (The Test of Early Reading Ability-Deaf or Hard of Hearing [TERA-D/HH] is an exception), instruments developed for children with normal hearing are often utilized to evaluate a child's reading readiness and reading skills. The disadvantages of using assessment instruments designed for children with normal hearing include (1) the items of the test may be too difficult for the children with hearing loss to complete and (2) it is difficult to assess how well a child is doing compared to the peer group comprised of children with hearing loss. On the other hand, if a child is in a mainstream or inclusion classroom, test scores may indicate how well he or she may be expected to perform in that setting and how well the child performs with respect to classmates who have normal hearing. Table 16-2 presents a sample of instruments used for assessing reading, as well as the grades (for normal hearing children) appropriate for testing and the areas of skill evaluated. These areas of skill include reading and language comprehension, phonology, syntax and semantics, decoding, phoneme awareness, alphabetic principles, letter knowledge, and concepts about print.

For children who are on the cusp of reading readiness, sometimes a teacher completes a simple checklist to assess preliteracy performance. For example, the teacher might indicate whether a child *never, sometimes,* or *always* demonstrates some of the following developmental benchmarks (adapted from Bodrova, Leong, Paynter, & Semenov, 2000):

- Holds a book upright and turns the pages of the book from front to back
- Pretends to read familiar books; joins in with predictable phrases (e.g., "I will huff and puff and blow your house down.")
- Reads environmental print (such as a McDonald's sign or a stop sign)
- Identifies letters in his or her name
- Tells a story when stimulated with a sequence of pictures
- Pretends or creates using language
- Listens responsively to narratives and books
- Tells stories

Table 16-2. A sample of assessments used to assess reading performance.

ASSESSMENT	GRADE	AREAS ASSESSED
Analytical Reading Inventory (6th Ed.) (Woods & Moe, 1999)	K, 1, 2, 3, and higher	Reading comprehension, language comprehension, decoding
Bader Reading and Language Inventory (3rd Ed.) (Bader, 1998)	Pre-K, K, 1, 2, 3, and higher	Reading comprehension, language comprehension, phonology, syntax, semantics, decoding, phoneme awareness, letter knowledge, concepts about print
Brigance Comprehensive Inventory of Basic Skills-Revised (CIBS-R) (Brigance, 1999)	Pre-K, K, 1, 2, 3, and higher	Reading comprehension, phonology, semantics, decoding, letter knowledge
Durrell Analysis of Reading Difficulty (3rd Ed.) (DAR) (Durrell & Catterson, 1980)	Pre-K, K, 1, 2, 3, and higher	Reading comprehension, language comprehension, semantics, decoding, phoneme awareness
GOALS: A Performance Based Measure of Achievement (Psychological Corp., 1994)	1, 2, 3, and higher	Reading comprehension, language comprehension
Gray Oral Reading Test-Diagnostic (GORT-D) (Bryant & Wiederholt, 1991)	K, 1, 2, 3, and higher	Reading comprehension, syntax, decoding
Kaufman Assessment Battery for Children (K-ABC) (Kaufman & Kaufman, 1983)	Pre-K, K, 1, 2, 3, and higher	Reading comprehension, semantics, decoding
Reading and Oral Language Assessment (ROLA) (Littcon Inc., 2000)	K, 1, 2, 3, and higher	Reading comprehension, language comprehension, decoding, lexical knowledge, phoneme awareness, letter knowledge, concepts about print
Signposts Early Literacy Battery and Pre-DRP Test (Touchstone Applied Science Associates, Inc., 2001)	K, 1, 2, and 3	Reading comprehension, language comprehension, syntax, semantics, decoding, phoneme awareness, letter knowledge
Test of Early Reading Ability-Deaf or Hard of Hearing (TERA-D/HH) (Reid, Hresko, Hammill, & Wiltshire, 1991)	Pre-K, K, 1, and 2	Letter knowledge, concepts about reading
Woodcock Diagnostic Reading Battery (WDRB) (Woodcock, 1997)	K, 1, 2, 3, and higher	Reading comprehension, semantics, decoding, letter knowledge
Woodcock-Johnson Psycho-Educational Battery (WJ-R) (Woodcock & Johnson, 1989)	K, 1, 2, 3, and higher	Reading comprehension, lexical knowledge

▪ SPEECH AND LANGUAGE THERAPY

Most children with significant hearing loss need abundant amounts of speech and language therapy. Speech and language skills often do not emerge spontaneously. Concerted attention over many years must be placed on developing skills if a child is to learn to speak and use English.

Still Holds True Today

In the early part of the 20th century, G. Sibley Haycock (1933) wrote a book about teaching speech to children who have significant hearing loss. This book had enormous influence in the time it was written, and it subsequently influenced the development of more modem curriculums (e.g., Ling, 1976). The goal of the program outlined in the book was to promote natural speech in deaf children. To this end, it was suggested that children be taught by such methods as will give to [their speech] the following characteristics:

- In general, the movements of the mechanisms involved must be correctly controlled and become, through practice and habit, more or less automatic. In particular, the breathing and the vocalization must be correct in method and controlled in action, and the consonants and the vowels must be easily and smoothly produced and correct as to sound, according to the locally accepted standard of pronunciation.
- The constituent phonetic elements composing words must be rendered with due regard to their relationship to one another.
- Words must be properly accented.
- Words in sentences must be given the measure of emphasis required by the meaning they are intended to convey.
- The speech must be duly phrased, and uttered with ease and fluency.
- The voice should express emotional quality.
- The rate of the speech must approximate to the normal.
- The speech must be duly phrased, and uttered with ease and fluency.
- The voice should express emotional quality.

- The rate of the speech must approximate to the normal.
- The sentences must be marked by a rise and fall of the voice, giving to the speech a certain amount of tunefulness. (p. 18)

These goals still are relevant to today's speech curricula.

Speech Therapy

Goals for a comprehensive speech-development program may include the following (Carney & Moeller, 1998, p. S62):

- Increase vocalizations that have appropriate timing characteristics and that require numerous vocal tract movements
- Expand phonetic and phonemic repertoires
- Establish link between audition and speech production
- Improve suprasegmental aspects of speech
- Increase speech intelligibility

Results from the speech evaluation are used to select therapy goals. The phonetic transcriptions of elicited and spontaneous speech may be used for phoneme and phonological error pattern analysis. Phonetic error analysis yields an inventory of sounds a child can produce, as well as a catalog of the child's deletions, substitutions, and distortions. Phonological error analysis reveals phonological process errors. These may include final consonant deletions, cluster reductions, and frontings. Therapy goals may focus on increasing a child's phonetic repertoire and on reducing phonological process errors. Auditory modeling is used extensively, sometimes in conjunction with a visual and tactile supplement.

Therapy curricula often differ according to the way speech is presented to the child and how feedback is provided. For instance, in an auditory approach, children may receive instructions and correction about their speech via the auditory modality primarily, although often, no attempt is made to limit children's use of nonauditory cues, such as natural facial cues. In a more visual approach, visual stimuli are presented purposefully to supplement the auditory signal. A visual program may entail the use of mirrors, Cued Speech, or graphic symbols that are paired with specific speech sounds or prosodic features.

Probably the most widely implemented speech therapy program based on an auditory approach was developed by Daniel Ling (1976). This program rests on the premise that there is a hierarchy of speech skills. The most effective and efficient way to learn how to talk is to learn skills in an appropriate sequence and to build on an existing skill to develop a new one. For instance, before a child can learn specific speech sounds, he or she must first learn to regulate voice level and pitch. A child should be able to speak homophenous syllable strings, such as *bee-bee-bee*, before being asked to speak heterogeneous strings, such as *bee-boo-bee-boo*.

Visual methods include the Northampton Charts, developed at Clark School for the Deaf in 1885 and updated in 1925. Sounds are associated with a letter, and the sounds are represented on charts, which are on display during the therapy session, and even in the classroom throughout the day. Visual methods also include the use of computer-based visual feedback systems, such as the IBM Speech Viewer (IBM, 1988). Computer-based visual aids may present a visual response to a child's production, indicating the "goodness" of production or overall accuracy. For instance, a child may sustain phonation into a microphone connected to the computer, and a balloon shown on the computer monitor is shown growing in size throughout the duration of phonation (Figure 16-11).

Language Therapy

Therapy goals in language development may include the following (Carney & Moeller, 1998):

- Increase communication between parent and child
- Promote an understanding of complex concepts and discourse units
- Enhance vocabulary growth
- Increase world knowledge
- Enhance self-expression

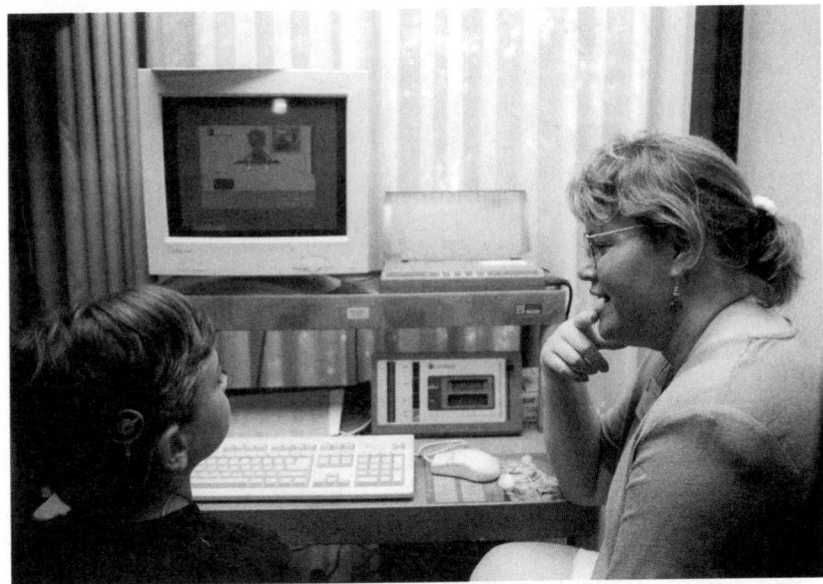

FIGURE 16-11. Computer-based visual aids are sometimes used during speech and language therapy *(Photograph by Kim Readmond, courtesy of the Central Institute for the Deaf)*

- Enhance growth in use of language syntax and pragmatics
- Develop narrative skills

A number of curricula have been developed for promoting language growth. Language curricula vary from highly structured to naturalistic. Most modern curricula advocate more naturalistic methods. Therapy goals often are based on information about the language development of normally hearing children, and goals are reinforced throughout the day, whether at school or at home (Figure 16-12).

Content, form, and pragmatics are addressed in the development of a language intervention plan. Special emphasis may be placed on vocabulary development if the child is younger, and children might be encouraged to use conjunctions, pronouns, and modals.

If a child is school age, concerted attention may be placed on the development of syntax and semantics. The speech-language pathologist may spend time observing the child in the classroom.

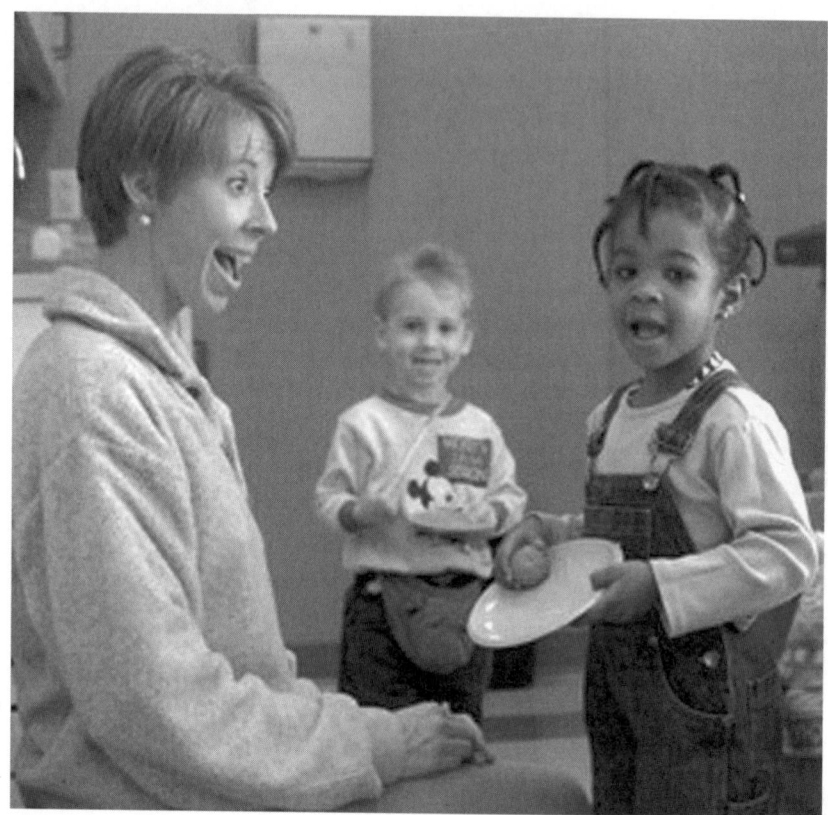

FIGURE 16-12. Naturalistic methods of language instruction include optimizing on everyday events (and structuring the environment so that events occur) to promote the growth of form, content, and pragmatics. In this encounter, a student is showing her teacher an apple on a plate. The teacher repeats the child's production of the word *apple* and expands on it by saying, "The apple is on the plate." Her goal is to fine-tune the child's understanding of the preposition, *on.* The teacher also expands the child's pragmatic skills by asking, "Please, may I have the apple?" [hence, demonstrating the proper use of the word, *please*], and when the preschooler gives it to her, the teacher responds by saying, "Thank you." [demonstrating the proper use of the word, *thank you*] *(Photograph by Kim Readmond, courtesy of the Central Institute for the Deaf)*

The speech-language pathologist then makes specific recommendations about how the classroom teacher might reinforce speech and language therapy goals in a naturalistic setting and incorporate goals into the academic curriculum. The classroom observation also may reveal specific language error patterns that the child is producing outside the therapy setting.

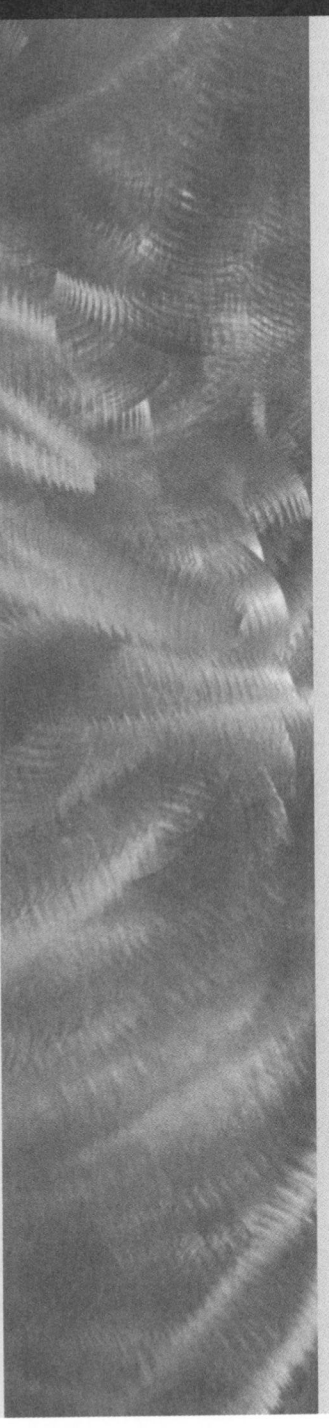

CASE STUDIES

In this section, writing samples are presented from a group of 10- and 11-year-old children. These children attend a private school for the deaf on a full-time basis. Their hearing losses range from severe-to-profound to profound.

The samples are characteristic of the writing skills demonstrated by a group of children of this age and with this degree of hearing loss, both in terms of variability in their skill level (e.g., although some wrote only a few sentences, others wrote complete paragraphs) and in the types of errors that they made. The class assignment was to describe the scene depicted in Figure 16-13. The children were shown this picture after their teacher read them a story about a girl and her purchase of a magic sled.

To summarize the story: A girl went to a store and bought a sled. She discovered that it was magic. Instead of walking up a snowy hill, the sled carried her upward.

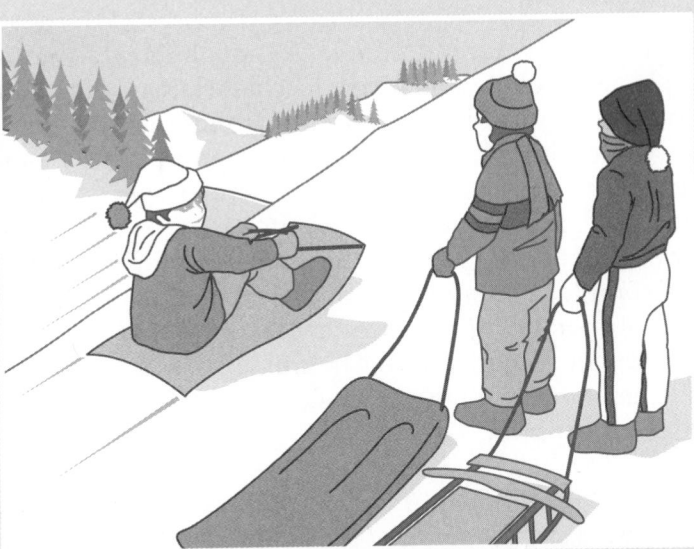

FIGURE 16-13. A picture like the one used to elicit the written language samples presented for the case studies of this chapter.

(continues)

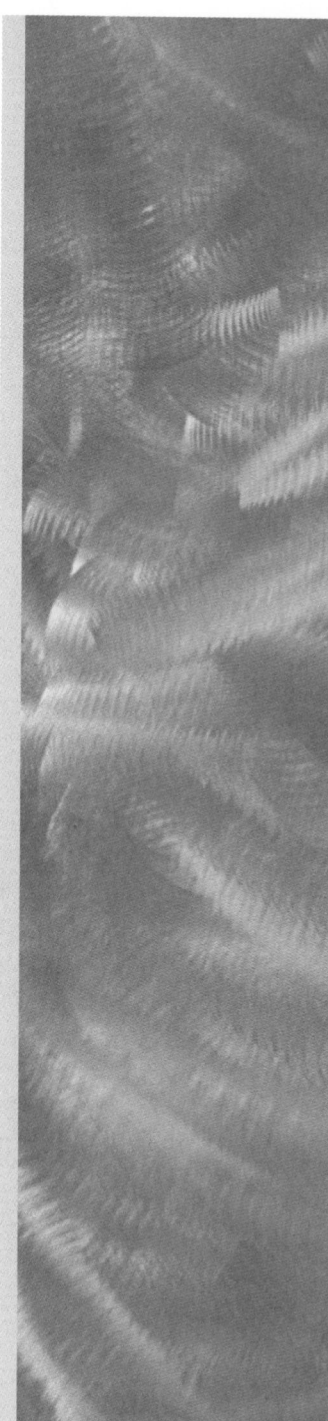

The figure shown after the story shows two boys watching in amazement, as a girl sleds upward instead of downward on the snowy hill.

The first sample was written by Michelle. Michelle wrote only two sentences:

> *The gril going up the hill.*
>
> *The boys look the gril going up the hill.*

Michelle described the key element of the picture: the girl was sledding upward and the boys were impressed enough by the action that they stopped and watched. She also used fairly complex syntactic structures, including two clauses strung together for the second sentence. Some of the errors include omission of the function word, *is*, in the first sentence, and the word, *at*, in the second sentence. She also misspelled the word, *girl.* She used the commonplace word, *going*, in lieu of the more descriptive word, *sledding.* Overall, the narrative tells little about the story that was read by the teacher.

Jelyyn wrote the second sample. Although Jelyyn's writing sample also included many errors characteristic of children who have significant hearing loss (including spelling errors, tense disagreement, omission of morphemes, omission of function words, run-on sentences, verb disagreement, and inappropriate change in verb tense), her narration of the story and of the accompanying picture was more complex and more informative than that of her classmate, Michelle. She also used more appropriate punctuation. However, notice how she missed writing about the key element of the story: the sled was magic, and hence able to glide uphill.

> *A girl name Tiffany. She walking by the stroe and she saw a macigi sleding and she went into the store and*

(continues)

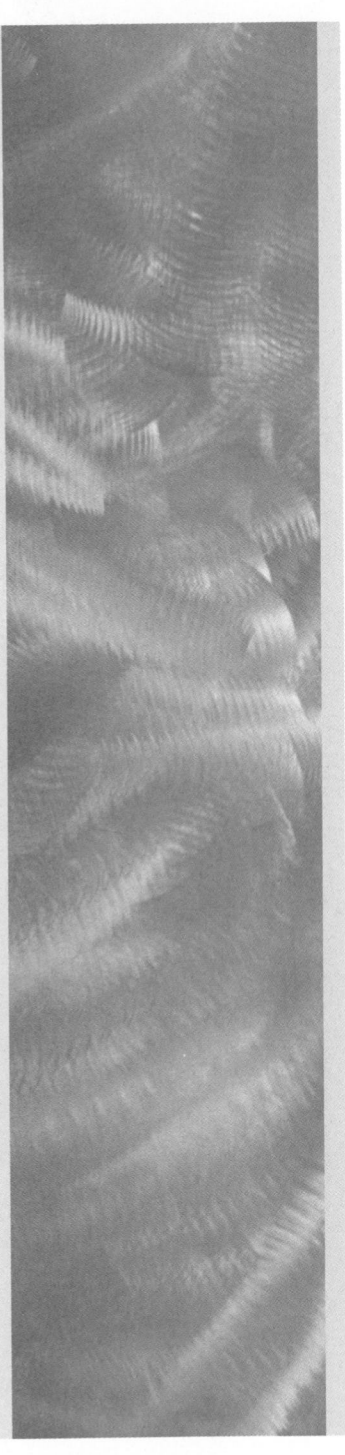

buy the macigi sleding and she can't wait to go sled down the hill. When she finish buy the sled. She was in a hurry. When she got home she put her snowpant on, hat, boots, mittens, scarft. And ran up the hill and she try to sleding down.

The next writing sample presents an example of how some children focus on an extraneous detail when they describe a pictorial scene. In addition, the paragraph's author, Shannon, failed to capitalize the first word of a sentence and committed some of the other errors demonstrated by Jelyyn in the preceding sample:

thay are snow outside. you cannt go slad way up. you can slad down in snow. the gril slad up in snow. the boys go walk up in snow. the wather is cold [extraneous detail].

The final sample presents what is technically the most narratively sound and grammatically correct paragraph of the four samples presented in this section. In writing it, the student, whose name is Allison, described the key elements of the story. Also, in the final sentence, she inserted dialog, which is a fairly advanced component in narrative writing. Grammatically, even though Allison did not use quotation marks and did not use a question mark where appropriate, she preceded the dialog with a comma (which was appropriate), and capitalized the first word. Other grammatical errors included the omission of function words and inappropriate changes in verb tense. Allison wrote:

It was winter time, and it was snowy in the picture. Dave, Kathy and Dan went sleding on big hill. They are tired to walk up on big hill but Kathy and her sled went up! Fanilly they get on top of hill. They ask her, How your sled went up

■ FINAL REMARKS

In this chapter, we considered speech and language development and, to a lesser extent, reading. Often, a primary concern of a speech and hearing professional who works with children is to foster growth in these areas. Speech and hearing professionals are often concerned with nurturing a child's social skills too. These social skills may include knowledge about how to behave politely, how to cooperate with peers, and how to follow rules. Many children who have hearing loss experience common social problems. These may include (Schum & Gfeller, 1994):

- A preference for playing with children younger than self
- Social isolation
- Naiveté about peer interests and customs
- Limited understanding about internal states such as feelings
- Difficulty in empathizing
- Feelings of frustration or intimidation during social interactions

Several useful discussions about the development of social skills are available in the literature, as are ways to alleviate such social difficulties as those just listed (Gfeller & Schum, 1994; Paul & Jackson, 1993; Schloss & Smith, 1990; Schum, 1991).

■ KEY CHAPTER POINTS

✔ Children with hearing loss may make characteristic speech errors, such as neutralizing vowels and omitting final consonants. These errors are primary factors in their overall low intelligibility levels.

✔ They often have problems in content, form, and pragmatics of language. For instance, they have reduced vocabulary and have mastered fewer syntactic structures than normally hearing children.

✔ Children who are hard-of-hearing often have difficulty in reading. Many deaf adults never attain better than a fourth grade reading level.

✔ Evidence suggests that receipt of a cochlear implant may enhance and accelerate speech, language, and literacy growth.

✔ A speech and language evaluation is performed in order to develop a hierarchy of speech-language therapy objectives.

▰ MULTIPLE CHOICE QUESTIONS

1. Typical segmental errors made by children who have profound deafness include:

    a. Breathiness

    b. Arhythmic speech patterns, characterized by abnormal syllable stress patterns

    c. Substitution of high vowels for low vowels

    d. Voicing confusions

2. On average, children who have profound hearing loss achieve about what level of intelligibility?

    a. 5%

    b. 20%

    c. 40%

    d. 60%

3. Which of the following is not a common error associated with vowel production by children who have significant hearing loss?

    a. Neutralization

    b. Diphthongization

    c. Shortening

    d. Nasalization

4. Of the following sounds, which one is most likely to be produced correctly by a talker who has a profound hearing loss?

    a. /b/

    b. /d/

    c. /g/

    d. /n/

5. Which of the following statements is most appropriate when describing the quality of speech produced by talkers who have significant hearing loss?

    a. It has a "sing-songy" quality.

    b. It sounds as if the talker is producing each sound or syllable or word as if it were an isolated unit.

    c. It sounds mechanical.

    d. It sounds like speech being produced at a distance.

6. Which is an example of a problem related to form?

    a. Restricted vocabulary, where words related to an entire concept may be unknown.

    b. A child asks a brand new acquaintance to lend her twenty dollars.

    c. A child sees a car driving by and says, "Car go fast."

    d. A child can understand the word *bank* when talking about a receptacle for money, but not when the word is used in reference to the ground flanking a river.

7. Which word is most likely to be learned first by a toddler who has a significant hearing loss?

    a. Bell

    b. Jealous

    c. Under

    d. Miss

8. When writing, a fourth grader who has significant hearing loss is likely:

    a. To omit function words such as *of* and *to*

    b. Under-use subject-verb-object sentence structures

    c. Follow too rigidly the narrative template of beginning, middle, and ending

    d. Over-use adverbs

9. Reading levels of high school graduates who have significant hearing loss and who use hearing aids:

    a. Hover around the seventh grade level

    b. Permit them to understand articles in *Time,* a periodical geared toward general U.S. readership.

    c. Barely allow them to read a local newspaper with un-
derstanding

    d. Have improved gradually during the past half century

10. Janice is a 3-year-old girl. She lost her hearing at the age of
2 months, following a severe viral infection. Seven months
ago, Janice received a cochlear implant. She is beginning to
articulate the following sounds accurately:

    a. Central vowels

    b. Front vowels

    c. Alveolars

    d. Palatals

11. When collecting a speech or language sample, it is important to:

    a. Make sure the child practices the sample several times
before it is collected for assessment purposes

    b. Collect a variety of measures, as children's perform-
ance may vary as a function of task type

    c. Use an aural/oral communication mode, especially if
you are interested in collecting a speech sample

    d. Remain unfamiliar to the child until you actually
begin testing, as talker familiarity may change how
well you understand the speech of the child

12. Which of the following factors probably has the least effect
on a child's speech intelligibility score?

    a. Listener experience

    b. Listening condition

    c. Speech materials

    d. A guardian present in the room when the sample is
collected

13. The speech therapy program developed by Daniel Ling is
based on:

    a. The premise that formal instruction precedes informal
instruction

    b. A hierarchy of speech skills

    c. The Northampton Chart

    d. Computer games, such as a balloon growing in size as
the child phonates into a microphone

14. Sometimes children who have significant hearing loss experience socialization issues. For example, they:
    a. May experience social isolation
    b. Prefer to avoid interacting with other children who have significant hearing loss, so not to appear a part of a minority
    c. Prefer the company of adults
    d. Experience excessive degrees of sympathy, as they can empathize with persons who face difficult situations

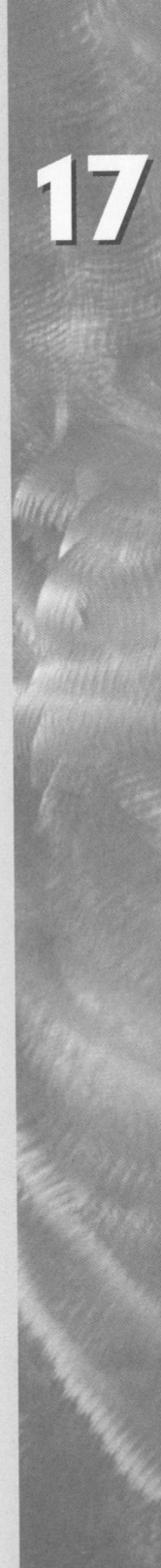

CHAPTER 17

Parent/Guardian-Centered Conversation and Language Instruction[1]

[1]Parts of Chapter 17 were adapted from *Let's Converse! A How-to Guide to Develop and Expand Conversational Skills of Children and Teenagers Who are Hearing Impaired* by N. Tye-Murray, 1994, Washington, DC: Alexander Graham Bell Association for the Deaf.

This chapter concerns the ways parents or children's primary caretakers may facilitate conversational interactions with their child. The guiding premise is that satisfying conversational interactions between children and their parents will nurture children's language and speech development and advance their social, emotional, and intellectual growth. The speech and hearing professional may play a significant role in helping parents learn how to support conversation and language development. In this chapter, we first consider language and then conversation, although there is really no clear distinction between the ways in which a parent fosters one versus the other.

When providing instruction to parents or guardians, it is important to remember that they know their child better than anyone, including all speech and hearing professionals. Your role is to provide information and empower parents to use their own talents, knowledge, and experiences to foster language growth and conversational skills. Communication patterns emerge in the context of the family system, and the most effective strategies for encouraging communication growth are those that are symbiotic with the family milieu.

■ PARENT-CENTERED LANGUAGE INTERVENTION

For younger children in particular, a clinician may spend time with a child's family, discussing ways to stimulate language practice in the home. Adults in a child's everyday life have a prime opportunity to stimulate a child's language production. The techniques listed in Figure 17-1 represent ways that parents can stimulate their child's language development. These techniques are simple for parents to implement yet are highly effective in expanding language competency. Speech and hearing professionals and other people who interact often with children who have hearing loss also may find these techniques helpful in stimulating their child's speech and language growth in both everyday and clinical settings.

Signaling Expectation

The first technique is to signal expectations. Wait for the child's response. During an interaction, often, after you say something, indicate that a response is expected, by tilting the head and rais-

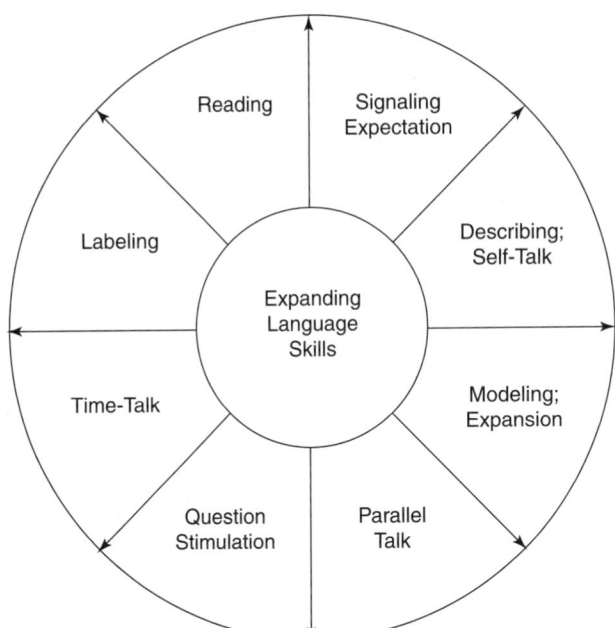

FIGURE 17-1. Language-stimulation techniques that parents and primary guardians can use to expand children's language skills.

ing eyebrows (Figure 17-2). This action is an effective means of generating a verbal response from the child. It also establishes a turn-taking pattern. For instance, a parent might say, "Hmmm, you have a block. I wonder what you are going to do with it." Then instead of continuing, she or he may look expectantly at the child, and wait for a reply.

Describing and Self-Talk

The second technique is called *describing* and self-talk. In implementing this technique, adults use an event or an idea the child is interested in and describe various aspects of it. Also, adults may use *self-talk,* and speak aloud about what they are doing or what they are thinking. In this way, they illustrate that language can be used to organize, analyze, and direct actions by thinking aloud through the process. For example, using the child's preferred communication mode, an adult may say, "I am unpacking my groceries. I'll take out the beef. Hmmm, let's have hamburgers tonight." The adult continues talking as she puts away the groceries, even though the child does not participate in a dialog.

Describing: an adult uses an event a child is interested in to talk about various aspects of the event.

In **self-talk,** adults talk aloud about what they are doing or thinking.

1. After asking a question, wait for an answer. Cock your head and look expectantly at your child.

2. Raise your eyebrows and look inquisitive.

3. Shrug your shoulders, holding your palms up.

4. Maintain visual contact as you wait for your child to respond.

5. Lean forward and look interested.

FIGURE 17-2. Different ways that a parent might signal expectation when interacting with a child. (Adapted from "Some ways to nurture children's conversational and language skills," by L. Spencer, 1994. In N. Tye-Murray (Ed.), *Let's converse! A how-to guide to develop and expand the conversational skills of children and teenagers who are hearing impaired* (pp. 51–84). Washington, DC: Alexander Graham Bell Association for the Deaf.)

Figure 17-3 presents media personalities who demonstrate self-talk and describing. In the following dialogue, a parent capitalizes on something that is happening in the backyard. Notice how the mother uses vocabulary appropriate for her child's age, which is 4 years. She uses language and vocabulary slightly more complex than his current language level. Joey has a receptive language level of age 3 years:

Joey: (touches a flower). "Flower."
Mother: "Yes, that flower is a daisy."

1. Martha Stewart

2. Emeril Lagasse (television chef)

3. (the late) Mr. Rogers (of *Mr. Rogers' Neighborhood*)

4. Bob Costas (sportscaster)

5. Mario Batali (television chef)

6. Bugs Bunny

FIGURE 17-3. Persons who present models of self-talk and description.

Joey:	"Daisy."
Mother:	"It has a yellow center."
Joey:	(touches the center of the daisy).
Mother:	"It has many white petals."
Joey:	(pulls on the flower).
Mother:	"You can pick some of the flowers. You can make a pretty bouquet."
Joey:	"Bouquet?"
Mother:	"Yes. Pick another flower. Many flowers make a bouquet." (picks two flowers).
Joey:	"Me too."
Mother:	"Yes, you can pick some flowers too."

In this example, the mother provides language to the ongoing activity and follows Joey's lead in describing what is happening.

Effective conversationalists talk about what they are doing and what they are thinking. They attend to the child's focus and talk about that, too. Even if their children do not understand every word, the context of the setting (e.g., putting away groceries; picking flowers in the garden) gives meaning to their words. Adults can act as if their children were participating in a conversation, just as mothers sometimes do when they talk to their infants who have normal hearing. For instance, mothers of babies make their remarks contingent on the infant's facial expressions and body gestures and unintelligible vocalizations and cooings. This kind of talking stimulates a child's language development, and it shows the child how conversation works. By conversing in this manner, the adult creates a phantom role for the child, and the child eventually develops the conversational skills to fulfill it.

One caveat must be appended to this discussion. When suggesting this technique, it is important that the adult does not interpret it to mean, "Talk, talk, talk." A nonending monologue is not the goal. It is essential when talking to children, that adults follow their focus of attention and talk about that focus and what is happening in a relaxed way. Also, pausing at appropriate intervals will give children time to think and an opportunity to contribute to the development and direction of the dialogue.

Here's an Example of How Describing and Self-Talk Can Promote Language and Literacy

In a book for parents, I included this example (Tye-Murray, 1994a):

"The importance of [describing and self-talk] can be demonstrated with a story about two children who have hearing impairments, Janet and Michelle. These two girls are in the same third grade class. On this particular afternoon, both girls are at home with their mothers, putting away groceries following a trip to the grocery store. Janet sits on the kitchen stool and watches her mother. Meanwhile, her mother industriously stacks cans in the cupboard. She puts away paper bags and washes fruit. For about 10 minutes, Janet and her mother do not converse. Eventually, Janet climbs off the stool and leaves.

Michelle also sits on a stool in her kitchen. Her mother says, "First, I'll put the cans away. They are in this sack. Let's see, I'll put the big cans on the bottom and the little ones on top." She puts the cans onto the shelf. "Oh," her mother says, "here are the peas. Looks like I already have some peas in the cupboard." The mother stops talking. During her pause, Michelle interjects, "Peas." Her mother smiles and responds to Michelle's remark, "You like peas? We have lots of them. Do you want some peas for dinner tonight?" Michelle stays in the kitchen and helps her mother start making soup.

The next day is Monday. The girls' teacher asks the class to write a story about two people, John and Jean. Given only the information about Janet and Michelle, consider which girl's story is likely to contain a greater variety of vocabulary words; which girl's story is likely to contain dialog between the two characters; who will have the least amount of difficulty in writing a story that flows smoothly from beginning to middle to end. Not all children with hearing impairments who interact with adults who talk a lot will become competent writers or conversationalists. However, it stands to reason that children who are exposed to language and conversation in everyday situations will more likely learn to converse then children who have not been similarly exposed. They also may learn to write and construct stories better. (p. 24)

Modeling and Expansion

Expansion: a language-stimulation technique in which an adult copies the meaning of a child's utterance but expands the grammar of the message.

When using a modeling or **expansion** language-stimulation technique, an adult copies the meaning of a child's utterances but modifies or expands the grammar of the message. For example a child might say, "Scissors." Her mother may then expand the utterance by saying, "You want the scissors. You can cut with the scissors." Some of the benefits of using modeling and expansion include (a) the child's message is reinforced, (b) new language structures are introduced, and (c) an imitation of the correct structure is prompted from the child. Table 17-1 presents five examples of modeling.

Parallel Talk

In using the technique of *parallel talk,* an adult matches language to an activity a child is performing. For example, as a child plays silently with a stuffed animal, an adult may use parallel talk and say, "You are holding the bear. Now you are feeding the bear. Oh, you hug the bear." This technique provides a model of language structures and also a commentary. It invites dialog. For example, the child may respond to the preceding remarks with, "Yes, this is my bear!"

Parallel talk: a language-stimulation technique in which an adult matches language to an activity a child is performing.

Question Stimulation

If used optimally, the use of questions is a potent means of stimulating language growth. Use of questions provides children with models of how to ask and answer questions. For example, a child may point to a bowl on the table and say, "Cereal?" A parent may respond, "Do you want some cereal?" and thereby provide a model of how to make a request. Although questions can be useful tools in promoting questions, a string of questions can

Table 17-1. Examples of language modeling. Modeling provides continuity in a conversation, especially when a child's utterance is incomplete. It also shows that the adult understands the child's remark(s), and it serves to expand the child's language competency. If done optimally, modeling will promote language development while still preserving the child's original intent.

CHILD'S REMARK	ADULT'S EXPANSION OF THE REMARK
"Bird."	"There's a bird in the tree."
"Ball."	"The ball is bouncing."
"Baby."	"You have a baby doll."
"Car."	"The car is very shiny."
"Star."	"Let's cut out the star with the scissors."

squelch a child's active participation. The Key Resources section suggests how parents might best use questions to provide children with language models and to stimulate language and conversational growth.

Time-Talk

Time-talk: a language-stimulation technique in which an adult purposely incorporates time-related language into the conversation.

The sixth language-stimulation technique is called **time-talk.** When using this strategy, link time words to events or routines that are significant to a child for the purpose of helping children develop the concepts and language of time. For example, adults can use time-talk and sequence events in their conversations, and use such time-related words as *before, during,* and *after.* A grandmother might say, "First, we will add sugar. Second, we will add an egg. Third, we will stir," demonstrating the use of time words, *first, second,* and *third.*

Table 17-2 presents time-related words for toddlers, young children, and older children and teenagers, and instances in which the words might be used. Incorporating time-related words into the daily routine or to significant events in the life of a family or class of children helps the child relate the words to meaningful time frames. In addition to expanding language skills, the introduction and reinforcement of time-related words helps the child develop abstract concepts of time passing and sequential patterning of events.

Labeling

Labeling: a language-stimulation technique in which an adult provides names to objects, actions, and events.

In using *labeling,* an adult provides names to objects, actions, and events. For instance, a child may pick up a toy cup. A parent might use labeling and comment, "That's a cup."

Reading

Regardless of a child's age, reading is one of the most effective and delightful ways to enrich language (Figure 17-4). From simple picture books designed to enrich vocabulary to full-scale novels and encyclopedias, by reading to and with a child, an adult will promote the development of vocabulary, syntax, se-

Table 17-2. Examples of time-related words for toddlers, children, and older children and teenagers, and instances in which they might be used.

AGE GROUP	WORDS	DAILY ROUTINE
Toddlers	*now, later*	Drawing pictures: "Now I'll draw a girl. Later, I'll draw a boy."
	morning, night	Playing with a doll: "It's morning. Time for the baby to wake up. . . . It's night time. Time for the baby to go to sleep."
Children	*today, tomorrow, yesterday*	Reviewing a calendar: "Tomorrow you have a soccer game. You had practice yesterday. You have practice today, too."
Older children and teenagers	*decade, century, millennium*	Studying space exploration during a history lesson: "Space exploration began in the second half of the last century. In the first few decades of this millennium, astronauts hope to reach Mars."

mantics, and pragmatics. Stories provide world and social information and models of conversation. For instance, through reading, a child learns there are other cultures and other families. The child learns social mores, what is considered courteous, what is considered rude, how to start a conversation, and how to end one. Reading is the key for unlocking a wealth of information, and is the cornerstone for achieving success in the academic setting. Parents and guardians should be encouraged to establish a daily reading routine, where they sit down with their child and enjoy reading a book together.

There are ways to maximize the benefits of reading. These include the following:

- Before reading the book, make predictions. If the book is a picture book, look at the pictures, and make comments like, *Let's look at the pictures first. What do you think is happening in this picture? What do you think is going to happen next? Why do you think that?*

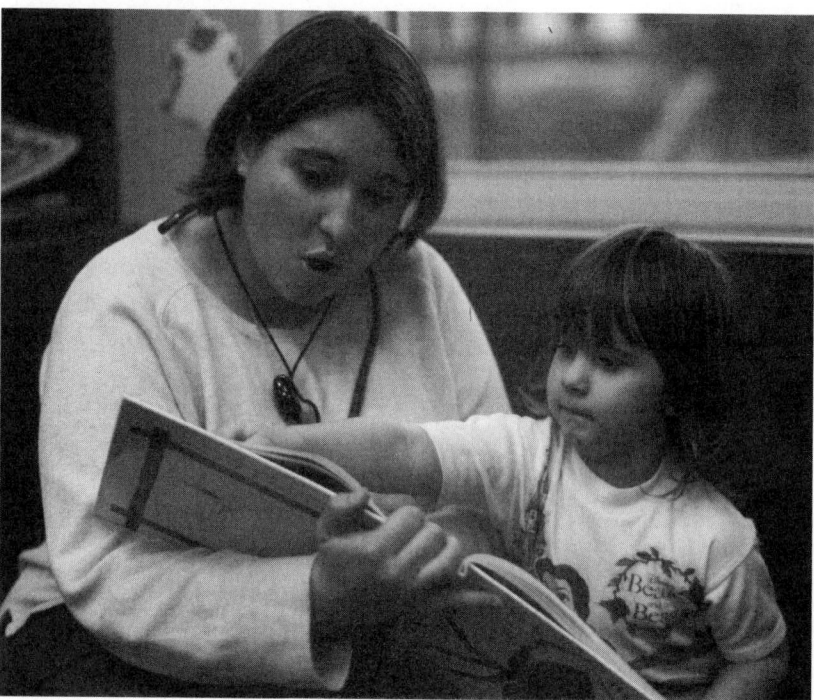

FIGURE 17-4. Sharing a book serves to expand a child's language and to develop conversational skills. In this picture, a parent is engaging her daughter in the reading activity by allowing her to turn the pages *(Photograph by Marcus Kosa, courtesy of the Central Institute of the Deaf)*

■ Talk about the story after you read it. Review what happened. *How do you think [main character] felt when this happened? What would you have done? Why do you think he did that?* Revisit the predictions that you made before reading the story. Ask questions like, *Were we right about this picture?* Make the story personally relevant to the child and to the family or to the class. *Has this ever happened to you?*

■ Expand on new information or new vocabulary that occurred or that will occur in the story. Introduce some of the new vocabulary and new information before you read the story. For example, you might say, *This story is about an octopus. Do you know what an octopus is? Here's a picture of an octopus.* Afterwards, if new words occurred in the story, make a point of using those words in subsequent conversation. If new information was presented, expand on it during conversation and in other contexts.

- Re-read favorite books. Let the child paraphrase the story along with the pictures, if the book is a storybook with pictures.
- Encourage literacy-related activities. Stage a play or dramatic event. Tell a story by drawing pictures. Pantomime a calamity, like climbing a footstool and falling off. These kind of activities develop a sense of narration and drama and an appreciation for storytelling and the nuances of daily life.

It will not be useful to simply hand a list to parents and say, "Try these at home." If possible, concomitant instruction should accompany these ideas. Parents may need explicit guidance in how to use language-stimulation techniques. Instruction can be provided in a variety of ways, ranging from less structured to more structured (Figure 17-5). You may find that even mainstream classroom teachers benefit from either less-structured or more-structured instruction in how to use language-stimulation techniques, particularly if they have a child who is hard-of-hearing in their classroom for the first time.

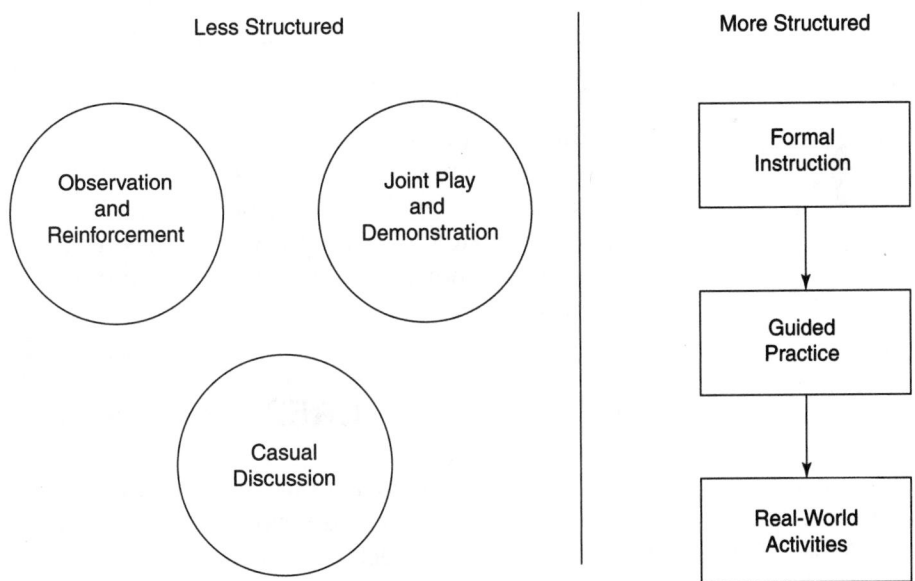

FIGURE 17-5. Two approaches for providing instruction to parents about language- and conversation-stimulation techniques.

■ LESS-STRUCTURED INSTRUCTION

Less-structured instruction: informal shaping of language-stimulation behaviors, often during play.

You might want to shape parents' language-stimulation behaviors in an informal manner, using **_less-structured instruction._** For example, you might observe parent and child as they engage in a conversation during a play session in the home or clinical setting. Afterward, you might say to the mother, "You seemed very attentive to Tim's focus of attention as you played with the Lego pieces. I like the way you named the colors of each piece he picked up." With this remark, you have given the mother positive reinforcement and provided instruction about how to increase vocabulary through the use of labeling. No doubt, such a remark would also serve to bolster her self-confidence and sense of satisfaction about the play session.

During an informal play session, a clinician also might join in with the parent (however, one must be careful not to take over the play session). The clinician might demonstrate language-expansion techniques and suggest additional activities. Parents can observe the effectiveness of a technique and realize that it probably is not beyond their abilities to implement it ("Hey, I can do that!").

Other less-structured activities may be casual discussions. For instance, a parent might ask you questions about language development, and you might discuss techniques informally.

In these less-structured kinds of interactions, it is extremely important that the clinician exercise tact and respect for the parent. Whenever possible, one should avoid being judgmental of the parent, critical, or negative. The goal is to empower and enable parents to facilitate language growth; criticism or an undue display of professional expertise will only sabotage a clinician's well-intentioned efforts.

■ MORE-STRUCTURED INSTRUCTION

More-structured instruction: formal or more systematic instruction for parents and caregivers in language-stimulation behaviors.

Instruction for parents or primary caregivers can be more structured and systematic, what is termed **_more-structured instruction._** In this case, a speech and hearing professional might provide formal instruction, guided learning, and real-world practice, just as in a communication strategies training program (Chapter 4). Instruction can occur in either a one-on-one setting or in a parent group forum.

Formal Instruction

During formal instruction, a clinician might begin by discussing each of the language-stimulation strategies and reviewing related examples. The clinician might provide audio- or videotaped examples of the strategies in use. For example, the first topic in Table 17-3 is signaling expectations. Two film clips might be shown to the parent group, the first where an adult signals low expectations that her child will communicate, as in the following interchange taken from the film transcript (from Spencer, 1994):

Child:	(Points toward crayons)
Mother:	"What are you pointing at?"
Child:	(Grabs a color)
Mother:	"You wanted the color. Here's some paper, too."
Mother:	"What are you drawing? It looks like a cat."
Child:	(Continues drawing)
Mother:	"Here is the black. You can color the tail black." (p. 52)

Table 17-3. Workbook exercises an aural rehabilitation specialist might give to parents so they may practice modeling and expansion.

Modeling and Expansion

On the lines below are some typical utterances a child might say. Beside each utterance, write your own expansion model.

Child's utterance	*Your expansion model*
1. "More."	_____
2. "Give."	_____
3. "Cup."	_____
4. "My turn."	_____

Possible expansions could include:

1. You want more juice.
2. Give the baby some juice.
3. Let's pour the juice in the cup.
4. It's your turn to pour.

In this first film clip, the mother asks questions, but does not expect her child to answer them. She does not pause and allow the child to initiate a remark. By providing the paper and crayon to her child, she has eliminated the need for him to ask for them. A second film clip demonstrates how an adult can signal higher expectations for communication, and thereby elicit more language from her child (Spencer, 1994):

Child:	(Points toward crayons)
Mother:	"What?" (looks around expectantly)
Child:	"Ka."
Mother:	"Color?"
Child:	"Cala."
Mother:	"Color. Green or black?" (waits)
Child:	"Bak."
Mother:	(Gives the child the black crayon . . . waits)
Child:	"Papa."
Mother:	"Paper—here's a big piece." (Holds paper up)
Child:	"Mine."
Mother:	"Draw me a picture." (pp. 52–53)

After parents view this second clip, parents and clinicians can talk about how the mother frequently pauses and allows time for her child to talk. She uses facial expressions that signal expectation for more information and establishes a turn-taking pattern.

Parental Influences

Parents' interaction styles may impinge on a child's development. A number of investigations have demonstrated that caregivers who interact with children who have a hearing loss behave differently than caregivers who interact with normally hearing children (Cole, 1993). They talk less, repeat themselves more often, provide fewer expansions, present shorter utterances, and present simpler grammatical structures. Interestingly, interaction styles correlate with language achievement. Language development has an inverse relationship with caregivers' use of imperatives and topic changes and with caregivers' frequency of negative remarks (Bromwich, 1981).

Audio- and videotaped examples are effective means of providing formal instruction about language nurturing. In the event no film clips are available, printed transcripts like the ones presented here can be discussed. Example transcripts for the other language-stimulation techniques appear in the Key Resources section at the end of the chapter.

Guided Practice

Means for providing guided practice include group discussions, role-playing, and self-critique. For example, in a group discussion, parents might share ideas about how they interest their children in using language in the home environment. They might reflect about how they interact with their child and discuss the techniques they use with one another.

Home-training programs can also provide guided-learning experiences. Parents may receive printed materials to read at home and workbook activities that provide guided-learning for the printed materials. An example of a workbook exercise that might be used in a home-training program appears in Table 17-3.

Real-World Activities

For real-world practice, the third component of a more structured program, parents might tape-record themselves while playing with their child at home and then review the tapes, checking to see whether they have implemented language-expansion techniques. This practice will help them be more mindful of their language-stimulation efforts and also will provide an opportunity to appreciate the success of their efforts.

When assigning a real-world practice activity, a clinician may want to adhere to the following guidelines (see Andrews & Andrews, 1990, p. 67):

- **The activity should be something already practiced and discussed.** It should address something that is relevant to a family and something that has been discussed between clinician and family.

- **An assignment should be given in rewarding contexts.** The clinician might say, "Susan seems to be learning the names of colors now that you are labeling them at home. You seem to be consistent with this. Now, this week, try to have her spontaneously name colors, perhaps by pausing and waiting for her to talk."
- **Ask the parent whether the assignment is possible, and whether it is appropriate.** We once asked a busy mother to follow a complex calendar of activities. After 3 days, she called us and began the conversation with, "I hate this—I just can't do it." Clearly, we should have talked to her more extensively beforehand and anticipated her concerns and minimized problems.
- **Demonstrate the assignment, and then ask the parent to try it, preferably with the child.** This step will ensure there is no confusion about the assignment and also will provide you with a first-hand look at how well the strategy works between parent and child, and it will let you know whether the assignment is appropriate.
- **Provide the assignment in writing.** This step will ensure there is no confusion as to what to do and will provide a back-up in case the parent forgets what you discussed.

Real-world practice might be monitored by asking parents to keep a journal about their communication interactions with their child on a daily basis for a set number of weeks. They also can complete daily checklists, indicating whether they consciously performed any of the techniques during that day.

FOSTERING LANGUAGE USE THROUGH CONVERSATION

Now that we have considered language-stimulation techniques and training activities for parents, we consider ways that parents can nurture conversational skills in their children and how they may learn to use repair strategies effectively. Procedures for providing instruction to parents are like those we just considered for encouraging language strategies. Both less-structured and more-structured procedures are appropriate, and some parents may benefit from formal instruction, guided learning, and real-world practice in developing their conversational skills and learning to use repair strategies in an optimal way.

The underlying premise for conversation-centered instruction is the belief that the best way for parents to stimulate language growth in the home is in the context of conversation. Conversations require children to use language for the purposes of expressing meaning and receiving messages, and to do so in situations that are relevant and motivating.

Although the importance of conversation between parent and child may seem self-evident, conversation does not always happen. Conversing requires effort, especially when conversing with a child who has hearing loss. Communication breakdowns occur frequently, and adults have to pay greater attention to how they phrase their messages and how they speak than they do when they talk to children who do not have hearing loss. At times, the conversations may not be rewarding to the adult and may provide little positive feedback. If the child does not understand their messages, and they do not understand their child's communicative intents, conversations may become frustrating. Yet, you should encourage adults to persevere in their conversations. Eventually, their efforts will motivate their children to learn language, to speak, and to engage in meaningful dialogue.

Table 17-4 lists some guidelines that a speech and hearing professional might review with parents. These guidelines concern ways to facilitate conversation with a child who has hearing loss. These are not rigid *do's* and *don'ts* of conversation but, if followed, often will stimulate a child to converse.

Table 17-4. Some conversational strategies for adults who interact with children who have hearing loss.

---

1. Allow your child to choose what to talk about, and respond to the communicative attempts.
2. Encourage your child to tell narratives and stories, and to give directions.
3. Organize your messages.
4. Speak with clear speech.
5. Speak positively and avoid critical language.
6. Do not overcontrol your conversations.

Allow a Child to Choose What to Talk About and Respond to His or Her Communicative Attempts

The phrase to remember when using this strategy is *stay attuned to the child.* An adult can observe the child's focus of attention and try to talk about what a child is doing and topics that interest the youngster. Remarks should be contingent on the child's utterances. For instance, if a child says, "This my car," a father can comment, "I bet the car can go fast." He probably should not respond, "Hand me that jeep over there." If a child is primarily nonverbal, and there are no spoken (or signed) remarks that invite a response, a conversational partner can acknowledge the child's facial expressions, gestures, and unintelligible vocalizations as if they were conversational turns. For example, a child's pointing finger may elicit the remark, "Oh, you want a block," from the child's parent.

Being together sharing time and attending to the child's focus of attention are often enough to encourage children to engage in conversation. However, specific activities such as puzzles, give-and-take games, and art can stimulate conversation. Figure 17-6 presents activities that can create a springboard for conversation between parents and infants and toddlers. Figures 17-7 and 17-8 present activities that may be appropriate for children and young teenagers, respectively.

---

1. Playing peek-a-boo

2. Playing "Where's the baby?"

3. Counting fingers and toes

4. Getting dressed

5. Playing with toys in the bathtub

6. Playing make-believe games

7. Going on an outing, such as to the zoo, playground, or swimming

---

FIGURE 17-6. Activities that can create a springboard for conversation between an adult and an infant or toddler.

1. Playing age-appropriate board games and computer games

2. Going on a scavenger hunt

3. Working on homework together

4. Putting a puzzle together

5. Decorating cookies

6. Working on an arts and crafts project

7. Looking through a photograph album, and identifying relatives or classmates and remembering past events

FIGURE 17-7. Activities that may create a springboard for conversation between an adult and a child.

1. Shopping together

2. Cooking dinner together

3. Visiting historical sites

4. Planning holiday celebrations

5. Discussing family history

6. Playing sports together

7. Discussing current events and magazines

FIGURE 17-8. Activities that may create a springboard for conversation between an adult and a young teenager.

Encourage a Child to Tell Narratives and Stories, and to Give Directions

Often when we engage in conversation, we share past experiences, we describe something, or we provide explanations. We tell stories about something that has happened to us or to someone else, or we predict a future experience. We take extended turns, where we speak several consecutive sentences that collectively have an internal cohesiveness. If children do not know how to take an extended turn, they will be constrained in their ability to participate in conversations.

The ability to tell a story may be a particularly important aspect of achieving conversational competency. In presenting a narrative, we usually describe a setting and the main characters, a theme or goal, episodes or events that develop the plot, and then we present a resolution. Many children with significant hearing loss experience difficulty in telling narratives. Their conversation often relates to concrete objects and often does not relate to absent objects or persons or abstractions. Difficulty with telling narratives limits children's potential to be active conversational partners and to take extended conversational turns.

The second suggested guideline pertains to the use of connected discourse in conversation. When something happens, or children seem excited about something, an adult might say, "Tell me about it." "Tell me more." or "Where did you go?" They can pause and give their children time to think and formulate their messages. Visual props, such as photographs or the drawing presented in Figure 17-9, can be used, as they are especially effective in helping children organize narratives. Visual props provide a concrete representation of what a child wants to talk about. The adult can encourage children to tell the *who, what, where, when,* and *why* as they refer back to the picture. When children tell only a part of the story, the adult can help them fill in the missing details by expanding on what the children have said (e.g., "The girl pinched him hard.") The adult can readily make acknowledgments (e.g., "I see."), show interest (e.g., "Really?"), and repeat some of what has been said (e.g., "He ate the French fry and then . . . ?"). If a child has difficulty constructing a narrative, the adult might present a model of a well-structured story.

Organize Your Messages

The third guideline requires adults to use meta-communication skills, and to think about *how* they will say *what* they are going to say. This guideline encourages adult conversational partners to organize their messages.

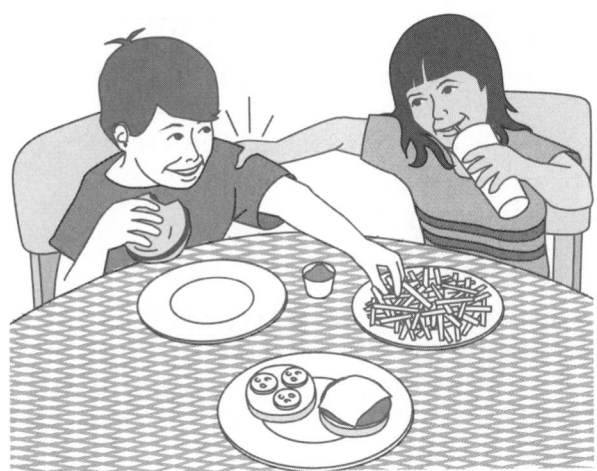

FIGURE 17-9. Children can tell a narrative about a picture portraying an event that happened to one or more of them. If the children have not had much practice in telling narratives, an adult might ask questions such as, "What is the boy eating?" and "What is the girl doing?" Afterward, the adult might summarize the event: "The boy and the girl were eating lunch. They had French fries, cheeseburgers, and chocolate shakes. The boy took the girl's French fry. The girl wanted him to stop. She pinched the boy." The children might then retell the story.

Principles of good message organization are presented in Figure 17-10. In general, well-*organized messages* are not ambiguous, verbose, or obscure. They are orderly in that ideas follow a logical sequence.

Two extremes of poor message organization are verbose messages and telegraphic messages. If a child with limited language skills asks, "Where's my sweater?" the child will more likely understand an adult who replies, "On the table," than an adult who instead says, "Even though I've asked you to hang up your sweater a million times, you left it on the top stairs." The first response is straightforward, whereas the second presents more information than the child can process, and an admonition to boot. Closely associated with verbosity is the problem of complex verbiage, which encompasses the use of convoluted syntax and dense semantics and many embedded clauses to interrelate ideas. An example of complex verbiage is the sentence, *The tennis shoes, which were dirty, are in the washing machine.* A better way to organize this message if speaking to a child who has limited

Organized messages: communications that are not wordy and do not use complex verbiage; terminology is precise and not ambiguous or obscure; orderly and logical sequence of ideas.

■ **Avoid verbosity and complex verbiage.**
"The present is on the front seat. I need to wrap it."
Rather than
"The present, which is on the front seat, needs to be wrapped."

■ **Avoid telegraphic speech.**
"The car keys are in my purse."
Rather than
"Keys in purse."

■ **Repeat important keywords and phrases.**
"Here is your cup. Please pour milk into the cup."
Rather than
"Here is your cup. Please pour milk into it."

■ **Use precise terminology.**
"The cookie is on the plate."
Rather than
"It's over there."

■ **Pause between your utterances. (Allow time for the child to think; both about what you have just said and about what to say next.)**
"I'm going to the park . . . Do you want to stay here?"
Rather than
"I'm going to the park, do you want to stay here?"

■ **Avoid run-on sentences.**
"First, we'll go to the field. Then we'll watch John play soccer. Then we might go out for lunch."
Rather than
"First, we'll go to the field and we'll watch John play soccer and then maybe afterwards we'll go out for lunch."

FIGURE 17-10. Principles of good message organization.

language skills would be to present it with two sentences: *The tennis shoes were dirty. I put them in the wash.*

Telegraphic speech is characterized by the omission of function words.

Telegraphic speech represents the opposite extreme of verbose speech and is a common mistake in message organization made by adults who communicate with their children using simultaneous communication. A child might ask, "Where's Bobby?" Her mother uses telegraphic speech when she responds, "Bobby go football." The mother has omitted important function words and has used inappropriate grammar. Not only does telegraphic speech open the door for communication breakdowns to occur (because the child might not understand the intended meaning), it also provides a deviant model of language to the child.

Speak With Clear Speech

When we engage in conversation, we often adopt a speaking style known as conversational speech. In conversational speech, some sounds may be combined together, and some sounds may be omitted. The following sentences represent conversational speech:

- *D'yeet yet?* For *Did you eat yet?*
- *Go'in fishin' 'morrow af'ernoon.* For *I'm going fishing tomorrow afternoon.*

Children who have hearing loss experience great difficulty in understanding conversational speech. They will understand more of the message if it is spoken with a speaking style known as clear speech (Schum, 1989). ***Clear speech*** is characterized by a somewhat slowed speaking rate and good (although not exaggerated) enunciation. Some sounds might be slightly longer than normal and more fully differentiated. Key words are emphasized, and pauses are inserted at clause boundaries. Examples of persons who speak with clear speech include:

Clear speech: using a somewhat slowed speaking rate and good but not exaggerated enunciation of words when conversing with someone with a hearing loss.

- An elementary school teacher
- A newscaster
- An airport employee who announces airline arrivals and departures
- A public radio broadcaster
- A politician
- Queen Elizabeth

Speak Positively and Avoid Critical Language

Almost any time an adult speaks, the individual has the option of using positive versus negative language. Using positive language means using words such as *can* rather than *can't*, *choose* rather than *have to*, and *will* rather than *won't*. For instance, instead of saying, "We can't go to the park today. It is raining," a parent might say, "We can stay inside and play a game." Figure 17-11 presents examples of positive versus negative language.

Example 1

A young child is building a tower of blocks. He is about to add another block to the teetering tower.

His father says (using negative language): "You can't add another block. The tower won't stay up."

His father says (using positive language): "Your tower is so tall!"

Example 2

A young teenager is in the kitchen. She quickly clears the table. She tells her mother she is going out.

The mother says (using negative language): "You can't leave for Sarah's house now. You must load the dishwasher."

The mother says (using positive language): "You can rinse the dishes. I'll wipe the table."

FIGURE 17-11. Examples of positive versus negative language.

Speaking positively extends beyond using positive language. As demonstrated by Figure 17-12, it also includes not being unduly critical. Many adults criticize or respond negatively more often when they interact with children who have hearing loss than when they interact with children who have normal hearing (e.g., Pipp Siegel & Biringen, 2000). Unfortunately, language development has an inverse relationship with adults' frequency of negative remarks. It is important for parents and guardians to remember that some children who encounter negativity when they attempt to communicate eventually stop trying to converse.

Do Not Over-Control Your Conversations

The final guideline is not to over-control a conversation with a child who has hearing loss. Table 17-5 presents examples of dialog that demonstrate over-controlling conversational moves and turns.

There are two possible (and not mutually exclusive) explanations as to why adults tend to over-control conversations when talking to children who have hearing loss. The first possibility is

---

Example 1

Child: "I forgot my books."

Adult: "You forgot your book again? I'm going to have to pin a note to your jacket."

Example 2

Child: "I spilled the milk."

Adult: (being unduly critical): "You made a mess. Why did you do that?"

Example 3

Child: "I don't like Teri any more."

Adult: (being unduly critical): "Teri is your friend. What's the matter with you?"

FIGURE 17-12. Examples of critical language.

that some adults want to provide abundant stimulation to compensate for the hearing loss. An undesirable outcome is that these adults become controlling, intrusive, and didactic. The second possibility relates to "learned helplessness." Because children experience difficulty in communicating their increasingly complex ideas and needs, some learn to be helpless. Learned helplessness is signaled by failure to initiate conversation and an inability to recognize that actions or remarks produce outcomes. Some adults respond to learned helplessness by taking control. In effect, they become the "chief" and the child becomes the "junior partner" in conversational interchanges.

Signs of over-controlling conversations include the following:

- A preponderance of your utterances are questions.
- Your child's reactions have little impact on what you say next.
- You label one object after another.
- You often correct your child's speech production and language and ask your child to imitate your model.
- You often change the topic of conversation.

Table 17–5. Examples of dialog in which an adult employed over-controlling behaviors during a conversation with a hard-of-hearing child.

Example 1

Child: "I read my book."

Adult: "Susan was looking for you."

Comment: Adults who over-control conversation often change the topic of conversation. For instance, an adult may not respond to a child's previous remark or attend to the child's focus of attention. When this happens frequently in the course of a conversation, the adult often becomes the "chief" and the child becomes a "junior partner" in the conversational interchange (Fey, Warr-Leeper, Webber, & Disher, 1988). In this interchange, the adult might have responded to the child's remark with, "We'll have to go to the library for another one." Such an acknowledgment might have opened the door for a discussion about what books to check out next.

Example 2

Child: "Red cup full."

Mother (originally responded): "Tom, say, "My cup is full.'"

Comment: Adults may over-control conversations when they too frequently correct a child's speech production and language. With her remark, the mother above is no longer conversing with her child, she is giving a language lesson. If corrections occur too frequently, children may become frustrated and may begin to ignore the conversational partner and withdraw from the conversation.

Example 1

Father: "What's in the bag?"

Daughter: "My papers."

Father: "Where did you get the bag?"

Daughter: "School."

Father: "What's that on it?"

Daughter: "My name."

Comment: In this conversation, the father was in complete control. He asked a rapid succession of questions while his daughter passively responded with one word answers. The answer to one question did not influence what the father said next. For instance, he would probably have asked, "What's that on it?" regardless of how his daughter had answered his previous question, "Where did you get the bag?" If he would have commented instead, "Your papers! You must have worked hard today," the daughter might have taken charge and told her father about her school work. In short, she may have become an active conversational partner, and spoken longer utterances.

Over-controlling conversational partners tend to ask an excessive number of questions. Although questions can be useful tools when starting a conversation, and even maintaining it, a string of questions can squelch a child's active participation. A child will more likely participate in a conversation if an adult makes comments and acknowledgments, in addition to asking questions. When making a comment, an adult introduces new information or new ideas. In making an acknowledgment, the adult acknowledges that she or he is paying attention (see Table 17-5).

Excessive labeling can be another sign of over-controlling a conversation. For instance, in a play session videotaped in our laboratory, a mother named every object on the table as she ate a snack with her child. She said, "Pickle. Green pickle. Sour pickle." When the child reached for a knife, she said, "Knife. Red knife," and then added, "Sandwich. Peanut butter sandwich." She rarely spoke a complete sentence. This excessive labeling probably stemmed from the mother's awareness of her son's limited vocabulary; he may understand only simple noun phrases. However, naming items, one after another, does not encourage the child to participate in conversation. He can only acknowledge that he recognizes the labels.

Another mother videotaped in our laboratory, and who communicated with her child with simultaneous communication, also labeled excessively when interacting with her son. In her case, she seemed to limit what she said so that her words matched her relatively limited sign vocabulary. Following is an excerpt from one interaction:

Mother: (Holds up a man made out of play dough). "A man."

Son: (Laughs.)

Mother: "A man. Pretty? Or funny? Which one?"

Son: "Huh?"

Mother: "Pretty man? Or funny man?"

Son: "Pretty."

This conversation would probably seem strange to a child who has normal hearing, and it probably seemed a little strange to this son who has hearing loss. The child's mother might have been a more effective conversational partner if she had used only speech when she did not know the signs. Then she would not have limited her conversation to a small set of noun and adjective labels.

Adults may over-control their conversations when they too frequently correct the child's speech production and language. For instance, one child we videotaped excitedly told his mother, "Blue car off." The mother immediately responded, "Kevin, say, 'The blue car fell off the table.'" With this remark, the mother took control of the conversation: The boy was no longer telling his story, the mother was giving a language lesson. Asking a child to imitate an adult model repeatedly may not only inhibit conversational dynamics and destroy spontaneity, it also may not be an effective way to nurture a child's language (and speech) development. The child may become frustrated or begin to ignore the adult. The child most likely will not remember the adult's corrections beyond the moment.

Finally, adults who over-control conversations sometimes change the topic of conversation with great frequency. One reason for this is due to the child's limited expressive skills. Adults change the topic of conversation to converse about something the adult can follow while the child talks or signs. This behavior is one reason adults often ask a lot of questions—they can reduce uncertainty by limiting the child's responses. Sometimes adults are insensitive to how quickly their children can process what they say, or how quickly they can absorb new information. Even children with normal hearing cannot switch from one topic of discussion to another quickly. When a hearing loss is present, children need even more time to make the transition from one topic to the next. Additional examples of over controlling conversations are presented in Figure 17-13, along with alternative versions.

Summary of Guidelines for Promoting Conversational Interactions

The six guidelines for promoting conversational interactions are simple to follow. In summary, adults might allow their children to select what to talk about, either by listening to their children or by attending to the children's focus of attention. They may model how to tell narratives and ask their children to tell them stories, encouraging them to follow a clear progression from beginning, to

Example 1

Child: "I read my book."

Adult (originally responded): "Susan was looking for you."

Adult (revised statement where adult does not change the topic of conversation): "We'll have to go to the library for another book."

Example 2

Adult: "Who was at the playground?"

Child: "Bob."

Adult (originally said): "When did you get home?"

Adult (revised statement where the adult is influenced by the child's response to her question, and does not ask another question): "I bet you two had fun."

Example 3

Child: "Red cup full."

Adult (originally responded): "Tom, say, 'My cup is full.'"

Adult (revised statement where the adult does not correct Tom's language, and expands on language): "So, your red cup is full! I'll stop pouring."

FIGURE 17-13. Examples of over-controlling conversations and alternative remarks.

middle, to end. Finally, effective conversational partners can learn to speak with organized messages and not over-control their conversations. As with the language techniques we just considered, you might present these strategies first with formal instruction, then guided practice, and finally, real-world instruction.

▬ PARENTAL USE OF REPAIR STRATEGIES

To have a successful conversation with their children, parents should be able to repair breakdowns in communication. Part of an aural rehabilitation plan for a child also may include providing training to parents about the use of repair strategies, both expressive and receptive. Repairing breakdowns in communication requires effort and patience on the part of conversational partners. However, the effective use of repair strategies can promote successful conversational interactions and lead to rewarding interchanges.

In Chapter 2, it was suggested that repair strategies provide explicit instruction to the communication partner (in the context of this chapter, a child) about what to do immediately following a communication breakdown. An expressive repair strategy can be used by an adult when the child has not understood the adult's message. A receptive repair strategy can be used when a parent does not understand something a child has said (or signed). In this section, we consider expressive and receptive repair strategies.

Expressive Repair Strategies

Communication breakdowns during conversation should never be considered the "fault" of either an adult or the child. However, adults can minimize the likelihood of communication breakdowns by considering their child's needs and abilities as they formulate their messages. A parent might ask him- or herself, "What are my child's cognitive abilities?" or "Does my child have the appropriate background knowledge and language level to understand this message?" The parent might attend to the child's emotional state (e.g., Is my child relaxed, angry, or tired?), and consider whether a message is supported by either linguistic or physical context. For example, does their message introduce a new topic? Is it supported by something concrete in the room? Finally, parents can ensure their child is aware of the *who* and the *what* of the message and ensure their messages are appropriate both for the child's linguistic sophistication and his or her communication mode.

During the initial phase of a communication strategies training program, you might want to discuss how parents know when their child does not recognize a message. A clinician will often emphasize that children with hearing impairment often respond just like children with normal hearing when they do not understand a message (Table 17-6). Children may appear inattentive, they may smile or respond inappropriately, or they may bluff

Table 17-6. Means by which children may signal a communication breakdown.

Children may demonstrate:

- Confused facial expressions
- Inattentiveness
- Disinterest
- Frustration
- Inappropriate responses
- Bluffing
- Use of verbal prompts ("What?" "Huh?")
- Body gestures (shoulder shrug; raised hands)
- Hesitation
- Smiling

---

and pretend to understand. In most cases (but not necessarily all), parents will want to respond to these signals of communication breakdown by using any one of the expressive repair strategies presented in Table 17-7.

REPEAT STRATEGY

When using the *repeat* repair strategy, parents simply repeat their original message, as in this interchange:

Parent:	"What did you do with your backpack?"
Child:	"Huh?"
Parent:	"What did you do with your backpack?"

Repeating a message might help a child recognize it; if he or she did not grasp it the first time around, hearing it a second time might be helpful. However, research suggests that other repair strategies may be more helpful, especially when several interchanges must occur before the child recognizes the parent's message.

REPHRASE STRATEGY

Perhaps one of the most remarkable aspects of human language is that we can say almost the same thing in many different ways. For

Table 17-7. Expressive repair strategies parents may use when their child does not recognize their message and examples of each.

Expressive Repair Strategies for Parents:

Repeat

Original sentence: *How are you?*

Repair strategy: *How are you?*

Rephrase

A. Substitute less visible words with more visible words.

B. Substitute words that are better specified by context.

C. Change sentence structure.
   Original sentence: *My soda can is on the table.*
   Repair strategy: *My pop is over there.*

Simplify

A. Use fewer words.

B. Use more commonplace words.

C. Use two sentences.
   Original sentence: *The yellow carton is in the closet.*
   Repair strategy: *The box is in the closet.*

Elaborate

A. Provide more information.

B. Repeat important keywords.
   Original sentence: *Marla called to ask about school.*
   Repair strategy: *Marla telephoned. Marla asked about school.*

Say a key word

Original sentence: *The kids are playing soccer.*

Repair strategy: Kids. *The kids are playing soccer.*

Choice-question (present a closed response set)

Original sentence: *Who was at the party?*

Repair strategy: *Was the whole class at the party?*

Build-from-the-known

Original sentence: *Take the lamp into the dining room.*

Repair strategy: *Here's the lamp. There's the dining room. Take the lamp into the dining room.*

Provide feedback

Original sentence: *Bring me the glove.*

Repair strategy: *Not the mug, the glove.*

example, the phrases, *Come to dinner, Time for supper,* and *Let's eat now* are equally effective in expressing the fact that it is time for a meal. Adults can exploit this characteristic of language to repair breakdowns in communication.

There are at least three ways to rephrase a message that has been misunderstood. The first way is to say words that are more visible on the face so the message is easier for the child to speechread. As we learned in Chapter 9, words that are visible on the face begin with sounds made with the lips pressed together (/p, b, m, w/), the upper lip pressing the lower teeth (/f, v/), or the tongue tip pressing the upper teeth (/θ/). Sounds that are not very visible on the face include sounds made within the mouth, such as /k, g, t, n, d/. So, instead of saying, "Good," you might say "Fine." Instead of saying "Carrot," you might say "Vegetable."

A second way to rephrase a message is to use words better specified by context. For instance, the sentence, *The SUV is in the driveway* may be easier to speechread than the sentence, *The car is in the driveway,* if the child sees there is a sports utility vehicle parked in the driveway.

A third way to rephrase a message is to use different sentence structure. For instance, *Let's go,* might be restructured to, *We should go.*

SIMPLIFY AND REDUCE STRATEGY

Message simplification may be accomplished by using more commonplace words, as in the following example:

Mrs. Linder: "I need some detergent."

Chris: "What?"

Mrs. Linder: "I need some soap."

When her son did not understand her message, Mrs. Linder substituted the more commonplace word *soap* for the less commonplace word *detergent.* Chris is more familiar with this word, and thus, more likely to recognize it. Table 17-8 presents other examples of substituting a less commonplace word with a more commonplace word.

Table 17-8. Words that can be substituted by more commonplace words when using a simplify repair strategy.

ORIGINAL WORD	SUBSTITUTED WORD
Jet	Plane
Sandals	Shoes
Navy (the color)	Blue
Ballet	Dance
Rose	Flower
Yacht	Boat
Cattle	Cows
Hornet	Bee
Briefcase	Bag
Market	Store

ELABORATE STRATEGY

When elaborating a message, key words are repeated more than once or additional information is provided. A mother might say, "Your book bag is hanging on the hook." When her daughter flashes her a confused look, she might elaborate by saying, "I carried your book bag to the garage. The book bag is hanging on a hook in the garage." In this instance, she repeated the key word, *book bag,* and she provided a little more information (i.e., the fact that she was the person who took the book bag to the garage).

REPEAT A KEY WORD STRATEGY

Repeating a key word establishes the topic of conversation and provides a context for recognizing subsequent words. This strategy is particularly effective in repairing breakdowns in communication if the talker has just changed the topic of conversation because the key word helps the child change his or her mind set (i.e., "I've got to think about something different now.") For example, an adult may initially say, "Let's ride our bikes in the park." When the young conversational partner cocks his head, the adult may indicate the topic of conversation. "Bikes," the adult might say. "Let's ride our bikes."

CHOICE-QUESTION STRATEGY

The choice-question repair strategy is effective when a child has not recognized a question. In the following example, a speech-language pathologist uses the choice-question repair strategy:

Speech-language pathologist:	"Which sticker do you want for your book?"
Sarah:	"Huh?"
Speech-language pathologist:	"Do you want a pony or a kitten sticker?"
Sarah:	"Pony."

The speech-language pathologist limited Sarah's responses to a closed set, a pony sticker or a kitten sticker. By using the choice-question repair strategy, she helped Sarah understand the question, and Sarah then responded to the message.

When using the choice-question repair strategy, it is important not to limit the child's response to either *yes* or *no* because the child then has an opportunity to bluff. For instance, the speech-language pathologist might have said, "Do you want the pony sticker?" Sarah then may have nodded her head, even if she did not understand the question, thereby creating the illusion of communication breakdown repair.

BUILD-FROM-THE-KNOWN STRATEGY

When building from the known, the adult starts with something the child knows or understands and then builds on that knowledge base. In the following example, Shane does not know the meaning of the word, *horizon.* As his father uses the build-from-the-known repair strategy, he also defines the meaning of the word. As such, this strategy is effective not only in repairing a communication breakdown, but also in expanding language.

Father:	"I see the boat on the horizon."
Shane:	"What?"
Father:	"There's a boat. The boat is far away. The boat is on the horizon."

PROVIDE FEEDBACK STRATEGY

The last expressive repair strategy is providing feedback. When a child indicates what part of the message he or she recognizes, the conversational partner provides feedback as to whether the child has recognized it correctly. A parent might say, "Give me the chocolate chip cookie. When the child points to a frosted cookie on the dessert tray, the parent might respond, "Not that one. I want the other cookie." The feedback repair strategy lets the child know whether he or she is on the right track in recognizing a message. It also lets the child know the adult is interested in making sure the message was recognized correctly.

Examples of each expressive repair strategy appear in Table 17-7.

Questions Parents Often Ask About Using Expressive Repair Strategies

1. What should I do if my child listens to only half of what I say before he starts to respond or he stops paying attention before I am through delivering my message?

Response: Indicate the length of your message, and use hand gestures to indicate where you are in the message as you deliver it. For instance, you might say, "There are three things we can do. (Holding up one finger) First, we can . . . (Holding up two fingers) Second, we can . . . This prepares the child for the length of the message and lets the youngster know where you are in your delivery.

Do not lecture or admonish your child. This certainly is not going to encourage a child to attend, nor will insisting that the child pay attention when he or she would rather be doing something else.

2. Which repair strategies should I use?

Response: No one repair strategy is appropriate for every situation. Usually a mixture of repair strategies is most effective. Your choice of repair strategies will depend in part on the age of your child and in part on your personal conversational style. For instance, elaborating a message may not be appropriate when the child is under 4 years of age. You may experi-

(continues)

ence problems rephrasing a message, so for *you*, repeating important key words might be a better repair strategy to use than the rephrase repair strategy.

Receptive Repair Strategies for Parents

Parents or guardians may tell you they feel comfortable in repairing communication breakdowns when their child does not understand something they say. The true difficulties arise when they do not understand their child's messages. In fact, the most valuable component of a communication strategies training program designed for parents may well be the component that deals with the use of receptive repair strategies.

Did You Say . . . ?

When you restate a message, you demonstrate that you are at least trying to understand it. You also provide a child with important information. By knowing what you recognized, the child can better supply the missing information. You might ask, "Did you say Jean is at the door?" The child can then indicate whether you have understood the message correctly. If you do not have a clue about what your child is talking about, you can focus on the child's nonverbal cues. For instance, if he or she talks quickly and with great animation, you might say, "You seem excited. Am I right?" In this instance, you have observed that something exciting has happened. Pinning a name to an emotional state not only helps to rectify breakdowns in communication, it also demonstrates that you recognize the child's feelings and that you have comprehended the nonverbal message. This can be a source of encouragement for the child to try to repair the communication breakdown.

When discussing receptive repair strategies with parents, it is again important to stress that communication breakdown is not the "fault" of either the parent or the child (e.g., "I wish I was better able to guess what my child means" or "I wish my child had better language"). However, parents can minimize difficulties by focusing attention on their children as they present a message, by paying attention to children's body movements and environmental and contextual clues and by relying on stored information about the conversational topic and their children.

REPEAT STRATEGY

Receptive repair strategies that might be reviewed during a communication strategies training program are outlined in Table 17-9. The first strategy is the *repeat* repair strategy. The adult asks the child to present the message again. Parents should be encouraged to use this strategy sparingly. If a parent continually asks, "What?" or says, "Tell me again," the child may become frustrated and simply say, "Never mind."

Table 17-9. Receptive repair strategies parents may use when they do not recognize their child's message.

Receptive Repair Strategies for Parents

Repeat: Ask the child to repeat the message.

Examples: *Tell me again.*

What did you say?

Repeat that please.

Tell me more: Encourage the child to provide more information.

Examples: *When did this happen?*

What happened next?

How do you feel about this?

Did you say . . . ?: Restate what they might have said.

Examples: *Did you say?*

I think you said. . . .

You seem excited. Am I right?

Tell me in a different way: Ask the child to change the delivery of the message.

Examples: *Show me.*

Please look at me so I can see your face.

Can you slow down a little?

TELL-ME-MORE STRATEGY

When using the tell-me-more strategy, the next strategy listed in Table 17-9, parents encourage their children to provide additional information, as in this example:

Child:	"Dana took dog boom."
Parent:	"When did she do that?"
Child:	"In there. It's mine!"
Parent:	"She has it now?"
Child:	"Yeah."

By using the tell-me-more receptive repair strategy, the parent gradually sorted out the problem by probing for more information.

DID YOU SAY . . . ? STRATEGY

A third receptive repair strategy is for adults to restate what they think they hear. When they restate a message, they are demonstrating that at least they are *trying* to understand it. Also, by knowing what the adult understood, the child can better provide the missing information. An adult might ask, "Did you say that Jean is here?" The child can then indicate whether the adult understood the message correctly.

If an adult has no clue what a child is talking about, then the adult can focus on the child's nonverbal cues. For instance, if a young boy talks slowly and with little energy, his mother might say, "You seem tired. Am I right?" In this instance, the mother has observed that the child feels sluggish. Pinning a name to an emotional and physical state not only helps rectify breakdowns in communication, it also demonstrates that the adult recognizes the child's feelings, and that the adult feels empathetic with them. Naming also teaches the child to identify his or her own emotions and helps the child acquire a vocabulary to describe them. Other ways to restate what a child has said include the following:

- "Did you say . . . ?"
- "I think you said . . . ."
- "You seem angry. Am I right?"

- "Let me see if I understand. You did . . . .
  Your sister did . . . ."
- (Repeat what you believe the child said, using rising intonation) "You dropped your books?"

TELL ME IN A DIFFERENT WAY STRATEGY

Finally, conversational partners can ask children to alter their delivery of messages. They may ask older children to write their messages down. They can ask younger children to draw a picture or act out what they mean.

Questions Parents Often Ask About Using Receptive Repair Strategies

1. How can I encourage family members and strangers to use receptive repair strategies with my child?

Response: Relatives and strangers often do not know what to do when they cannot recognize the speech of a child who has a hearing impairment. Sometimes they pretend to understand. Alternatively, they may begin to address all of their remarks to you, and expect you to act as a go-between. Sometimes you can instruct relatives about how to use receptive repair strategies, although this is not always possible or successful. The most straightforward way to handle this problem is to teach children to repair breakdowns in communication themselves. Children must learn to take social responsibility for signaling the occurrence of breakdowns and develop effective skills to rectify them.

2. Should I try to understand everything my child says?

Response: Quite simply, the answer to this question is *no.* Excessive use of receptive repair strategies may lead to your overcontrolling the conversation. When interacting with a child who has a significant hearing impairment, you must be willing to conjecture and accept ambiguity, and occasionally endure puzzlement about what your child is attempting to express. If you halt the conversation too many times to confirm a message, your child may become increasingly passive and withdrawn from the conversational interchange. Rely on intelligent guessing sometimes, and allow the child to have some unhindered turns in a conversation before you intervene to confirm the child's message.

There is a potential danger in providing language and conversation training to parents and guardians, and a case study that we consider in this section reveals it. Sometimes adults become so wrapped up in their role as language teacher and conversational partner that they lose sight of their role as parent and caretaker. They may experience difficulty in relaxing and may begin to feel their child's successes will only be realized through their own unrelenting efforts as a teacher. Luterman (1987, p. 17) presents a poignant example from an interview with a set of parents from his case load, who are reminiscing about their experiences with raising a child who had a significant hearing loss:

> Mother: "The one thing we didn't do was live in the present. That was one thing we didn't do enough of. There was always one more goal, one more word to be learned. There was always so much to be done."

> Father: "The goals drove us. We accepted our roles and we lost a lot of fun. We treated it as work. You know it was an unending job. It wasn't any eight to five. We were instructing the kid twenty-four hours a day. And, you could run yourself out of energy."

Two parents from our case load, Mrs. Summerwell and Mrs. Thomas were both mothers of 4-year-old children at the time we knew them. Both parents were keen to provide a good language model for their children and to promote conversational competency. Although both mothers used many of the language and conversation stimulating techniques described in this chapter, one mother could not relax when she interacted with her daughter, and thus, realized less success in promoting conversation (and also, in reaping the rewards of a comfortable mother-daughter relationship). Prior to the videotape session summarized here, she

(continues)

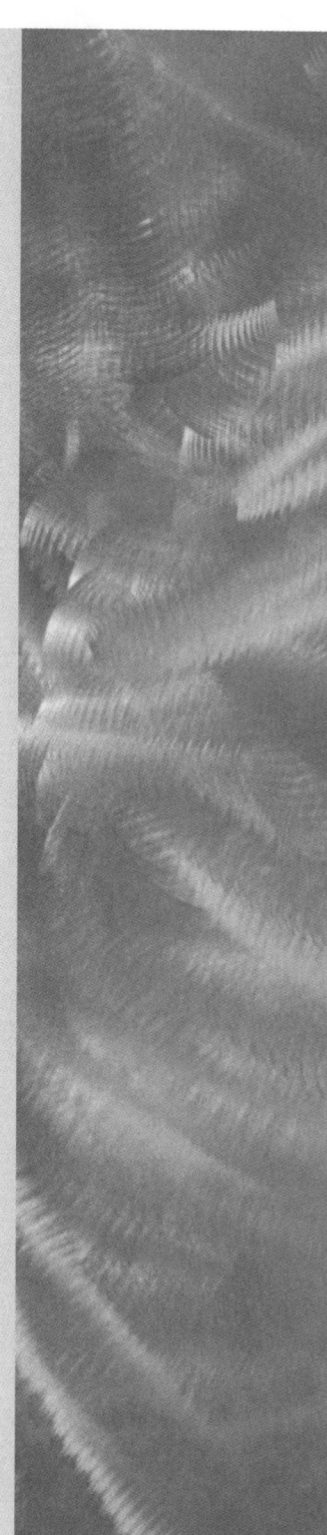

made the off-the-cuff comment, "I used to be a happy-go-lucky person before Julie was born. Now I am wound up all the time." Indeed, Mrs. Summerwell did seem anxious and tense. In the play session we videotaped, we asked her to make shapes with play dough along with her daughter Julie.

Mrs. Summerwell first formed an "O" with a lump of the play dough and held it up to her mouth and said, "Oh, oh, oh." She then shaped an "E", and said, "Eeeeeee, eeee, eeee." She banged the play knife against the table and said, "Tap, tap, tap. Listen, tap, tap, tap." She labeled everything: "Julie, here's a can; box, here's the box; Look! A French fry. Here's a French fry!" The frenetic activity continued for 20 minutes. During this time, Julie became reluctant to look at her mother. Throughout their play session, Mrs. Summerwell never relaxed, and little Julie sensed this.

In contrast to Mrs. Summerwell, Mrs. Thomas is a case study of a parent who presented a more relaxed model of a conversational partner. In the same type of videotaped play session, Mrs. Thomas formed an "O" with a lump of play dough. When her son seemed uninterested, this mother surprised him by hanging the play dough "O" on the end of her nose and then pretended it was not there. In other words, she relaxed and had fun.

Providing language stimulation and appropriate conversational models is important, and it is encouraging when adults can do this occasionally within the context of children's daily routine. However, when taken to the extreme, children can begin to feel their days are a never-ending lesson or test session. Sometimes children shut down. They become reluctant to make eye contact, and they do not attend to a person who is talking, because the person is probably trying to teach or test them. Parents' over-responding to their children's efforts to converse may actually serve to discourage communication. For example, at one point in the play session described previously, Mrs. Summerwell exclaimed, "Yes, Julie! Blue, that's blue! You said blue!" when Julie pointed to a lump of blue play dough and said,

(continues)

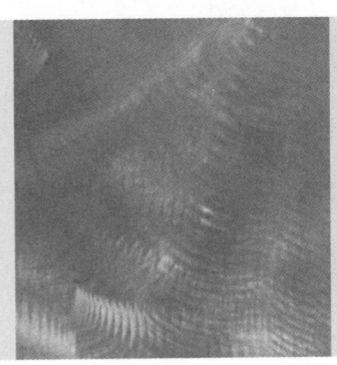

"Blu-uuue." This overblown response suggested that Mrs. Summerwell expected less, and so Julie might provide less the next time.

When encouraging parents and guardians to stimulate language growth and conversation, never lose sight of the importance of parent and child playing simply for the sake of having fun and enjoying each other's company.

FINAL REMARKS

In this chapter, we have just scratched the surface of ways parents can promote language and conversational skills in their children. We have considered how adults can communicate so children will attend to what they say, and how they may listen and respond so children will want to communicate and be able to communicate. The discussion has been confined to language and the mechanics of conversation. However, to converse effectively and to learn language, children must also have world knowledge. Some children experience difficulty when engaging in conversations because they lack a base of information about the world and about how people function in the world. This reduced knowledge base limits what they can understand and what they can talk about. Gfeller and Schum (1994) presented a program that describes how parents and other adults in a child's life can facilitate the acquisition of general world information, as well as information about the community, family culture, and the mass media.

Family Dynamics

A parent-centered program may touch on the subject of discipline and the hard-of-hearing child. Families often need understanding and support from a clinician, and this requires that the clinician understands the dynamics of the family. Sometimes, the following family dynamics may be in place:

Regardless of the cause of the child's hearing loss, parents find themselves needing to give the deaf child much of their

(continues)

time and attention. Siblings become aware of this inequity and often feel resentful and jealous of their hearing-impaired sibling. There is a great variability in how parents interact with their deaf child. Some parents state they have the same expectations in terms of behavior and achievement for both their deaf and hearing children. They set limits and enforce consequences for inappropriate behavior; many parents have difficulty in achieving this. Two factors get in the way. Foremost is communication. It is often easier for the parent to do the task than to spend the time getting the child's attention and making sure the task is understood and then completed. Less obvious are the emotions the parents have toward the child. The parent may feel as though the child has suffered enough and places less demands on the child. The child gets out of doing what siblings are expected to do. This often affects the personality of the child, who may grow up always expecting special treatment. (Kravitz & Selekman, 1992, p. 593)

KEY CHAPTER POINTS

✔ Parents and caregivers can use a variety of techniques to promote language growth. These include modeling and expansion, parallel talk, question simulation, time-talk, labeling, and reading.

✔ Questions should be asked judiciously. An ineffective use of questions can lead to adults over-controlling their conversations with children.

✔ An adult who engages effectively in self-talk and describing while interacting with a child often capitalizes on something that is happening in the environment, using vocabulary and language that is slightly more complex than a child's current language level.

✔ Some of the benefits of using modeling techniques are that a child's message is reinforced, new language structures are introduced or expanded, and the child has an opportunity to imitate a correct model.

✔ There are many ways to maximize the benefits of reading to a child, including the techniques of making predictions, talking about the story after reading it, and re-reading.

✔ Instruction for parents and guardians may be either less structured or more structured.

✔ Enjoyable conversational interactions are some of the most effective means to promote language growth in children. Parents and caregivers can learn techniques that will facilitate conversation. These techniques include responding to communicative intents and avoiding the use of critical or negative language.

✔ Clear speech is characterized by somewhat slowed speaking rate and precise enunciation.

✔ Parents can learn to use expressive and receptive repair strategies to rectify communication breakdowns.

MULTIPLE CHOICE QUESTIONS

1. Tommy Eiten says, "Car." His mother says, "The car goes around." Her remark is best described as an example of:
   a. Modeling and expansion
   b. Parallel talk
   c. Signaling expectation
   d. Self-talk

2. Which of the following is not true about question stimulation?
   a. It stimulates language growth.
   b. It is symptomatic of parents losing control of a conversation.
   c. It may provide a springboard for conversation.
   d. It can stifle conversation.

3. When we engage in conversation, we share past experiences, we describe something, or we provide explanations. For this reason, children should be encouraged to:
   a. Tell narratives
   b. Memorize story passages
   c. Watch television
   d. Follow directions

4. One common reason parents might over-control conversations is that:

    a. They enjoy playing the role of "chief" to their child's role of "junior partner."

    b. They know what information they want to know, so they ask too many questions.

    c. Their children have developed "learned-helplessness."

    d. They believe children should learn the names of the objects in their environment.

5. Guided learning is a component of:

    a. Parallel talk

    b. Formal instruction

    c. Language stimulation

    d. Conversational modeling

6. Clear speech is:

    a. How most people talk when telling a narrative

    b. Characterized by unambiguous language

    c. Characterized by precise enunciation and the prolongation of some sounds

    d. The name of a speech-language therapy intervention program

7. One way to use the Elaborate repair strategy is to:

    a. Use more commonplace words

    b. Break a long sentence into two short sentences

    c. Repeat important keywords, while providing more information

    d. Speak a keyword

8. You say, "The cattle are in the barn." Your child shrugs and shakes his head. You then say, "The cows are in the barn." This repair strategy is an example of:

    a. Keyword

    b. Simplification

    c. Building-from-the-known

    d. Repeat

9. An effective conversational strategy adults can use when talking to children, and one that promotes language development is to:

   a. Correct language errors

   b. Treat the child as a phantom conversational partner in instances where the child has minimal language and speech

   c. Change the topic of conversation to one that is familiar

   d. Limit language and vocabulary to structures and words known to be familiar to the child

10. One danger in providing instruction to parents and guardians about how to stimulate language and conversation is:

   a. They may begin to experience difficulty in relaxing when interacting with their child.

   b. They might assume they are the experts in the area of speech and language development in their child.

   c. They may exhibit signs of "learned-helplessness."

   d. They might lose their confidence in their own judgment as parents.

KEY RESOURCES

Asking Questions

Although questions can be useful tools in promoting questions, a string of questions can squelch a child's active participation in a conversation. A child will more likely participate in a conversation if an adult makes comments and acknowledgments in addition to asking questions. When making a comment, the adult introduces new information or new ideas. In making an acknowledgment, the adult acknowledges that he or she is paying attention and understands what the child is saying. Ways to ask questions effectively include the five guidelines listed next. An aural-rehabilitation specialist might review these guidelines with parents, and provide examples during a discussion about how to foster a child's language growth through conversation.

1. **Do not ask questions with a right answer in mind.** Be willing to accept a variety of responses. If you are willing only to accept

a particular response, your child will perceive you have a blueprint for the conversation in mind, and the child's task is to identify and follow it.

2. **If you are asking a series of questions, allow your next question to be influenced by the child's response to a previous question.** Children must know you are listening to what they have to say and that they are helping direct the conversation. In short, your next question should be contingent on your child's response to your previous question.

3. **Do not be in a hurry to answer your own questions.** A child needs time to recognize your words and to formulate a reply. Be patient in waiting for a response. Avoid asking questions in this way: "Who gave you the Valentine's card? I bet Susan gave it to you."

4. **Do not limit your questions to those that can be answered with a yes-no response.** *Yes-no* questions require minimal involvement on a child's part. *Wh-questions* (who, what, where, when, why) are more likely to result in a child's active participation in the conversation. If you use a *yes-no* question, try pairing it with a *wh-question*. For example, "What did you do today? (pause, and if no response) Did you have gym class?"

5. **Avoid asking rote questions that require a pat response.** A child should have an opportunity to provide a response that develops the conversation. Do not ask questions in this way: "You went to the movie? Did you see the big screen? Was the room dark?" The answer is "Of course!" to all three questions.

Research supports this discussion. A group of investigators analyzed conversational interactions between 16 elementary school teachers and their deaf students (Wood, Wood, Griffiths, Howarth, & Howarth, 1986). They transcribed every word a teacher and student said during a conversation (they used oral/aural communication) and then coded their utterances. When the teachers asked questions, students usually answered them and then stopped. Only for 14% of the questions did children elaborate their responses, and they rarely initiated additional conversation. The fewer the questions asked by a teacher during a conversation, the more likely a child was to elaborate an answer and to speak in longer utterances throughout the conversation. In short, children talked more when their teachers questioned less. A general rule that may be useful is this:

Questions should not be avoided entirely. They should be integrated into the conversation with other comments and acknowledgments and used occasionally for modeling purposes.

Transcripts for Instructing Adults About Language-Stimulation Techniques

Technique: Describing

Child:	(picking up toy car) "My."
Adult:	"You are picking up your car."
Child:	"Car."
Adult:	"That's a race car."
Child:	(pushes car along the floor)
Adult:	"See how fast the car goes. Look, it hit the chair!"

Technique: Self-talk (providing an ongoing commentary)

Adult:	"I am looking for my keys. Hmmm, I thought I put them in my purse. No, they are not here. Maybe they are in the drawer. I will open it. Yes, here they are. Phew, I am relieved to find them."

Technique: Modeling and Expansion

Child:	"Bowl."
Adult:	"You want a cereal bowl. Here it is."
Child:	"Dah."
Adult:	"Pudding. Let's put the pudding in the bowl."

Technique: Parallel talk

Child:	(Playing with bean-bag stuffed animals)
Adult:	"The tiger is hiding under the box. I wonder who he is hiding from."
Child:	(Moves toy cat toward box)
Adult:	"The cat is looking for the tiger. Maybe they are playing hide-and-seek."
Child:	(Throws box off toy tiger)
Adult:	"He found him! The cat found the tiger."

Technique: Question stimulation (question-stimulation phrases are in italics)

Child:	"Dah?"
Adult:	"Do you want the cookie?"
Child:	"My cookie."
Adult:	"No, that's not your cookie. *Whose cookie is this? Whose cookie?*"
Child:	"Who cookie?"
Adult:	"That's Daddy's cookie."

Technique: Time-talk (time-related words are in italics)

Adult:	(looking at scrap book) "Here are the new pictures. Here is a picture of our jack-o-lantern."
Child:	"Halloween."
Adult:	"Yes, Halloween was *last week*. We made a jack-o-lantern."
Child:	"I want Halloween now."
Adult:	"*Today?* No, we have to *wait a whole year*. Halloween won't come again until *next year*."

Techniques: Labeling

Child:	"Dah."
Adult:	"Crayon."
Child:	"Blue."
Adult:	"Here's the blue crayon."

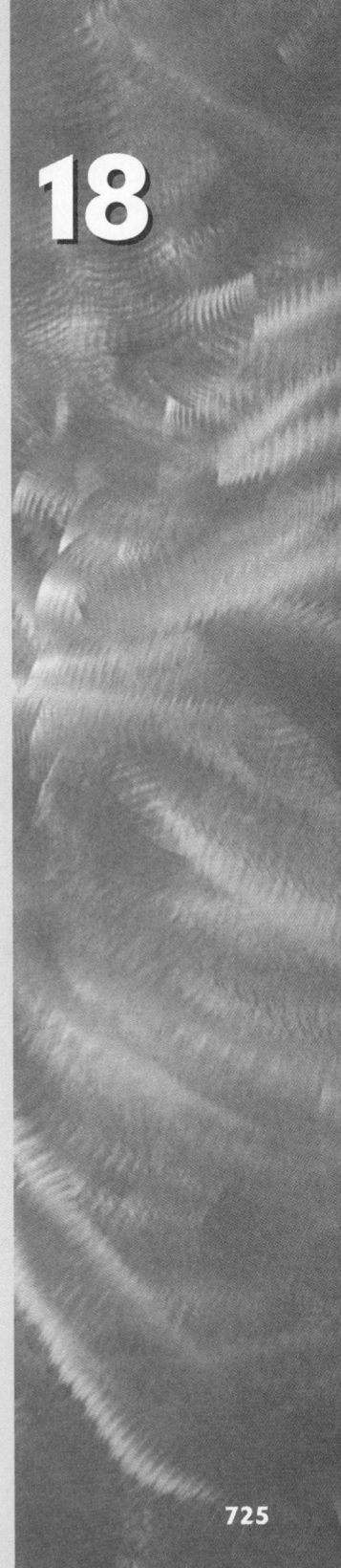

CHAPTER 18

Management of Cochlear Implants in Children[1]

TOPICS

[1]Parts of this chapter are from "Aural Rehabilitation and Patient Management" by N. Tye-Murray, 1993a. In R. S. Tyler (Ed.), *Cochlear Implants: Audiological Foundations* (pp. 87–144). Clifton Park, NY: Delmar Learning.

Children and their families require support and assistance from a variety of professionals before and after the child receives a cochlear implant. In this chapter we consider the support and aural rehabilitation that speech and hearing professionals provide during and following the implantation process.

Who Makes the Decision About Getting a Cochlear Implant?

When the child is very young, the parents are responsible for making the decision as to whether a child will be a candidate for cochlear implantation and receives an implant once the implant team has determined that the child is an appropriate candidate. They also are responsible for ensuring the child uses the cochlear implant following the implantation surgery and ensuring the child receives appropriate aural rehabilitation services. Your role as a speech and hearing professional is to assist in determining whether the child is an appropriate candidate. If candidacy is affirmed, then you may provide additional information and counseling to parents that will assist them in making a decision.

When the child is older, he or she also participates in the decision as to whether to receive a cochlear implant. If the child is a young teenager, careful consideration must be given to the youth's expectations and desires. If the adolescent is not committed to making the cochlear implant a successful endeavor, he or she will not likely receive benefit. Negative peer pressure and a desire to identify with the Deaf Culture are some reasons why older children may not want a cochlear implant. Moreover, a disinterest in acquiring speech and listening skills, and a firm commitment to sign, might dissuade older children and adolescents.

■ OVERVIEW

A cochlear implant service delivery model usually includes seven components. These components are summarized in Table 18-1. They are: initial contact, preimplant counseling, formal evaluation, surgery, fitting, follow-up evaluation, and aural rehabilitation.

Table 18-1. Seven stages of the cochlear implant process and the professionals who may be involved with each stage.

STAGE	PROFESSIONAL(S)	DESCRIPTION
Initial contact	Clinical coordinator	Family receives general information about cochlear implants and candidacy; child may be scheduled for an appointment at the cochlear implant center
Preimplant counseling	Speech and hearing professional (usually an audiologist)	Family and child (and educator) receive specific information about candidacy, benefits, commitments, and costs and are asked to consider such issues as culture and communication mode
Formal evaluation	Audiologist, surgeon, speech-language pathologist, psychologist, educator	Perform medical, hearing, speech, language, and psychological evaluation to determine candidacy, and evaluate the educational environment and adequacy for support of auditory skill development
Surgery	Surgeon	The internal hardware of the cochlear implant is implanted
Fitting/tune-up	Audiologist	The device is fitted on the child and a map is created; parents (and child) receive instruction about care and maintenance
Follow-up	Audiologist and other members of the cochlear implant team	Any problems are explored, and new developments about cochlear implants are reviewed with the family
Aural rehabilitation	Speech and hearing professionals in both the medical and educational centers and educators	The child receives long-term speech perception training and speech and language therapy

The key members of a *cochlear implant team* who interact with the child and family are also indicated for each component. The team minimally is comprised of a clinical coordinator, an audiologist, and a surgeon. It usually includes a speech-language pathologist, a psychologist, an educator or an aural rehabilitation specialist.

Cochlear implant team: key members include an otolaryngologist, audiologist, speech-language pathologist, psychologist, educator, and/or aural rehabilitation specialist.

■ INITIAL CONTACT

The first step toward obtaining a cochlear implant is taken by a child's parents or primary caregivers. They may have read a newspaper article or talked to a speech and hearing professional or teacher and desire more information about cochlear implants and candidacy. The parents may have observed other children in their child's classroom who use cochlear implants and been impressed by their progress. A parent might contact the clinical coordinator at the cochlear implant center and ask questions like those listed in Table 18-2.

The clinical coordinator sends printed materials and schedules an appointment for a preliminary counseling session or formal evaluation. The printed materials may cover the following topics in a cursory fashion: the functions of a cochlear implant, how the cochlear implant differs from a hearing aid, who is a cochlear implant candidate, the reasons why some children may receive more benefit than others, the kinds of benefits that can be expected, and the limitations of a cochlear implant.

Table 18-2. Questions parents may ask during the initial contact.

- Is my child an appropriate candidate?
- How does a cochlear implant work? How does it differ from a hearing aid?
- Will the cochlear implant help my child to talk and hear better?
- Can a cochlear implant electrocute my child? Is it dangerous to use?
- Can my child still play sports if he or she gets one?
- How old does my child need to be?
- Will the cochlear implant lost my child's entire lifetime? What happens if it "wears out"?
- Is the cochlear implant waterproof? Will my child be able to take a bath or shower?
- What happens if my child gets hit in the head?
- How often do the devices break?
- How much do they cost? Will my insurance pay for it?
- What's involved in obtaining a cochlear implant?
- Will my child still need to change communication mode? Is signing allowed with a cochlear implant?
- Will my child have to go to a special school for implanted children?
- Are cochlear implants hard to take care of?

PRELIMINARY COUNSELING

Counseling for the family, and child if he or she is old enough to understand the candidacy process, is critical. If the child is in an educational setting, then the child's teacher is often invited to the preliminary counseling session. The educator should be an integral part in the implant process. The educator can provide information about how the child performs in the school setting and ultimately will play a major role in ensuring the child receives optimal benefit from the device.

The Role of the Educator

Receipt of a cochlear implant is just a first step in an aural rehabilitation plan. Postimplant aural rehabilitation in an educational setting is an important subsequent step.

The educator plays an essential role in maximizing the child's benefits from using a device. The Network of Educators of Children with Cochlear Implants (NECCI), a professional organization of speech and hearing professionals and educators, has created guidelines that delineate the role of the educator in the cochlear implant process (Nevins & Chute, 1996). Some of these guidelines suggest the following.

- An educator who is familiar with aural rehabilitation should be involved in every stage of the cochlear implant process, from preimplant counseling to formal evaluation to follow-up and aural rehabilitation.
- An educator can provide a bridge of communication between the child's family, the cochlear-implant center, and the educational setting. Networking and clear communication among the significant people in a child's life are the most effective means to optimize his or her effective use of the cochlear implant.
- All children who receive a cochlear implant require an intensive and long-term program of aural rehabilitation provided in the context of a child's educational program. The educator must play a primary role in coordinating aural rehabilitation services and in providing speech, language, and listening practice in the context of the classroom routine. (If a commitment to an intensive program of auditory skill development is not in place, then the child likely will receive little benefit from the cochlear implant.)

Counseling provides information about obtaining, maintaining, and using a cochlear implant, and for maximizing its benefits. Counseling is ongoing and occurs throughout the cochlear implant process. At one time or another, every member of the cochlear implant team provides counseling. Whether child and family members are at the stage of determining candidacy or of planning aural rehabilitation, they must be aware of what is happening and what will happen, they must be prepared for a variety of outcomes, and they must feel as if they are contributing to the decisions that concern them.

Although counseling is ongoing, a block of time usually is set aside for preliminary counseling, either before or after the formal evaluation. This counseling session is most often conducted by an audiologist. The topics included in the preliminary counseling session are summarized in Table 18-3. In the following discussion, we consider what a speech and hearing professional might tell the family about each of these topics. Families might be encouraged to visit the Web sites of cochlear implant manufacturers. The Key Resources list addresses.

Audiological and Medical Candidacy Qualifications

The speech and hearing professional reviews audiological and medical candidacy criteria. All children who receive a cochlear implant must have a severe-to-profound bilateral sensorineural hearing loss. They should show limited progress in the development of auditory skills. What constitutes "limited progress" is open to interpretation, and its criteria is dependent on the implant candidate's age and maturity. If a child is able to perform speech tests (which happens at about 4 or 5 years old), then the child will be tested while he or she wears optimally fitted hearing aids. The tests typically include single-word tests, such as the

Table 18-3. Topics that often are reviewed during the preliminary counseling session.

- Audiological and medical candidacy qualifications
- Cochlear implant hardware
- Costs
- Realistic expectations
- Commitments
- Cultural considerations
- Communication mode

Lexical Neighborhood Test (LNT) that we considered in Chapter 6. Children who identify words with greater than 30% accuracy are typically not considered appropriate for receiving a cochlear implant. For younger children unable to perform standardized tests of speech recognition, the evaluation of auditory skills and ability to benefit from the use of hearing aids might be performed through the use of parent questionnaires and more informal measures of speech recognition.

All children should have a trial period with appropriate amplification before being considered as a cochlear implant candidate. This trial period should last 10 weeks or longer to ensure that the cochlear implant is the only viable means of providing usable residual hearing to the child. If the child appears to be acquiring speech and language skills with the use of a hearing aid, then candidacy should be questioned.

The exception to this trial-period policy pertains to the child who has incurred a hearing loss following meningitis. Ossification of the cochlea often occurs after such an infection. If computerized axial tomography (a CAT scan) indicates ossification, then the trial period might be shortened or even bypassed.

The Food and Drug Administration approved the Cochlear Corporation's cochlear implant for implantation in children as young as 12 months of age. The evaluation process may begin before the baby reaches the age of 1 year. (Figure 18-1).

Scientific data show a correlation between duration of deafness and benefit, with children who receive cochlear implants after a short period of deafness performing better on measures of speech perception than those who receive one after a longer period (Tyler, 1993). In addition, researchers have found that children who receive a cochlear implant at a younger age show better development in their speech, language, and listening skills than children who receive a cochlear implant at an older age (e.g., Kileny, Zwolan, & Ashbaugh, 2001; Svirsky, Robbins, Kirk, Pisoni, & Miyamoto, 2000). For these reasons, more children below the age of 2 years are receiving cochlear implants than ever before. An increasingly frequent scenario goes as follows. A baby is identified as having a significant hearing loss during a newborn screening test in the newborn nursery. The hearing loss is confirmed in a subsequent diagnostic session in which an ABR is performed. The

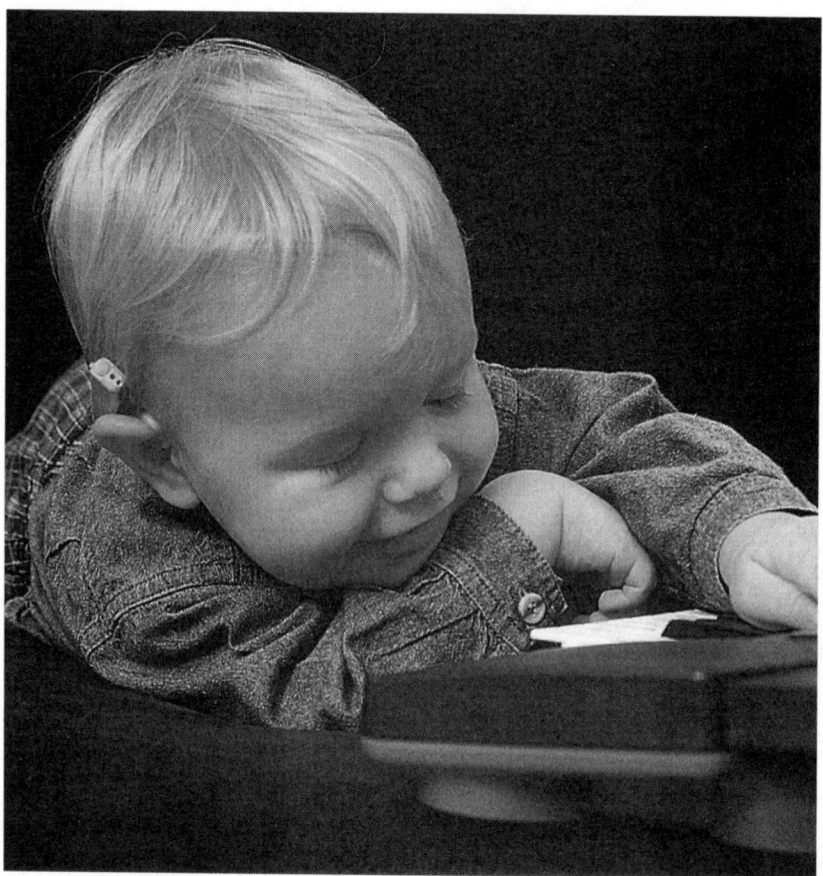

FIGURE 18-1. Research suggests that the younger a child is at the time of implantation, the greater the advantage afforded for speech, language, and auditory development. (Photograph by Med-El, with permission)

baby is fit with hearing aids shortly thereafter and provided with optimal opportunity to develop auditory skills. If the child fails to progress in auditory skills development, then the child receives a cochlear implant at the age of 1 year.

Good general health, no chronic ear disease, and an unobstructed cochlea are often prerequisites for most cochlear implant surgeries. The child should not have recently experienced otitis media or other middle ear pathology. If the hearing loss is related to auditory neuropathy or other lesions of the acoustic nerve or central auditory pathway, implantation typically is not recommended. The presence of other disabilities, such as blindness or mental retardation, may require special consideration but does not necessarily preclude implantation.

In addition to a general physical, the child often receives a head computed tomographic (CT) scan. The CT scan provides a visual scan of the cochlea and reveals any cochlear anomalies or structural features that might preclude or complicate the implanting of an electrode into the spirals of the cochlea. Although children with cochlear malformations have received cochlear implants (Harker, Vanderheiden, Veazey, Gentile, & McCleary, 1999), and have demonstrated benefit, it is optimal that the cochlea be shaped normally for full insertion of the electrode array to occur.

The Cochlear Implant Hardware

A brief overview of the cochlear implant hardware is important so that the family will appreciate what the device will look like, how it will be worn, and what will be involved in maintaining it in good working order. This information can be established with the aid of photographs like that shown in Figure 18-2 and by letting the family and child meet other young cochlear implant users.

When cochlear implants were first approved for children by the Food and Drug Administration (FDA) in 1990, the devices included speech processors about the size of an oversized deck of cards. This speech processor could be worn in a variety of ways, including in a chest harness or a fanny pack. New developments have led to miniaturization of the speech processor, so that most children wear their speech processors behind their ear, in a fashion similar to a behind-the-ear hearing aid (although very young children sometimes use body-worn processors because they are easier to monitor and pose less risk of damage or loss).

Costs and Reimbursements

Costs and reimbursement issues are discussed in great detail prior to implantation. The cochlear implant and surgery are expensive. Costs include coverage for the formal evaluation, hospitalization, surgery; the device itself, fitting, follow-up visits, and aural rehabilitation. The family should expect some expenses related to cochlear implant maintenance annually because problems with

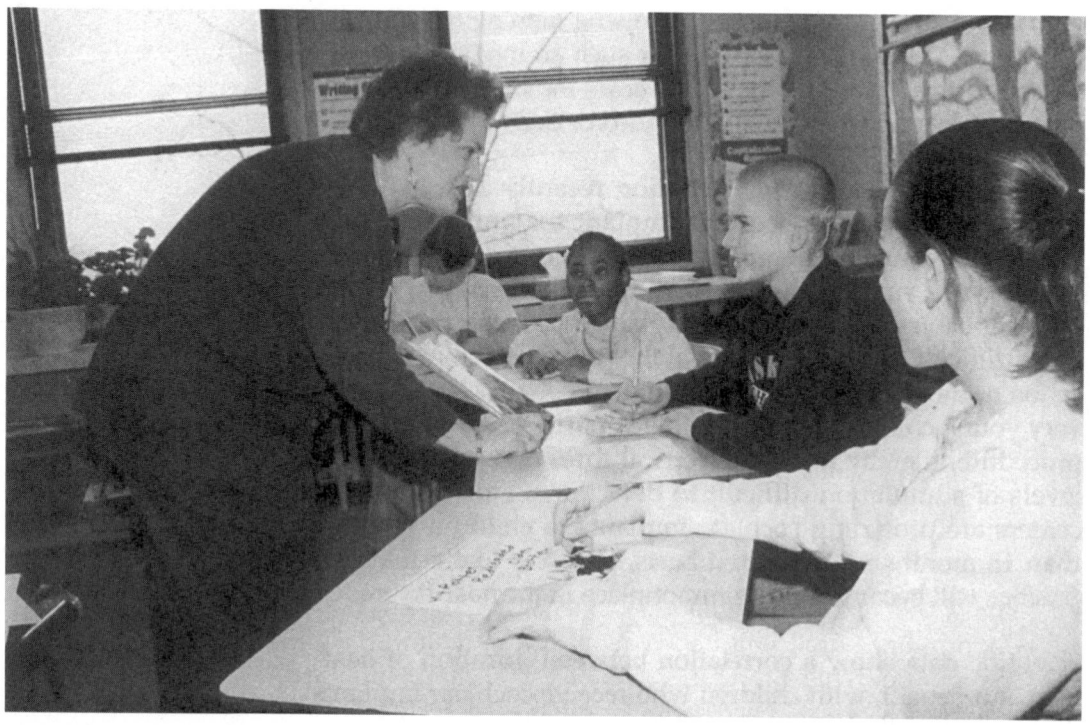

FIGURE 18-2. A child wearing a cochlear implant. Parents and child should have an appreciation of how the child will wear the cochlear implant and what it will look like before the cochlear implant surgery. (Photograph by Kim Readmond, courtesy of the Central Institute for the Deaf)

the device hardware are not uncommon. For instance, a microphone may have to be replaced frequently, especially with very young users who are physically active.

In some instances, the family's medical insurance policy will pay for some costs related to obtaining a cochlear implant. Because many policies are negotiated individually, and benefits change periodically, it is difficult to generalize with accuracy how much of the total costs might be covered by any particular policy. Preauthorization of insurance benefits should be obtained from the provider before significant costs are incurred. The clinical coordinator and the family usually share responsibility for obtaining preauthorization.

Insurance policies can be classified as private, state, or federal plans. Private insurance companies (with the exception of many Health Maintenance Organizations [HMOs]) have been the most cooperative in approving coverage of cochlear implants, although there is considerable variability in the extent of authorized benefits. Medicaid, which is jointly funded by the state and federal governments, provides some coverage (for those who cannot afford health insurance) in some states. Finally, federal programs such as Champus (designed for retired and disabled military personnel and their dependents) may pay for some fraction of the costs incurred for cochlear implantation,

Realistic Expectations

The family and child must develop realistic expectations about what the cochlear implant will provide. Otherwise, they may suffer disappointment and frustration and even a sense of betrayal after the child receives the device. Unmet expectations will dampen enthusiasm to participate in follow-up visits and aural rehabilitation and may even lead to nonuse of the cochlear implant.

All members of the cochlear implant team help the candidate and family members develop realistic expectations, beginning with the clinical coordinator during the initial contact. During the preliminary counseling session, the family's expectations are further probed and corrected when necessary. The speech and hearing professional who conducts the preliminary counseling session makes it clear the child will always have a hearing deficit. The cochlear implant is a communication aid and not a bionic ear that will provide normal hearing. The audiologist also explains in laymen's terms how other young users perform.

A questionnaire might be administered to sample family member's expectations about possible benefits of using a device. If responses indicate the presence of unrealistic expectations (e.g., a parent may indicate, *A cochlear implant will solve the difficulties I have in communicating with my child*, or *My child is going to begin talking shortly after he gets one of these devices*), you will want to work with the family before continuing to cochlear implant surgery.

Ways to establish realistic expectations include the provision of opportunities for parents to talk with a variety of other parents of young cochlear implant users, some of whom receive more and some of whom receive less benefit from their devices. Scientific data about children's performance with a cochlear implant over time also might be shared with parents; data should indicate the best and poorest performance of groups of children and average performance. Data about listening, speech, and language might be discussed (see Chapter 16 for examples of databases). When presenting research findings, it is important to do so in a way that is comprehensible and accessible to the parents.

The speech and hearing professional might summarize the following information for parents: First, parents should understand that a number of factors influence a child's performance with a cochlear implant. A child with a postlingual hearing loss will exhibit better listening abilities than one with a prelingual hearing loss, at least for several years following implantation. Children who are under 5 years of age at the time of implantation are more likely to benefit than older children, especially children who are older than 10 years. A child who has a hearing loss of short duration likely will show greater benefit than one who has a loss of long duration. The support system provided by the family, the status of the auditory nerve and cochlea, the child's personality and interest in communicating with speech, communication mode, and the quality and quantity of aural rehabilitation are other factors that affect amount of benefit.

With these foregoing qualifications, the speech and hearing professional might summarize what we know about the performance of children, on average, heretofore. Most children who have prelingual hearing losses and who receive a cochlear implant achieve sound awareness and speech reading enhancement when using their cochlear implants. Moreover, most children achieve improvement in their speech and language performance. Those who receive a great deal of benefit achieve open-set word recognition and speak clearly enough that most people understand what they say (Chapter 16). Performance on measures of speech and language tend to improve over time, and many children do not demonstrate a plateau in their skill development, even after 5 or more years of cochlear implant use.

One potential pitfall in establishing realistic expectations is that parents may come to expect too little and never challenge their child to listen. Some parents are delighted that, on receiving a cochlear implant, their child begins to respond to environmental sounds and to recognize his or her own name. They do not expect the child to utilize the electrical signal as a means of enhancing speechreading performance, nor for speech listening, even when audiological testing indicates good benefit from the device. To some extent, parents—and teachers—can limit a child's performance by their own limited expectations.

Commitments

Receiving a cochlear implant requires tremendous commitment from the family and child in terms of time, effort, and money. It is important that the magnitude of these commitments is fully comprehended before the family proceeds with implantation.

The child (and parents) must return to the cochlear implant center periodically for device adjustments and audiological evaluation. During the first year of cochlear implant use, return trips may number six or more. They usually occur at least annually thereafter. A visit to the cochlear implant center may require that the parent take leave from work and that the family allocate funds for travel and perhaps lodging, if the cochlear implant center is far from the home.

Parents usually must maintain the device. They must learn how to determine when the device is malfunctioning and how to perform minor repairs, such as replacing a cord. They must have the financial means to replace nonfunctioning hardware. The parents typically are responsible for handling the device (e.g., placing it on the body, turning it on, and adjusting the level) and storing the device when it is not in use. Unless the child is older, the parents must assume responsibility for ensuring the child wears the device during all waking hours at the appropriate settings. They may need to instruct the child's teacher about how to handle it.

Receipt of a cochlear implant marks the beginning of an aural rehabilitation process that may last for years. The family must ensure the child has a stimulating auditory environment in both the home and in the school. Ideally, family members should be willing to direct the child's attention toward sounds in the home environment and label them and consistently integrate speech into their communication mode.

Most aural rehabilitation programs for young cochlear implant users involve parents. Although an involved family does not necessarily guarantee a successful cochlear implant user, a child probably will not be a successful user without one. Involved parents demonstrate all or many of the following behaviors. They:

- Ensure the child wears the cochlear implant regularly
- Ensure the cochlear implant is in good working order
- Provide consistent auditory speech stimulation and a good language model in everyday settings
- Stimulate the child's speech and language production
- Engage their child frequently in conversation
- Maintain regular contact with school personnel
- Participate in the development and implementation of the child's educational program

During the preimplant counseling session, a clinician will stress the importance of parental involvement.

Social Considerations

Parents of cochlear implant candidates need to be aware of the controversy surrounding implantation in children. Many members of the Deaf Community discourage cochlear implantation for young prelingually deaf children. Some have suggested that a cochlear implant may prevent or delay a child from becoming acculturated as a member of the Deaf Community. After receiving a cochlear implant, the child may not learn ASL or socialize with members of the Deaf Community because of the necessity of intense auditory stimulation and an emphasis on oral/aural communication skills during childhood. On the other hand, the child may not develop the oral/aural skills that would allow him or her to integrate easily into the hearing world. A cochlear implant also may delay the parents' acceptance of the child's hearing loss.

The debate about whether children should be implanted erupted around 1990, when the FDA approved the marketing of multichannel cochlear implants for implantation in children as young as 2 years of age. At that time, in response to the FDA decision, the National Association for the Deaf (NAD) issued a position statement, that included the denouncement:

> The NAD deplores the decision of the Food and Drug Administration which was unsound scientifically, procedurally, and ethically.

The statement went on to call for the FDA to withdraw marketing approval. Similar anger about implant use in children was expressed in a 1994 *New York Times Magazine* article. The reporter (Solomon, 1994), after inter-viewing numerous members of the Deaf Culture, offered this opinion:

> Cochlear implants remind me, more than anything else, of sex-change surgery. Are transsexuals really members of their chosen sex? Well, they look like that other sex, take on the roles of that other sex, and so on, but they do not have all those internal workings of the other sex, and cannot create children in the organic fashion of members of the chosen sex. Cochlear implants do not allow you to hear, but rather to do something that looks like hearing. (p. 1)

In June, 1997, the *Washington Post* published an indepth article dealing with Deaf Culture and the anger of its members directed toward cochlear implants and toward those who view deafness as a pathology rather than a culture. The reporter summarized current views of children who use cochlear implants, as well as the view that children should be raised by members of their *culture* rather than members of their *family:*

> Deaf Culture activists maintain that those children [who use cochlear implants] are sure to be failures—deprived of the dignity of their deafness and yet never accepted as full members of the hearing world. They say that choosing to implant children is irresponsible, done for the convenience of hearing parents. At the very least, they argue, deaf children should be allowed to wait to make the choice themselves. They recommend that deaf children be raised by the deaf community, using American Sign Language, in one of 85 residential schools scattered across the country. Trying to "fix" a deaf child, they say, is like trying to "fix" someone because he or she speaks Japanese. (Arana-Ward, 1997, p. 8)

Although the issue of how the use of cochlear implants and the celebration of Deaf Culture will co-exist continues to evolve, there does appear to be some changes in how various constituencies view the use of cochlear implants by very young children. For example, the NAD issued a revised position statement on cochlear implants in October, 2000. This statement recognizes that cochlear

implants are being used and are part of the explosion of techno-
logical developments (such as closed captioning, hearing aids,
email, and other listening systems) that have enhanced communication for deaf persons. The statement recognizes the rights of parents to make decisions about implantation on behalf of their own
children. The statement emphasizes the wellness model "upon
which the physical and psychosocial integrity of deaf children and
adults is based" (p. 2) and notes that many such individuals live a
well-integrated and healthy life without benefit of technological
listening aids. If parents decide to have their child receive cochlear
implantation, the statement urges them to include sign language
as part of the child's early development.

Many parents are aware of the controversy surrounding cochlear
implantation, even before contacting a cochlear implant center.
One role of the speech and hearing professional may be to provide
parents with additional information about the controversy and to
provide support whether they opt for or against implantation.
Moreover, they can provide parents with concrete data about how
children develop and learn with a cochlear implant, data that may
serve to counteract excessive negative publicity.

Professionals at many cochlear implant centers encourage parents
to meet deaf adults who use ASL. These interactions may help
parents appreciate the rich culture afforded by the Deaf Community (and may even lead them to reconsider their decision for
cochlear implantation). If their child proves not to benefit much
after receiving a cochlear implant, parents' awareness of the Deaf
Community may mollify unrealized hopes.

Communication Mode

A cochlear implant need not affect communication mode, especially during the first year. For instance, if parents and child communicate using simultaneous communication prior to the child's
receiving a cochlear implant, they usually continue using simultaneous communication afterward.

Although communication mode often does not change, this is
not to say that communication is inconsequential to progress
with a cochlear implant. Data suggest (see Chapter 16) that children who are in an educational setting that utilizes aural/oral

communication excel in their speech and listening skills, as compared to children who are in a simultaneous communication classroom placement. In addition, children who use primarily ASL tend to receive little benefit from use of an implant.

■ FORMAL EVALUATION

The formal evaluation includes extensive audiological testing and medical examination It may last from 1 to 5 days. It always includes audiological teaching and a medical examination and often includes a psychological and educational evaluation.

Audiological Testing

The audiological testing usually occurs first. The test battery usually includes unaided threshold testing, aided threshold testing, speech recognition testing, and impedance testing. If the child is under the age of 5 years, testing also includes auditory brain stem response audiometry.

Tests of speech recognition must indicate that the child receives limited benefit from a conventional hearing aid. The tests used to determine benefit from hearing-aid use vary as a function of the child's age and language skills. Tests that may be used to determine speech recognition skills include the CID Early Speech Perception (ESP) Tests (Moog & Geers, 1990), the Northwestern University Children's Perception of Speech (NU-CHIPS) test (Elliott & Katz, 1980), and the Word Intelligibility by Picture Identification (WIPI) test (Ross & Lerman, 1971).

Medical Examination

The medical examination includes a medical history and physical examination to assess general health and to determine whether the child can undergo general anesthesia. A CT scan of the temporal bone of the skull determines the status of the inner ear. Ideally, the cochlea should be structurally normal, although as noted, there have been reports that children with cochlear deformities have been implanted successfully. It is desirable that the cochlea be free of bone growth. However, there have been instances in which existing bone growth has been removed during the surgery and the patient subsequently received benefit from the cochlear implant. If the otologist determines that medical reasons exist that preclude implantation of an electrode (such as a cochlea structural anomaly), the remainder of the formal evaluation is canceled. If the child is found to have otitis media, then surgery will not be considered until the condition is resolved.

Language and Speech Evaluation

A speech-language pathologist evaluates the child's language and speech skills. Typically, these measures are not used for determining candidacy, although the language measures may indicate whether the child can participate in the cochlear implant fitting process. Grossly delayed language is cause for concern. This situation may indicate the child is not receiving sufficient language stimulation in the home or school environment, which does not bode well for successful cochlear implant use. The language measures may help the audiologist select language-appropriate tests for measuring the child's hearing abilities. Both the language and speech measures can be used to design an aural rehabilitation program following surgery and may indicate secondary benefits of implantation.

Psychological and Educational Evaluation

Two other professionals often are involved in the formal evaluation. An educator often participates and may be a member of the cochlear implant team or may be from the child's educational setting. The educator evaluates the child's educational placement and considers whether there is adequate support for auditory skill development. The educator also may evaluate a child's academic achievement, although performance on these measures may not greatly influence candidacy decisions.

The psychologist may determine whether additional conditions that are disabling are present, such as mental retardation or attention deficit disorder. The psychologist also may help to evaluate whether the family has realistic expectations about the benefits of implantation.

Decision

Once the child has passed through each stage of the formal evaluation, the members of the cochlear implant team meet and discuss their test results. The parents often are invited to this meeting. If the child meets the audiological and medical criteria, realistic expectations are present, and the child has a home and school environment that supports auditory and speech skills, then implantation is usually recommended. It then falls on the parents to decide whether their child will proceed to the next stage of the process—surgery.

A number of factors can cloud a decision about candidacy. These include the presence of any of the following:

- Emotional disturbance in the child or family members
- Severe behavioral problems
- An unwillingness to commit time or effort on the family's (or child's) part toward making the cochlear implant a successful communication aid
- Unrealistic expectations
- A child's inability to participate in the fitting procedure (say because of limited language or reduced cognitive functioning)
- The presence of other disabilities, such as impaired vision, that cannot be corrected

There are no cookbook procedures to follow when confounding factors are present. Usually, a decision is reached after much discussion among the team members, the family, the child, and, often, an educator.

■ SURGERY

Once a child's candidacy is established, surgery is scheduled. Cochlear implant surgery requires general anesthesia and lasts about 2–3 hours. Afterward, the child may spend 1 to 2 nights in the hospital, or surgery might be performed as an outpatient procedure.

Regardless of the counseling that has occurred beforehand, children and their families often feel anxious before the surgery. Some worry about the anesthesia, potential surgical complications, the aftermath of surgery, and whether their child will receive benefit from the device. Some parents may experience guilt for inflicting a surgical procedure on their child. As a speech and hearing professional, you will want to recognize and acknowledge these feelings and provide additional counseling when necessary.

During surgery, the hair around the incision is shaved, then a post-auricular incision is made. The surgeon creates a small depression in the mastoid bone, which will cradle the receiver against the skull. Then the surgeon drills through the mastoid bone and inserts the electrode array into the cochlea. Once the receiver is secured to the skull, the incision is stitched closed.

The stitches are removed about 2 weeks following surgery. The child may return to school as soon as he or she feels capable of attending, usually within a week of surgery.

Some risks associated with surgery include:

- Risks related to general anesthesia.
- The surgery is performed in the vicinity of the facial nerve, so there is a remote possibility that temporary or permanent facial paralysis may occur.
- The surgical site may become infected; in extreme cases, removal of the device may be necessary.
- Temporary pain in the wound may follow surgery.
- Nausea or slight vertigo may occur for a few days.
- There is a slight risk of taste disturbances, such as a metallic taste.
- Residual hearing in the ear to be implanted will most likely be sacrificed (although with improvements in the technology and surgical procedures, this is not always the case).
- A possible association between cochlear implants and meningitis may exist.

THE COCHLEAR IMPLANT FITTING

Cochlear implant fitting: the process of programming the implant's speech processor.

Map: the program established for the speech processor.

The child returns to the cochlear implant center about 4 to 6 weeks following surgery for the *cochlear implant fitting.* The external components are placed on the child and adjusted so the child can wear them comfortably. The audiologist then adjusts the stimulus parameters of the speech processor, which determine the signals delivered to the electrodes in the electrode array. The program that is established for the speech processor is called a *map.* The

Preparing for the Big Day

The first cochlear implant fitting session is usually the source of both excitement and anxiety for parents and their child. Some children may be frightened and not know what to expect. They may be aware of their parents' hopes and anxieties and might find this state of affairs stressful. In preparation for the first tune-up session:

- Avoid a big build-up. Otherwise, the anticipation may be nerve-wracking for both parents and the child.
- Leave siblings, grandparents and friends at home. It is usually better if just the parents are present.
- Bring along a few of the child's noise-making toys. Once the speech processor is programmed, the child will be able to hear moderately soft sounds. A noise-making toy is a good way to introduce the child to sound.
- Counsel and prepare friends and family, especially grandparents, that the tune-up is only the first stage of the child's implant experience. The child must learn that sound is meaningful before he or she will respond to it; this may take months of time and practice.

process for establishing a map may be called *mapping* or a *tune-up*. Many cochlear implants interface with a personal computer for the tune-up process (Figure 18-3).

The time necessary to fit and map a cochlear implant varies, depending on the maturity and cooperation of the child. A young child must learn to detect when sound is present and to indicate when it is soft and comfortably loud. Initial thresholds may be high, and maximum current levels may be low; these may change as the child becomes accustomed to hearing. In addition, due to a limited attention span, only a few electrodes may be programmed during the initial fitting session. Although most children can use their cochlear implant after one or two fittings, an optimum fitting may require several months.

When the device is activated, the prelingually deaf child may show no response to sound. Other responses include fright, surprise,

Mapping: another term used to describe the process for establishing a map.

Tune-up: the process for establishing a map.

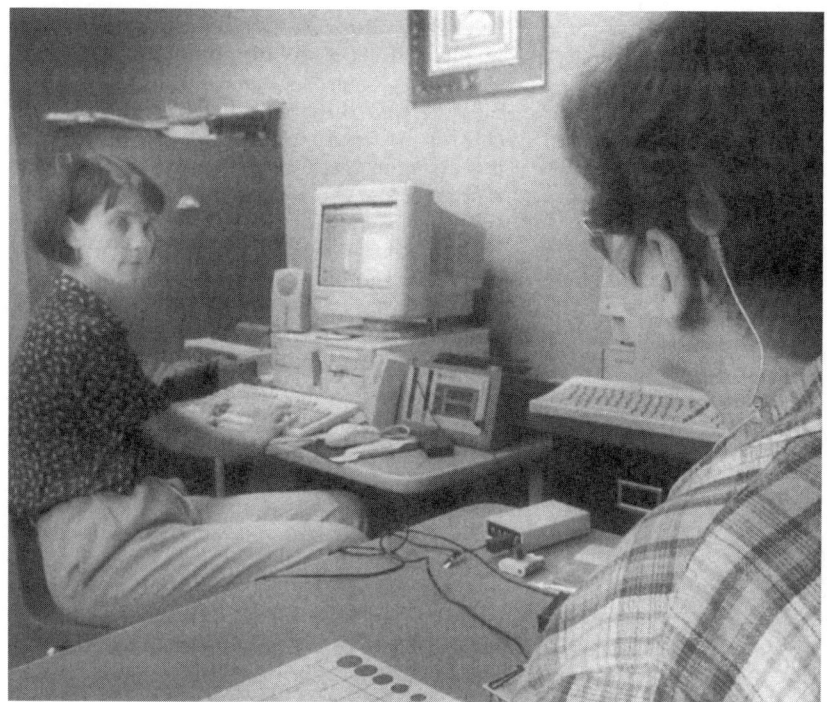

FIGURE 18-3. An audiologist may use a personal computer when establishing a map for a cochlear implant. (Photograph by Marcus Kosa, courtesy of the Central Institute for the Deaf)

rejection, distress, or wonderment. Some children report a sensation in the neck or head.

The speech processor is mapped specifically to the child's needs and responses to sound. The components of establishing a map include setting threshold levels, setting comfort levels, and "flagging," or turning off, electrodes that are problematic. The map is set so that each electrode presents stimulation strong enough that the child is aware of sound, but not so loud as to cause discomfort. Responses are obtained using pediatric hearing evaluation techniques appropriate to a child's age (e.g., Behavioral Observation Audiometry, Visual Reinforcement Audiometry, or Play Audiometry). During the initial mapping session, an audiologist will seek to determine:

- The type of electrode stimulation to use; for example, some cochlear implants have processors that may be set to stimulate the electrodes simultaneously (all channels stimulated at the same time), partially simultaneously (some channels at the same time, some in sequence) or non-simultaneously (all channels in sequence). In addition, the rate of stimulation and the pattern of stimulation may be varied. Selection of the stimulation pattern will vary with children, and there is no one best pattern for all children.

- The volume setting.
- The sensitivity setting.
- Program choices (more than one map may be set in a speech processor).
- Locks and controls (to prevent a child from changing settings inadvertently).

Speech-Processing Strategies and Interleaved Sampling

Cochlear implants include a speech-processing strategy, which is housed in the hardware that is either worn on the body or behind the ear. The speech-processing strategy is a code for converting the acoustic signal into electrical pulses. The electrical pulses are then passed onto the electrode array. Low pitch sensations are elicited when electrodes at the apex of the cochlea are stimulated, while high pitch sensations are elicited when electrodes at the base are stimulated. When the signal is speech, low-pitched sounds such as /m/ result in stimulation of apical electrodes while high-pitched sounds such as /s/ result in stimulation of basal electrodes. The perceived loudness of sound is determined by the amplitude of the stimulus current.

In Chapter 7, it was noted that many speech-processing strategies utilize an interleaved sampling approach (also called *continuous interleaved sampling*), where trains of electrical pulses are delivered across the electrode array in a non-overlapping (non-simultaneous) sequence. Thus only one electrode receives stimulation at any one time. When programming the speech processor, the audiologist may set a number of parameters within the interleaved sampling approach so that speech recognition will be maximized for the particular child. Some of these parameters include:

- **Pulse rate:** The pulse rate refers to how many pulses per second are delivered to each electrode in the electrode array. As a general rule of thumb, faster pulse rates are associated with better speech recognition performance because the stimulation pattern better encodes fine temporal variations in the speech signal. However, there are some exceptions to this rule.
- **Stimulation order:** Stimulation order refers to the sequence in which the electrodes receive stimulation. For example, electrodes may receive stimulation in an apex-to-base order or in a base-to-apex order. Electrodes may receive stimulation in a "staggered" order, so that non-adjacent electrodes receive sequential electrical pulses. The reason that staggered stimulation is used is to maximize the spatial separation between stimulated electrodes, and presumably, to limit channel interaction (so that one group of neurons doesn't receive stimulation from two different electrodes carrying two different sequences of pulses).
- **Compression function:** The acoustic amplitudes of the signal are compressed to fit within the patient's electrical dynamic range.

Parent Instruction

Before leaving the cochlear implant center, parents receive instruction about how to handle the device. Mecklenburg et al. (1990)

How Do You Establish a Map?

Most cochlear implant maps are established by programming the following parameters:

- **Dynamic range:** In adjusting the speech processor, each electrode in the electrode array (Chapter 6) is programmed

(continues)

according to the threshold of stimulation and maximum acceptable loudness level. The difference between these two current levels defines a *dynamic range.* An *electrical threshold (T-level)* is the amount of current that must be passed through an electrode so the child is just aware of a sound sensation. *Maximum comfort level (C-level)* is the maximum current level that can be introduced before the individual experiences discomfort. The thresholds and maximum comfort levels will vary among electrodes and between children as a function of neuronal survival in the auditory nerve.

- Loudness balancing. Through *loudness balancing,* the speech processor is programmed so stimulation across electrodes preserves the loudness contour of the speech signal. This step is often difficult to perform with children They must judge the relative loudness of signals presented to different electrodes in the cochlear implant electrode array (see Chapter 6). If the electrodes are not balanced, the child might experience occasional popping sounds and may not hear some speech information.

- Pitch and pitch ranking: Electrodes situated near the basal end of the cochlea are programmed to represent the high-frequency range and those near the apical end represent the low-frequency range. This representation matches the tonotopic organization of the cochlea. *Pitch ranking* determines the ability to discriminate pitch from the basal to the apical electrodes. During pitch ranking, two electrodes are stimulated, one right after the other. The child's task is to indicate which stimulus pulse has a higher or lower pitch. As with loudness balancing, this too can be a difficult task for small children to perform.

Dynamic range: the difference between the threshold of stimulation and maximum acceptable loudness.

Electrical threshold: the amount of current that must be passed through an electrode so that the wearer is just aware of a sound sensation.

T-level: another term used for threshold.

Maximum comfort level: the maximum current level that can be introduced before the implant wearer experiences discomfort.

Loudness balancing: programming the speech processor so that stimulation follows the loudness contour of the incoming speech signal.

Pitch ranking determines the ability to discriminate pitch from stimulation of the basal to apical electrodes.

presented a list of topics that are reviewed, and these still hold true today. These are:

- How is the speech processor turned on and off?
- How are the batteries changed?
- How long should the batteries last?
- Can rechargeable batteries be used?

- How is the speech processor tested to see if it's working properly?
- What does the sensitivity control do?
- Can the speech processor be repaired?
- How can the speech processor be connected to a radio-frequency or infrared transmission system?
- How can the telephone signal be fed into the speech processor? (p. 214)

Additional topics of instruction include the warranty, how to put the device on and take it off, how to troubleshoot the device, and how to perform minor repairs. Simple ways that parents may use to troubleshoot the device and ensure proper functioning include the following:

- Perform a listening check, with Ling's (1976) Five/Six-Sounds Test (described later), to ensure the child is receiving sound appropriately
- If the device is not working, check to see if cords are plugged in backwards, if a cord is cracked or broken, if a battery is inserted improperly, if the battery is dead, or if battery contacts are dirty.
- Ensure the device is kept away from moisture and humidity.
- Encourage the child to tell an adult when the device is not functioning properly. For example, is the sound off? Does it sound muffled? Is there a popping sound?

A schedule for when the child will wear the cochlear implant is established. The child begins by wearing the device in a quiet environment. After a period from 1 week to 2 months, the cochlear implant usually is worn during all waking hours. Parents usually are responsible for enforcing the schedule. Exceptions to regular use include the following:

- The hardware is in danger of falling off or being damaged, as when the child is playing outside or participating in gym class.
- The hardware is in danger of getting wet. The child may not wear it outside in the rain or when using the drinking fountain. Cochlear implants are not waterproof.

■ FOLLOW-UP VISITS

After the first year of cochlear implant use, the child returns to the cochlear implant center annually (or more often). Audiological evaluation indicates whether the cochlear implant is functioning properly and whether performance has changed. Decreased performance is cause for concern because it may signal problems with the device or physiological changes in the auditory system. The audiologist may adjust the speech processor to enhance performance. During the annual visit, the family is advised whether the manufacturer has made new software or other options available for the cochlear implant and the child may be provided with an opportunity to try them.

Children should return to the cochlear implant center whenever problems arise that cannot be fixed by a minor repair. These problems include:

- An intermittent signal
- Facial stimulation
- A change in sound quality
- Cessation of sound
- An abnormal popping or squeaking

Sometimes, children will not be aware of changes in their device functioning or will not know how to verbalize that a change has occurred. Parents should be alerted to red flags that may signal a problem. For instance, if a child no longer responds to the sounds he or she once heard, the device may be malfunctioning. Ling's Five Sounds Test (Ling, 1988) may be administered daily for the purpose of assessing whether a child's hearing capacity has changed. For this test, the parent or educator vocalizes the sounds *oo, ee, ah, sh,* and *ss* (and sometimes *m*), with mouth hidden from the child's view. The child's task is to indicate when the sounds are presented, say by clapping. Thus, a parent might say, "Shhh," and the child claps. If the child suddenly is unable to detect a sound that was previously audible, then there is reason to suspect a device problem.

Another indicator of a malfunction includes a change in the child's frequency of vocalization, voice quality, or articulation accuracy, suggesting that he or she is less able to self-monitor his or her speaking. For example, if a parent of a young child remarks, "He seems so quiet lately. He doesn't hum the way he used to," or "He suddenly sounds monotone," then there is reason to suspect a device problem.

■ AURAL REHABILITATION

Listening and speech skills do not emerge spontaneously as a result of children receiving cochlear implants and then being exposed to conversation in their everyday environments. A concerted, deliberate rehabilitation effort is required before they learn to utilize the electrical signal from the cochlear implant for the purpose of speech recognition and speech and language acquisition. The aural rehabilitation plan must include participation by the parents, speech and hearing professionals, and educators.

Parents

The aural rehabilitation specialist usually describes informal speech recognition training activities for the parents and child to perform at home. For example, a game of musical chairs can encourage the development of sound detection skills in the young child. Table 18-4 presents sample activities parents might perform during the daily routine. These kinds of activities can provide the child with successful listening experiences and promote skill growth.

Speech and Hearing Professionals and Educators

Most aural rehabilitation programs extend beyond the boundaries of the family. Speech and hearing professionals and educators play a primary role in helping children develop listening, speech, and language skills once they have been fitted with their cochlear implants.

An ideal therapy plan integrates auditory goals with goals for speech production, language acquisition, and classroom curriculum. For instance Nevins and Chute (1996) suggested specific procedures for incorporating listening practice into daily classroom

Table 18-4. Routine activities or familiar activities that parents can capitalize on in providing listening practice for their children.

The speech and hearing professional may interact with parents and prepare lists of routine activities they perform regularly with their child in the home environment. They then may discuss how they can incorporate listening practice into these activities. A sample list may include the following:

- **Getting dressed in the morning.** The child will listen and discriminate between the words *pants* and *sweatshirt*.
- **Setting the table.** The child will discriminate auditorily between the words *fork* and *napkin*.
- **Playing favorite games.** The child will discriminate between the words *yellow* and *blue* while playing the game of Candyland.
- **Playing quietly.** The child will respond to his or her name when a parent calls.

---

routines as well as lessons of science, social studies, reading, language, and other school subjects. The daily roll call may provide opportunity for practice in auditory name recognition. In a science unit, closed sets of vocabulary about the weather can be presented in an audition-only mode; for example, a teacher might say with his or her mouth hidden *clouds* or *lightning* or *thunderstorm,* three words that differ in prosodic pattern (p. 149). The child would be expected to discriminate among the three words.

Administrative support from the child's special education program is essential in case management. This is because there is a critical need for networking among family, classroom teachers, audiologists, speech-language pathologists, and additional cochlear-implant and educational team members. School personnel should be encouraged to call members of the cochlear implant center with any questions or comments. Collaborative meetings between education staff and cochlear implant staff are sometimes held via telephone or face-to-face to establish information-exchange networks.

Although each child's pattern of progress is individual, the level of therapy should remain high for a prolonged interval, even as long as 5 years or more. The speech and hearing professional has the unique challenge of maintaining the child's interest and motivation to achieve goals over years of therapy.

Other roles of the speech and hearing professional in an educational setting include the following:

- To provide information about the cochlear implant and how it works
- To evaluate the child's speech and listening performance in the school environment
- To provide a school inservice to other professionals in the child's school
- To provide instruction to the classroom teacher about how to troubleshoot the device

CASE STUDY 1

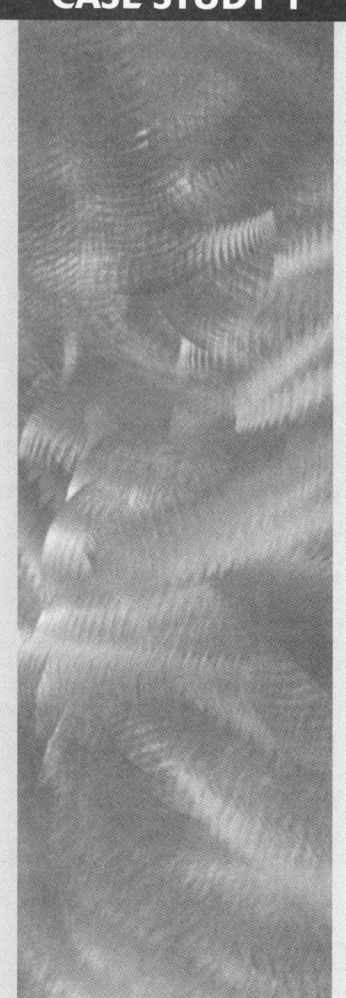

This case study provides an example of some of the issues that must be considered when determining cochlear implant candidacy.

Janet Dooley was diagnosed with a bilateral profound hearing loss at 10 months of age. The etiology was unknown. She has worn hearing aids for 4 months, and has been participating in a parent-infant program that utilizes simultaneous communication. Janet has not developed any spoken language, but has developed a sign vocabulary of five words. Her parents are hopeful that a cochlear implant will accelerate her language development and stimulate her speech production. The following issues should be addressed:

- **Confirmation of hearing status.** An audiologist should perform an extensive audiological assessment, including ABRs, OAEs, and behavioral audiometry. It is important that accurate information about the magnitude of the hearing loss is available, and it must be determined whether Janet is receiving optimal benefit from the hearing aid.
- **Evaluation of changes in speech and language.** A comprehensive spoken language assessment should be performed to determine how well Janet is progressing with her hearing aid. A determination can be made as to whether her aided hearing is allowing her

(continues)

to acquire oral communication skills. If she is showing little progress, she may be an appropriate candidate.

- **Review of educational placement.** Her current parent-infant program should be examined to determine whether it affords adequate auditory speech stimulation. If it does not, the parents may wish to reconsider placement. The fact that she has shown little progress in her speech skills and language in her current placement suggests that it may not be an optimum placement.
- **Medical examination.** Impedance testing and an otoscopic examination should be performed to evaluate the health of the middle ear. A CT scan can determine whether the cochlea is normal on either side of the head. A comprehensive medical examination should be performed to rule out any other contraindications to cochlear implant surgery.
- **Development of realistic expectations.** Janet's parents should be briefed about benefit with a cochlear implant. They can be advised that hearing, speech, and language may not be any better with a cochlear implant than with a hearing aid.

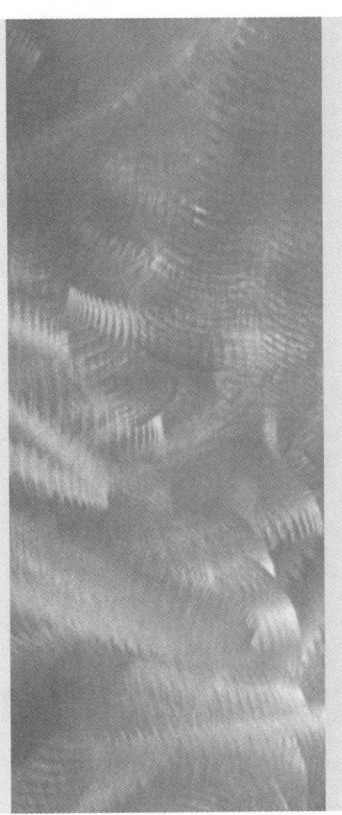

CASE STUDY 2

This case study, provided by Cherow and Boswell (1999, p. 25), demonstrates how a child progressed from using hearing aids to receiving a cochlear implant:

" 'Hope Johnson was referred for audiologic testing at Arkansas Children's Hospital in Little Rock at 9 months of age because of recurring otitis media. Her initial behavioral auditory threshold responses were very elevated and she had abnormal tympanograms,' recalled Patti Martin, director of Audiology and Speech-Language Pathology at Arkansas Children's Hospital. Following PE tube placement, she came back for an audiologic evaluation. 'We did behavioral testing, tympanometry, auditory brain response (ABR) and

(continues)

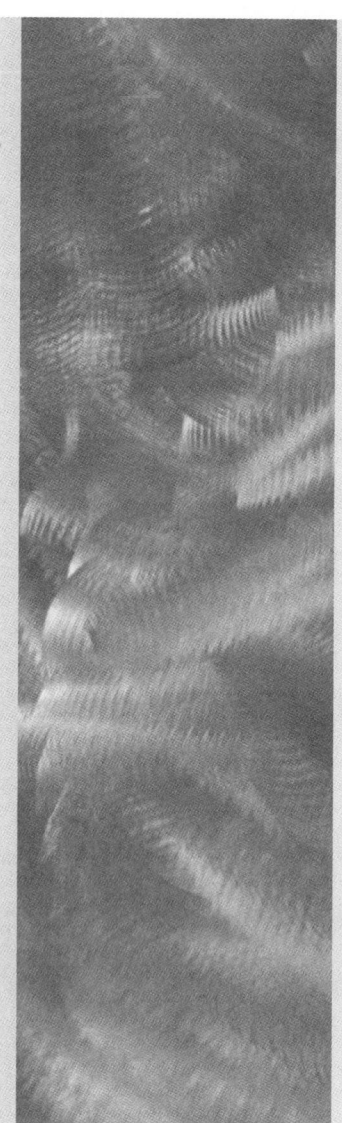

otoacoustic emission (OAE) testing, which indicated a severe-to-profound bilateral sensorineural hearing loss in the 80 dB–120 dB range.' A subsequent audiologic testing using the cross-check principle confirmed the diagnosis.

Martin fitted Hope with hearing aids with an integrated FM system that she used when she entered preschool 2 days a week at the Child Enrichment Center at Children's Hospital. Martin also provided an in-service to Hope's preschool teachers and staff, explaining how to use the FM system effectively.

As Martin continued to work with Hope and her family, performing audiologic evaluations every 2 to 3 months, she noticed a gradual progression in Hope's hearing loss. When tests showed a complete loss of hearing in Hope's right ear and a corner audiogram in her left, Martin suggested the possibility of a cochlear implant, providing the family with information to make the decision and putting them in contact with other families whose child had received a cochlear implant. 'Hope didn't have functional hearing for speech. We felt that the cochlear implant would minimally increase awareness of all environmental sounds,'" Martin said.

After Hope's surgery, the cochlear implant team met with her every few weeks. As Hope approaches her second birthday, with her cochlear implant she has a 30 dB threshold across all frequencies and responds to soft environmental sounds. 'The most exciting thing is her response to us and our voices,' says Hope's mother Sarah. 'Her receptive language skills are growing by the day.'"

▬ FINAL REMARKS

Speech perception training and speech-language therapy curricula for children who use cochlear implants are, for the most part, not much different in content and organization that those that are appropriate for use with children who use hearing aids. For instance, the techniques and hierarchy of objectives described in Chapters 8 and 10 for auditory training and speechreading training, respectively, are appropriate for children who use either type of listening device. Perhaps the greatest difference you will note when working with children who use the two types of listening devices is that, on average, children who use cochlear implants progress faster in their skill acquisition than children with similar hearing losses who use hearing aids. They also progress farther. Thus, a child who uses a cochlear implant may perform open-set word recognition exercises in an auditory training program curriculum, whereas a child who uses a hearing aid may advance only to closed-set word recognition exercises. Moreover, children may require less structured language teaching techniques, and instead, may progress with more naturalistic, real-world language instruction than their counterparts who use hearing aids.

■ KEY CHAPTER POINTS

- ✔ The cochlear implant service delivery model often has seven key components: initial contact, preimplant counseling, formal evaluation, surgery, fitting, follow-up evaluation, and aural rehabilitation.
- ✔ Once candidacy is determined, parents are responsible for making the decision about whether the child will receive a cochlear implant.
- ✔ The preliminary counseling session may occur before or after the formal evaluation. Counseling is critical for the parents and child. They receive information about obtaining, maintaining, and using a cochlear implant, and for maximizing its benefits. Often, the child's educator plays an important role during this stage of the process.
- ✔ Typically, children must be at least 12 months of age before receiving a cochlear implant and have a severe-to-profound bilateral hearing loss, although there are exceptions. They should be healthy and ideally have no other disabilities other than deafness.
- ✔ Receiving a cochlear implant requires a tremendous commitment from the family and the child, in terms of money, time, and effort. The family needs to be aware of these commitments and be willing to become intimately involved in the aural rehabilitation plan.
- ✔ It is important for parents to develop realistic expectations before the cochlear implant surgery. Some parents view the cochlear implant as a "bionic ear" and have inordinately, high hopes about what the device can do for their child. These parents may be disappointed by a child's initial results with a cochlear implant and may even become disinterested in postimplant aural rehabilitation.

✔ Cochlear implantation for children has been a controversial issue for many years. Parents need to be aware of the fact that many members of the Deaf Community disapprove of cochlear implants for children, and parents should have some appreciation of the reasons underlying this disapproval. They should also be familiar with data indicating the benefits of cochlear implant use.

✔ Although many children do not change their mode of communication after receiving a cochlear implant, they will receive little benefit if there is not a firm commitment to auditory and speech development in the home and school settings. Children who use primarily ASL likely will receive minimal benefit from receiving a cochlear implant.

✔ During the fitting or tune-up, a map is established for the cochlear implant speech processor. The length of time necessary to fit a child varies and is contingent on the child's maturity and cooperation.

✔ A concerted aural rehabilitation effort must follow receipt of a cochlear implant. Children need intensive speech perception training and speech and language therapy after they begin to use a cochlear implant and for many years thereafter. The curricula appropriate for young cochlear implant users are often similar to those that are appropriate for hearing-aid users who are of similar age, although language instruction may be less formal and more naturalistic.

■■■ MULTIPLE CHOICE QUESTIONS

1. Criteria for implanting children include the following:
   a. The child is at least 2 years of age.
   b. The child does not use simultaneous communication.
   c. The child has had a trial period with bilateral hearing aids.
   d. The parents are not members of the Deaf Culture.

2. Counseling about the cochlear implant occurs during:
   a. Preliminary contact
   b. Candidacy consideration
   c. Aural rehabilitation
   d. Every stage of the implant process

3. Jenny Sayers is 11 months old. Five months ago an ABR confirmed the presence of a profound bilateral hearing loss. She has worn hearing aids for the last 2 months. Her mother is about to enroll her in a parent-infant program. She will likely receive a cochlear implant when:

   a. She turns 12 months old next month

   b. After it is demonstrated she is not developing auditory skills as a result of her involvement in the aural rehabilitation program

   c. After a second ABR is performed

   d. At the age of 2 years

4. Which of the following statements is false?

   a. A child who has a cochlear anomaly is not a candidate for cochlear implantation.

   b. A child who uses ASL is not as likely to benefit from receipt of a cochlear implant than a child who uses a different mode of communication.

   c. Parents should have minimal expectations about the potential benefits of cochlear implantation.

   d. A child who has a severe-to-profound bilateral sensorineural hearing loss may be considered as a candidate for a cochlear implant, even if he or she is over the age of 5 years.

5. Cultural considerations in relation to the decision about whether a child should receive a cochlear implantation pertain to issues of:

   a. Deaf Culture and the use of ASL

   b. Ethnic background

   c. Family's socioeconomic status

   d. Family support

6. The cochlear implant tune-up is:

   a. The process for establishing a map

   b. The program in the speech processor

   c. Fitting the device to the child's ear

   d. The difference between a child's threshold and maximum comfort level

7. Ling's Five Sounds Test is comprised of the following sounds:

   a. Mmm, bah, ah, fah, gah

   b. Oo, ee, ah, sh, ss

   c. Mmm, ee, ah, gah, tah

   d. Oo, ee, uu, oe, ow

8. Which of the following statements is false?

   a. On receiving a cochlear implant, the child must begin immediately to use aural/oral communication or he or she will receive minimal benefit from the device.

   b. If a child continues to use ASL, he or she will not receive optimal benefit from the device.

   c. The family must learn how to nurture auditory and speech skills.

   d. The child's teacher may receive an inservice from a member of the cochlear implant team.

KEY RESOURCES

Cochlear Implant Manufacturers' Web Site Addresses

Advanced Bionics—Clarion
http://www.cochlearimplant.com

Cochlear Corporation—Nucleus
http://www.cochlear.com

MED-EL—Combi 4+
http://www.medel.com

AllHear—AllHear single channel implant
http://www.allhear.com

Antwerp Bionic Systems—Laura
http://ubcaserv.ubca.uia.ac.be/en_site/index.html

MXM Laboratories—Digisonic
http://www.mxmlab.com/digisonic/index.html

Appendix: Answers to Multiple Choice Questions

CHAPTER 1

1. c
2. d
3. a
4. b

CHAPTER 2

1. a
2. d
3. d
4. c
5. b
6. a
7. d

CHAPTER 3

1. a
2. b
3. d
4. d
5. b
6. b
7. c
8. a
9. d

CHAPTER 4

1. c
2. a
3. d
4. b
5. b
6. d
7. a
8. c
9. b

CHAPTER 5

1. a
2. c
3. a
4. c
5. b
6. c
7. c
8. d

CHAPTER 6

1. c
2. b
3. a
4. b
5. a
6. d
7. a
8. b
9. c

CHAPTER 7

1. b
2. d
3. b
4. a
5. c
6. b
7. d
8. c

9. a
10. c
11. a
12. c
13. d
14. c
15. a

CHAPTER 8

1. c
2. a
3. a
4. b
5. d
6. d
7. b
8. a
9. b

CHAPTER 9

1. c
2. c
3. a
4. b
5. d
6. a
7. c
8. d
9. b

CHAPTER 10

1. a
2. b
3. c
4. a
5. c
6. d

CHAPTER 11

1. a
2. b
3. d
4. a
5. b
6. d
7. b
8. c
9. d
10. c
11. a

CHAPTER 12

1. a
2. b
3. d
4. c
5. c
6. c
7. a
8. b

9. c
10. a
11. a
12. b
13. d
14. b

CHAPTER 13

1. c
2. a
3. d
4. c
5. d
6. b
7. c
8. c
9. a
10. c
11. c
12. b

CHAPTER 14

1. d
2. c
3. b
4. c
5. a
6. a
7. b
8. d

9. c
10. b
11. d
12. b
13. a
14. c
15. a
16. b

CHAPTER 15

1. c
2. c
3. a
4. b
5. d
6. a
7. d
8. c
9. b
10. b
11. d
12. b

CHAPTER 16

1. d
2. b
3. c
4. b
5. d
6. c

7. a
8. a
9. c
10. a
11. b
12. d
13. b
14. a

CHAPTER 17

1. a
2. b
3. a
4. c
5. b
6. c
7. c
8. b
9. b
10. a

CHAPTER 18

1. c
2. d
3. b
4. c
5. a
6. a
7. b
8. a

Glossary

Terms used in this text and other terms related to aural rehabilitation.

AAA: American Academy of Audiology.

AARP: American Association of Retired Persons.

ABR: Auditory brainstem response.

Acceptance: The final stage of adjustment to a hearing loss in which the patient realizes that life goes on, albeit differently.

Acoupedic approach: A comprehensive habilitation program for infants and their families that emphasizes auditory training without formal lipreading instruction.

Acoustic cue: Acoustic information in a segment of speech that conveys phonetic information.

Acoustic feedback: Sound produced when the amplified sound from a device receiver is picked up again by the microphone and reamplified; a high-pitched squeal.

Acoustic feedback cancellation: A feature that avoids the annoying squeal produced by hearing aids when the microphone picks up the amplified sound from the hearing aid and reamplifies it.

Acquired hearing loss: Hearing loss that is acquired after birth.

Action level: Noise exposure level at which a worker must be enrolled in an occupational hearing conservation program; OSHA defines this level as 85 dBA for an average of 8 hours per day.

Acute otitis media: Inflammation of the middle ear that lasts for 3 weeks or less.

ADA: Americans with Disabilities Act; Academy of Dispensing Audiologists.

Adaptive and attending strategies: Methods of counteracting maladaptive behaviors that stem from hearing loss.

Adjacency pairs: Linked speaking turns.

Adventitious hearing loss: Hearing loss occurring after birth.

Aggressive conversational style: Conversational style characteristic of some persons who have hearing loss, characterized by hostility, belligerence, and bad attitude.

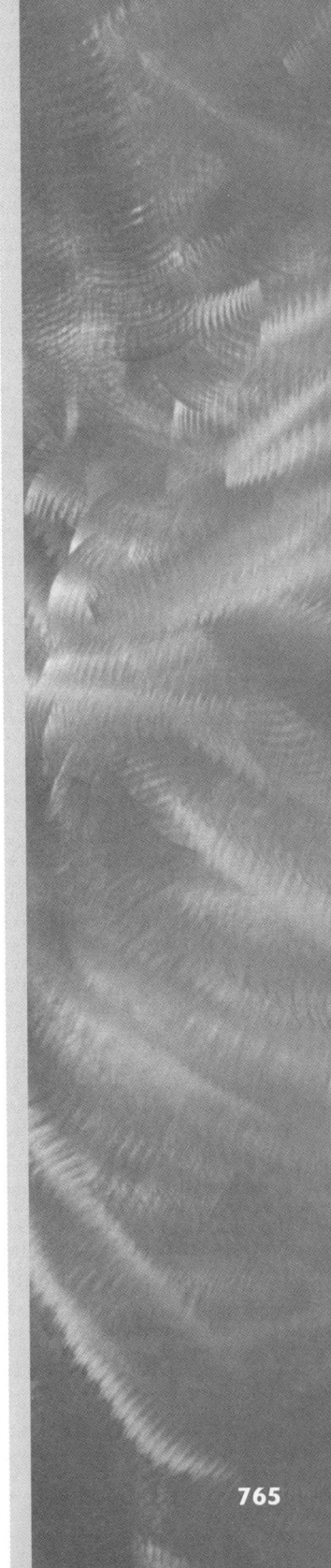

Aided thresholds: Hearing thresholds obtained from a patient using hearing aids, indicated by an "A" on the audiogram.

Air-bone gap: The difference between air- and bone-conduction thresholds; a difference may indicate a conductive component in the hearing loss.

Air conduction: Sound travels through the air, enters the external auditory canal, and progresses through the middle ear, inner ear, and then to the brain; air conduction thresholds are represented by "O" (right ear) and "X" (left ear) on the audiogram.

ALD: Assistive listening device; may be hard-wired or wireless; designed to enhance detection and recognition of environmental sounds and speech.

ALGO: An automated ABR screening device used for screening newborns.

Alleles: The different possible codes of a gene.

Altered speech: Human speech that is recorded and then altered in some manner.

Alzheimer's disease: Dementia, characterized by progressive neuronal degeneration and mental deterioration.

Ambient noise: Noise in a listening environment.

American Academy of Audiology: AAA; professional society for audiologists, founded in 1988.

American Association of Retired Persons: AARP; Consumer group for persons over the age of 50 years.

American National Standards Institute: ANSI; group that determines standards for measuring instruments, including audiometers.

American Sign Language: ASL; a manual system of communication used by members of the Deaf Culture in the United States; sometimes referred to as Ameslan.

American Speech-Language-Hearing Association: ASHA; professional organization of speech and hearing professionals, including speech-language pathologists, audiologists, and speech and hearing scientists.

American Tinnitus Association: ATA; consumer organization for persons who have tinnitus.

Americans with Disabilities Act: ADA; United States law enacted in 1990 to provide equal access to persons with disabilities.

Amplification: Provision of increased intensity of sound.

Amplifier: Equipment that increases the intensity of sound.

Analytic speechreading training: An instructional method that focuses the student's attention on speechreading individual speech units.

Anger and **guilt:** Stages that sometimes follow depression in adjusting to a hearing loss.

Anomaly: A structure that is irregular or deviates from the norm, such as a cochlear anomaly.

Anoxia: Deficiency or absence of oxygen in the bodily tissues.

Anticipatory strategies: Methods of preparing for a communication interaction.

Aperiodic: Not occurring at regular intervals; not periodic.

Apgar score: A numeric value between 1 and 10 assigned to a newborn to describe physical status at birth; determined by the baby's color, heart rate, respiration, muscle tone, and responsiveness.

Articulation: Movement and positioning of the oral cavity structures, including tongue tip, tongue body, jaw, and lips, during speech production.

ASHA: American Speech-Language-Hearing Association.

Assertive conversational style: Conversational style used by some persons with hearing loss, characterized by a respect for the rights of others and assuming responsibility for the success of the conversational interaction.

Assistive listening device: ALD; instrument designed to provide awareness or identification of environmental signals and speech and to improve signal-to-noise ratios; usually includes a microphone and a receiver.

ATA: American Tinnitus Association.

Attack time: The time between when a signal begins to the onset of its steady-state amplified value.

Attention deficit disorder: ADD; cognitive deficit that limits an individual's ability to pay attention and stay focused on a task; may involve restlessness, distractibility, and hyperactivity.

Audible: Loud enough to be heard.

Audiogram: A graphic representation of hearing thresholds as a function of stimulus frequency.

Audiologic rehabilitation: Term often used synonymously with aural rehabilitation or aural habilitation; sometimes may entail greater emphasis on the provision and follow-up of listening devices and less emphasis on communication strategies training and speech perception training.

Audiologist: Allied health care professional who has academic accreditation in the practice of audiology; professional who provides an array of services related to hearing evaluation and rehabilitation.

Audiometer: Electronic instrument used for the measurement of hearing sensitivity.

Audiometric zero: Lowest sound pressure level that can just be detected by an average adult ear at any particular frequency; designated as 0 dB Hearing Level (HL) on an audiogram.

Audiovisual: Speech that is presented to both the auditory and visual modalities.

Audition: Hearing.

Audition-only: Presentation of only an auditory signal in testing.

Audition-plus-vision: Presentation of both auditory and visual signals simultaneously, as in speechreading.

Auditorily: With audition.

Auditory: Pertaining to hearing.

Auditory brainstem implant: ABI; implant that has an electrode that implants to the juncture of the eighth cranial nerve and the cochlear nucleus in the brainstem; provides crude sound awareness.

Auditory brainstem response: ABR; auditory evoked potential that originates from the eighth cranial nerve and is generated by electrical stimulation of the cochlea via an electrode.

Auditory canal: External auditory meatus.

Auditory feedback: One's own speech signal that is heard while speaking.

Auditory memory: Acquisition, storage, and retrieval of auditory sound patterns in both short-term and long-term form.

Auditory neuropathy: Condition where the patient has a pure-tone audiogram that shows any degree of hearing loss, from mild to profound, and shows normal OAEs. ABRs are either absent or degraded.

Auditory-only: Speech that is presented to only the auditory modality.

Auditory training: Instruction designed to maximize an individual's use of residual hearing by means of both formal and informal listening practice.

Auditory-verbal therapy: An educational approach in which technology, techniques, and strategies are used to enable children to listen and understand spoken language, with a primary emphasis on the auditory modality for learning.

Aural habilitation: Sometimes used synonymously with aural rehabilitation; intervention for persons who have not developed listening, speech, and language skills; may include diagnosis of communication and hearing-related difficulties, speech perception training, speech and language therapy, manual communication, and educational management.

Aural/oral communication: The language used by persons with normal hearing.

Aural/oral method: An instructional method used to teach children with significant hearing loss using hearing, speechreading, and spoken language, but not manual communication.

Aural rehabilitation: Intervention aimed at minimizing and alleviating the communication difficulties associated with hearing loss; may include diagnosis of hearing loss and communication handicap, amplification, counseling, communication strategies training, speech perception training, family instruction, speech-language therapy, and educational management.

Auricle: Pinna; external or outer ear.

Automatic gain control: AGC; nonlinear hearing aid compression circuitry that changes gain as signal level changes or limits the output of the hearing aid when the level reaches a specified value.

Autosomal dominant: One parent passes a dominant allele to the child; the probability of the trait being expressed in the child is 50%.

Autosomal recessive inheritance: Transmission of genetic characteristics in which both parents must pass on the genetic characteristic.

Autosome: Any of the 22 pairs of 23 chromosome pairs not related to determination of gender.

Background noise: Extraneous noise that masks the acoustic signal of interest.

Battery: A cell that provides electrical power.

Behavioral audiometry: Pure-tone and speech audiometry that requires a behavioral response from the patient.

Behavioral/observational audiometry: BOA; method of testing a child's hearing in which the tester presents a sound stimulus and observes the child's behavior for change.

Behind-the-ear hearing aid: BTE; a hearing aid worn over the pinna and coupled to the ear canal by means of an earmold.

Bilateral: On both sides; involving both ears.

Bilingual/bicultural model: Teaching children with significant hearing loss ASL as their first language and then later English in school as they develop reading and writing skills.

Binaural: For both ears.

Binaural advantage: The advantage of using both ears instead of one, such as better hearing thresholds and enhanced listening in the presence of background noise.

Binaural amplification: Use of a hearing aid in each ear.

Binaural squelch: Improvement in listening in noise when wearing two hearing aids instead of one, resulting in a 2–3 dB improvement in signal-to-noise ratio.

Body hearing aid: A hearing aid worn on the body; includes a box worn on the torso and a cord connecting to an ear-level receiver.

Bone conduction: Transmission of sound through the bones in the body, particularly the skull.

Bone-conductor: Vibrator or oscillator that is used to transmit sound to the bones of the skull by means of vibration.

BTE: Behind-the-ear hearing aid.

CAD: Central auditory disorder.

Carrier phrase: In speech audiometry, a phrase that precedes the target word, such as, "Say the word _____."

Cataract: Progressive retinal disorder that entails a clouding of the lens; causes blurred vision and impairs contrast sensitivity.

CAT scan: Computerized axial tomography scan.

Center-based program: Program wherein children attend therapy for a designated number of hours per week.

Central auditory disorder: CAD; functional auditory disorder that is centered in the brainstem or cortex, and not the peripheral hearing system (outer, middle, or inner ear).

Cerumen: Ear wax.

Chromosome pair: The basic unit of genes; structures carrying the genes of a cell and made up of a single strand of DNA.

Chronic: Of long-standing duration.

Chronological age: Age of an individual referenced to birth.

CIC: Completely-in-the-canal hearing aid.

Circuit: A combination of electronic components that conveys electronic current.

Circuitry: The parts of an electric circuit.

Classroom acoustics: The background noise and reverberation properties characteristic of a classroom, determined by the size and surfaces of the room, the sound sources inside and outside, furnishings, people, and other factors.

Clear speech: Speech that is at a moderately loud conversational level, characterized by precise but not exaggerated articulation, pausing at appropriate linguistic boundaries, and somewhat slow speaking rate; often used to increase the message recognition of hard-of-hearing listeners.

Closed captioning: Printed text or printed dialog that corresponds to the auditory speech signal from a television program or movie.

Closed-ended questions: Questions used to gather quantitative information.

Closed-set: A stimulus or response set that contains a fixed number of items, known to the patient.

CNT: Could not test.

Coarticulation: The influence of one phoneme on either a preceding or succeeding phoneme.

Cochlear implant: Device implanted in the skull that permits persons with deafness to receive stimulation of the auditory mechanism; typically comprised of a microphone, a speech processor, and an electrode array inserted into the cochlea; directly stimulates the auditory nerve by means of electrical current.

Cochlear implant mapping: Process of programming the implant's speech processor.

Cochlear-implant team: Group of professionals who are part of the cochlear implant process; usually includes an otolaryngologist, audiologist, and clinical coordinator and may include an educator, aural rehabilitation specialist, speech-language pathologist, psychologist, and/or social worker.

Cochlear nucleus: Cluster of cell bodies in the brain stem where the nerve fibers leading from the cochlea enter and synapse.

Comer audiogram: An audiogram that displays a profound hearing loss, with thresholds measurable only in the low frequencies.

Comfortable loudness level: Intensity level that is comfortable to listen to sound.

Communication: The act of exchanging messages; may entail the use of speech, sign, writing, or hand gestures.

Communication breakdown: Instance in the course of a conversation when one participant does not recognize the message presented by another.

Communication disorder: An impairment in one's ability to communicate.

Communication handicap: Psychosocial disadvantages that result from hearing loss, including the limitations that occur in performing the activities of everyday life.

Communication partner: Person with whom one engages in conversation.

Communication strategies training: Instruction provided to a person with hearing loss or the person's frequent communication partner that pertains to communication strategies and the management of communication difficulties.

Communication strategy: A course of action taken to enhance communication.

Completely-in-the-canal (CIC) hearing aid: An aid that fits entirely within the external ear canal.

Comprehension: A higher level of auditory skill development characterized by an ability to understand spoken messages.

Compressed speech: Speech that has had segments removed and then has been compressed in such a way that the frequency composition remains intact.

Compression (in hearing aid circuitry): Nonlinear amplifier gain used to determine and limit output gain as a function of input gain.

Compression ratio: The ratio in decibels between the acoustic input to a hearing-aid amplifier and its auditory output.

Computerized axial tomography: CAT; a computer-generated picture of a section of the brain compiled from sectional radiographs obtained from the same plane.

Concha: The bowl-like depression of the outer ear that forms the mouth of the external ear canal.

Conditioned play audiometry: Method of testing children 2.5 years and older in which the child is trained to perform a task in response to presentation of a sound.

Conductive hearing loss: Hearing loss that stems from an impairment in the outer or middle ear and that does not involve the inner ear.

Configuration: Refers to the extent of hearing loss at each frequency and gives an overall description to the hearing loss.

Congenital: Present at birth.

Congenital hearing loss: Hearing loss that exists at or dates from birth; reduced hearing sensitivity related to pre- or perinatal causes.

Congruence with self: The first tenet of person-centered counseling in which clinicians act as themselves in interactions with patients and do not assume a facade of professionalism.

Consonant-vowel-consonant: CVC; a monosyllabic word structure; CVCs often are used as stimuli in isolated-word speech-recognition tests.

Construct validity: Statistical term meaning the extent to which a test measures what it is supposed to measure, usually a trait or skill (e.g., speech perception).

Constructive strategy: Tactic designed to optimize the listening environment for communication; a kind of facilitative strategy.

Content validity: Statistical term meaning the extent to which a test adequately samples what it is supposed to measure.

Contextual information: Linguistic support available for identifying a target word, phrase, or sentence.

Continuous discourse tracking: CDT; aural rehabilitation technique in which the receiver (listener) attempts to repeat verbatim text that is presented by a sender (speaker); performance is summarized as the number of words repeated per minute.

Conversational fluency: Relates to how smoothly conversation unfolds and is reflected by the time spent in repairing communication breakdowns, the exchange of information and ideas, and the sharing of speaking time.

Conversational rules: Implicit rules that guide the conduct of participants engaged in conversation.

Conversational turn: During the course of a conversation, the period during which a participant delivers a contribution to the conversation.

Critical period: The early years of a child's or animal's life in which the language and vocal patterns of the individual's species are acquired most easily.

Cued Speech: A system for enhancing speech-reading; hand configurations are placed at different mouth and throat positions to distinguish between similar visual speech patterns.

CVC: Consonant-Vowel-Consonant syllable.

Cycling: In speech perception training, coming back to a training objective that has been achieved with some success in order to provide reinforcement and additional learning.

DAC: Digital-to-analog conversion.

DAI: Direct audio input.

Daily log: A procedure for assessing conversational fluency and communication handicap, in which respondents perform a self-monitoring procedure about behaviors of interest and provide self-reports; usually completed more than once, over a set period of time.

dB: Decibel.

Deaf: Having minimal or no hearing.

Deaf Culture: A subculture in society that shares a common language (American Sign Language), beliefs, customs, arts, history, and folklore; primarily comprised of individuals who have prelingual deafness.

Decibel: Logarithmic unit of sound pressure; 1/10th of a Bel; unit for expressing sound intensity.

Delayed-onset hereditary hearing loss: Hearing is normal at birth, then declines later in life as a result of a hereditary disorder.

Dementia: Progressive loss of cognitive function.

Depression: Often follows denial in reaching acceptance of a hearing loss.

Describing: An adult uses an event a child is interested in to talk about various aspects of the event.

Detection: The ability to recognize when a sound is present and when it is absent.

Developmental delay: Lagging behind in development relative to age-matched peers.

Diabetic retinopathy: Results from longstanding diabetes, causing blurred and distorted vision in the central visual field and sometimes a detached retina.

Digital hearing aid: Hearing aid that utilizes digital technology to process the signal.

Digital processing: Done by a hearing aid that converts the signal from analog to digital form, processes the signal to achieve a target, then converts the signal back to analog form.

Direct audio input: DAI; hard-wired connection that leads directly from the sound source to the hearing aid or other listening device.

Directional microphone: Microphone that is more sensitive to sound originating from in front of the hearing-aid user than from behind.

Disability: A loss of function.

Discourse: Communication of thoughts by use of language.

Discrimination: In speech-perception training, the ability to distinguish one stimulus from another; in speech-recognition testing, sometimes used to refer to word-recognition ability.

Disorder: An abnormality in functioning.

Dissonance theory: Theory concerning situations in which one's self-perceptions do not coincide with reality.

Distortion: Undesirable change in the audio signal.

DNA: Deoxyribonucleic acid; molecules that carry genetic instructions.

DNT: Did not test.

Dominant hereditary hearing loss: Hearing loss that stems from a genetic characteristic on at least one gene of a pair.

Dominating conversational behaviors: Characteristic of an aggressive conversational style; includes taking extended speaking turns, frequent interruptions, and abrupt topic changes.

Dri-aid kit: A small package used to keep moisture out of the internal components of listening devices.

Drill activity: Repeated exercises and rote activities.

DSP: Digital signal processing.

DSP hearing aid: Hearing aid that utilizes digital signal processing; signal is converted from an analog to digital signal, the signal is manipulated according to a processing algorithm, and then the signal is converted back into an analog signal.

Dynamic range: The difference in decibels between an individual's threshold of sensitivity for a sound and the level at which the sound becomes uncomfortably loud.

Dysfunction: Abnormal function.

EAR plugs: Etymotic Applied Research plugs; provide ear protection.

Ear protection: Term used to refer to hearing protectors such as ear plugs and ear muffs.

Earache: Pain in the ear.

Earhook: The curved apparatus of a behind-the-ear hearing aid and some other types of listening devices that connects the device case to the earmold, and hooks over the pinna.

Earmold: A device that fits into the concha and directs sound from the earhook of a listening device to the ear canal.

Earmold acoustics: The influence of the earmold's configuration and structure, such as bore length and venting, on the acoustic properties of the sound delivered to the tympanic membrane by a listening device.

Earmold bore: A hole in the earmold through which an amplified audio signal travels.

Earmold impression: Cast made of the concha and ear canal.

Earmold vent: A canal drilled in the earmold for the purpose of aeration or alteration of the audio signal.

Earmuffs: A kind of ear protection, made of earcups that seal around the ear for the purpose of sound attenuation.

Earplug: A kind of ear protection, consisting of a material that is inserted into the ear canal for the purpose of sound attenuation.

Effective gain: Difference in decibels between a patient's aided and unaided thresholds.

Effusion: In the middle ear, exudation of body fluid from the middle ear membranous walls as a result of inflammation.

Eighth cranial nerve: The cranial nerve consisting of an auditory and vestibular branch.

Electrical threshold: The amount of current that must be passed through an electrode so that the cochlear implant user is just aware of sound sensation.

Electroacoustic: Related to the conversion of an acoustic signal to an electrical signal or an electrical signal to an acoustic signal.

Electrode: Metal ball or plate through which electrical stimulation is applied to the body or electrical energy is measured.

Electrode array: Electrodes placed in pairs on a carrier wire and inserted into the cochlea; component of a cochlear implant.

Emotional acceptance and adjustment counseling: Explores individuals' reactions to loss of hearing.

Empathetic understanding: Third tenet of person-centered counseling. The counselor listens to the patient's concerns and feelings about a hearing problem, reflects them back to the patient, and helps the patient identify solutions.

ENT: Ear, nose, and throat.

Equivalent lists: In speech recognition testing, test lists that contain items that are presumed to be equally difficult to recognize.

Evoked potential: Electrical activity generated in the brain in response to a sensory stimulus.

Expanded speech: Recorded speech that is altered by duplicating small segments of the signal so that the speech sounds as if it were produced with a slow speaking rate; no additional spectral information is introduced.

Expansion: Language-stimulation technique in which an adult copies the meaning of a child's utterance but modifies or expands the grammar of the message.

Expressive repair strategy: Tactic taken by an individual when a communication partner has not understood one of his or her messages.

Extended repair: Many repair strategies are needed to mend a communication breakdown.

External auditory meatus: External ear canal.

External ear canal: The canal of the outer ear leading from the concha to the tympanic membrane.

Eyeglass hearing aid: Style of hearing aid in which the hearing aid is housed in the temple piece of a pair of eyeglasses.

f_0: Fundamental frequency.

F1: First formant.

F2: Second formant

Facilitative strategy: A strategy used to facilitate communication; includes means taken to instruct the talker, structure the listening environment, enhance the structure of the received message, and affect the speech recognition performance of the individual using the strategy.

Familial deafness: Deafness reoccurring in members of the same family.

Favorable seating for speechreading: Includes being close enough to see the talker's lip movements, being able to see the talker full-face rather than in profile, and having the talker's face well lit.

FDA: Food and Drug Administration.

Fetal alcohol syndrome: Syndrome found in children whose mothers abused alcohol while the child was in utero; children who have the syndrome may have mental retardation, low birth weight, unusual eye spacing, chronic otitis media, and sensorineural hearing loss.

Filter: In listening devices, a component that differentially amplifies and attenuates certain bands of frequencies in the incoming signal.

Filtered speech: Speech that has been passed through filter banks for the purpose of removing or amplifying frequency bands in the signal.

Fingerspelling: A kind of manual communication in which words are spelled letter-by-letter using standard hand configurations.

5-dB rule: Noise protection rule that specifies that the intensity level of a sound can be increased by 5 dB for every 50% reduction in the length of presentation of the sound.

Flat audiogram: Audiogram configuration in which the thresholds across frequencies are similar.

Fluctuating hearing loss: Hearing loss that varies in magnitude over time.

FM: Frequency modulation.

FM auditory trainer: Classroom assistive listening device in which the teacher wears a microphone and the signal is transmitted to the student(s) by means of frequency modulated radio waves.

FM boot: A small boot-like device worn on the bottom of a user's hearing aid that contains an FM receiver; used as part of an FM assistive listening device.

Food and Drug Administration: FDA; U.S. government agency that oversees the regulation of medical devices such as hearing aids and cochlear implants.

Formal instruction: The first stage in a communication-strategies training program, in which individuals receive information about various types of communication strategies and other appropriate listening and speaking behaviors.

Formal training: In reference to speech perception training, highly structured activities that may involve drill, usually scheduled to occur during designated times of the day, either in a one-on-one lesson format or in a small group.

Formant: A resonance in the vocal tract that results in some frequencies in the speech signal having more energy than other frequencies.

Formant 1: The first frequency band above the fundamental frequency that demonstrates high energy in the speech signal.

Formant 2: The second frequency band above the fundamental frequency that demonstrates high energy in the speech signal.

Formant transition: Segment in the speech signal that displays rapid change in the frequency or spectral composition of the formants.

Frequency: The number of regularly repeated events in a given unit of time; usually measured in *cycles* per second and *ex* pressed in Hertz (Hz).

Frequency modulation (FM): The process of creating a complex signal by means of sinusoidally varying a carrier wave frequency.

Frequency of usage: A measure indicating how often a particular word occurs during everyday conversation.

Frequency response: Output characteristics of a listening device; denoted as gain as a function of frequency.

Frequent communication partner: A particular person with whom another often converses; often a family member.

Fricative: Speech sound generated by creating turbulent airflow through a constriction in the oral cavity.

Full-on gain: Hearing aid setting that results in the maximum acoustic output.

Functional gain: Difference in decibels between unaided and aided thresholds.

Fundamental frequency: F_0; in speech, the lowest frequency in the speech output; voice pitch.

Gain: In hearing aids, the difference in decibels between the input level of an acoustic signal and the output level.

Gain/frequency response: The difference between the amplitude of the input signal and the amplitude of the output signal across frequencies.

Gene: DNA structure that is the unit of heredity.

Genetic: Concerning heredity.

Genetic counseling: Providing information to prospective parents about the likelihood of an inherited condition or disorder in their children.

Genotype: The genetic make-up of an individual.

Geriatric: Concerning the aging process.

Glaucoma: Caused by the malfunction of the eye's drainage system that results in irreversible damage to the optic nerve.

Group discussion: A meeting that provides a forum for class members to discuss communication issues.

Guided learning: The second stage in a communication strategies training program, in which individuals use conversational strategies in a structured setting.

Habilitation: Program or intervention aimed at the initial development of skills and abilities.

HAE: Hearing aid evaluation.

HAO: Hearing aid orientation.

Hair cells: Sensory cells in the cochlea that attach to the nerve endings of the eighth cranial nerve.

Handicap: Obstacles to everyday functioning that result from a disability.

Hard-of-hearing: HOH; having a hearing loss; usually not used to refer to a profound hearing loss.

Hard-wired assistive listening devices: Directly connected by wires.

Head shadow: Attenuation of sound to one ear because of the presence of the head between the ear and the sound source.

Headphone: Earphone.

Hearing aid: An electronic listening device designed to amplify and deliver sound from the environment to the listener; includes a microphone, amplifier, and receiver.

Hearing aid evaluation: HAE; procedure wherein an appropriate hearing aid is selected for an individual.

Hearing aid orientation: HAO; process of instructing a patient (and a patient's family member) to handle, use, and maintain a new hearing aid.

Hearing-aid test box: An off-the-ear determination of SSPL-90 in which the hearing aid is connected to a 2-cc coupler to stimulate the human ear canal, an input signal that sweeps the frequencies at 90 dB SPL is input, and the aid's output is measured.

Hearing conservation: Prevention or reduction of hearing loss through a program of identifying and minimizing risk, monitoring hearing sensitivity, education, and providing protection from noise exposure.

Hearing disability: Functional limitations imposed on an individual as a result of hearing loss.

Hearing disorder: A disturbance of the auditory structures and/or auditory functioning.

Hearing handicap: Difficulties in everyday functioning that arise as a result of hearing loss.

Hearing impairment: Abnormal or reduced hearing sensitivity; hearing loss.

Hearing level: HL; decibel level referenced to audiometric zero.

Hearing loss: Abnormal or reduced hearing sensitivity; hearing impairment.

Hearing loss, mild: Hearing thresholds between 25 and 40 dB HL.

Hearing loss, moderate: Hearing thresholds between 40 and 55 dB HL.

Hearing loss, moderate-to-severe: Hearing thresholds between 55 and 70 dB HL.

Hearing loss, severe: Hearing thresholds between 70 and 90 dB HL.

Hearing loss, profound: Hearing loss greater than 90 dB HL.

Hearing protection: Devices designed to minimize the risk of noise-induced hearing loss.

Hearing threshold: Level of intensity at which a sound is just audible to an individual.

Heterozygous: Having two different alleles of the same gene.

High-pass filtered speech: Speech that has been passed through filter banks, leaving the higher but not the lower frequencies.

HL: Hearing level.

Holistic: An approach to speechreading that incorporates several methods and includes the child in setting goals.

HMO: Health maintenance organization.

Home-based program: An early interventionist visits the infant's home and provides instruction for the child and parents.

Homophenes: Words that look identical on the mouth.

Homozygous: Having two identical alleles of the same gene; the same allele is inherited from both parents.

Identification: The ability to label auditory stimuli.

IEP: Individualized educational plan.

IFSP: Individualized family service plan.

Impairment: Reduced or abnormal function.

Impedance audiometry: Battery of measures designed to assess middle ear functioning, including tympanometry and acoustic reflex threshold determination; immittance audiometry.

Impression: Cast made of the concha and/or ear canal for the purpose of creating an earmold or a hearing aid.

Impulse noise: A burst of sound, as produced by a gunshot or an explosion; has an instantaneous rise time and short duration.

Incidence: Frequency of occurrence.

Inclusion: Integrates all students and activities into the daily routine of the general education classroom.

Individualized education plan: IEP; federally mandated plan for providing education to children with disabilities, updated once a year.

Individualized family service plan: IFSP; federally mandated plan for the education of preschool children with an emphasis on family involvement, updated annually.

Individuals with Disabilities Education Act: IDEA; U.S. Public Laws 94-142 and 99-457, which mandate free and appropriate education for all children with disabilities over the age of 3 years, and encourages services for children below 3 years of age.

Induction loop system: A length of wire surrounding the circumference of a room or table that conducts electrical energy from an amplifier, and thus creates a magnetic field; the current flow from an induction loop can induce the telecoil in a hearing aid to providing amplified sound to the user.

Industrial audiometry: Assessment of hearing at regular intervals for the purpose of assessing the effects of noise exposure, as well as the measurement of industrial noise levels.

Informal training: In reference to speech perception training, activities that occur during the daily routine, often incorporated into other activities, such as conversation or academic learning.

Informational counseling: Includes imparting information about the hearing loss and the benefits and limitations of amplification.

Infrared system: Assistive listening device that broadcasts from the sound source to a receiver/amplifier by means of infrared light waves.

Inner ear: Part of the hearing mechanism that houses the structures for hearing and balance and includes the cochlea, vestibules, and semicircular canals.

Input signal: Acoustic signal that enters a listening device.

Insertion gain: Hearing aid gain.

Instructional strategy: Instruction provided to a communication partner so that the person converses in a way that maximizes the hard-of-hearing person's recognition of messages and minimizes the possibility of communication breakdown; a kind of facilitative communication strategy.

Intelligibility: The degree to which speech can be recognized.

Interactive behavior: The use of cooperative conversational tactics, consistent with an assistive conversational style.

Interactive communication behaviors: Consistent with an assertive conversational style; Includes a sharing of responsibility for advancing a topic of conversation, choosing what to talk about, showing interest, and responding to remarks appropriately.

Interdisciplinary team: A group of professionals with different expertise working together for the purpose of providing assessment and intervention in a coordinated and cooperative fashion.

Interleave: To interweave patterns of signals.

Interleave pulsatile stimulation: A cochlear implant processing strategy whereby trains of pulses are delivered across electrodes in the electrode array in a nonsimultaneous fashion.

Internal components: Components of a cochlear implant that are implanted within the skull.

Intervention program: For children, this includes family counseling, hearing-aid fitting, selection of appropriate assistive listening devices, speech perception training, and other aspects of a child's educational and rehabilitation program.

Interview: An assessment procedure to assess conversational fluency and communication handicap, in which individuals talk about their conversational problems and consider possible reasons as to why communication breakdowns happen.

In-the-canal hearing aid: ITC; hearing aid that fits in the external ear canal, with only a partial filling of the concha.

In-the-ear hearing aid: ITE; hearing aid that fits into the concha of the ear.

Intraural: Between the two ears.

Ipsilateral: Pertaining to the same side.

ITC hearing aid: In-the-canal hearing aid.

ITE hearing aid: In-the-ear hearing aid.

Itinerant teachers: Teachers who work in several schools, providing support services to children who are deaf or hard-of-hearing and their teachers.

JND: just noticeable difference.

Just noticeable difference: JND; the smallest increment of stimulus change in which the stimulus can be perceived as different; difference limen.

K-AMP circuit: Hearing-aid circuit designed to provide more gain for moderate-level sound, no gain for high-intensity sound, and compression limiting for the highest level sound; also often provides more amplification for high frequencies.

Kinesthetic: Relating to the perception of movement, position, and tension of body parts.

Kneepoint: Point on an input-output function of a hearing aid where compression is activated.

Labeling: A language-stimulation technique in which an adult provides names to objects, actions, and events.

Language: Complex system of symbols that are used in a rule-governed fashion for the purpose of communication.

LDL: Loudness discomfort level.

Learning disability: LD; a lack of ability in an area of learning that is inconsistent with an individual's cognitive capacity and is not a result of a deficit in sensory, motor, or emotional disorder.

Learning effect: Performance on a test improves as a function of familiarity with the test procedures and test items and not because of a change in ability.

Less-structured instruction: Informal shaping of language-stimulation behavior, often during play.

Level: Intensity of sound.

Lexical: Concerning the lexicon.

Lexical neighbors: Words that are phonemically (or visually) similar.

Lexicon: All of the units of meaning, such as words and morphemes, in a given language.

Life factors: Conditions that help define one's life, such as relationships, family, and vocation.

Life stages: Ranges in which a hearing loss may have a different impact.

Limited set: The response items in a stimulus or response set are limited by situational or contextual cues, for example, words related to summer.

Linear amplification: Hearing aid amplification system in which there is a one-to-one correspondence between the input and output until the maximum output level is reached.

Linked adjacency pairs: Two remarks that often are linked in conversation, as when one communication partner asks, "How are you?" and another responds, "Fine, thank you."

Lipreading: The process of recognizing speech using only the visual speech signal and other visual cues, such as facial expression.

Listening check: Informal assessment of whether a listening device is functioning appropriately.

Live-voice testing: Stimuli in a test of speech recognition are presented by a talker in real time.

Localization: The ability to locate the source of a sound in space due to the normal ear's sensitivity to interaural differences in phase and intensity.

Loudness: Perception of the intensity of a sound.

Loudness balancing: Programming the speech processor so that stimulation follows the loudness contour of the incoming speed signal.

Loudness comfort level: Level at which sound is perceived to be comfortably loud.

Loudness discomfort level: LDL; level at which sound is perceived to be uncomfortably loud.

Loudness summation: A summing of the signals received by each ear, resulting in a 3-dB advantage for binaural over monaural hearing.

Low-pass filtered speech: Speech that has been passed through filter banks, leaving the lower, but not the higher, frequencies.

Lucite: Material often used for constructing earmolds.

Macular degeneration: Progressive loss of both reading vision and distance vision.

Magnetic loop: Induction loop.

Mainstream classrooms: Deaf or hard-of-hearing children attend classes with their normally hearing peers.

Mainstreaming: Reassignment of children with disabilities from a special education classroom to a classroom in the regular school environment.

Maladaptive strategy: Inappropriate behavioral mechanisms for coping with the difficulties caused in conversation by hearing loss, such as avoidance behavior.

Managed care: A health care reimbursement plan in which an organization intercedes between patient and provider and determines the kind and extent of services that will be provided.

Manner of articulation: Classification of a speech sound as a function of how it is produced in the oral cavity (e.g., glide).

Manual alphabet: Series of hand configurations that correspond to each letter in the alphabet; used to fingerspell words in manual communication.

Manual communication: Communication modes that entail the use of fingerspelling, signs, and gestures.

Manually coded English: A form of communication in which manual signs correspond to English words.

Map: Specifications of threshold, suprathreshold, and frequency by which the speech processor of a cochlear implant processes the speech signal and delivers it in electrical form to the electrodes in the electrode array.

Mapping: Another term used to describe the process for establishing a map.

Masker: For tinnitus, an electronic listening device that delivers low-level noise to the ear for the purpose of masking the presence of tinnitus.

Masking: Noise that interferes with the perception of another sound.

Maximum comfort level: The maximum current level that can be introduced before the implant wearer experiences discomfort.

Maximum power output (MPO): maximum level intensity that a hearing aid can produce; SSPL.

MCL: Most comfortable loudness.

Mean length speaking turn: MLT; used in the assessment of conversational interactions, computed by determining the average number of words a person speaks during a set number of conversational turns.

Mean length turn ratio (MLT ratio): The ratio of the MLTs of two speakers in a conversation.

Meningitis: A common cause of childhood deafness caused by bacterial or viral inflammation of the meninges.

Mental age: Intellectual age.

Mental health problem: Psychopathology or clusters of other acute chronic symptoms.

Mental retardation: Intellectual function is below normal range.

Message-tailoring strategy: Phrasing one's remarks in a way that constrains the responses of a communication partner; a kind of facilitative communication strategy.

Metalinguistic: To think about and attend to the use of language.

Microphone: Transducer that converts an audio signal into an electronic signal.

Middle ear: Portion of the hearing mechanism extending from the tympanic membrane to the oval window of the cochlea; includes the ossicles and middle ear cavity.

Mimetic: Imitating or copying the movements.

Mixed hearing loss: A hearing loss that has a conductive and sensorineural component.

Mobile unit: A mobile van that is equipped to screen hearing; used for educational and on-site industrial hearing screening programs.

Modality: Any of the five senses, including audition and vision.

Modeling: An instructor demonstrates a desired behavior and a student attempts to imitate it.

Monaural: Concerning one ear.

Monosyllabic word: A word comprised of one syllable.

Morpheme: Smallest unit of language that conveys meaning.

Most comfortable loudness: MCL; level at which sound is most comfortable for a listener, usually measured in dB HL.

Multiband compression: A method of shaping the loudness growth of a signal to maximize speech for the listener using different degrees of compression and output limiting for different frequencies.

Multichannel: More than one channel of information; often used to describe cochlear implants that present different channels of information to different regions of the cochlea.

Multidisciplinary team: A group of professionals with different expertise contributing to the assessment, intervention, and management program for a particular individual.

Multiple channels: A hearing aid that filters the signal into frequency bands so that some bands (usually the high-frequency bands) can receive more gain than others.

Multiple-memory hearing aid: A hearing aid that can be programmed to process the speech signal in more than one way, so that the user can adjust the processing strategy for different listening environments.

Multisensory approach: Educational approach for deaf children that emphasizes the use of vision, residual hearing, and sometimes touch to enhance communication.

Myringitis: Inflammation of the tympanic membrane.

NAD: National Association of the Deaf.

National Association of the Deaf: NAD; advocacy group for members of the Deaf Culture.

NECCI: Network of Educators of Children with Cochlear Implants.

Neckloop: A transducer worn around the neck as part of an FM assistive device system, consisting of a cord from a receiver; transmits signals via magnetic induction to the telecoil of the user's hearing aid.

Neonatal: Concerning the first 4 weeks of life.

Network of Educators of Children with Cochlear Implants: NECCI; professional organization of speech and hearing professionals and educators who are involved with children who receive and use cochlear implants.

NIHL: Noise-induced hearing loss.

Noise: Unwanted sound.

Noise exposure: Level of noise and duration of exposure.

Noise-induced hearing loss: NIHL; sensorineural hearing loss that is the result of exposure to excessive levels of sound; auditory trauma caused by loud sound and resulting in permanent hearing loss.

Noise-induced permanent threshold shift: NIPTS; permanent decrease in an individual's hearing thresholds as a result of exposure to excessive sound levels.

Noise-induced temporary threshold shift: NITTS; transient shift in an individual's hearing thresholds as a result of exposure

to excessive sound levels; temporary threshold shift.

Noise reduction: The difference in sound pressure level (SPL) of a noise, measured at two different locations.

Noninteractive communication behaviors: Characteristic of a passive conversational style; includes failure to contribute to the development of a conversational topic, minimal response to turn-taking signals, and a proclivity to bluff.

Nonlinear amplification: Amplification system that does not provide a one-to-one correspondence between input and output at all input levels.

Nonsense syllable: Single syllable of speech that has no meaning.

Nonspecific repair strategy: A repair strategy used to repair a communication breakdown that does not provide specific instruction to the communication partner about what to do next: *what, huh, pardon.*

Nonsyndromic hearing loss: A hearing loss that has no other associated findings.

Norm: Standards derived from a sample of the population of interest, thought to represent typical values of the characteristic under study or test.

NR: No response.

OAE: Otoacoustic emission.

Objective: Physically measurable.

Occlusion effect: Enhancement of the level of low-frequency sound in bone-conducted signals as a result of occlusion of the ear canal.

Occupational hearing loss: Noise-induced hearing loss incurred on the job.

Occupational Safety and Health Act: U.S. federal legislation passed in 1970 to ensure safe and healthy work environments; resulted in the establishment of OSHA, NIOSH, and OSHRC.

Occupational Safety and Health Administration: OSHA; Federal agency that regulates occupational health and safety hazards and establishes and enforces minimum standards for industrial hearing conservation programs.

OHCP: Occupational hearing conservation program.

Omnidirectional microphone: Microphone that is sensitive to sound coming from all directions.

On-off control: A small switch that moves back and forth to turn the hearing aid off when not in use and on when needed; may be incorporated into the volume wheel.

Open-ended questions: Questions that elicit qualitative information.

Open-set: Testing or training task that does not provide a set of choices to the patient.

Oral interpreter: A professional who silently repeats a talker's message as it is spoken, so that a hard-of-hearing person may lipread the message.

Oralism: Method of instruction for deaf children that emphasizes spoken language skills to the exclusion of manual communication.

Organized messages: Communications that are not wordy and do not use complex verbiage; terminology is precise.

OSHA: Occupational Safety and Health Administration.

Ossification: A conversion of tissue into bone.

Otitis media: Inflammation of the middle ear.

Oto: Otolaryngology.

Otoacoustic emission: OAE; low-level sound emitted by the cochlear spontaneously on presentation of an auditory stimulus.

Otolaryngologist: Physician who specializes in the diagnosis and treatment of diseases and conditions of the ear, nose, and throat.

Otologist: Physician who specializes in the diagnosis and treatment of diseases and conditions of the ear.

Otoscope: Instrument for visual examination of the external ear and tympanic membrane.

Ototoxic: Having a poisonous effect on the structures of the ear, particularly the hair cells in the cochlea and vestibular organs.

Outer ear: Peripheral part of the auditory mechanism that includes the pinna, the concha, the external auditory canal, and lateral wall of the tympanic membrane.

Output: Energy or information exiting from a listening device.

Output limiting: Limiting the output of a listening device by means of peak-clipping or compression.

Output stage: The process signal is boosted.

Parallel talk: A language-stimulation technique, wherein an adult matches language to an activity a child is performing.

Passive conversational style: Conversational style of some persons who have hearing loss, characterized by withdrawal from conversation, frequent bluffing, and avoidance of social interactions.

Patient orientation: An orientation centered on the patient's background, current status, needs, and wants, on which the design and delivery of rehabilitative services are based.

Peak-clipping: A method of limiting hearing aid output in which a constant or linear amount of gain is provided across a range of input levels until it reaches a saturation level at which the amplifier begins to "clip" off the peaks of the signal.

Perilingual: Hearing loss acquired during the stage of spoken language acquisition.

Perinatal: During birth.

Personal FM trainer: A listening device in which the speaker wears a wireless microphone and the speech is frequency modulated on radio waves transmitted through the room to the listener, who wears a receiver.

Phenotype: Visible expression of a genotype of an individual.

Phoneme: A speech sound.

Phonetic alphabet: Symbols that represent the sound of a spoken language.

Phonetically balanced word lists: PB word lists; sets of words that contain speech sounds with the same frequency of occurrence as in everyday conversation.

Pinna: Auricle; the cartilaginous structures of the outer ear.

Pitch ranking: Determines the ability to discriminate pitch from stimulation of the basal to apical electrodes.

PL 101-336: Americans with Disabilities Act (ADA) of 1990.

PL 101-431: Television Decoder Circuitry Act of 1990.

PL 94-142: Individuals with Disabilities Education Act of 1975.

Place of articulation: Classification of a speech sound according to where in the vocal tract it is produced (e.g., bilabial).

Play audiometry: Behavioral method for testing the hearing thresholds of young children, in which correct identification of a stimulus presentation is rewarded by allowing the child to perform a play-oriented activity.

Plosive: Stop-consonant speech sound that is produced by creating an oral cavity closure, building air pressure behind the closure, and then releasing it (e.g., /p, t, k/).

Postlingual: Hearing loss incurred after the acquisition of spoken language.

Postnatal: After birth.

Pragmatics: The study of how language is used.

Preamplifier stage: The signal from the microphone is amplified.

Predicament: The "sum of all pertinent aspects of client state and situation, including disorders, impairments, disabilities, handicaps, environments, demands, resources, attitudes, behaviors, and so on." Hyde & Riko, 1994, p. 351

Prelingual: Hearing loss incurred before the acquisition of spoken language.

Prenatal: Before birth.

Presbycusis: Age-related hearing loss.

Prescribed gain: Gain and frequency response of a hearing aid that are determined by use of a prescriptive formula.

Prescription procedures: Fitting hearing aids by using a formula to calculate the desired gain and frequency response.

Prescriptive hearing-aid fitting: Strategy for fitting hearing aids by using a formula to calculate the desired gain and frequency response; formula incorporates pure-tone audiometric thresholds and, usually, information about uncomfortable loudness levels.

Probe microphone: Microphone transducer that is inserted into the external ear canal for the purpose of measuring sound near the tympanic membrane.

Processing strategy: Strategy used by cochlear implants to determine how the input signal is processed, including the degree of amplification of different frequency bands and the manner in which the signal is delivered by different electrodes in the electrode array; process used to transform the speech signal into a pattern of electrical stimulation.

Program: The setting of a speech processor or hearing aid according to the user's measured thresholds, comfort levels, and other subjective responses to stimulation.

Programmability: In a hearing aid it means that several parameters of the instrument, such as gain, are controlled by a computer.

Programmable hearing aid: Hearing aid in which several parameters of the instrument, such as gain, are under computer control.

Progressive hearing loss: Advancing; occurring over time.

Prosodic cues: Cues provided by intonation, rate, and duration of speech sounds.

Prosody: Suprasegmental aspects of the speech signal, including fluctuations in voice pitch, rhythm, rate, intensity, and stress patterns; intonation.

Psychic costs: Nonmonetary costs that relate to psychosocial well-being.

PTA: Pure-tone average.

Pure-tone average: PTA: Average of hearing thresholds at 500 Hz, 1000 Hz, and 2000 Hz.

Quest?AR: A structured communication procedure used to assess communication difficulties.

Questionnaires: A procedure to assess conversational fluency and communication handicap, in which respondents provide subjective information about their listening and communication difficulties.

Rational acceptance and adjustment counseling: Counseling that focuses on the permanency of the hearing loss and concrete means of managing communication problems.

Reactive: Self-monitoring can provide reactive procedure as it may influence how a person uses communication behaviors and strategies.

Real-ear gain: Gain of a hearing aid at the tympanic membrane, measured with a probe-microphone; the difference between the SPL in the external ear canal and the SPL at the field reference point for a specified sound field.

Real-ear measures: The use of a probe microphone to measure hearing aid gain and frequency response delivered by a hearing aid at the tympanic membrane.

Real-time captioning: Captioning of a person's speech in real-time using computer technology.

Real-world practice: The third stage in a communication strategies training exercise, practice of a new skill or behavior in an everyday environment.

Receiver: Component that converts electrical energy into acoustic energy, as in a hearing aid; or component of an FM system worn by the listener that receives FM signals from a transmitter; or individual who receives a message from a sender.

Receptive repair strategy: Tactic taken by an individual when he or she has not understood a message presented by a communication partner.

Recorded stimuli: Test items presented via a tape recorder or a compact disc player.

Rehabilitation: Intervention designed for the reteaching of particular skills.

Reinforcement: Something desirable, such as a sticker or privilege, provided to a student after he or she performs a training activity or behaves in a desired manner.

Release time: The time it takes for an amplifier to return to its steady state after a loud sound ends.

Relay system: System used by persons with significant hearing loss to use the telephone; individual contacts a relay operator who serves to transmit messages between caller and person called by means of teletype and/or voice.

Reliability: Extent to which a test yields similar results with repeated administration.

Remote control: Hand-held device that permits adjustments in the volume or changes in the program of a programmable hearing aid.

Repair strategies: Tactics implemented by a participant in a conversation to rectify breakdowns in communication.

Residual hearing: The hearing remaining in a person who has hearing loss.

Resource rooms: Provide instruction in particular areas for children who spend part of their day in regular classrooms.

Reverberation: Prolongation of an auditory signal by multiple reflections in a closed environment; amount of echo in an enclosed space.

Role-play: Individuals participate in hypothetical real-world situations.

Round window: Membrane covered opening between the middle ear space and the scala tympani section of the cochlea in the inner ear.

S/N ratio: Signal-to-noise ratio.

Sales orientation: An orientation to providing rehabilitation services in which emphasis is placed on persuading the patient to pursue and procure services, interventions, and listening devices.

Saturation level: Point at which an amplifier no longer provides an increase in output compared to input.

Saturation sound pressure level (SSPL): The maximum sound pressure level that can be delivered by a hearing aid with its volume full-on.

Screening: The use of tests that are quick and easy to administer to a large group for the purpose of identifying individuals who require further diagnostic testing.

SDT: Speech detection threshold.

Seeing Essential English: SEE1; a manual communication system that incorporates some signs of American Sign Language and some English syntax.

Segmental errors: Pertaining to the sounds of speech.

Self-concept: How persons view themselves.

Self-contained classrooms: Those that contain only deaf or hard-of-hearing children.

Self Help for Hard of Hearing People: SHHH; organization for adults who have hearing loss.

Self-sufficiency and independence: Whether a person can conduct day-to-day activities without undue reliance on others.

Self-talk: Language-stimulation technique in which an adult describes what he or she is doing or thinking for the purpose of promoting language development in a child.

Semantic: Related to meaning, and the relationship between units of language and their referents.

Sender: Individual who presents a message, as opposed to a *receiver.*

Senile: Related to old age.

Sensation level: SL; the intensity level of a sound in dB expressed in reference to the individual's threshold for the sound.

Sensorineural hearing loss: SNHL; hearing loss with a cochlear or retrocochlear origin.

Sign interpreter: A professional who translates spoken English into a form of signed English or ASL, or vice versa.

Sign language: System of manual communication in which hand configurations, positions, and movements are used to express concepts and linguistic information.

Signal processing: Manipulation of various parameters of the signal.

Signal-processing stage: The signal is manipulated to enhance or extract component information.

Signal-to-noise ratio: S/N ratio; the level of a signal relative to a background of noise, usually expressed in dB.

Signed English: Manual communication system that utilizes English word order and syntax.

Signing Exact English: SEE2; a simplified version of Seeing Essential English.

Silica gel: Agent that absorbs moisture, often used in the storage of hearing aids.

Simple amplification systems: Systems that merely amplify the audio signal so that it is more audible to a person with hearing loss.

Simultaneous communication: Educational approach used with individuals with severe and profound hearing loss that integrates aural/oral communication and manual communication; total communication.

SL: Sensational level.

SLP: Speech-language pathologist.

SNHL: Sensorineural hearing loss.

Sociolinguistics: The branch of linguistics that concerns the effects of social and cultural differences within a language community on its use of language and conversational patterns.

Sound awareness: The most basic auditory skill level; awareness of when a sound is present and when it is not.

Sound discrimination: A basic auditory skill level in which the listener is able to tell whether two sounds are different or the same.

Sound field: A free-field environment where sound is propagated.

Sound field testing: Determination of hearing sensitivity or speech recognition ability with the stimuli presented through loudspeakers, often used in pediatric testing or hearing-aid evaluations.

Sound level: The intensity of a sound expressed in decibels.

Sound level meter: An instrument designed to measure the intensity of sound in dB according to an accepted standard.

Sound pressure level: SPL; magnitude of sound energy relative to a reference pressure, 0.0002 dynes/cm^2.

Sound-proof: Impenetrable by acoustic energy.

Specific repair strategy: Repair strategy used to rectify a communication breakdown that provides explicit instruction to the communication partner about what to do next.

Speech: Coordination of respiration, phonation, articulation, and resonation for the purpose of producing spoken language.

Speech audiometry: Measurement of speech listening skills, including speech awareness and speech recognition.

Speech discrimination score: The percentage of nonsyllabic words presented at a comfortable listening level that can be correctly repeated.

Speech-language pathology: Professional discipline related to the study, diagnosis, and treatment of speech and language disorders.

Speech processor: The component of a cochlear implant where the input signal is modified for presentation to the electrodes in the electrode array.

Speech reception threshold: SRT; threshold level for speech recognition, that is the lowest presentation level for spondee words at which 50% can be identified correctly.

Speech recognition: The ability to perceive and identify speech units.

Speechreading: Speech recognition using auditory and visual cues.

Speechreading enhancement: The difference or ratio between speech recognition performance in an audition-only condition and an audition-plus-vision condition.

Spiral ganglion: Comprised of the nuclei of the nerve fibers that connect to the hair cells and meet in the central core (which is called the *modiolus*) of the cochlea.

SPL: Sound pressure level.

Spondee: Two-syllable word with equal stress on each syllable.

Spondee threshold: ST; speech reception threshold.

SRT: Speech reception threshold.

SSPL-90 curve: Saturation sound pressure level 90; electroacoustic assessment of a hearing aid's maximum level of output signal, expressed as a frequency response curve to a

90 dB signal, with the hearing aid volume control set to full-on.

ST: Speech threshold.

Stage of life: Phases in the life cycle, including childhood, young adulthood, middle age, and old age.

Stimulus: Something that can evoke or elicit a response.

Stop consonant: Plosive; speech sound produced by building up air pressure behind a closure in the oral cavity and then releasing it (e.g., /p, t, k/).

Structured communication interaction: Simulated conversation that reflects some of the communication difficulties a person with hearing loss may experience during everyday conversation; for example, TOPICON.

Sudden hearing loss: Hearing loss that is incurred suddenly; acute and rapid onset.

Suprasegmental errors: Prosodic aspects of speech; variations in pitch, rate, intensity, and duration superimposed on phonemes and words.

Syndrome: Collection of conditions that co-occur as a result from a single cause and constitute a distinct clinical entity.

Syntax: Word order in a given language.

Synthesized speech: Speech generated by computer.

T-switch: Telecoil switch.

Tactile aid: Vibrotactile aid; aid that transduces sound to vibration and delivers it to the skin for the purpose of sound awareness and gross sound identification.

Target gain: In hearing-aid fitting, the prescribed gain for each frequency against which the actual hearing-aid output is compared.

TDD: Telecommunication device for the deaf.

Telecoil: T coil; induction coil often in a hearing aid that receives electromagnetic signals from a telephone or a loop amplification system.

Telecoil switch: T-switch; switch on a hearing aid that activates the telecoil.

Telecommunication device for the deaf: TDD; TT (text telephone); TTY; telephone device for persons with deafness or significant hearing loss in which messages are typed on a keyboard; transmitted over telephone wires, and displayed on a small monitor screen.

Telegraphic speech: Spoken language patterns that are characterized by the omission of function words and, sometimes, incorrect word order.

Telephone amplifier: Assistive listening device that increases the intensity of a Signal emanating from a telephone receiver.

Television Decoder Circuitry Act: U.S. Public Law 101-336 of 1990; act that requires all televisions with a 13-inch diagonal screen or wider to contain circuitry necessary for closed captioning.

Temperament: Stable personality traits.

Temporary threshold shift: TTS; transient hearing loss following exposure to excessive noise.

Test-retest reliability: Measure of test consistency from one presentation to the next.

Text telephones: Consist of a telephone, a keyboard, and a message display screen. The telephone handset fits into the terminal cradle. Both parties communicate by typing their messages.

3-dB rule: Time-intensity tradeoff that states for every 50% decrease in noise-exposure, a 3 dB-A increase in noise level is permitted without increasing the risk of noise-induced hearing loss.

Threshold: Level at which sound can be detected only 50% of the time.

Threshold shift: Change in hearing sensitivity expressed in dB.

Time-compressed speech: Speech that has been accelerated by means of removing segments from the waveform and compressing the remaining segments together, without changing its frequency composition.

Time-talk: A language-stimulation techniques wherein an adult purposely incorporates time-related language into conversation.

Time-weighted average: TWA; index of daily noise exposure that is the product of durations of exposure relative to the allowable durations of exposure for a particular sound level.

Tinnitus: Sensation of noise in the head without an external cause.

Tinnitus masker: Electronic hearing aid that generates and outputs noise at low levels for the purpose of masking an individual's tinnitus.

T-level: Another term used for threshold.

TOPICON: An example of a structured communication interaction activity.

Transmitter: A device that emits electromagnetic rays; a component of an FM system that modulates the frequency of a radio signal in an audio frequency signal and transmits the waves through air to an amplifier/receiver.

TT: Text telephone; TDD.

TTS: Temporary threshold shift.

TTY: Teletypewriter; less-frequently used term than TDD or TT.

Tune-up: Mapping; establishing a map for a cochlear implant speech processor.

TWA: Time-weighted average.

Tx: Therapy or treatment.

Tympanogram: Graph of middle ear immittance as a function of air pressure in the external auditory canal.

UCL: Uncomfortable loudness.

UL: Uncomfortable level.

ULL: Uncomfortable loudness level.

Uncomfortable level: UL; level at which sound is judged to be so loud as to be uncomfortable to the listener.

Uncomfortable loudness level: ULL; UCL; intensity level at which a listener judges a sound to be uncomfortably loud; loudness discomfort level.

Unconditional positive regard: The second tenet of person-centered counseling, in which clinicians assume that patients know best and assume that they have the inner resources to overcome their conversation difficulties.

Underserved: A group of patients receiving less than ideal services.

Unilateral: Pertaining to one side.

Unisensory approach: Use of only residual hearing to receive spoken messages.

Unserved: Refers to a group of patients in need of but not receiving services.

Use gain: Amount of gain provided by a hearing aid when the volume control is set where it is commonly used.

Vent: Bore drilled into an earmold that permits the passage of sound and air; used for aeration of the external auditory canal or for acoustic modification of the amplified sound.

Vertigo: Dizziness, including a sensation of spinning or whirling.

Vibratory pagers: Instead of emitting audible beeps, the pager vibrates against the user to signal a call.

Vibrotactile: Pertaining to the detection of vibrations through the sense of touch.

Vibrotactile hearing aid: An assistive listening device that converts acoustic energy into vibratory patterns that are delivered to the skin.

Videotaped scenarios: Videotaped examples of communication interactions, which may include use of communications strategies and language-stimulation techniques.

Viseme: Groups of speech sounds that appear identical on the lips (e.g., /p, m, b/).

Vision only: Presentation of only a visual stimulus in testing.

Visual alerting systems: Assistive devices that include alarm clocks, doorbells, and smoke detectors in which the alerting mechanism is a flashing light.

Visual reinforcement audiometry: VRA; audiometric technique used with young children in which a correct response to a stimulus presentation is reinforced by a visual reward, such as the activation of a lighted toy.

Voicing: Classification of a speech sound according to whether it is produced with or without voice (e.g., /b/ versus /p/).

Volume control: Manual or automatic control used to adjust the output of a listening device.

Vowel formants: Resonances in the vocal tract that cause some frequencies to have more energy than other frequencies.

VRA: Visual reinforcement audiometry.

WATCH: A brief communication strategies training program.

Weighting scale: Sound level meter filtering network, in which the measurement of one band of frequencies is emphasized over another (e.g., dBA scale).

White noise: Noise having energy at all frequencies audible to the human ear.

Wide-band noise: White noise.

Wireless system: An assistive listening device in which wires are not necessary to connect the sound source to the listener; includes FM and infrared systems.

Word recognition: Ability to perceive and identify a word.

Word-recognition score: Percent words correct.

X-linked: Refers to the mother carrying a recessive allele for a trait on the sex chromosomes, which is not expressed in female progeny but is passed to males.

References

Abrahamson, J. (1991). Teaching coping strategies: A client education approach to aural rehabilitation. *Journal of the Academy of Rehabilitative Audiology, 24*, 43–54.

Alcantara, J. I., Cowan, R. S. C., Blamey, P. J., & Clark, G. M. (1990). A comparison of two training strategies for speech recognition with an electrotactile speech processor. *Journal of Speech and Hearing Research, 33*, 195–204.

Allen, T. E. (1986). Patterns of academic achievement among hearing impaired students: 1974 and 1983. In A. N. Schildroth & M. A. Karchmer (Eds.), *Deaf children in America* (pp. 161–206). San Diego, CA: College-Hill Press.

Alpiner, J. G., & Garstecki, D. C. (1996). Audiologic rehabilitation for adults: Assessment and management. In R. L. Schow & M. A. Nerbonne (Eds.), *Introduction to audiologic rehabilitation* (3rd ed., pp. 361–412). Needham Heights, MA: Allyn & Bacon.

American Speech-Language-Hearing Association (ASHA) (2002). Knowledge and skills required for the practice of audiologic/aural rehabilitation: Executive summary. *ASHA Supplement 22.*

Anders, G. (1997). Doctors learn to bridge cultural gaps. *The Wall Street Journal* Sep. 4, n177.

Andersson, G., Melin, L., Lindberg, P., & Scott, B. (1995). Development of a short scale for self-assessment of experiences of hearing loss: The hearing coping assessment. *Scandinavian Audiology, 24*, 147–154.

Andersson, U., Lyxell, B., Rönnberg, J., & Spens, K. E. (2001). Cognitive correlates of visual speech understanding in hearing-impaired individuals. *Journal of Deaf Studies and Deaf Education, 6*, 103–115.

Andrews, J. R., & Andrews, M. A. (1990). *Family based treatment in communication disorders: A systemic approach.* Sandwich, IL: Janelle Publications.

Anita, S. D., Stinson, M. S., & Gaustad, M. G. (2002). Developing membership in the education of deaf and hard-of-hearing students in inclusive settings. *Journal of Deaf Studies and Deaf Education, 7*, 214–229.

Arana-Ward, M. (1997). As technology advances, a bitter debate divides the deaf. *Washington Post*, May 11, A1.

Arehart, K. H., Yoshinaga-Itano, C., Thomson, V., Gabbard, S. A., & Brown, A. S. (1998). State of the states: The status of universal newborn hearing screening, assessment, and intervention systems in 16 states. *American Journal of Audiology, 7*, 101–114.

Arlinger, S., Billermark, E., Oberg, M., Lunner, T., & Hellgren, J. (1998). Clinical trial of a digital hearing aid. *Scandinavian Audiology, 27*, 51–61.

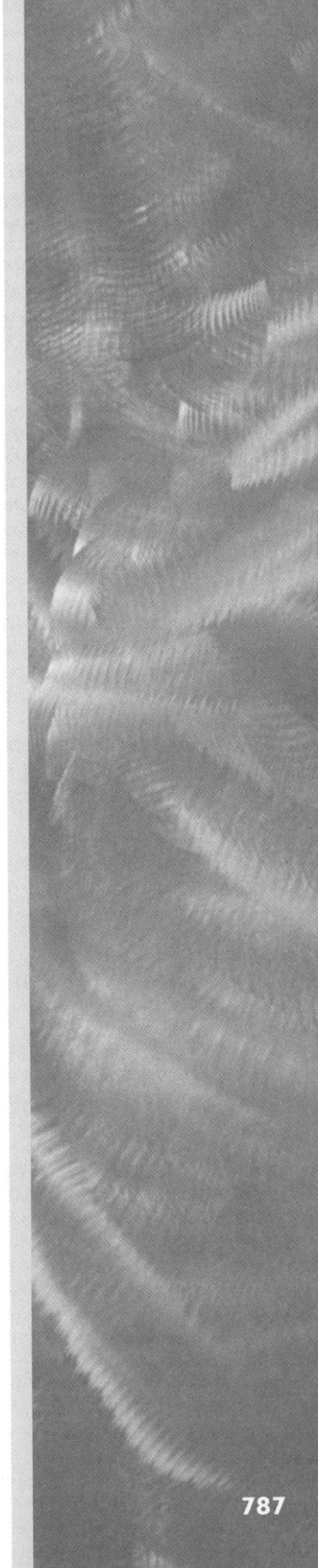

Armstrong, T. L. (1991). *The relationship between gender and psychological distress in hard-of-hearing people.* Paper presented to the American Public Health Association, Washington, D.C.

Arnold, P., & Hill, F. (2001). Bisensory augmentation: A speechreading advantage when speech is clearly audible and intact. *British Journal of Psychology, 92,* 339–355.

ASHA Leader (2002). Data snapshot and quick facts. *ASHA Leader, 7,* 10, 32.

ASHA Leader (2002). Focus on multiculturalism: Data snapshots. *ASHA Leader, 7,* 32.

Axelsson, A., & Ringdahl, A. (1989). Tinnitus: A study of its prevalence and characteristics. *British Journal of Audiology, 23,* 53–62.

Bader, L. A. (1998). *Bader reading and language inventory* (3rd Ed.). Upper Saddle River, MN: Prentice Hall.

Baker, C. (1993). *Foundations of bilingual education and bilingualism.* Clevedon, Avon, U.K.: Multicultural Matters.

Bamford, J. and Saunders, E. (1985). *Hearing impairment, auditory perception, and language disability.* London: Edward Arnold.

Barcham, L. J., & Stephens, S. D. (1980). The use of an open-ended problems questionnaire in auditory rehabilitation. *British Journal of Audiology, 14,* 49–54.

Beck, A. T., & Emery, G. (1985). *Anxiety disorders and phobias.* New York: Basic Books.

Bellis, T. J. (1996). *Assessment and management of central auditory processing disorders in the educational setting: From science to practice.* Clifton Park, NY: Delmar Learning.

Bench, J., & Bamford, J. (1979). *Speech-hearing tests and the spoken language of hearing-impaired children.* London: Academic Press.

Benitez, L., & Speaks, C. (1968). A test of speech intelligibility in the Spanish language. *International Audiology, 7,* 16–22.

Benson, V., & Marano, M. A. (1998). *Current estimates from the National Health Interview Survey, 1995.* National Center for Health Statistics. *Vital Health Stat 10* [1991].)

Bentler, R. A., & Kramer, S. E. (2000). Guidelines for choosing a self-report outcome measure. *Ear and Hearing, 21,* 37S–49S.

Berger, K. W. (1972). *Speechreading: Principles and methods.* Baltimore, MD: National Education Press.

Berko, J. (1984). The child's learning of English morphology. *Word, 14,* 150–177.

Bernstein, L. E., Auer, E. T., & Tucker, P. E. (2001). Enhanced speechreading in deaf adults: Can short-term training/practice close the gap for hearing adults? *Journal of Speech, Language, and Hearing Research, 44,* 5–18.

Bernstein, L. E., Demorest, M. E., Coulter, D. C., & O'Connell, M. P. (1991). Lipreading sentences with vibrotactile vocoders: Performance of normal-hearing and hearing-impaired subjects. *Journal of the Acoustical Society of America, 90,* 2971–2984.

Berry, J. A., Gold, S. L., Frederick, E. A., Gray, W. C., & Staecker, H. (2002). Patient-based outcomes in patients with primary tinnitus undergoing tinnitus retraining therapy. *Archives of Otolaryngology—Head and Neck Surgery, 128,* 1153–1157.

Berry, S. (1981). *Written language syntax test.* Washington, DC: Gallaudet College Press.

Bess, F. H. (2000). The role of generic health-related quality of life measures in establishing audiological rehabilitation. *Ear and Hearing, 21,* 74S–79S.

Bilger, R. C., Nuetzel, J. M., Rabinowitz, W. M., & Rzeczkowski, C. (1984). Standardization of a test of speech perception in noise. *Journal of Speech and Hearing Research, 27,* 32–48.

Binnie, C.A. (1991). New perspectives in audiological rehabilitation. In G. A. Studebaker, F. H. Bess, & L. B. Beck (Eds.), The Vanderbilt Health-aid Report II (pp. 233–243). Parkton, MD: York Press.

Binzer, S. M., Mauze, E., Tye-Murray, N., Heydebrand, G., & Skinner, M. (Submitted). Attitudes, conversational skills, and problem-management of cochlear implant users and their partners following a group psychosocial intervention.

Blamey, P. J., & Alcantara, J. I. (1994). Research in auditory training. *Journal of the Academy of Rehabilitative Audiology, 27*(Suppl.), 161–192.

Blood, G. W., Blood, I. M., & Danhauer, J. L. (1978). Listeners' impression of normal-hearing and hearing-impaired children. *Journal of Communication Disorders, 11,* 513–518.

Bloom, S. (1999). Marketing to baby boomers: Challenges and opportunities are greater than ever. *Hearing Journal, 52,* 23–30.

Bodrova, E., Leong, D. J., Paynter, D. E., & Semenov, D. (2000). *A framework for early literacy instruction: Aligning standards to developmental accomplishments and student behaviors.* Aurora, CO: Mid-continent Research for Education and Learning.

Boettcher, F. A. (2002). Presbycusis and the auditory brainstem response. *Journal of Speech-Language-Hearing Research, 45,* 1249–1262.

Boothroyd, A. (1984). Auditory perception of speech contrasts by subjects with sensorineural hearing loss. *Journal of Speech and Hearing Research, 27,* 134–144.

Boothroyd, A. (1991). Assessment of speech perception capacity in profoundly deaf children. *The American Journal of Otology, 12*(Suppl.), 67–72.

Boothroyd, A., Hanin, L., & Hnath-Chisholm, T. (1985). *The CUNY sentence test.* New York, NY: City University of New York.

Borg, E. (2000). Ecological aspects of auditory rehabilitation. *Acta Otolaryngol, 120,* 234–241.

Borg, E., Danermark, B., & Borg, B. (2002). Behavioural awareness, interaction and counseling education in audiological rehabilitation: Development of methods and application in a pilot study. *International Journal of Audiology, 41,* 308–322.

Brackett, D. (1990). Developing an individualized education program for the mainstreamed hearing-impaired student. In M. Ross (Ed.), *Hearing-impaired children in the mainstream* (pp. 81–94). Parkton, MD: York Press.

Brainerd, S. H., & Frankel, B. G. (1985). The relationship between audiometric and self-report measures of hearing handicap. *Ear and Hearing, 6,* 89–92.

Brigance, A. H. (1999). *Brigance comprehensive inventory of basic skills-revised (CIBS-R).* North Billerica, MA: Curriculum Associates.

Broadcaster. (1991). *Cochlear Implants in children: A position paper of the National Association of the Deaf.* Silver Springs, MD: National Association of the Deaf.

Bromwich, R. (1981). *Working with parents and infants: An interactional approach.* Baltimore, MD: University Park Press.

Brooks, D. N. (1979). Counseling and its effect on hearing aid use. *Scandinavian Audiology, 8,* 101–107.

Brooks, D. N. (1990). Measures for the assessment of hearing aid provision and rehabilitation. *British Journal of Audiology, 24,* 229–233.

Bryant, B., & Wiederhold, J. L. (1991). *Gray oral reading test-diagnostic (GORT-D).* Austin, TX: Pro-Ed.

Caissie, R., & Rockwell, E. (1994). Communication difficulties experienced by nursing home residents with a hearing loss during conversation with staff members. *Journal of Speech-Language Pathology and Audiology, 18,* 127–134.

Campbell, R. (1998). How brains see speech: The cortical localization of speechreading in hearing people. In R. Campbell, B. Dodd, & D. Burnham (Eds.), *Hearing by eye II* (pp. 177–194). East Sussex, UK: Psychology Press.

Carney, A., & Moeller, M. P. (1998). Treatment efficacy: Hearing loss in children. *Journal of Speech, Language, and Hearing Research, 41*(Suppl.), S61–S84.

Carrow, E. (1973). *Test for auditory comprehension of language.* Lamar, TX: Learning Concepts.

Cassie, R. (2002). Conversational topic shifting and its effect on communication breakdowns. *The Volta Review, 102,* 45–56.

Cassie, R., & Gibson, C. L. (1997). The effectiveness of repair strategies used by people with hearing losses and their conversational partners. *The Volta Review, 99,* 203–218.

Castle, D. (1988). The oral interpreter. *Volta Review, 90,* 307–313.

Ceasar, L. G., & Williams, D. R. (2002). Socioculture and the delivery of health care: Who gets what and why. *ASHA Leader, 7,* 6–8.

Centers for Disease Control and Prevention. (2001). Trends in vision and hearing among older Americans. *Aging Trends, 2,* 1–8.

Cherow, E., & Boswell, S. (1999). Pediatric audiology: Poised for the future. *ASHA* (May/June), 24–30.

Cherry, R., & Rubinstein, A. (1988). Speechreading instruction for adults: Issues and practices. *Volta Review, 90,* 289–306.

Chessman, M. G. (1997). Speech perception by elderly listeners: Basic knowledge and implications for audiology. *Journal of Speech-Language Pathology and Audiology, 21.*

Cienkowski, K. M., & Carney, A. E. (2002). Auditory-visual speech perception and aging. *Ear and Hearing, 23,* 439–449.

Ciocci, S., & Baran, J. (1998). The use of conversational repair strategies by children who are deaf. *American Annals of the Deaf, 143,* 235–245.

Citron, D. (2000). Counseling and orientation toward amplification. In M. Valente, H. Hosford-Dunn, & R. J. Roseser, *Audiology treatment,* (pp. 459–488). New York: Thieme.

Clark, J. G. (1994). Understanding, building and maintaining relationships with patients. *Effective counseling in audiology: Perspectives and practice* (pp. 18–37). Englewood Cliffs, NJ: PrenticeHall.

Clark, T. (1994). SKI*HI: Applications for home-based intervention. In J. Rousch & N. Matkin (Eds.), *Infants and toddlers with hearing loss: Family-centered assessment and intervention* (pp. 237–251). Baltimore, MD: York Press.

Code of Ethics. (1984). In W. H. Northcott (Ed.), *Oral interpreting: Principles and practices* (pp. 266–269). Baltimore, MD: University Park Press.

Cole, E. B. (1993). *Listening and talking: A guide to promoting spoken language in young hearing-impaired children.* Washington, DC: Alexander Graham Bell Association for the Deaf.

Coles, R. R. A. (1984). Epidemiology of tinnitus: (1) Prevalence. *Journal of Laryngology and Otology* (Suppl.), *9,* 7–15.

Compton, C. L. (1995). Selecting what's best for the individual. In R. S. Tyler & D. J. Schum (Eds.), *Assistive devices for persons with hearing impairment* (pp. 224–250). Needham Heights, Md: Allyn & Bacon.

Comstock, C. L., & Martin, F. N. (1984). A children's Spanish word discrimination test for non-Spanish-speaking clinicians. *Ear and Hearing, 14* (5), 164–170.

Cornett, R. O. (1967). Cued speech. *American Annals of the Deaf, 112,* 313.

Cowie, R., & Douglas-Cowie, E. (1992). *Postlingually acquired deafness: Speech deterioration and the wider consequences.* New York: Mouton de Gruyter.

Cox, R. M., & Alexander, G. C. (1991). Hearing aid benefit in everyday environments. *Ear and Hearing, 12,* 127–139.

Cox, R. M. & Alexander, G. C. (1995). The abbreviated profile of hearing aid benefit. *Ear and Hearing, 16,* 176–183.

Cox, R. M., & Alexander, G. C. (1999). Measuring satisfaction with amplification in daily life: The SADL scale. *Ear and Hearing, 20,* 306–320.

Cox, R. M., Alexander, G. C., & Gilmore, C. (1987). Development of the connected speech test (CST), *Ear and Hearing, 9,* 198–207.

Cox, R. M., & Gilmore, C. (1990). Development of the profile of hearing aid performance (PHAP). *Journal of Speech and Hearing Research, 33,* 343–357.

Cox, R. M., Gilmore, C. G., & Alexander, G. C. (1991). Comparison of two questionnaires for patient-assessed hearing aid benefit. *Journal of the American Academy of Audiology, 2,* 134–145.

Cox, R. M., & Rivera, I. M. (1992). Predictability and reliability of hearing aid benefit measured using the PHAP. *Journal of the American Academy of Audiology, 3,* 242–254.

Craig, W. N. (1964). Effects of preschool training on the development of reading and lipreading skills of deaf children. *American Annals of the Deaf, 109,* 280–296.

Crandell, C. C., & Smaldino, J. J. (1995). An update of classroom acoustics for children with hearing impairment. *Volta Review, 97,* 4–12.

Crandell, C. C., & Smaldino, J. J. (2000). Classroom acoustics for children with normal hearing and with hearing impairment. *Language, Speech, and Hearing Services in Schools, 31,* 362–370.

Cunningham, W. R., & Brookbank, J. W. (1988). *Gerontology: The psychology, biology, and sociology of aging.* New York: Harper and Row.

Dagenais, P., & Critz-Crosby, P. (1992). Comparing tongue positioning by normal hearing and hearing-impaired children during vowel production. *Journal of Speech and Hearing Research, 35,* 5–44.

Daly, N., Bench, J., & Chappell, H. (1996). Gender differences in speechreadability. *Journal of the Academy of Rehabilitative Audiology, 29,* 27–40.

Dancer, J. (2001). Arkansas tinnitus survey reflects national picture. *Advance for Speech-Language Pathologists and Audiologists,* Sept. 10, 10–11.

Dancer, J., & Gener. J. (1999). Survey on the use of adult hearing assessment scales. *Hearing Review; 6, 26,* 35.

Dancer, J., Krain, M., Thompson, C., Davis, P., & Glenn, J. (1994). A cross-sectional investigation of speechreading in adults: Effects of gender, practice, and education. *Volta Review, 96,* 31–40.

Danhauer, J. L., Johnson, C. E., Kasten, R. N., & Brimacombe, J. A. (1985, March). The hearing aid effect: Summary, conclusions and recommendations. *The Hearing Journal,* 12–14.

Davis, A., & Refaie, A. E. (2000). Epidemiology of tinnitus. In R. Tyler (Ed.), *Tinnitus handbook* (pp. 1–23). Clifton Park, NY: Delmar Learning.

Davis, H., & Silverman, R. (1978). *Hearing and deafness* (4th ed.). New York: Holt Rinehart, and Winston.

DeFillipo, C. L., & Scott, B. L. (1978). A method for hearing and evaluating the reception of ongoing speech. *Journal of the Acoustical Society of America, 63,* 1186–1192.

DeFillipo, C. L., Sims, D. G., & Gottermeier, L. (1995). Linking visual and kinesthetic imagery in lipreading instruction. *Journal of Speech and Hearing Research, 38,* 244–256.

Demorest, M. E., & Erdman, S. A. (1987). Development of the communication profile for the hearing impaired. *Journal of Speech and Hearing Disorders, 52,* 129–143.

Demorest, M. E., & Walden, B. E. (1984). Psychometric principles in the selection, interpretation, and evaluation of communication self-assessment inventories. *Journal of Speech and Hearing Disorders, 54,* 180–188.

Deno, E. (1970). The cascade of special education services. *Exceptional Children, 39,* 495.

Dillon, H., Birtles, G., & Lovegrove, R. (1999). Measuring the outcomes of a national rehabilitation program: Normative data for the client oriented scale of improvement (COSI) and the hearing aid user's questionnaire (HAUQ). *Journal of the American Academy of Audiology, 10,* 67–79.

Dillon, H., James, A., & Ginis, J. (1997). Client oriented scale of improvement (COSI) and its relationship to several other measurements of benefit and satisfaction provided by hearing aids. *Journal of the American Academy of Audiology, 8,* 27–43.

Dorman, M. (1993). Speech perception by adults. In R. S. Tyler (Ed.), *Cochlear implants: Audiological foundations* (pp. 145–190). Clifton Park, NY: Delmar Learning.

Dowell, R., Brown, A., & Mecklenburg, D. (1990). Clinical assessment of implanted deaf adults. In G. Clark, Y. Tong, & J. Patrick (Eds.), *Cochlear prostheses* (pp. 193–206). Edinburgh: Churchill Livingstone.

Downs, M. (1974). Deafness management quotient (DMQ). *Hearing and Speech News, 42,* 26–28.

Dunn, L., & Dunn, L. (1981). *Peabody picture vocabulary test-revised.* Circle Pines, MN: American Guidance Service.

Dunst, C. (1985). Rethinking early intervention. *Analysis and Intervention in Developmental Disabilities, 5,* 165–201.

Durrell, D., & Catterson, J. (1980). *Durrell analysis of reading difficulty* (3rd Ed.). San Antonio, TX: Harcourt Brace Educational Measurement.

Edgerton, B. J., & Danhauer, J. L. (1979). *Clinical implications of speech discrimination testing using nonsense stimuli.* Baltimore, MD: University Park Press.

Elfenbein, J. (1994). Communication breakdowns in conversations: Child-initiated repair strategies. In N. Tye-Murray (Ed.), *Let's converse: A how-to guide to develop and expand the conversational skills of children and teenagers who are hearing impaired* (pp. 123–146).

Washington DC: Alexander Graham Bell Association for the Deaf.

Elliott, L., & Katz, D. (1980). *Development of a new children's test of speech discrimination.* St. Louis, MO: Audiotec.

Ellis, A., & Grieger, R. (1977). *Handbook of rational-emotive therapy.* New York: Springer.

Engen, E., & Engen, T. (1983). *Rhode Island test of language structure manual.* Baltimore, MD: University Park Press.

English, K., Mendel, L. L., Rojeski, T., & Hornak, J. (1999). Counseling in audiology, or learning to listen: Pre- and post-measures from an audiology counseling course. *American Journal of Audiology, 8,* 34–39.

Erber, N. P. (1974). Visual perception of speech by deaf children: Recent developments and continuing needs. *Journal of Speech and Hearing Disorders, 39,* 178–185.

Erber, N. P. (1982). *Auditory training.* Washington, DC: Alexander Graham Bell Association for the Deaf.

Erber, N. P. (1985). *Telephone communication and hearing impairment.* San Diego: College-Hill Press.

Erber, N. P. (1988). *Communication therapy for hearing impaired adults.* Abbotsford, Victoria: Clavis Publishing.

Erber, N. P. (1996). *Communication therapy for adults with sensory loss* (2nd ed.). Melbourne, Australia: Clavis Publishing.

Erber, N. P. (1998). Dyalog: A computer-based measure of conversational performance. *Journal of the Academy of Rehabilitative Audiology, 31,* 69–76.

Erber, N. P., & Lind, C. (1994). Communication therapy: Theory and practice. *Journal of the Academy of Rehabilitative Audiology, 27*(Suppl.), 267–287.

Erber, N. P. & Yelland, J. (1998). CONAN: A system for analysis of temporal factors in conversation. *Journal of Academy of Rehabilitative Audiology, 31,* 77–86.

Erdman, S. A. (2000). Counseling hearing impaired adults. In J. Alpiner & P. McCarthy (Eds.), *Rehabilitative audiology: Children and adults* (3rd ed., pp. 435–470). Baltimore, MD: Williams and Wilkins.

Erdman, S. A. (1994). Self-assessment: From research focus to research tool. *Journal of the Academy of Rehabilitative Audiology, 27*(Suppl.), 67–92.

Erler, S. F., & Garstecki, D. C. (in press). Hearing loss-and hearing-related stigma: Perceptions of women with age-normal hearing. *American Journal of Audiology.*

Ertmer, D. J., Leonard, J. S., & Pachuilo, M. L. (2002). Communication intervention for children with cochlear implants: Two case studies. *Language, Speech, and Hearing Services in Schools, 33,* 205–217.

Estabrooks, W. (1994). *Auditory-verbal therapy.* Washington, DC: Alexander Graham Bell Association for the Deaf.

Farrimond, T. (1959). Age differences in the ability to use visual codes in auditory communication. *Language and Speech, 2,* 179.

Feinmesser, M., Tell, L., & Levi, H. (1982). Follow-up of 40,000 infants screened for hearing defect. *Audiology, 21,* 197–203.

Fey, M. E., Warr-Leeper, G., Webber, S. A., & Disher, L. M. (1988). Repairing children's repairs: Evaluation and facilitation of children's clarification requests and responses. *Topics in Language Disorders, 8,* 63–84.

Flexor, C. (1999). *Facilitating hearing and listening in young children* (2nd ed). Clifton Park, NY: Delmar Learning.

Flexor, C. (1997). Sound-field FM systems: Questions most often asked about classroom amplification. *Hearsay, 11,* 514.

Forner, L., & Hixon, T. (1977). Respiratory kinematics in profoundly hearing-impaired speakers. *Journal of Speech and Hearing Research, 66,* 373–408.

Fryauf Bertschy, H., Tyler, R., Kelsay, D., Gantz, B., & Woodworth, B. (1997). Cochlear implant use by prelingually deafened children: The influences of age at implant and length of device use. *Journal of Speech Hearing Language Research, 40,* 183–199.

Gagné, J. P., Dinon, D., & Parsons, J. (1991). An evaluation of CAST: A computer-aided speechreading training program. *Journal of Speech and Hearing Research, 34*, 213–221.

Gagné, J. P., & Jennings, M. B. (2000). Audiological rehabilitation intervention services for adults with acquired hearing impairment. In M. Valente, H. Hosford-Dunn, & R. J. Roeser (Eds.), *Audiology treatment* (pp. 547–579), New York: Thieme.

Gagné, J. P., McDuff, S., & Getty, L. (1999). Some limitations of evaluative investigations based solely on normed outcome measures. *Journal of the American Academy of Audiology, 10*, 46–62.

Gagné, J. P., Stelmacovich, P., & Yovetich, W. (1991). Reactions to requests for clarification used by hearing-impaired individuals. *Volta Review, 93*, 129–143.

Gagné, J. P., Tugby, K. G., & Michoud, J. (1991). Development of a speechreading test on the utilization of contextual cues (STUCC): Preliminary findings with normal-hearing subjects. *Journal of the Academy of Rehabilitative Audiology, 24*, 157–170.

Gagné, J. P., & Wyllie, K. M. (1989). Relative effectiveness of three repair strategies on the visual-identification of misperceived words. *Ear and Hearing, 10*, 368–374.

Garahan, M. B., Waller, J. A., Houghton, M., Tisdale, W. A., & Runge, C. F. (1992). Hearing loss prevalence and management in nursing home residents. *Journal of the American Geriatric Society, 40*, 130–134.

Garstecki, D. C., & Erler, S. F. (1998). Hearing loss, control, and demographic factors influencing hearing aid use among older adults. *Journal of Speech, Language, and Hearing Research, 41*, 527–537.

Garstecki, D. C., & Erler, S. F. (1999). Older adult performance on the communication profile for the hearing impaired: Gender difference. *Journal of Speech, Language, and Hearing Research, 42*, 785–796.

Gatehouse, S. (1999). Glasgow hearing aid benefit profile: Derivation and validation of a client-centered outcome measure for hearing aid services. *Journal of American Academy of Audiology, 10*, 80–103.

Geers, A. (2003). Predictors of reading skill development in children with early cochlear implantation. *Ear and Hearing, 24*, 59S–68S.

Geers, A., & Brenner, C. (2003). Background and educational characteristics of prelingually deaf children. *Ear and Hearing, 24*, 2S–14S.

Geers, A. E., & Moog, J. S. (1987). Predicting spoken language acquisition in profoundly deaf children. *Journal of Speech and Hearing Disorders, 52*, 84–94.

Geers, A. E., & Moog, J. S. (1992). Speech perception and production skills of students with impaired hearing from oral and total communication education settings. *Journal of Speech and Hearing Research, 35*, 1384–1393.

Geers, A., Nicholas, G. G., & Sedey, A. L. (2003). Language skills of children with early cochlear implantation. *Ear and Hearing, 24*, 46S–58S.

Getty, L., & Hétu, R. (1991). Development of a rehabilitation program for people affected with occupational hearing loss. *Audiology, 30*, 317–329.

Gfeller, K., & Schum, R. (1994). Requisites for conversation: Engendering world knowledge. In N. Tye-Murray (Ed.), *Let's converse: A how-to-guide to develop and expand conversational skills of children and teenagers who are hearing impaired* (pp. 177–212). Washington, DC: Alexander Graham Bell Association for the Deaf.

Gfeller, K., Mehr, M. A., and Witt, S. (2001). Aural rehabilitation of music perception and enjoyment of adult cochlear implant users. Paper presented at the Academy of Rehabilitative Audiology Summer Institute, Vancouver, British Columbia.

Giolas, T. G. and Kaplan, H. (1997). Special populations. *Seminars in Hearing, 18*, 199–214.

Giolas, T. G., Owens, E., Lamb, S. H., & Schubert, E. D. (1979). Hearing performance inventory. *Journal of Speech and Hearing Disorders, 44*, 169–195.

Gitles, T. (1999). Re-inventing the profession: the relationship model of hearing care. *The Hearing Journal, 52*, 53–56.

Givens, G. D., & Greenfeld, D. (1982). Revision behaviors of normal and hearing-impaired children. *Ear and Hearing, 3,* 274–279.

Glennon, S. L. (1990). Homework activities for social skills training. In P. J. Schloss & M. A. Smith (Eds.), *Teaching social skills to hearing-impaired students* (pp. 85–90). Washington, DC: Alexander Graham Bell Association for the Deaf.

Golding-Meadow, S., & Mayberry, R. I. (2001). How do profoundly deaf children learn to read? *Learning Disabilities Research and Practice, 16,* 222–229.

Goldman, R., & Fristoe, M. (1969). *Test of Articulation.* Circle Pines, MN: American Guidance Service.

Goodale, C. (2003). Redefining the baby boomer image. *Advance for Audiologists, 5,* 51–52.

Gordon-Salant, S. (1987). Consonant recognition and confusion patterns among elderly hearing-impaired subjects. *Ear and Hearing, 8,* 270–276.

Green, K. (1998). The use of auditory and visual information during phonetic processing: Implications for theories of speech perception. In R. Campbell, B. Dodd, & D. Burnham (Eds.), *Hearing by eye II* (pp. 3–26). East Sussex, UK: Psychology Press Ltd.

Greenberg, M. (1983). Family stress and child competence: The effects of early intervention for families with deaf infants. *American Annals of the Deaf, 128,* 407–417.

Greenberg, M. T., Calderson, R., & Kusche, C. (1984). Early intervention using simultaneous communication with deaf infants: The effects on communicative development. *Child Development, 55,* 607–616.

Greenburg, J. H., & Jenkins, J. J. (1964). Studies in the psychological correlates of the sound system of American English. *Word, 20,* 157–177.

Greenstein, J. (1975). *Methods of fostering language development in deaf infants: Final report (BBB00581).* Washington, DC: Bureau of Education for the Handicapped (DHEW/OE).

Groher, M. E. (1989). Modifications in assessment and treatment for the communicatively impaired elderly. In R. Hull & K. Griffin (Eds.), *Communication disorders in aging* (pp. 50–72). Newbury Park, CA: Sage.

Hale, S., & Myerson, J. (1996). Experimental evidence for differential slowing in the lexical and nonlexical domains. *Aging, Neuropsychology, and Aging, 3,* 154–165.

Hallam, R. S., & Brooks, D. N. (1996). Development of the hearing attitudes in rehabilitation questionnaire (HARQ). *British Journal of Audiology, 30,* 199–213.

Hallberg, L. R-M. (1998). Evaluation of a Swedish version of the Hearing Disabilities and Handicaps Scale, based on a clinical sample of 101 men with noise-induced hearing loss. *Scandinavian Audiology, 27,* 21–29.

Hallberg, L. R-M. (1996). Occupational hearing loss: Coping and family life. *Scandinavian Audiology, 25,* 25–33.

Hallberg, L. R.-M. (1999). Hearing impairment, coping, and consequences on family life. *Journal of the Academy of Rehabilitative Audiology, 32,* 45–59.

Hallberg, L. R-M., & Barennas, M. L. (1993). Living with a male with noise-induced hearing loss: Experiences from the perspective of spouses. *British Journal of Audiology, 27,* 253–261.

Hanin, L. (1988). *The effects of experience and linguistic context on speechreading.* Unpublished doctoral dissertation, The City University Graduate School, New York, NY.

Hanratty, V., & Lawlor, D. A. (2000). Effective management of the elderly hearing impaired: A review. *Journal of Public Health Medicine, 22,* 512–517.

Hansen, D., & Howard, S. R. (1992). *Facilitating early language.* Vero Beach, FL: The Speech Bin.

Harker, L. A., Vanderheiden, S., Veazey, D., Gentile, N., & McCleary, E. (1999). Multichannel cochlear implantation in children with large vestibular aqueduct syndrome. *Annals of Otology, Rhinology, and Laryngology, 108,* 39–43.

Haskins, H. (1949). *A phonetically balanced test of speech discrimination for children.* Unpublished master's thesis, Northwestern University, Evanston, IL.

Hasenstab, M. S., & Tobey, E. A. (1991). Language development in children receiving Nucleus multichannel cochlear implants. *Ear and Hearing, 12*, 55S–65S.

Haycock, G. S. (1933). *The teaching of speech.* Washington DC: Alexander Graham Bell Association for the Deaf.

Hazard, W. R., Andrews, R., Bierman, E. L., & Blass, J. P. (1990). *Principles of geriatric medicine and gerontology* (2nd ed.). New York: McGraw Hill.

Hazell, J. W. (1990). Tinnitus, III: The practical management of sensorineural tinnitus. *Journal of Otolaryngology, 19*, 11–18.

Hearing Journal, The. (1991). A timeline of the hearing industry. *The Hearing Journal, 50*, 54–72.

Hear-It Organization (2003). Costly for the individual—expensive for society. *http://www. press.hear-it.org.*

Heider, F., & Heider, G. (1940). An experimental investigation of lip reading. *Psychological Monographs, 232*, 1–153.

Heller, P. J. (1990). Psycho-educational assessment. In M. Ross (Ed.), *Hearing-impaired children in the mainstream* (pp. 45–60). Baltimore, MD: York Press.

Hergils, L. and Hergils, A. (2000). Universal neonatal hearing screening—parental attitudes and concern. *British Journal of Audiology, 34*, 321–327.

Hétu, R. (1996). The stigma attached to hearing impairment. *Scandinavian Audiology, 43*, 12–24.

Hétu, R., & Getty, L. (1991). Development of a rehabilitation program for people affected with occupational hearing loss. *Audiology, 30*, 305–316.

Hétu, R., Betty, L., Philibert, L., Desilets, F., Noble, W., & Stephens, D. (1994). Development of a clinical tool for the measurement of the severity of hearing disabilities and handicaps. *Journal of Speech-Language Pathology and Audiology (French), 18*, 82–95.

Hétu, R., Reverin, L., Getty, L., Lalande, N. M., & St-Cyr, C. (1990). The reluctance to acknowledge hearing difficulties among hearing-impaired workers. *British Journal of Audiology, 24*, 265–276.

Heydebrand, G., Binzer, S., Mauzé, E., Tye-Murray, N., & Skinner, M. (Submitted). The efficacy of a cognitive-behavioral group intervention for adult cochlear implant recipients in improving communication and coping skills.

High, W. S., Fairbanks, G., and Glorig, A. (1964). Scale for self-assessment of hearing handicap. *Journal of Speech and Hearing Disorders, 29*, 215–230.

Hines, J. (2000). Communication problems of hearing-impaired patients. *Nursing Standard, 14*, 33–37.

Hirsch, H. V. B., & Spinelli, D. N. (1970). Visual experience modifies distribution of horizontally and vertically oriented receptive fields in cats. *Science, 168*, 869–871.

Hirsh, I. J., Davis, H., Silverman, S. R., Reynolds, E. G., Eldert, E., & Benson, R. W. (1952). Development of materials for speech audiometry. *Journal of Speech and Hearing Disorders, 17*, 321–337.

Hnath-Chisolm, T. E., Laipply, E., & Boothroyd, A. (1998). Age-related changes on a children's test of sensory-level speech perception capacity. *Journal of Speech, Language, and Hearing Research, 41*, 94–106.

Hogan, A. (2001). *Hearing rehabilitation for deafened adults: A psychosocial approach.* Philadelphia: Whurr Publishers.

Holmes, A. (1995). Hearing aids and the older adult. In S. A. Lesner & P. B. Kricos, (Eds.), *Hearing care for the older adult: Audiologic rehabilitation* (pp. 59–74). Boston: Butterworth-Heinemann.

Honnell, S., Dancer, J., & Gentry, B. (1991). Age and speechreading performance in relation to percent correct, eyeblinks, and written responses. *Volta Review, 93*, 207–231.

Hoover, B. M. (2001). Hearing aid fitting in infants. *The Volta Review, 102*, 57–73.

Houle, C. O. (1997). *Governing boards.* San Francisco, CA: Jossey-Bass Publishers.

Hull, R. H. (1995). *Hearing in aging.* Clifton Park, NY: Delmar Learning.

Hull, R. H. (1997). Hearing loss in older adulthood. In R. H. Hull (Ed.), *Aural rehabilitation: Serving children and adults* (3rd ed., pp. 373–392), Clifton Park, NY: Delmar Learning.

Hull, R. H., & Griffin, K. (1992). *Communication disorders in aging.* Beverly Hills, CA: Sage.

Humes, L. E. (1996). Speech understanding in the elderly. *Journal of the American Academy of Audiology, 7,* 161–167.

Hutton, C. L. (1980). Responses to a Hearing Problem Inventory. *Journal of the Academy of Rehabilitative Audiology, 13,* 133–154.

Huttunen, K. H. (2001). Educational needs of speech and language therapists in the field of audiology. *Scandinavian Audiology, 30,* 88–89.

Hyde, M. L., & Riko, K. (1994). A decision-analytic approach to audiological rehabilitation. *Journal of Rehabilitative Audiology, 27,* 337–374.

IBM. (1988). IBM Personal System/2 Independence Series. *Speech Viewer Application Software User's Guide.* Boca Raton, FL: IBM.

Israelite, N., Ower, J., & Goldstein, G. (2002). Hard-of-hearing adolescents and identity construction: Influences of school experiences, peers, and teachers. *Journal of Deaf Studies and Deaf Education, 7,* 134–148.

Itoh, M., Horii, Y., Daniloff, R., & Binnie, C. (1982). Selected aerodynamic characteristics of deaf individuals' various speech and nonspeech tasks. *Folia Phoniatrica, 34,* 191–209.

Jackson, P. L. (1992). A psychological and economic profile of the hearing impaired and deaf. In R. H. Hull (Ed.) *Aural rehabilitation* (2nd ed., pp. 42–49). Clifton Park, NY: Delmar Learning.

Janota, J. (1999). Otitis media. *ASHA* (May/June), 48.

Jastreboff, P. J. (1990). Phantom auditory perception (tinnitus): Mechanisms of generation and perception. *Neuroscience Research, 8,* 221–254.

Jastreboff, P. J. (2000). Tinnitus habituation therapy (THT) and tinnitus retraining therapy (TRT). In R. Tyler (Ed.), *Tinnitus handbook* (pp. 357–376). Clifton Park, NY: Delmar Learning.

Jastreboff, P. J., Gray, W. C., & Gold, S. L. (1996). Neurophysiological approach to tinnitus patients. *American Journal of Otology, 17,* 236–240.

Jeffers, J., & Barley, M. (1971). *Speechreading (lipreading).* Springfield, IL: Charles C. Thomas.

Jenkins, L., Myerson, J., Joerding, J. A., & Hale, S. (2000). Converging evidence that visuospatial cognition is more age-sensitive than verbal cognition. *Psychology and Aging, 15,* 157–175.

Jennings, M. B. (1993). *Aural rehabilitation curriculum series: Hearing help class II: Coping with hearing loss.* Toronto: Canadian Hearing Society.

Jensema, C., & Trybus, R. (1978). *Communication patterns and educational achievement of hearing impaired students* (Series T, No. 2). Washington, DC: Gallaudet College, Office of Demographic Studies.

Jerger, J., Chmiel, R., Wilson, N., Luchi, R. (1995). Hearing impairment in older adults: new concepts. *Journal of American Geriatrics, 43,* 928–935.

Jerger, J., Speaks, C., & Trammell, J. L. (1968). A new approach to speech audiometry. *Journal of Speech and Hearing Disorders, 33,* 318–329.

Jerram, J. C., & Purdy, S. C. (2001). Technology, expectations, and adjustment to hearing loss: Predictions of hearing-aid outcome. *Journal of the American Academy of Audiology, 12,* 64–75.

Jimenez-Sanchez, C., & Anita, S. (1999). Team-teaching in an integrated classroom: Perceptions of deaf and hearing teachers. *Journal of Deaf Studies and Deaf Education, 4,* 215–224.

John, J., & Howarth, J. (1976). The effect of time distortions on the intelligibility of deaf children's speech. *Language and Speech, 8,* 127–134.

Johnson, D. D. (1975). Communication characteristics of NTID students. *Journal of the Academy of Rehabilitative Audiology, 8,* 17–32.

Johnson, S. M., & Wilhite, G. (1971). Self-observation as an agent of behavioral change. *Behavior Therapy, 2,* 488–497.

Joint Committee on Infant Hearing (1994). 1994 Position statement. *International Journal of Pediatric Otorhinolaryngology, 32,* 265–274.

Joint Committee on Infant Hearing (2000). 2000 Position statement, principles, and guidelines for early hearing detection and intervention programs. *Pediatrics, 106,* 798–817.

Jones, L., Kyle, J., & Wood, P. (1987). *Words apart: Losing your hearing as an adult.* New York: Tavistock Publications.

Kaplan, H. (1996). Assistive devices for the elderly. *Journal of the American Academy of Audiology, 7,* 203–211.

Kaplan, H., Bally, S. J., & Brandt, F. (1995). Revised communication self-assessment scale inventory for deaf adults (CSDA). *Journal of the American Academy of Audiology, 6,* 311–329.

Kaplan, H., Bally, S., Brandt, F., Busacco, D., & Pray, J. (1997). Communications scale for older adults (CSOA). *Journal of the American Academy of Audiology, 8,* 203–217.

Kaplan, H., Bally, S. J., & Garretson, C. (1985). *Speechreading: A way to improve understanding.* Washington DC: Gallaudet University Press.

Kaplan, H., Feeley, J., & Brown, J. (1978). A modified Denver scale: Test-retest reliability. *Journal of the Academy of Rehabilitation Audiology, 11,* 15–32.

Kaufman, A., & Kaufman, N. (1983). *Kaufman assessment battery for children (K-ABC).* Circle Pines, MN: American Guidance Service, Inc.

Kaufman, L. (1979). *Perception: The world transformed.* New York: Oxford University Press.

Keats, B. J. B. (2002). Genes and syndromic hearing loss. *Journal of Communication Disorders, 35,* 355–366.

Kentish, R. C., Crocker, S. R., & McKenna, L. (2000). Children's experience of tinnitus: A preliminary survey of children presenting to a psychology department. *British Journal of Audiology, 34,* 335–340.

Kerr, P. C., & Cowie, R. I. D. (1997). Acquired deafness: A multi-dimensional experience. *British Journal of Audiology, 31,* 177–188.

Kileny, P. R., Zwolan, T. A., Ashbaugh, C. (2001). The influence of age at implantation on performance with a cochlear implant in children. *Otology and Neurotology, 22,* 42–46.

Killion, M. C., & Villchur, E. (1993). Kessler was right—partly: But SIN test shows some aids improve hearing in noise. *Hearing Journal, 46,* 31–35.

Kinsella-Meier, M. A. (1996). The process of communication therapy. In M. J. Mosely and S. J. Bally (Eds.), *Communication therapy: An integrated approach to aural rehabilitation* (pp. 3–23). Washington, DC: Gallaudet University Press.

Kirchner, R., & Peterson, R. (1980). Multiple impairments among noninstitutionalized blind and visually impaired persons. *Journal of Visual Impairment and Blindness, 74,* 42–44.

Kirk, K. I. (1998). Assessing speech perception in listeners with cochlear implants: The development of the Lexical Neighborhood Tests. *Volta Review, 100,* 63–86.

Kirk, K. I., Miyamoto, R. T., Ying, E. A., Perdew, A. E., & Zuganelis, H. (2002). Cochlear implantation in young children: Effects of age at implantation and communication mode. *Volta Review, 102,* 123–126.

Kirk, K. I., Pisoni, D. B., & Osberger, M. J. (1995). Lexical effects on spoken word recognition by pediatric cochlear implant users. *Ear and Hearing, 16,* 470–481.

Kirkwood, D. H. (2002). Caring for our youngest patients: A unique opportunity and challenge. *The Hearing Journal, 55,* 3.

Kishon-Rabin, L., & Henkin, Y. (2000). Age-related changes in the visual perception of phonologically significant contrasts. *British Journal of Audiology, 34,* 363–374.

Knutson, J. F., & Lansing, C. R. (1990). The relationship between communication problems and psychological difficulties in persons with profound acquired hearing loss. *Journal of Speech and Hearing Disorders, 55,* 656–664.

Kochkin, S. (1992). MarkeTrak III: Higher hearing aid sales don't signal better market penetration. *The Hearing Journal, 45,* 47–54.

Kochkin, S. (1997). Professional forum. *Hearing Health, 13,* 21–22.

Kochkin, S. (1999). Baby boomers spur growth in potential market, but penetration rate declines. *Hearing Journal, 52,* 33–48.

Kochkin, S. (2000). MarkeTrakV: Why my hearing aids are in the drawer: The consumer perspective. *Hearing Journal, 53*(2), 34–42.

Kotler, P. H., & Andreasen, A. R. (1996). *Strategic marketing for nonprofit organizations* (5th ed.). Upper Saddle River, NJ: Prentice-Hall.

Kozak, V. J. and Brooks, B. M. (2001). *Baby talk: Helping your hearing-impaired baby list and talk.* St. Louis, MO: Central Institute for the Deaf.

Kramer, S. E., Kapteyn, T. S., & Festen, J. M. (1998). The self-reporting handicapping effect of hearing disabilities. *Audiology, 37,* 302–310.

Kramer, S. E., Kapteyn, T. S., Festern, J. M., & Tobi, H. (1995). Factors in subjective hearing disability. *Audiology, 34,* 167–199.

Kramer, S. E., Kapteyn, T. S., Festen, J. M., & Tobi, H. (1996). The relationships between self-reported hearing disability and measurements of auditory disability. *Audiology, 35,* 277–287.

Kraus, N., McGee, T., Carrell, T., King, C., Tremblay, K., & Nicol, T. (1995). Central auditory system plasticity associated with speech discrimination training. *Journal of Cognitive Neuroscience, 7,* 25–32.

Kravitz, L., & Selekman, J. (1992). Understanding hearing loss in children. *Pediatric Nursing, 18,* 591–594.

Kretschmer, R., & Kretschmer, L. (1978). *Language development and intervention with the hearing impaired.* Baltimore, MD: University Park Press.

Kricos, P. B., & Holmes, A. E. (1996). Efficacy of audiologic rehabilitation for older adults. *Journal of the American Academy of Audiology, 7,* 219–229.

Kricos, P. B., & Lesner, S. A. (1995). *Hearing care for the older adult: Audiologic rehabilitation.* Boston, MA: Butterworth-Heinemann.

Kricos, P. B., Lesner, S. A., Sandridge, S. A., & Yanke, R. B. (1987). Perceived benefits of amplification as a function of central auditory status in the elderly. *Ear and Hearing, 8,* 337–342.

Kuhl, P. K., & Meltzoff, A. N. (1982). The bimodal perception of speech in infancy. *Science, 218,* 1138–1141.

Lach, R., Ling, D., Ling, L., & Ship, N. (1970). Early speech development in deaf infants. *American Annals of the Deaf, 115,* 522–526.

Lachs, L., Pisoni, D. B., & Kirk, K. I. (2001). Use of audiovisual information in speech perception by prelingually deaf children with cochlear implants: A first report. *Ear and Hearing, 22,* 236–251.

Lansing, C. R., & Davis, J. M. (1988). Early versus delayed speech perception training for adult cochlear implant users: Initial results. *Journal of the Academy of Rehabilitative Audiology, 21,* 29–41.

Lansing, C. R., & Helgeson, C. L. (1995). Priming the visual recognition of spoken words. *Journal of Speech and Hearing Research, 38,* 1377–1386.

Lansing, C. R., & McConkie, G. W. (1999). Attention to facial regions in segmental and prosodic visual speech perception tasks. *Journal of Speech, Language, and Hearing Research, 42,* 526–539.

Lee, L. (1974). *Developmental sentence analysis.* Evanston, IL: Northwestern University Press.

Leigh, I. W. (1999). Inclusive education and personal development. *Journal of Deaf Studies and Deaf Education, 4,* 236–245.

Lesner, K., Sandridge, S., & Kricos, P. (1987). Training influences on visual consonant and sentence recognition. *Ear and Hearing, 8,* 283–287.

Lesner, S. (1996). Group hearing care for older adults. In P. Kricos & S. Lesner (Eds.), *Hearing care for the older adult: Audiologic rehabilitation* (pp. 203–277). Newton, MA: Butterworth-Heinemann.

Levitt, H. (1987). *Fundamental speech skills test.* New York: City University of New York.

Levitt, H., McGarr, N. S., & Geffner, D. (Eds.). (1987). *Development of language and communication skills in hearing-impaired children.* Washington, DC: ASHA.

Lindblade, D. D., & McDonald, M. (1995). Removing communication barriers for the hearing-impaired elderly. *Medsurgery Nursing, 4,* 370–385.

Ling, D. (1976). *Speech and the hearing-impaired child: Theory and practice.* Washington, DC: Alexander Graham Bell Association for the Deaf.

Litconn, Inc. (2000). *Reading and oral language assessment (ROLA).* Fresno, CA: LitConn, Inc.

Luce, P. A. (1986). A computational analysis of uniqueness points in auditory word recognition. *Perception and Psychophysics, 39,* 155–159.

Luce, P. A., & Pisoni, D. B. (1998). Recognizing spoken words: The neighborhood activation model. *Ear and Hearing, 19,* 1–36.

Luterman, D. (1987). *Deafness in the family.* Washington, DC: Alexander Graham Bell Association for the Deaf.

Luterman, D. (1996). Listening with the third ear. *Hearing Instruments, 47,* 12.

Luterman, D. (2001). *Counseling parents of hearing-impaired children* (4th ed.). Boston, MA: Little, Brown.

Luterman, D., & Kurtzer-White, E. (1999). Identifying hearing loss: Parents' needs. *American Journal of Audiology, 8,* 13–18.

Luterman, D., & Kurtzer-White, E. (1998). Letter to the editor. *ASHA Leader.*

Luterman, D., & Ross, M. (1991). *When your child is deaf.* Parkton, MD: York Press.

Luxford, W. M., & Brackmann, D. E. (1985). The history of cochlear implants. In R. F. Gray (Ed.), *Cochlear implants* (pp. 1–26). San Diego, CA: College-Hill Press.

Lyxell, B. (1994). Skilled speechreading: A single-case study. *Scandinavian Journal of Audiology, 35,* 212–219.

Madell, J. R. (2000). Counseling for diagnosis and management of auditory disorders in infants, children, and adults. In M. Valente, H. Hosford-Dunn, & R. J. Roeser (Eds.), *Audiology treatment* (pp. 291–305). New York: Thieme.

Maki-Torkko, E., Brorsson, B., Davis, A., Mair, W., Myhre, K., Parving, A., Roine, R. Rosenhall, U., Sorri, M., & Stilven, S. (2001). Hearing impairment among adults—Extent of the problem and scientific evidence on the outcome of hearing aid rehabilitation. *Scandinavian Audiology, 30,* 8–15.

Markides, A. (1970). The speech of deaf and partially hearing children with special reference to factors affecting intelligibility. *British Journal of Disordered Communication, 5,* 126–140.

Marler, P. (1989). Learning by instinct: Birdsong. *Asha, 31,* 75–79.

Marmor, G., & Petitito, L. (1979). Simultaneous communication in the classroom: How well is English grammar represented? In W.

Tokoe (Ed.), *Sign language studies.* Silver Spring, MD: Linstok Press.

Marschark, M., Young, A., & Lukomski, J. (2002). Perspectives in inclusion. *Journal of Deaf Studies and Deaf Education, 7,* 187–188.

Martin, R. (2004). Wear your hearing aids or your brain will rust. *The Hearing Journal, 57,* 46.

Mauzé, E., & Frederick, E. (1995). *Communication-based aural rehabilitation class for hearing-impaired adults.* St. Louis, MO: Central Institute for the Deaf.

McCullough, J. A., & Wilson, R. H. (2001). Performance on a Spanish picture-identification task using a multimedia format. *Journal of the American Academy of Audiology, 12,* 254–260.

McCullough, J. A., Wilson, R. H., Birck, J. D., & Anderson, L. G. (1995). A multimedia approach for estimating speech recognition of multilingual clients. *American Journal of Audiology, 3,* 19–22.

McFadden, K. (1982). *Tinnitus: Facts, theories, and treatments.* Washington, DC: National Academy Press.

McFall, R. M. (1970). Effects of self-monitoring on normal smoking behavior. *Journal of Consulting and Clinical Psychology, 35,* 135–142.

McGarr, N. (1987). Communication skills of hearing-impaired children in schools for the deaf. In H. Levitt, N. McGarr, & D. Geffner (Eds.), *Development of language and communication in hearing-impaired children. ASHA Monographs, 26,* 91–107.

McGarr, N., & Lofqvist, A. (1982). Obstruent production in hearing-impaired speakers: Interarticulator timing and acoustics. *Journal of the Acoustical Society of America, 72,* 34–42.

McGuire, R. (2002). Marketing to the baby boomer. *The Hearing Review,* September, 44–46.

McGurk, H., & MacDonald, J. (1976). Hearing lips and seeing voices. *Nature, 264,* 746–748.

McKenna, L. (1987). Goal planning in audiological rehabilitation. *British Journal of Audiology, 21,* 5–11.

Mecklenburg, D., Dowell, R., and Brown, A. (1990). Aural rehabilitation for children. In

G. Clark, Y. Tong, and J. Patrick (Eds.), *Cochlear Protheses* (p. 214). Edinburgh: Churchill Livingstone.

Mendel, L., & Danhauer, J. (1997). *Audiologic evaluation and management and speech perception assessment.* San Diego: Singular Publishing Group.

Messina, J. J., & Messina, C. M. (2004). The Federal Laws Governing Education for Exceptional Students. Retrieved February 11, 2004, from *http://www.copying.org/involvepar/laws.htm.*

Metz, D., Whitehead, R., & Whitehead, B. (1984). Mechanics of vocal fold vibration and laryngeal articulatory gestures produced by hearing-impaired speakers. *Journal of Speech and Hearing Research, 27,* 62–69.

Miller, D. A., & Fredrickson, J. M. (2000). Implantable hearing aids. In M. Valente, H. Hosford-Dunn, & R. J. Roeser (Eds.), *Audiology treatment* (pp. 489–510). New York: Thieme.

Miller, G. A., & Nicely, P. E. (1955). An analysis of perceptual confusions among some English consonants. *Journal of the Acoustical Society of America, 27,* 338–352.

Miyamoto, R., Houston, D., & Kirk, K. (2002). Early cochlear implantation in congenitally deaf children. *Audiology Today* (Special Issue), 35–40.

Mize, J., & Wigley, H. (2002). *Hearing the truth about pediatric audiology.* Paper presented at the American Speech-Language-Hearing Association Convention, Atlanta, GA.

Moeller, M. P., Coufal, K. L., Hixson, P. K. (1990). The efficacy of speech-language pathology intervention: Hearing-impaired children. *Seminars in Hearing, 11,* 227–240.

Monsen, R. (1976). The production of English stop consonants in the speech of deaf children. *Journal of Phonetics, 4,* 29–42.

Monsen, R. (1978). Toward measuring how well hearing-impaired children speak. *Journal of Speech and Hearing Research, 21,* 197–219.

Monsen, R. (1981). A usable test for the speech intelligibility of deaf talkers. *American Annals of the Deaf, 126,* 845–852.

Montgomery, A. A. (1994). WATCH: A practical approach to brief auditory rehabilitation. *The Hearing Journal, 10,* 10–55.

Montgomery, A., & Demorest, M. (1988). Issues and developments in the evaluation of speechreading. *Volta Review, 90,* 119–148.

Moog, J. (1988). *The CID phonetic inventory.* St. Louis, MO: Central Institute for the Deaf.

Moog, J., Biedenstein, J., & Davidson, L. (1995). *The SPICE.* St. Louis, MO: Central Institute for the Deaf.

Moog, J., & Geers, A. (1979). *Grammatical analysis of elicited language: simple sentence level.* St. Louis, MO: Central Institute for the Deaf.

Moog, J., & Geers, A. (1990). *Early speech perception test.* St. Louis, MO: Central Institute for the Deaf.

Moog, J. S., Kozak, V. J., & Geers, A. (1983). *Grammatical analysis of elicited language (GAEL-p).* St. Louis, MO: Central Institute for the Deaf.

Most, T. (2002). The use of repair strategies by children with and without hearing impairment. *Language, Speech, and Hearing in Schools, 33,* 112–123.

Mueller, H. G. (1994). CIC hearing aids: What is their impact on the occlusion effect? *The Hearing Journal, 47,* 29–30, 32–35.

Mueller, H. G., & Bender, D. (1988). Reasons for obtaining hearing aids: Do they relate to subsequent benefit? [Abstract]. *Corti's Organ, 11.*

Mueller, H. G., Bryant, M., Brown, W., & Budinger, A. (1991). Hearing aid selection for high-frequency hearing loss. In G. Studebaker, F. Bess, & L. Beck (Eds.), *The Vanderbilt Hearing-Aid Report II* (pp. 35–51). Parkton, MD: York Press.

Mueller, H. G. (2001). Speech audiometry and hearing aid fittings: Going steady or casual acquaintances? *The Hearing Journal, 54,* 19–29.

Mueller, H. G., & Grimes, A. (1987). Amplification systems for the hearing impaired. In J. G. Alpiner & P. A. McCarthy (Eds.), *Rehabilitative audiology: Children and adults* (pp. 116–162). Baltimore, MD: Williams and Wilkins.

Mueller, H. G., & Palmer, C. V. (1998). The profile of aided loudness: A new "PAL" for 98. *The Hearing Journal, 51,* 10–19.

Mulrow, C., Aguilar, C., & Endicott, J. (1990). Association between hearing impairment and the quality of life of elderly individuals. *Journal of the American Geriatric Society, 38,* 45–50.

Musselman, C., Wilson, A., & Lindsay, P. (1988). Effects of early intervention on hearing-impaired children. *Exceptional Children, 55,* 222–228.

National Association for the Deaf (2000). *NAD Position Statement on Cochlear Implants.* http://www.nad.org/infocenter/newsroom/positions/CochlearImplants.html.

National Center for Health Statistics (1987). *Current estimates from the National Health Interview Survey: United States, 1987.* (Vital and Health Statistics. Series 10). Washington, DC: United States Government Printing Office.

National Center for Health Statistics (1994). Data from the National Health Interview Survey, Series 10, Number 188.

National Council on Aging (1999). *The consequences of untreated hearing loss in older persons.* Washington, DC: Author.

National Institutes of Deafness and Communication Disorders (2002). Report of the ad hoc committee on epidemiology and statistics in communication.

National Dissemination Center for Children with Disabilities (2003). Deafness and hearing loss. Disability Fact Sheet, No. 3, October.

Nevins, M. E., & Chute, P. M. (1996). *Children with cochlear implants in educational settings.* Clifton Park, NY: Delmar Learning.

Newby, H. A., & Popelka, G. R. (1992). *Audiology* (6th ed.). Englewood Cliffs, NJ: Prentice-Hall.

Newman, C. W., Weinstein, B. E., Jacobson, G. P., & Hug, G. A. (1990). The hearing handicap inventory for adults: Psychometric adequacy and audiometric correlates. *Ear and Hearing, 11,* 430–433.

Nidday, K. J., & Elfenbein, J. L. (1991). The effects of visual barriers used during auditory training on sound transmission. *Journal of Speech and Hearing Research, 34,* 694–696.

Nilsson, M., Soli, S. D., & Sullivan, J. A. (1994). Development of the hearing in noise test for the measurement of speech reception threshold in quiet and in noise. *Journal of the Acoustical Society of America, 95,* 1085–1099.

Niskar, A. S., Kieszak, S. M., Holmes, A., Esteban, E., Rubin, C., & Brody, D. J. (1998). Prevalence of hearing loss among children 6 to 19 years of age. *Journal of the American Medical Association, 279,* 1071–1075.

Nix, G. W. (1983). How total is total communication? *Journal of British Association for Teachers of the Deaf, 7,* 177–181.

Noble, W. (1996). What is psychosocial approach to hearing loss? *Scandinavian Audiology, 25,* 6–11.

Northcott, W. H. (1990). Mainstreaming: Roots and wings. In M. Ross (Ed.), *Hearing-impaired children in the mainstream* (pp. 1–26). Parkton, MD: York Press.

Northern, J., & Beyer, C. M. (1999). Reducing hearing aid returns through patient education. *Audiology Today, 11,* 10–11.

Northern, J., & Downs, M. (1984). *Hearing in children.* Baltimore, MD: Lippincott, Williams, & Wilkins.

Northern, J., & Downs, M. P. (1991). *Hearing in children* (4th ed.). Baltimore, MD: Williams and Wilkins.

Nussbaum, J. F., Thompson, T., & Robinson, J. D. (1989). *Communication and aging.* New York: Harper and Row.

Osberger, M. J., & Fischer, L. M. (2000). Preoperative predictors of postoperative implant performance in children. *Annals of Otology, Rhinology, and Laryngology, 109,* 44–46.

Osberger, M. J., Robbins, A. M., Todd, S. L., & Riley, A. I. (1994). Speech and intelligibility of children with cochlear implants. *The Volta Review, 96,* 169–180.

Palmer, C. V., Mueller, H. G., & Moriarty, M. (1999). Profile of aided loudness: A validation procedure. *The Hearing Journal, 52,* 34–42.

Parving, A. (1985). Hearing disorders in childhood: Some procedures for detection, identification and diagnostic evaluation. *Pediatric Otorhinolaryngology, 9,* 31–57.

Pascoe, D. P. (1991). *Hearing aids: Who needs them?* St. Louis, MO: Big Bend Books.

Pascoe, D. P. (1995). Post-fitting and rehabilitative management of the adult hearing-aid user. In

R. E. Sandlin (Ed.), *Handbook of hearing aid amplification* (Vol. 2, pp. 61–86). Clifton Park, NY: Delmar Learning.

Paul, P. V., & Jackson, D. W. (1993). *Toward a psychology of deafness.* Boston, MA: Allyn & Bacon.

Paul, R. G., & Cox, R. M. (1995). Measuring hearing aid benefit with the APHAB: Is this as good as it gets? *American Journal of Audiology, 4,* 10–13.

Pederson, K. E., Rosenthal, U., & Moller, M. B. (1991). Longitudinal study of changes in speech perception between 70 and 81 years of age. *Audiology, 30,* 201–211.

Pichora-Fuller, M. K. (1997). Language comprehension in older listeners. *Journal of Speech-Language Pathology and Audiology, 21,* 125–142.

Pipp-Siegel, S., & Biringen, Z. (2000). Assessing the quality of relationships between parents and children: The emotional availability scales. *The Volta Review, 100,* 237–249.

Plath, P. (1991). Speech recognition in the elderly. *Acta Otolaryngology, 476*(Suppl.), 127–130.

Pollack, D. (1970). *Educational audiology for the limited hearing infant.* Springfield, IL: Charles C. Thomas.

Pratt, S. R., & Tye-Murray, N. (1997). Speech impairment secondary to hearing loss. In M. McNeil (Ed.), *The clinical management of sensorimotor speech disorders* (pp. 345–387). New York: Thieme Medical Publishers.

Prendergast, S. G., & Kelley, L. A. (2002). Aural rehab services: Survey reports who offers which ones and how often. *The Hearing Journal, 55,* 30–35.

Psychological Corp. (1994). *GOALS: A performance based measure of achievement.* San Antonio, TX: Psychological Corp.

Quigley, S. P., & Kretschmer, R. E. (1982). *The education of deaf children.* Austin, TX: Pro-Ed.

Quigley, S. P., Monranelli, D. S. & Wilbur, R. B. (1976). Some aspects of the verb system in the language of deaf students. *Journal of Speech and Hearing Research, 19,* 536–550.

Quigley, S. P., & Paul, P. V. (1984). *Language and deafness.* London, England: Croom Helm.

Quittner, A., & Steck, J. (1989, November). *Impact of hearing loss on child development and family adjustment.* Paper presented at the meeting of the American Speech-Language-Hearing Association, St. Louis, MO.

Reich, G. E. (2000). American Tinnitus Association and self-help groups. In R. Tyler (Ed.), *Tinnitus handbook* (pp. 419–436). Clifton Park, NY: Delmar Learning.

Reid, K., Hresko, W., Hammill, D., & Wiltshire, S. (1991). *Test of early reading ability—Deaf and hard of hearing (TERA-D/HH).* Austin, TX: Pro-Ed.

Reisberg, D., McLean, J., & Goldfield, A. (1987). Easy to hear but hard to understand: A speechreading advantage with intact stimuli. In R. Campbell & B. Dodd (Eds.), *Hearing by eye: The psychology of lip-reading* (pp. 97–113). London, UK: Erlbaum.

Reynell, J. K. (1977). *Reynell development language scale.* Windsor, Ontario: NFER Publishing.

Ries, P. W. (1991). The demography of hearing loss. In H. Orlans (Ed.) *Adjustment to adult hearing loss* (2nd ed., pp. 3–22), Clifton Park, NY: Delmar Learning.

Ringdahl, A., Eriksson-Mangold, M., & Andersson, G. (1998). Psychometric evaluation of the Gothenburg profile for measurement of experienced hearing disability and handicap: Applications with new hearing aid candidates and experienced hearing aid users. *British Journal of Audiology, 32,* 375–385.

Robards-Armstrong, C., & Stone, H. E. (1994). Research in audiological rehabilitation: Current and future directions, the consumer's perspective. *Journal of the Academy of Rehabilitative Audiology, 27*(Suppl.), 25–46.

Robb, M., & Pang-Ching, G. (1992). Relative timing characteristics of hearing-impaired speakers. *Journal of the Acoustical Society of America, 91,* 2954–2960.

Robbins, A. M., Renshaw, J. J., Miyamoto, R. T., Osberger, M. J., & Pope, M. L. (1988). Minimal pairs test, Indianapolis: Indiana University School of Medicine.

Robinson, L. F., & Reis, H. T. (1989). The effects of interruption, gender, and status on interpersonal perceptions. *Journal of Nonverbal Behavior, 13,* 141–151.

Rogers, C. R. (1980). *A way of being.* Boston: Houghton Mifflin.

Rönnberg, J., Andersson, J., Samuelsson, S. Södderfeldt, B., Lyxell, B., & Risberg, J. (1999). A speechreading expert: The case of MM. *Journal of Speech-Language-Hearing Research, 42,* 5–20.

Rosen, S. M., Fourcin, A. J., & Moore, B. C. J. (1981). Voice pitch as an aid to lipreading. *Nature, 291,* 150–152.

Rosenberg, G. (1998). FM sound field research identifies benefits for students and teachers. *Educational Audiology Review, 15,* 6–8.

Ross, M. (1990). Definitions and descriptions. In J. Davis (Ed.), *Our forgotten children: Hard of hearing pupils in the schools.* Washington, DC: Self Help for Hard of Hearing People, Inc.

Ross, M., & Lerman, J. (1971). *Word intelligibility by picture identification.* Pittsburgh, PA: Stanwix House.

Rothman, H. (1976). A spectrographic investigation of consonant-vowel transitions in the speech of deaf adults. *Phonetica, 4,* 129–136.

Roush, J. (1994). Strengthening family–professional relations: Advice from parents. In J. Rousch & N. D. Matkin (Eds.), *Infants and toddlers with hearing loss* (pp. 337–350). Baltimore, MD: York Press.

Roush, J., & McWilliam, R. (1990). A new challenge for pediatric audiology: Public Law 99-457. *Journal of the American Academy of Audiology, 1,* 196–208.

Rubinstein, A., & Boothroyd, A. (1987). Effects of two approaches to auditory training on speech recognition by hearing-impaired adults. *Journal of Speech and Hearing Research, 30,* 153–160.

Rubinstein, A., Cherry, R., Hecht, P., & Idler, C. (2000). Anticipatory strategy training: Implications for the postlingually hearing-impaired adult. *Journal of the American Academy of Audiology, 11,* 52–55.

Salthouse, T. A. (1994). The aging of working memory. *Neuropsychology, 8,* 535–543.

Samar, V., & Metz, D. (1988). Criterion validity of speech intelligibility rating-scale procedures for the hearing-impaired population. *Journal of Speech and Hearing Research, 31,* 307–316.

Samar, V. J., & Sims, D. G. (1983). Visual evoked response correlates of speechreading performance in normal-hearing adults: A replication and factor analytic extension. *Journal of Speech and Hearing Research, 26,* 2–9.

Scarborough, H. (1990). Index of productive syntax. *Applied Psycholinguistics, 11,* 122.

Scheetz, N. (1993). *Orientation to deafness.* Needham Heights, MA: Allyn & Bacon.

Schlesinger, H., & Acree, M. (1984). Antecedents to achievement and adjustment in deaf adolescents: A longitudinal study of deaf children. In G. B. Anderson & D. Watson (Eds.), *The habilitation and rehabilitation of deaf adolescents* (pp. 48–61). Washington, DC: The National Academy of Gallaudet College.

Schloss, P. J., & Smith, M. A. (1990). *Teaching social skills to hearing-impaired students.* Washington, DC: Alexander Graham Bell Association for the Deaf.

Schneider, B. (1997). Psychoacoustics and aging: Implications for everyday listening. *Journal of Speech-Language Pathology and Audiology, 21,* 111–124.

Schow, R. L. (2001). A standardized AR battery for dispensers is proposed. *The Hearing Journal,* 10–20.

Schow, R., & Nerbonne, M. (1980). Hearing levels among elderly nursing home residents. *Journal of Speech and Hearing Disorders, 45,* 124–132.

Schow, R. I., & Nerbonne, M. A. (1982). Communication screening profile: Use with elderly adults. *Ear and Hearing, 3,* 135–147.

Schulz, J. H. (1992). *The economics of aging* (5th ed.). New York: Auburn.

Schum, D. J. (1989). *Clear and conversational speech by untrained talkers: Intelligibility.* Paper presented at the American Speech-Language-Hearing Association, Seattle, WA.

Schum, D. J. (1999). Perceived hearing aid benefit in relation to perceived needs. *Journal of the American Academy of Audiology, 10,* 40–45.

Schum, L. K., & Tye-Murray, N. (1995). Alerting and assistive systems: Counseling implications for cochlear implant users. In R. S. Tyler & D. J. Schum (Eds.), *Assistive devices for persons with hearing impairment* (pp. 86–122). Needham Heights, MA: Allyn & Bacon.

Schum, R., & Gfeller, K. (1994). Requisites for conversation: Engendering social skills. In N. Tye-Murray (Ed.), *Let's converse: A how-to-guide to develop and expand conversational skills of children and teenagers who are hearing impaired* (pp. 147–176). Washington, DC: Alexander Graham Bell Association for the Deaf.

Schum, R. L. (1991). Communication and social growth: A developmental model of social behavior in deaf children. *Ear and Hearing, 12,* 320–327.

Secord, W. (1981). *T-MAC: Test of minimal articulation competence.* Columbus, OH: Charles E. Merrill.

Seyfried, D. N., & Kricos, P. B. (1996). Language and speech of the deaf and hard of hearing. In R. L. Schow & M. A. Nerbonne (Eds.), *Introduction to audiologic rehabilitation* (3rd Ed. pp. 168–228). Boston, MA: Allyn & Bacon.

Shatner, W. (1997). Sound of silence. *People Magazine, 47,* 153–155.

Shepherd, D. (1982). Visual-neural correlates of speech-reading ability in normal-hearing adults: Reliability. *Journal of Speech and Hearing Research, 25,* 521–527.

Shepherd, D. C., DeLavergne, R. W., Frueh, F. X., & Colbridge, C. (1977). Visual-neural correlate of speech-reading abilities in normal-hearing adults. *Journal of Speech and Hearing Research, 20,* 752–765.

Shimon, D. A. (1992). *Coping with hearing loss and hearing aids.* Clifton Park, NY: Delmar Learning.

Shultz, D., & Mowry, R. B. (1995). Older adults in long-term care facilities. In P. B. Kricos & S. A. Lesner (Eds.), *Hearing care for the older adults: Audiologic rehabilitation* (pp. 167–179). Newton, MA: Butterworth-Heinemann.

Siebein, G. W., Gold, M. A., Siebein, G. W., & Ermann, M. G. (2000). Ten ways to provide a high-quality acoustical environment in schools. *Language, Speech, and Hearing Services in Schools, 31,* 376–384.

Silverman, R. S., & Hirsh, I. (1955). Problems related to the use of speech in clinical audiometry. *Annals of Otology, Rhinology, and Laryngology, 64,* 1234–1244.

Sims, D., Dorn, C., Clark, C., Bryant, L., & Mumford, B. (2002). *New developments in computer assisted speechreading and auditory training.* Paper presented at the American Speech-Language-Hearing Association, Atlanta, GA.

Sims, D., & Gottermeier, L. (2000). Computer applications in audiologic rehabilitation. In J. G. Alpiner & P. A. McCarthy (Eds.), *Rehabilitative audiology: Children and adults,* (3rd Ed., pp. 556–571). Baltimore: Lippincott Williams and Wilkins.

Sininger, Y. S. (2002). Otoacoustic emissions in the diagnosis of hearing disorder in infants. *Hearing Journal, 55,* 22–26.

Skinner, B. F. (1953). *Science and human behavior.* New York: Macmillan.

Skinner, B. F. (1971). *Beyond freedom and dignity.* New York: Knopf.

Smith, C. (1975). Residual hearing and speech production in the deaf. *Journal of Speech and Hearing Research, 19,* 795–811.

Solomon, A. (1994). Defiantly deaf. The New York Times Magazine, August 28, 38–45 and 62–66.

Sommers, M., Tye-Murray, N., & Spehar, B. (Submitted). *Auditory-visual perception and visual enhancement in normal-hearing younger and older adults.*

Sommers, M., Tye-Murray, N., & Spehar, B. (2002). *Audiovisual integration and age.* Poster presented at the Acoustical Society of America, Cancun, Mexico.

Sorkin, D. (2002). Cochlear implant candidacy and outcomes: 2002 update. *Hearing Loss,* July/August, 12–17.

Speaks, C., & Jerger, J. (1965). Performance-intensity characteristics of synthetic sentences. *Journal of Speech and Hearing Research, 9,* 305–312.

Speaks, C. S., Jerger, J., & Trammell, J. (1970). Measurement of hearing handicap. *Journal of Speech and Hearing Research, 13,* 768–776.

Spencer, L. (1994). Some ways to nurture children's conversational and language skills. In N. Tye-Murray (Ed.), *Let's converse: A how-to guide to develop and expand the conversational skills of children and teenagers who are hearing impaired* (pp. 51–84). Washington, DC: Alexander Graham Bell Association for the Deaf.

Spencer, L., Tomblin, J. B., & Gantz, B. J. (1997). Reading skills in children with multichannel cochlear implant experience. *Volta Review, 99,* 193–202.

Sptizer, J. B. (1997). Cochlear implant and other options for persons with profound impairment. In H. T. Tobin (Ed.), *Practical hearing aid selection and fitting* (pp. 121–132). Washington, DC: Department of Veterans Affairs.

Stach, B. A. (2000). *Comprehensive dictionary of audiology* (2nd Ed.). Clifton Park, NY: Delmar Learning.

Stapells, D. R. (2002). The tone-evoked ABR: Why it's the measure of choice for young infants. *The Hearing Journal, 55,* 14–18.

Stephens, D. (1996). Hearing rehabilitation in a psychosocial framework. *Scandinavian Audiology, 25,* 57–66.

Stephens, D., & Hétu, R. (1991). Impairment, disability, and handicap in audiology: Towards a consensus. *Audiology, 30,* 185–200.

Stephens, S. D., Jaworski, A., Kerr, P., & Zhao, F. (1998). Use of patient-specific estimates in patient evaluation and rehabilitation. *Scandinavian Audiology Supplement, 49,* 61–68.

Stephens, S. D., Jaworski, A., Lewis, P., & Aslan, S. (1999). An analysis of the communication tactics used by hearing-impaired adults. *British Journal of Audiology, 33,* 17–27.

Stinson, M. S., & Anita, S. D. (1999). Considerations in educating deaf and hard-of-hearing students in inclusive settings. *Journal of Deaf Studies and Deaf Education, 4,* 163–175.

Stoel-Gammon, C. (1988). Prelinguistic vocalizations of hearing-impaired and normally hearing subjects: A comparison of consonantal inventories. *Journal of Speech and Hearing Disorders, 53,* 302–315.

Stouffer, J. L., & Tyler, R. S. (1990). Characterization of tinnitus by tinnitus patients. *Journal of Speech and Hearing Disorders, 55,* 439–453.

Stout, G., & Windel, J. (1992). *Developmental approach to successful listening II.* Englewood, CO: Resource Point.

Strawbridge, W. J., Cohen, R. D., Shema, S. J., & Kaplan, G. A. (1996). Successful aging: Predictors and associated activities. *American Journal of Epidemiology, 144,* 135–141.

Subtelny, J. D., Orlando, N. A., & Whitehead, R. L. (1981). *Speech and voice characteristics of the deaf.* Washington, DC: Alexander Graham Bell Association for the Deaf.

Summerfield, Q. (1989). Visual perception of phonetic gestures. In I. G. Mattingly (Ed.), *Modularity and the motor theory of speech perception* (pp. 117–137). Hillsdale, NJ: Laurence Erbaum Associates.

Summerfield, Q. (1992). Lipreading and audiovisual speech perception. *Phil. Royal Society of London, 71–78.*

Sutherland, G. (1995). Increasing consumer acceptance of assistive devices. In R. S. Tyler & D. J. Schum (Eds.), *Assistive devices for persons with hearing impairment* (pp. 251–266). Needham Heights, MA: Allyn & Bacon.

Svirsky, M. A., Chute, P. M., Green, J., Bollard, P., & Miyamoto, R. T. (2002). Language development in children who are prelingually deaf who have used the SPEAK or CIS stimulation strategies. *Volta Review, 102,* 199–214.

Svirsky, M., Robbins, A. M., Kirk, K. I., Pisoni, D. B., & Miyamoto, R. T. (2000). Language development in profoundly deaf children with cochlear implants. *Psychological Science, 11,* 153–158.

Sweetow, R., & Barrager, D. (1980). Quality of comprehensive audiological care: A survey of parents of hearing-impaired children. *ASHA, 22,* 841–847.

Tannahill, J. C. (1979). The Hearing handicap scale as a measure of hearing aid benefit. *Journal of Speech and Hearing Disorders, 44,* 91–99.

Taylor, B., & Hansen, V. (2002). To change the industry, we must change, part 1. *The Hearing Review, 9,* 28–56.

Taylor, K. S., & Jurma, W. E. (1999). Study suggests that group rehabilitation increases benefit of hearing aid fittings. *The Hearing Journal, 52,* 48–54.

Teele, D., Klein, J., & Rosner, B. (1989). Epidemiology of otitis media during the first seven years of life in children in greater Boston. *Journal of Infectious Diseases, 160,* 83–94.

Thorn, F., & Thorn, S. (1989). Speechreading with reduced vision: A problem of aging. *Journal of Optometry Society of America, 6,* 491–499.

Tillman, T. W., & Carhart, R. (1966). *An expanded test for speech discrimination utilizing CNC monosyllabic words: Northwestern University auditory test no. 6.* [Technical Report No. SAM-TR-6655. USAF School of Aerospace Medicine]. San Antonio, TX: Brooks Air Force Base.

Tobey, E., Geers, A., Brenner, C., Altuna, D., & Gabbert, G. (2003). Factors associated with speech production skills in children implanted by age five. *Ear and Hearing, 24,* 36S–45S.

Tomaski, S. M., & Grundfast, K. M. (1999). A stepwise approach to the diagnosis and treatment of hereditary hearing loss. *Pediatric Clinics of North America, 1,* 35–49.

Tomblin, J. B., Spencer, L., Flock, S., Tyler, R., & Gantz, B. (1999). A comparison of language achievement in children with cochlear implants and children using hearing aids. *Journal of Speech, Language, and Hearing Research, 42,* 497–509.

Tomoeda, C. K., & Bayles, K. A. (2002). Cultivating cultural competence in the workplace, classroom, and clinic. *ASHA Leader, 7,* 4–17.

Tong, Y. C., Busby, P. A., & Clark, G. M. (1988). Perceptual studies on cochlear implant patients with early onset of profound hearing impairment prior to normal development of auditory, speech, and language skills. *Journal of the Acoustical Society of America, 84,* 951–962.

Touchstone Applied Science Associates (2001). *Signposts early literacy battery and pre-DRP test.* Brewster, NY: Touchstone Applied Science Associations, Inc.

Traynor, R. M. (1995). Financial and marketing considerations in the rehabilitation of older adults. In P. B. Kricos & S. A. Lesner (Eds.), *Hearing care for the older adults: Audiologic rehabilitation* (pp. 185–202). Newton, MA: Butterworth-Heinemann.

Tremblay, K. L., & Kraus, N. (2002). Auditory training induces asymmetrical changes in cortical neural activity. *Journal of Speech, Language, and Hearing Research, 45,* 564–572.

Tremblay, K. L., Kraus, N., Carell, T., & McGee, T. (1997). Central auditory system plasticity: Generalization to novel stimuli following listening training. *Journal of the Acoustical Society of America, 102,* 3762–3773.

Trybus, R. J., & Krachmer, M. A. (1977). School achievement scores of hearing-impaired children: National data on achievement status and growth patterns. *American Annals of the Deaf, 122,* 62–69.

Trychin, S. (1987a). *Did I do that?* [manual]. Washington, DC: Gallaudet University Press.

Trychin, S. (1987b). *Did I do that?* [videotape]. Washington, DC: Gallaudet University Press.

Trychin, S. (1988). *So that's the problem!* Washington, DC: Gallaudet University Press.

Trychin, S. (1994). Helping people cope with hearing loss. In J. G. Clark & F. N. Martin (Eds.), *Effective counseling in audiology: Perspectives and practice* (pp. 247–277). Englewood Cliffs, NJ: Simon and Schuster.

Trychin, S., & Wright, F. (1989). *Is that what you think?* Washington, DC: Gallaudet University Press.

Tullos, D. C. (1990). Strategies for assessing and training social skills-facilitator behavior. In P. J. Schloss & M. A. Smith (Eds.), *Teaching social skills to hearing-impaired students* (pp. 45–57). Washington, DC: Alexander Graham Bell Association for the Deaf.

Tye-Murray, N. (1987). Effects of vowel context on the articulatory closure postures of deaf speakers. *Journal of Speech and Hearing Research, 30,* 90–104.

Tye-Murray, N. (1991). The establishment of open articulatory postures by deaf and hearing talkers. *Journal of Speech and Hearing Research, 34,* 453–459.

Tye-Murray, N. (1991a). Repair strategy usage by hearing-impaired adults and changes following communication therapy. *Journal of Speech and Hearing Research, 34,* 921–928.

Tye-Murray, N. (1992a). Communication therapy. In N. Tye-Murray (Ed.), *Children with cochlear implants: A handbook for parents, teachers and speech and hearing professionals* (pp. 137–168). Washington, DC: Alexander Graham Bell Association for the Deaf.

Tye-Murray, N. (1992b). Auditory training. In N. Tye-Murray (Ed.), *Children with cochlear implants: A handbook for parents, teachers and speech and hearing professionals* (pp. 91–114). Washington, DC: Alexander Graham Bell Association for the Deaf.

Tye-Murray, N. (1992c). Speechreading training. In N. Tye-Murray (Ed.), *Children with cochlear implants: A handbook for parents, teachers and speech and hearing professionals* (pp. 115–136). Washington, DC: Alexander Graham Bell Association for the Deaf.

Tye-Murray, N. (1992d). Teaching speech perception skills: General guidelines. In N. Tye-Murray (Ed.), *Children with cochlear implants: A handbook for parents, teachers and speech and hearing professionals* (pp. 79–90). Washington, DC: Alexander Graham Bell Association for the Deaf.

Tye-Murray, N. (1992e). Preparing for communication interactions: The value of anticipatory strategies for adults with hearing impairment. *Journal of Speech and Hearing Research, 35,* 430–435.

Tye-Murray, N. (1993a). Aural rehabilitation and patient management. *Cochlear implants: Audiological foundations.* (pp. 87–144). Clifton Park, NY: Delmar Learning.

Tye-Murray, N. (1993b). *Communication training for hearing-impaired children and teenagers: Speechreading, listening, and using repair strategies.* Austin, TX: Pro-Ed.

Tye-Murray, N. (1994a). Some conversation strategies for adults who interact with hard-of-hearing children. In N. Tye-Murray (Ed.), *Let's converse! A how-to guide to develop and expand the conversational skills of children and teenagers who are hearing impaired* (pp. 11–50). Washington, DC: Alexander Graham Bell Association for the Deaf.

Tye-Murray, N. (1994b). Communication breakdowns in conversations: Adult-initiated repair strategies. In N. Tye-Murray (Ed.), *Let's converse! A how-to guide to develop and expand the conversational skills of children and teenagers who are hearing impaired* (pp. 85–121). Washington, DC: Alexander Graham Bell Association for the Deaf.

Tye-Murray, N. (1994c). Communication therapy. In N. Tye-Murray (Ed.), *Let's converse! A how-to guide to develop and expand the conversational skills of children and teenagers who are hearing impaired* (pp. 137–168). Washington, DC: Alexander Graham Bell Association for the Deaf.

Tye-Murray, N. (1997). *Communication strategies training for older adults and teenagers.* Austin, TX: Pro-Ed.

Tye-Murray, N. (2002a). *Conversation made easy: Speechreading and conversation training for individuals who have hearing loss (adults and teenagers).* St. Louis, MO: Central Institute for the Deaf.

Tye-Murray, N. (2002b). *Conversation made easy: Speechreading and conversation training for individuals who have hearing loss (children).* St. Louis, MO: Central Institute for the Deaf.

Tye-Murray, N. (2003). Conversational fluency in children who use cochlear implants. *Ear and Hearing, (24),* 82S–90S.

Tye-Murray, N., & Folkins, J. (1990). Jaw and lip movements of deaf talkers producing utterances with known stress patterns. *Journal of the Acoustical Society of America, 87,* 2675–2683.

Tye-Murray, N., & Fryauf-Bertschy, H. (1992). Auditory training. In N. Tye-Murray (Ed.), *Children with cochlear implants: A handbook for parents, teachers and speech and hearing professionals.* Washington, DC: Alexander Graham Bell Association for the Deaf.

Tye-Murray, N., & Geers, A. (2002). *The Children's audiovisual enhancement speech test (CHIVE).* St. Louis, MO: Central Institute for the Deaf.

Tye-Murray, N., & Kelsey, D. R. (1993). Communication therapy for parents of cochlear implant users. *Volta Review, 95,* 21–32.

Tye-Murray, N., Knutson, J. F., & Lemke, J. (1993). Assessment of communication strategies use: Questionnaires and daily diaries. *Seminars in Hearing, 14,* 338–353.

Tye-Murray, N., Purdy, S. C., & Woodworth, G. (1992). The reported use of communication strategies by members of SHHH and its relationship to client, talker, and situational variables. *Journal of Speech and Hearing Research, 35,* 708–717.

Tye-Murray, N., Purdy, S. C., Woodworth, G., & Tyler, R. S. (1990). Effects of repair strategies on visual identification of sentences. *Journal of Speech and Hearing Disorders, 55,* 621–627.

Tye-Murray, N., Sommers, M., & Spehar, B. (Submitted). *Gender effects in lipreading.*

Tye-Murray, N., Spencer, L., & Woodworth, G. (1995). Acquisition of speech by children who have prolonged cochlear implant experience. *Journal of Speech and Hearing Research, 38,* 327–337.

Tye-Murray, N., Tomblin, B., & Spencer, L., November (1997). *Speech and language acquisition over time in children with cochlear implants.* Paper presented at the American Speech-Language Hearing Convention. Boston, MA.

Tye-Murray, N., & Witt, S. (1996). Conversational moves and conversational styles of adult cochlear-implant users. *Journal of the Academy of Rehabilitative Audiology, 29,* 11–25.

Tye-Murray, N., Witt, S., & Castelloe, J. (1996). Initial evaluation of an interactive test of sentence gist recognition. *Journal of the American Academy of Audiology, 7,* 396–405.

Tye-Murray, N., Witt, S., & Schum, L. (1995). Effects of talker familiarity on communication breakdown in conversation with adult cochlear-implant users. *Ear and Hearing, 16,* 459–469.

Tye-Murray, N., Witt, S., Schum, L., & Sobaski, C. (1995). Communication breakdowns: Partner contingencies and partner reactions. *Journal of the Academy of Rehabilitative Audiology, 25,* 1–27.

Tye-Murray, N., Zimmermann, G., & Folkins, J. (1987). Movement timing in deaf and hearing speakers: Comparison of phonetically heterogeneous syllable strings. *Journal of Speech and Hearing Research, 30,* 411–417.

Tyler, R. S. (1993). Speech perception by children. In R. Tyler (Ed.), *Cochlear implants: Audiological foundations* (pp. 191–256). San Diego, CA: Singular Publishing Group.

Tyler, R. S., Fryauf-Bertschy, H., & Kelsay, D. (1991). *Audiovisual feature test for young children.* Iowa City: The University of Iowa Hospitals and Clinics.

Tyler, R. S., Fryauf-Bertschy, H., & Kelsay, D. (1991). *A closed-set speech perception test for hearing-impaired children.* Iowa City, IA: University of Iowa.

Tyler, R. S., Preece, J., & Tye-Murray, N. (1986). *The Iowa phoneme and sentence tests.* Iowa City: The University of Iowa Hospitals and Clinics.

Tyler, R. S., and Baker, L. J. (1983). Difficulties experienced by tinnitus sufferers. *Journal of Speech and Hearing Disorders, 48,* 150–154.

U.S. Bureau of the Census. (1997). *Statistical abstract of the United States 1996.* Washington, DC: U. S. Government Printing Office.

U.S. Department of Commerce Bureau of the Census (1984). *Statistical abstract of the U.S.* Washington, D.C.: Government Printing Office.

U.S. Department of Commerce Bureau of the Census. (1986). *Statistical abstract of the U.S.* (106th ed.). Washington, DC: Government Printing Office.

U.S. Public Health Service. (1990). *Healthy people 2000.* Washington, DC: Government Printing Office.

VandenBrink, R. H. S. (1995). Attitude and illness behaviour in hearing impaired elderly. Thesis. University of Groningen, The Netherlands.

Van Hecke, M. (1994). Emotional responses to hearing loss. In J. G. Clark and F. N. Martin (Eds.) *Effective counseling in Audiology: Perspectives and practice.* Englewood Cliffs, NJ: Prentice-Hall Inc., 92–115.

Van Uden, A. (1988). Interrelating reception and expression in speechreading training. *Volta Review, 90,* 261–272.

Ventry, I., & Weinstein, B. (1982). The hearing inventory for the elderly: A new tool. *Ear and Hearing, 3,* 128.

Ventry, I., & Weinstein, B. (1983). Identification of elderly people with hearing problems. *Asha, 25,* 37–47.

Vergara, K. C., & Miskiel, L. W. (1994). CHATS: *The Miami cochlear implant, auditory and tactile skills curriculum.* Miami, FL: Intelligent Hearing Systems.

Vernon, J. A., & Meikle, M. B. (2000). Tinnitus masking. In R. Tyler (Ed.), *Tinnitus handbook* (pp. 313–356). Clifton Park, NY: Delmar Learning.

Vinding, T. (1989). Age-related macular degeneration: Macular changes, prevalence, and sex ratio. *Acta Ophthalmology, 67,* 609–616.

Voeks, S., Gallagher, C., Langer, E., & Drinka, P. (1990). Hearing loss in the nursing home: An institutional issue. *Journal of the American Geriatrics Society, 38,* 141–145.

Voelker, C. (1938). An experimental study of the comparative rate of utterances of deaf and normal-hearing speakers. *American Annals of the Deaf, 83,* 274–284.

Von Hapsburg, D., & Peña, E. D. (2002). Understanding bilingualism and its impact on speech audiometry. *Journal of Speech, Language, and Hearing Research, 45,* 202–213.

Vonlanthen, A. (2000). *Hearing instrument technology for the hearing healthcare professional* (2nd Ed.). Clifton Park, NY: Delmar Learning.

Walden, B. E., Demorest, M. E., & Helper, E. L. (1984). Test-retest reliability of the hearing handicap inventory for the elderly. *Ear and Hearing, 7,* 295–299.

Walden, B. E., Erdman, S. A., Montgomery, A. A., Schwartz, D. M., & Prosek, R. A. (1981). Effects of training on the visual recognition of consonants. *Journal of Speech and Hearing Research, 20,* 130–145.

Walden, B. E., Prosek, R. A., Montgomery, A. A., Scherr, C. K., & Jones, C. J. (1977). Effects of training on the visual recognition of consonants. *Journal of Speech and Hearing Research, 20,* 130–145.

Waltzman, S., Cohen, N., Gomolin, R., Green, J., Shapiro, W., Brackett, D., & Zara, C. (1997). Perception and production results in children implanted between 2 and 5 years of age. *Advances in OtoRhino-Laryngology, 52,* 177–180.

Wayner, D. S., & Abrahamson, M. A. (1996). *Learning to hear again: An audiologic rehabilitation curriculum guide.* Austin, TX: Hear Again.

Wayner, D. S., & Abrahamson, M. A. (1998). *Learning to hear again with a cochlear implant: An audiologic rehabilitation curriculum guide.* Austin, TX: Hear Again.

Weinstein, B. E. (1991). The quantification of hearing aid benefit in the elderly: The role of self-assessment measures. *Acta Otolaryngology, 476*(Suppl.), 257–261.

Weinstein, B. E., Spitzer, J. B., & Ventry, I. M. (1986). Test-retest reliability of the hearing handicap inventory for the elderly. *Ear and Hearing, 7,* 295–299.

Weinstein, B. E., & Ventry, I. M. (1983). Audiometric correlates of the hearing handicap inventory for the elderly. *Journal of Speech and Hearing Disorders, 48,* 379–384.

Weisleder, P., & Hodgson, W. R. (1980). Evaluation of four Spanish word-recognition-ability lists. *Ear and Hearing, 1,* 387–393.

Weisleder, P., & Hodgson, W. R. (1989). Evaluation of four Spanish word-recognition-ability lists. *Ear and Hearing, 10,* 387–393.

White, S. (1984). *Antecedents of language functioning in the deaf: Implications for early intervention. Project summary* (EDD0001). Washington, DC: U.S. Department of Education.

White, S., & White, R. (1987). The effects of hearing status of the family and age of intervention on reception and expressive oral language skills in hearing-impaired infants. In H. Levitt, N. S. McGarr, & D. Geffner (Eds.), *Development of language and communication skills in hearing-impaired children.* Washington, DC: ASHA.

Widen, J. E., & O'Grady, G. M. (2002). Using visual reinforcement audiometry in the assessment of hearing in infants. *The Hearing Journal, 55,* 28–36.

Williams-Scott, B., & Kipila, E. (1987). Cued speech: A professional point of view. In S. Schwartz (Ed.), *Choices in deafness; A parent's guide.* Washington, DC: Woodbine House.

Williamson, J. D., & Fried, M. D. (1996). Characterization of older adults who attribute functional decrements to "old age." *Journal of the American Geriatrics Society, 44,* 1429–1434.

Willott, J. F. (1996). Anatomic and physiologic aging: A behavioral neuroscience perspective. *Journal of the American Academy of Audiology, 7,* 141–151.

Wilson, P. H., & Henry, J. L. (2000). Psychological management of tinnitus. In R. S. Tyler (Ed.), *Tinnitus handbook* (pp. 263–280). Clifton Park, NY: Delmar Learning.

Wingfield, A., Stine, E. A., Lahar, C. J., & Aberdden, J. S. (1988). Does the capacity of working memory change with age? *Experimental Aging Research, 14,* 103–107.

Witt, S. (1997). *Effectiveness of an intensive aural rehabilitation program for adult cochlear implant users; A demonstration project.* Unpublished master's thesis. University of Iowa, Iowa City.

Wolff, A. B., & Harkins, J. E. (1986). Multihandicapped students. In A. N. Schildroth & M. A. Karchmer (Eds.), *Deaf children in America* (pp. 55–82). San Diego, CA: College-Hill Press.

Wood, E., & Sandsone, S. C. (2000). *American government: A complete coursebook.* Wilmington, MA: Houghton Mifflin.

Wood, D., Wood, H., Griffiths, A., & Howarth, I. (1986). *Teaching and talking with deaf children.* New York: John Wiley and Sons.

Woodcock, R. (1997). *Woodcock diagnostic reading battery (WDRB).* Itasca, IL: Riverside Publishing Company.

Woodcock, R., & Johnson, M. B. (1989). *Woodcock-Johnson psycho-educational battery (WJ-R).* Itasca, IL: Riverside Publishing Company.

Woods, M. L., & Moe, A. (1999). *Analytical reading inventory* (6th Ed.). Columbus, OH: Merrill Education (Prentice Hall).

Woodward, M. F., & Barber, C. G. (1960). Phoneme perception in lipreading. *Journal of Speech and Hearing Research, 17,* 212–222.

World Health Organization. (1999). Beta-2 draft, Short Version.

World Health Organization. (WHO) (2000). *International classification of functioning, disability, and health.* Geneva, Switzerland: World Health Organization.

Wylde, M. A. (1982). The remediation process: Psychologic and counseling aspects. In J. G. Alpiner (Ed.), *Handbook of adult rehabilitation audiology* (2nd Ed.). Baltimore, MD: Williams and Wilkins.

Yoshinaga-Itano, C. (1988). Speechreading instruction for children. *Volta Review, 90,* 241–260.

Yoshinaga-Itano, C., & Downey, D. M. (1996). Development of school-aged deaf, hard-of-hearing and normally hearing students' written language. *Volta Review, 98,* 3–7.

Yoshinaga-Itano, C., & Gravel, J. S. (2001). The evidence for universal newborn hearing screening. *American Journal of Audiology, 10,* 62–64.

Yoshingaga-Itano, C., Sedey, A., Coulter, D. K., and Mehl, A. L. (1998). Language of early and later identified children with hearing loss. *Pediatrics, 102,* 1161–1171.

Yoshinaga-Itano, C., Snyder, L. S., & Mayberry, R. (1996). How deaf and normally hearing students convey meaning within and between written sentences. *Volta Review, 98,* 9–38.

Zones, J., Estes, C., & Binney, E. (1987). Gender, public policy and the oldest old. *Aging Society, 7,* 275–302.

Index

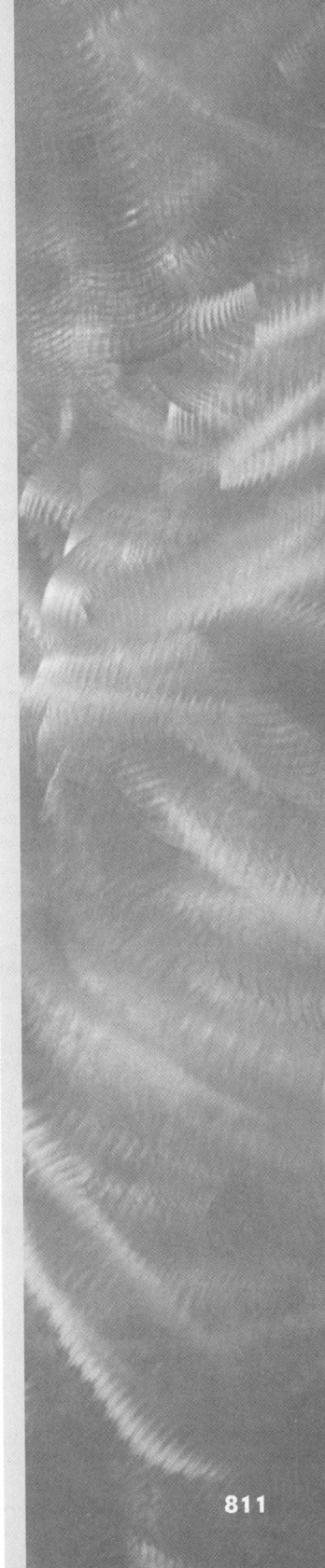